BIO-IMPLANT INTERFACE

Improving Biomaterials and Tissue Reactions

Jan Eirik Ellingsen
S. Petter Lyngstadaas

CRC PRESS

Boca Raton London New York Washington, D.C.

Library of Congress Cataloging-in-Publication Data

Bio-implant interface : improving biomaterials and tissue reactions / edited by Jan Eirik Ellingsen, S. Petter Lyngstadaas.

p. cm.

ISBN 0-8493-1474-7

1. Biomedical materials. 2. Artificial organs. 3. Transplantation of organs, tissues, etc. I. Ellingsen, Jan Eirik. II. Lyngstadaas, S. Petter.

R857.M3 B476 2003

610′.284—dc21 2002191162

Direct all inquiries to CRC Press LLC, 2000 N.W. Corporate Blvd., Boca Raton, Florida 33431.

Visit the CRC Press Web site at www.crcpress.com

International Standard Book Number 0-8493-1474-7

Library of Congress Card Number 2002191162

Printed in the United States of America 1 2 3 4 5 6 7 8 9 0

Printed on acid-free paper

Preface

Implanted biomaterials represent rapidly increasing treatment modalities for replacement of anatomical structures like bones and teeth and for restoring lost body functions. Optimal mechanical and biological functioning of implanted materials is of utmost importance for the outcome of such treatments, especially in the fields of implant dentistry and orthopedic and plastic surgery where the biomechanical, biochemical, functional, and esthetic demands on the implanted material are extreme. A good clinical outcome is based on several aspects of the combination (integration) of biological and material sciences and tissue engineering. The rapid progress of modern biomaterial medicine continuously challenges clinicians and scientists alike in the pursuit for new and better designs that will improve biocompatibility and patient responses to implants. The state of the art in biomaterial medicine is continuously changing and improving in combination with technological advances in biology and material science.

The authors of this book, all renowned scientists in their fields, gathered on the *M/S Nordnorge* and sailed the coast of Norway while reviewing and discussing the individual topics now included in this book.

The aim of this work is to present state-of-the-art knowledge of the important interface between materials and living tissue. Its main focus is the interaction of tissues and biomaterials. Controlling and patterning of bio-implant interface reactions are expected to exert tremendous impact on future designs and prospects for implant treatment. Strategies for controlling this intriguing interface are going to arise from a fusion of clinical expertise with several scientific fields including implant design, biomechanics, surface topography, chemistry, matrix biology, cell biology, molecular biology, and synthetic biomaterials design.

It is our hope that this book will update the readers in this important aspect of patient-oriented basic science and initiate and stimulate further work in this important biomedical field. We also hope that such work will eventually benefit the many patients who now remain untreated or suffer poor outcomes.

Jan Eirik Ellingsen
Staale Petter Lyngstadaas

Editors

Jan Eirik Ellingsen earned a D.D.S. in 1982 and a Ph.D. in 1985 and qualified as a clinical specialist in prosthetic dentistry in 1991. He became an associate professor in the department of prosthetic dentistry 1986 and held a position as specialist dentist in that same department from 1991 until 1993. He was appointed professor in dentistry at University of Oslo in 1993 and has served as director of the Oral Research Laboratory since 1996.

His research activity has focused on surface reactions to teeth and biomaterials. In particular, the mechanisms of regeneration and binding of bone tissue to biomaterials following implantation have been given much attention. He has been heading a project on engineering of biomaterial surfaces for improved tissue response. The group is now focusing on chemical, electrochemical, and biological methods for experimental surface modifications of biomaterials for improving the regeneration of the tissue and integration of the biomaterial.

Staale Petter Lyngstadaas earned a B.E. in biochemistry in 1984, a D.D.S. in 1991, and a Ph.D. in 1995 with a thesis on molecular biology and extracellular matrix biomineralization in tooth formation. From 1996 to 1997, he held a fellowship in oral pathology. He became an associate professor in oral pathology in 1997, and later in 2000, in biomaterials research. He was appointed professor of biomaterials in 2001.

His main research interests have focused on the development of the craniofacial complex, including teeth, dental ligaments, alveolar bones, and jawbones. Combining insight in developmental biology and molecular biology with experience from pathology and biomaterials science, he studied mechanisms that operate during development, repair, and regeneration of hard tissues. Much of his work has centered on the formation of extracellular matrix and how the matrix influences growth and guides repair, regeneration, and biomineralization processes in hard tissues. Moreover, he is engaged in designing bioactive biomaterials based on extracellular matrix biology to improve the performance of implants by controlling tissue responses and tissue integration of the implanted materials.

Contributors

Tomas Albrektsson, M.D., Ph.D., O.Dhc. Department of Biomaterials, Göteborg University, Göteborg, Sweden

P. Mark Bartold School of Dentistry, University of Adelaide, Adelaide, Australia, p.bartold@mailbox.uq.edu.au

Elia Beniash Feinberg School of Medicine, Northwestern University, Evanston, Illinois

Jean-Pierre Bernard School of Dental Medicine, University of Geneva, Geneva, Switzerland

Steven J. Brookes Leeds Dental Institute, University of Leeds, Leeds, U.K.

Donald M. Brunette Faculty of Dentistry, University of British Columbia, Vancouver, British Columbia, Canada, brunette@interchange.ubc.ca

Babak Chehroudi Faculty of Dentistry, University of British Columbia, Vancouver, British Columbia, Canada

Lyndon F. Cooper, D.D.S., Ph.D. University of North Carolina, Chapel Hill, North Carolina, Lyndon_Cooper@dentistry.unc.edu

Paul Coulthard Oral and Maxillofacial Surgery, University Dental Hospital of Manchester, Manchester, U.K.

John E. Davies Faculties of Dentistry and Medicine, University of Toronto, Toronto, Ontario, Canada, davies@ecf.utoronto.ca

Björn Delin, D.D.S. Astra Tech AB, Mölndal, Sweden, bjorn.delin@astratech.com

Jan Eirik Ellingsen Faculty of Dentistry, University of Oslo, Oslo, Norway, janee@odont.uio.no

Marco Esposito Institute for Surgical Sciences, Göteborg University, Göteborg, Sweden, marco.esposito@odontologi.gu.se

Stina Gestrelius Biora AB, Malmö, Sweden, stina.gestrelius@biora.com

Jeannette Glass-Brudzinski Faculty of Dentistry, University of British Columbia, Vancouver, British Columbia, Canada

Stig Hansson, Ph.D. Astra Tech, Mölndal, Sweden, stig.hansson@tech.se.astra.com

Jeffrey D. Hartgerink Feinberg School of Medicine, Northwestern University, Evanston, Illinois

Arne Hensteen-Pettersen Scandinavian Institute of Dental Materials, Haslum, Norway, ahp@niom.no

John A. Jansen, D.D.S., Ph.D. University Medical Center, University of Nijmegen, Nijmegen, The Netherlands, j.jansen@dent.kun.nl

Carina B. Johansson, Ph.D. Department of Biomaterials, Göteborg University, Göteborg, Sweden

John C. Keller, Ph.D. Dows Institute for Dental Research, University of Iowa, Iowa City, Iowa

Ali Khakbaznejad Faculty of Dentistry, University of British Columbia, Vancouver, British Columbia, Canada

Jennifer Kirkham Leeds Dental Institute, University of Leeds, Leeds, U.K.

Staale Petter Lyngstadaas Faculty of Dentistry, University of Oslo, Oslo, Norway, spl@odont.uio.no

Ronald Midura, Ph.D. The Cleveland Clinic Foundation, Cleveland, Ohio

Hiroshi Murakami Aichi-Gakuin University, Nagoya, Japan

Hans-Georg Neumann DOT GmbH, Rostock, Germany

Michael L. Paine Dental School, University of Southern California, Los Angeles, California, paine@hsc.usc.edu

Jun Y. Park University of Toronto, Toronto, Ontario, Canada

Hiran Perinpanayagam, D.D.S., M.S. Dows Institute for Dental Research, University of Iowa, Iowa City, Iowa

Daniel Perrin Odontology Department, CHU, Dijon, France

Robert M. Pilliar, B.A.Sc., Ph.D. Faculty of Dentistry, University of Toronto, Toronto, Ontario, Canada, bob.pilliar@utoronto.ca

Colin Robinson Leeds Dental Institute, University of Leeds, Leeds, U.K., ORL6CR@ORALBIO.LEEDS.AC.UK

Galen Schneider, D.D.S., Ph.D. Dows Institute for Dental Research, University of Iowa, Iowa City, Iowa

Mitsuru Shimonishi Faculty of Dentistry, Tohoku University, Sendai, Japan

Roger C. Shore Leeds Dental Institute, University of Leeds, Leeds, U.K.

Ivan Slaby Biora AB, Malmö, Sweden

D. Alistair Smith Department of Physics and Astronomy, University of Leeds, Leeds, U.K.

Eli D. Sone Feinberg School of Medicine, Northwestern University, Evanston, Illinois

Malcolm L. Snead School of Dentistry, University of Southern California, Los Angeles, California, mlsnead@hsc.usc.edu

Axel Spahr Periodontology and Pedodontics, University of Ulm, Ulm, Germany

Clark M. Stanford, D.D.S., Ph.D. Dows Institute for Dental Research, University of Iowa, Iowa City, Iowa, Clark-Stanford@uiowa.edu

Samuel I. Stupp Feinberg School of Medicine, Northwestern University, Evanston, Illinois, s-stupp@northwestern.edu

Serge Szmukler-Moncler Salpétrière Hospital, University of Paris, Paris, France, ssm@bluewin.ch

Masanori Takekawa Faculty of Dentistry, University of British Columbia, Vancouver, British Columbia, Canada

Pentti Tengvall Laboratory of Applied Physics, Linköping University, Linköping, Sweden, pet@ifm.liu.se

Petra J. ter Brugge University Medical Center, University of Nijmegen, Nijmegen, The Netherlands

Marcus Textor Biomaterials and Biosensor Surface Group, Swiss Federal Institute of Technology, Schlieren, Switzerland, textor@surface.mat.ethz.ch

Irma Thesleff Institute of Biotechnology, University of Helsinki, Helsinki, Finland, irma.thesleff@helsinki.fi

Peter Thomsen, M.D., Ph.D., F.B.S.E. Department of Biomaterials, Göteborg University, Göteborg, Sweden, peter.thomsen@biomaterials.gu.se

Samuele Tosatti Swiss Federal Institute of Technology, Laboratory for Surface Science and Technology, Schlieren, Switzerland

Mark Tummers Institute of Biotechnology, University of Helsinki, Helsinki, Finland

Edwin van der Wal Debye Institute, University of Utrecht, Utrecht, The Netherlands

Arjen M. Vredenberg Debye Institute, University of Utrecht, Utrecht, The Netherlands

Ann Wennerberg, L.D.S., Ph.D. Department of Prosthetic Dentistry, Göteborg University, Göteborg, Sweden, ann.wennerberg@biomaterials.gu.se

Marco Wieland Institut Straumann AG, Waldenburg, Switzerland

David F. Williams Department of Clinical Engineering, University of Liverpool, Liverpool, U.K., dfw@liverpool.ac.uk

Joop G.C. Wolke University Medical Center, University of Nijmegen, Nijmegen, The Netherlands

Jennifer C. Wong Dental School, University of Southern California, Los Angeles, California

Simon R. Wood Leeds Dental Institute, University of Leeds, Leeds, U.K.

Helen V. Worthington Oral Health and Development, University Dental Hospital of Manchester, Manchester, U.K.

Yin Xiao School of Dentistry, University of Queensland, Brisbane, Australia

Peter Zeggel DOT GmbH, Rostock, Germany

Acknowledgments

The editors would like to express their thanks to the people who made this book a reality. The assistance of Siv Jamtøya, the secretary at the Oral Research Laboratory, Institute of Clinical Dentistry, University of Oslo, has been invaluable to this project. Her enthusiastic work in planning and handling the logistics during the workshop on the *M/S Nordnorge* and, in particular, her input in the process of editing the manuscripts were vital factors in the production of this book.

The editors would also like to thank Astra Tech AB for financial support that made it possible to gather scientists from many nations on a ship on the coast of Norway to focus on the past, present, and future of the bio-implant interface.

The editors also take this opportunity to thank all the contributors to this book. Without their willingness to share their knowledge, it would not have been possible to realize this book.

The publisher, CRC Press, Susan Farmer, Marsha Hecht, and Jamie Sigal are acknowledged for their significant contributions to this effort.

Finally, we want to thank our families for their support and patience during the production of this book.

Contents

Section I Success and Failure of Bone–Implant Attachments: An Evidence-Based Approach

1 **Role of Implant Surface Properties on the Clinical Outcome of Osseointegrated Oral Implant Therapy: An Evidence-Based Approach** 3
Marco Esposito, Helen V. Worthington, Paul Coulthard, Ann Wennerberg, and Peter Thomsen

Section II Can Implant Macro Design and Micro Texturing Improve Bone Response?

2 **Toward an Optimized Dental Implant Design** 29
Stig Hansson

3 **Implant Surface Design for Development and Maintenance of Osseointegration** 43
Robert M. Pilliar

4 **Bone Response to Surface Roughness: Measurements and Results from Experimental and Clinical Studies** 59
Ann Wennerberg and Tomas Albrektsson

5 **From Microroughness to Resorbable Bioactive Coatings** 73
Serge Szmukler-Moncler, Peter Zeggel, Daniel Perrin, Jean-Pierre Bernard, and Hans-Georg Neumann

Section III Cell and Tissue Reactions to Biomaterials

6 **Improving the Bio-Implant Interface by Controlling Cell Behavior Using Surface Topography** 103
Donald M. Brunette, Ali Khakbaznejad, Masanori Takekawa, Mitsuru Shimonishi, Hiroshi Murakami, Marco Wieland, Babak Chehroudi, Jeannette Glass-Brudzinski, and Marcus Textor

7 **Osteoblast Response to Pure Titanium and Titanium Alloy** 123
Michael L. Paine and Jennifer C. Wong

8 **Biomedical Implant Surface Topography and Its Effects on Osteoblast Differentiation *In Vitro*** 141
Clark M. Stanford, Galen Schneider, Hiran Perinpanayagam, John C. Keller, and Ronald Midura

9 **Cellular Interactions at Commercially Pure Titanium Implants** 165
Lyndon F. Cooper

10 **A Selection of Oral Implant Materials Based on Experimental Studies** 183
Peter Thomsen and Carina B. Johansson

11 **Possibilities of Improving Implants and Regenerating Dentoalveolar Tissues by Tissue Engineering Using Stem Cells and Growth Factors** 205
Irma Thesleff and Mark Tummers

12 **Critical Issues in Endosseous Peri-Implant Wound Healing** 219
John E. Davies and Jun Y. Park

Section IV Extracellular Matrix Biology and Biomineralization in Bone Formation and Implant Integration

13 **Initiation and Modulation of Crystal Growth in Skeletal Tissues: Role of Extracellular Matrix** 231
Colin Robinson, Roger, C. Shore, Simon R. Wood, Steven J. Brookes, D. Alistair Smith, and Jennifer Kirkham

14 **Use of a Matrix Scaffold for Tissue Engineering and Bone Regeneration** 247
P. Mark Bartold and Yin Xiao

15 **Inducing Bone Growth Using Extracellular Matrix Proteins** 261
Staale Petter Lyngstadaas, Jan Eirik Ellingsen, Axel Spahr, and Ivan Slaby

Section V Surface Chemistry, Biochemistry, and Molecules: How Do They Interact with Biological Environment?

16 How Surfaces Interact with the Biological Environment...... 285
Pentti Tengvall

17 Osteocapacities of Calcium Phosphate Ceramics 305
John A. Jansen, Petra J. ter Brugge, Edwin van der Wal, Arjen M. Vredenberg, and Joop G.C. Wolke

18 Increasing Biocompatibility by Chemical Modification of Titanium Surfaces 323
Jan Eirik Ellingsen and Staale Petter Lyngstadaas

19 Use Of Molecular Assembly Techniques for Tailoring Chemical Properties of Smooth and Rough Titanium Surfaces 341
Marcus Textor, Samuele Tosatti, Marco Wieland, and Donald M. Brunette

Section VI Development and Application of Scientific Data: Regulatory and Commercial Aspects

20 Development and Application of Scientific Data: Do Industry and Academia Have Different Scientific Perspectives? 369
Björn Delin

21 Medical Devices: Regulatory Perspectives and Aspects of Regulatory Risk Management 373
Stina Gestrelius and Arne Hensten-Pettersen

Section VII Inventive Forward Looks: Where Do We Go from Here?

22 Self-Assembling and Biomimetic Biomaterials 393
Samuel I. Stupp, Elia Beniash, Jeffrey D. Hartgerink, and Eli D. Sone

23 The Inert–Bioactivity Conundrum 407
David F. Williams

24 Enhancing the Processes of Discovery and Innovation for Optimal Host Response at Implant Surfaces 431
Malcolm L. Snead

Index 441

Section I

Success and Failure of Bone–Implant Attachments: An Evidence-Based Approach

1

Role of Implant Surface Properties on the Clinical Outcome of Osseointegrated Oral Implant Therapy: An Evidence-Based Approach

Marco Esposito, Helen V. Worthington, Paul Coulthard, Ann Wennerberg, and Peter Thomsen

CONTENTS

1.1 Introduction 4
1.2 Materials and Methods 5
  1.2.1 Search Strategy for Identification of RCTs 6
  1.2.2 Study Selection, Quality Assessment, and Data Extraction 6
  1.2.3 Data Synthesis 8
  1.2.4 Descriptions of Studies 8
  1.2.5 Methodological Quality of Included Studies 9
  1.2.6 Implant Characteristics 9
1.3 Results 15
  1.3.1 Astra versus Brånemark Implants 15
  1.3.2 Astra versus ITI Implants 17
  1.3.3 Brånemark versus IMZ Implants 17
  1.3.4 Brånemark versus ITI Implants 18
  1.3.5 IMZ versus ITI Implants 18
  1.3.6 Steri-Oss versus Southern Implants 18
1.4 Discussion 19
1.5 Conclusions 21
Acknowledgments 21
References 22

0-8493-1474-7/03/$0.00+$1.50

1.1 Introduction

Osseointegrated oral implants are available in different materials, body shapes, diameters, lengths, platforms, surface properties, and coatings. In particular, implant surface modifications and coatings have been subjected to aggressive marketing aimed at establishing the superiority of a given surface over the others. In implant research, the word *machined* has been used frequently to describe a turned, milled, or polished surface. However, a machined surface can be any object produced by a machine. Surfaces produced by electrodischarge, polishing, grinding, honing, and sand blasting are all examples of machined surfaces.[1] Thus, an implant surface requires a more precise description.

Numerous surface modifications have been developed and are currently used with the aim of enhancing clinical performance, including turned, blasted, acid-etched, porous-sintered, oxidized, plasma-sprayed, hydroxyapatite-coated surfaces, and combinations of these procedures. It has been estimated that dentists can choose from more than 1300 types of implants that vary in form, material, dimension, surface properties, and interface geometry.[2]

It is therefore important to know whether certain surface modifications or particular materials will improve clinical results and provide the best available treatment. In recent years, the concept of evidence-based practice has become popular.[3–5] The concept implies the integration of the individual experience of a clinician with the best available evidence from systematic research.[6]

Various study designs can be used to investigate specific scientific hypotheses. The ideal study design should be chosen on the basis of parameters to be evaluated. The consensus is that a randomized controlled clinical trial (RCT) is the preferred design to answer questions on the effectiveness of therapeutic intervention.[7,8] Every clinical trial intended to evaluate treatment effectiveness is comparative. Appropriate controls must be included because the only way to assess effectiveness is to compare differences in outcomes between a test group in which the intervention under investigation is administered and a control group in which another intervention or no intervention is delivered. Obviously, the control population should not be different from the test population. Test and control groups should be as similar as possible with the exception of the administered treatment.

The best way to ensure this similarity in groups to be compared is randomization. RCT participants are randomly selected to receive or not receive one or more treatments to be compared. Randomization allows all participants the same chances of assignment to a study group and investigators are prevented from influencing the course of a study by systematically including patients with different prognoses into a certain group. Randomization, if done properly, reduces the risk of serious imbalance in unknown but important factors that can influence the results of a trial.[9] No other study design allows investigators to balance these unknown factors.

Like all studies, RCTs are open to bias if not correctly conducted.[10] In addition, an RCT with an inadequate number of patients (i.e., inadequate statistical power) may be unable to detect a significant difference in interventions even if a difference exists. It has been recently shown that RCTs on oral implants seldom included statistical power calculations[11] and other means must be used to identify the most effective interventions.

One accepted way to overcome this problem is to combine data from different trials if they address similar comparisons and report the same outcome measures. In particular, systematic reviews (SRs) are used to assess the quality of RCTs and, when possible, combine results of different RCTs to reach more reliable conclusions.[8,12] SRs have clearly formulated hypotheses and employ systematic and explicit methods to identify, select, and critically appraise relevant clinical research. Data from original trials are collected, analyzed, and, if possible, summarized in order to produce more precise estimates of the intervention effects than those derived from individual trials.[8,12] SRs, if not properly conducted, may lead to erroneous conclusions.[13–15] It is therefore important that SRs are conducted according to the highest scientific standards.[16]

The QUOROM statement[16] provides guidelines on how to improve the reporting of SRs and meta-analyses of RCTs. Such guidelines will improve not only the reporting, but will also increase the awareness of what is required to conduct a good quality SR.

The aim of this chapter is to assess possible differences in performance among various root-formed osseointegrated implant types with respect to surface characteristics, materials, and shapes of implants. This was done by conducting a Cochrane systematic review (http://www.update-software.com/ccweb/cochrane/cc-broch.htm)[12,17] with the Cochrane Oral Health Group (http://www.cochrane-oral.man.ac.uk/).

1.2 Materials and Methods

All RCTs of root-form osseointegrated oral implants comparing different implant types (surface properties, materials, and shapes) having minimal follow-up periods of 1 year in function were considered for this review. Studies reporting on bone grafting, guided bone regeneration procedures, and placement of implants in freshly extracted tooth sockets were not considered. Endpoints were 1, 3, and 5 years. Longer follow-up periods may be considered in the future.

The following true or primary outcome measures[8] were considered in this review:

1. **Biological implant failure**, defined as implant mobility and removal of stable implants dictated by progressive marginal bone loss.[18,19] Biological failures were grouped as early (failure to estab-

lish osseointegration) and late (failure to maintain established osseointegration). Failures occurring before bridge placement or, in the case of immediate or early loaded implants, soon after (weeks or a few months) prosthesis insertion, were considered early failures.

2. **Mechanical implant failure**, defined as implant fracture and all other mechanical complications not allowing use of the implants.

The surrogate or secondary outcome measure[8] was the appearance of marginal bone level changes on intraoral radiographs taken with the paralleling technique.

1.2.1 Search Strategy for Identification of RCTs

To identify trials on oral implants included or considered for this review, detailed search strategies were developed for each database searched. These were based on the search strategy developed for MEDLINE (Table 1.1) and revised appropriately for each database. The searched databases were:

1. Cochrane Oral Health Group Specialised Register
2. Cochrane Controlled Trials Register, Cochrane Library Issue 1, 2002
3. MEDLINE (1966 through May 2002)
4. EMBASE (1974 through May 2002)

The following journals were hand-searched by the Cochrane Collaboration or by one of the authors as being important for this review: *British Journal of Oral and Maxillofacial Surgery, Clinical Implant Dentistry and Related Research, Clinical Oral Implants Research, Implant Dentistry, International Journal of Oral and Maxillofacial Implants, International Journal of Oral and Maxillofacial Surgery, International Journal of Periodontics and Restorative Dentistry, International Journal of Prosthodontics, Journal of the American Dental Association, Journal of Biomedical Materials Research, Journal of Clinical Periodontology, Journal of Dental Research, Journal of Oral Implantology, Journal of Oral and Maxillofacial Surgery, Journal of Periodontology,* and the *Journal of Prosthetic Dentistry.*

The bibliographies of identified RCTs and review articles were checked for studies beyond the listed journals. PubMed was independently searched using the "related articles" feature. Personal references were also searched. Correspondence was conducted with professional contacts, authors of identified RCTs, and 55 oral implant manufacturers in attempts to identify unpublished or ongoing studies. No language restrictions were applied.

1.2.2 Study Selection, Quality Assessment, and Data Extraction

The titles and abstracts (when available) of all reports identified were scanned independently by two reviewers (ME and PC). For studies appear-

TABLE 1.1

Search Strategy Used in Medline Database to Identify Trials on Oral Implants

#1 randomized controlled trial.pt.
#2 controlled clinical trial.pt.
#3 randomized controlled trials.sh.
#4 random allocation.sh.
#5 double blind method.sh.
#6 single blind method.sh.
#7 latin square.ti,ab.
#8 crossover.ti,ab.
#9 (split adj (mouth or plot)).ti,ab.
#10 or/1–9
#11 (ANIMAL not HUMAN).sh.
#12 10 not 11
#13 clinical trial.pt.
#14 exp clinical trials/
#15 (clin$ adj25 trial$).ti,ab.
#16 ((singl$ or doubl$ or trebl$ or tripl$) adj25 (blind$ or mask$)).ti,ab.
#17 placebos.sh.
#18 placebo$.ti,ab.
#19 random$.ti,ab.
#20 research design.sh.
#21 or/13–20
#22 21 not 11
#23 22 not 12
#24 12 or 22
#25 exp Dental Implants/
#26 exp Dental Implantation/or dental implantation.mp.
#27 exp Dental Prosthesis, Implant-Supported/
#28 ((osseointegrated adj implant$) and (dental or oral)).mp. [mp = title, abstract, registry number word, mesh subject heading]
#29 dental implant$.mp. [mp = title, abstract, registry number word, mesh subject heading]
#30 (implant$ adj5 dent$).mp. [mp = title, abstract, registry number word, mesh subject heading]
#31 dental-implant$.mp. [mp = title, abstract, registry number word, mesh subject heading]
#32 (((overdenture$ or crown$ or bridge$ or prosthesis or prostheses or restoration$) adj10 (Dental or oral)) and implant$).mp. [mp = title, abstract, registry number word, mesh subject heading]
#33 "implant supported dental prosthesis".mp. [mp = title, abstract, registry number word, mesh subject heading]
#34 ("blade implant$" and (dental or oral)).mp. [mp = title, abstract, registry number word, mesh subject heading]
#35 ((endosseous adj5 implant$) and (dental or oral)).mp. [mp = title, abstract, registry number word, mesh subject heading]
#36 ((dental or oral) adj5 implant$).mp. [mp = title, abstract, registry number word, mesh subject heading]
#37 25 or 26 or 27 or 28 or 29 or 30 or 32 or 33 or 34 or 35 or 36
#38 24 and 37

ing to meet the inclusion criteria and those whose titles or abstracts were insufficient to enable the reviewers to make a clear decision, full reports were obtained. The full reports obtained from all electronic and other methods of searching were assessed independently by ME and PC to determine whether the studies met the inclusion criteria. Disagreements were resolved by discussion. All studies meeting the inclusion criteria then underwent validity assessment and data extraction.

Quality assessment of the included trials was undertaken independently and in duplicate by ME and PC. Three main quality criteria were examined: allocation concealment, blindness of patients and outcome assessors, and the completeness of reporting on follow-up. Further quality assessments were carried out to assess the definition of exclusion and inclusion criteria, adequate definition of success criteria, and comparability of control and treatment groups at entry. The quality assessment criteria were pilot-tested using several articles.

Data were extracted by ME and HW independently using specially designed data extraction forms. The forms were tested on several papers and modified as required before use. All disagreements were discussed and a third reviewer (PC) consulted where necessary. All authors were contacted to obtain clarification or missing information. Data were excluded until further clarification was available if agreement could not be reached.

For each trial, the following data were recorded: year of publication, country of origin, source of study funding, details about participants including demographic characteristics, details of types of interventions, and details of outcomes reported including methods of assessment and time intervals.

1.2.3 Data Synthesis

For dichotomous outcomes, the estimates of effects of interventions were expressed as relative risks together with 95% confidence intervals. For continuous outcomes, mean differences and 95% confidence intervals were used to summarize the data. Meta-analyses were to be attempted only when studies comparing similar interventions reported the same outcome measures.

1.2.4 Descriptions of Studies

Of the 30 eligible articles[20–49] reporting data of 14 different trials, we excluded 23 articles,[20,21,23–25,27,28,31–40,42,43,46–49] representing 9 trials due to problems with the data presented (Table 1.2). Of the five trials included (seven articles)[22,26,29,30,41,44,45] (Table 1.3), two were conducted in Sweden,[29,30,41] one in Finland,[22] one in New Zealand,[44,45] and one in The Netherlands.[26] All five trials had parallel group study designs. Four trials[22,26,29,30,44,45] received support from industry. Four were conducted at university dental clinics and one in a hospital.[29,30] All studies included adults.

Biological and mechanical failures and bone level measurements were recorded in all studies. However, in one trial,[41] peri-implant bone level measurements were partly performed on panoramic radiographs and were not included in the present analyses. In another trial,[26] insufficient data on bone level assessment were presented and the authors were not able to supply the required data. All trials reported on implants functionally

TABLE 1.2

Excluded Studies

Study	Reason for Exclusion
Friberg 1992[20]	Classified as not RCT based on author's reply
Geertman 1996[46] and Meijer 2000[47]	Data from two RCTs combined; separate data requested; no replies to letters
Boerrigter 1997[48] and Meijer 2000[49]	Number of enrolled patients unclear; no replies to letters
Jones 1997[21] and 1999[31]	Classified as not RCT; no reply to letter
Karlsson 1998[27] and Gotfredsen 2001[40]	Not all patients participated in split-mouth study; author's reply failed to clarify issue
Veteran studies (1997–2000)[23–25,28,32–38]	Unable to extract meaningful data due to extreme complexity of study design; no replies to letters
van Steenberghe 2000[39]	Split-mouth design; no patient-based paired standard deviation in report; we could have used data on implant failure (only one), but did not know how it was recorded; no reply to letter
Khang 2001[42]	Split-mouth study with unequal number of implants randomly allocated to patients; no reply to letter
Roccuzzo 2001[43]	Time of implant loading was confounded with implant type; mobile implants not considered failures

loaded for 1 year. One trial[45] included 2-year data and two trials presented 3-year data.[30,41]

1.2.5 Methodological Quality of Included Studies

The methods of randomization and allocation concealment were considered unclear for all trials despite author clarifications, with one exception.[26] According to information provided by the authors, the randomization procedure of this trial[26] was not concealed. No clarification was obtained for one trial.[41] It was not possible to blind the patients and outcome assessors to the interventions in all the included trials because the different shapes of implants and abutments were easily recognizable. However, in one trial,[29,30] an independent assessor made the radiographic evaluations. The reporting of withdrawals was not adequate for one trial.[26] However, an author of the study supplied the missing information. Only one study[29] undertook *a priori* calculation for the sample size to detect a true difference of 0.4 mm in marginal bone levels. The percent agreement and kappa scores of the two raters were 100%, 1.00 for allocation concealment and 60%, 0.38 for withdrawals.

1.2.6 Implant Characteristics

Six different implant types were compared. The surface roughness of each of the six implants was measured with an optical profilometer using confocal

TABLE 1.3

Interventions and Outcomes of Included Studies

Study and Duration	Intervention	Outcome
Batenburg[26] (1 year)	Brånemark® (Nobel Biocare AB, Göteborg, Sweden) submerged turned titanium screws versus ITI® (Institut Straumann AG, Waldenburg, Switzerland) nonsubmerged hollow plasma-sprayed titanium screws versus IMZ® (Friedrichsfeld AG, Mannheim, Germany) submerged titanium plasma-sprayed in totally edentulous mandibles supporting overdentures on 2 implants	Periotest and tapping the implant with superstructures removed; sensibility of lip and chin; marginal bone level changes on standardized intraoral radiographs; plaque accumulation; calculus; bleeding on probing; mucosa score; probing pocket depth; mucosa recession; width of attached peri-implant mucosa; 1-year data used
Åstrand 1999[29] (1 year) and Engquist 2002[30] (3 years)	Astra® (Astra Tech AB, Mölndal, Sweden) TiOblast submerged titanium screws versus Brånemark® (Nobel Biocare AB, Göteborg, Sweden) Mark II type submerged turned titanium screws in totally edentulous patients supporting fixed bridges	Pain from implant region; implant stability tested with superstructure removed; bridge survival; marginal bone level changes on standardized intraoral radiographs; plaque accumulation; bleeding on probing; operation time; mechanical complications; peri-implant infections with bone loss; presence or absence of attached peri-implant mucosa; 1- and 3-year data used
Moberg 2001[41] (3 years)	Brånemark® (Nobel Biocare AB, Göteborg, Sweden) Mark II type submerged turned titanium screws versus ITI® (Institut Straumann AG, Waldenburg, Switzerland) nonsubmerged hollow plasma-sprayed titanium screws in totally edentulous mandibles supporting fixed bridges	Periotest and tapping implant with superstructures removed at 3 years; marginal bone level changes on intraoral and panoramic radiographs; plaque accumulation; marginal bleeding; probing pocket depths; tightness of screws; sensory changes; treatment time; patient satisfaction; mechanical and biological complications; peri-implant infections with bone loss; 1- and 3-year data used
Kemppainen 1997[22] (1 year)	Astra® (Astra Tech AB, Mölndal, Sweden) TiOblast submerged titanium screws versus ITI® (Institut Straumann AG, Waldenburg, Switzerland) nonsubmerged hollow plasma-sprayed titanium screws and cylinders for single tooth replacement	Implant stability; marginal bone level changes on standardized intraoral radiographs; plaque accumulation; gingival index; probing pocket depth; 1-year data used
Tawse-Smith 2001[44] (1 year) and 2002[45] (2 years)	Steri-Oss® (Steri-Oss, Yorba Linda, California, U.S.) nonsubmerged acid-etched titanium screws HL series, 3.8 mm in diameter versus Southern® (Southern Implants Ltd, Irene, South Africa) nonsubmerged sand-blasted acid-etched titanium screws conventionally loaded at 12 weeks or early loaded at 6 weeks with mandibular overdentures on 2 implants	Periotest; marginal bone level changes on standardized intraoral radiographs; bridge survival; plaque accumulation; modified sulcus bleeding index; probing pocket depth; width of keratinized mucosa; 1-year data used

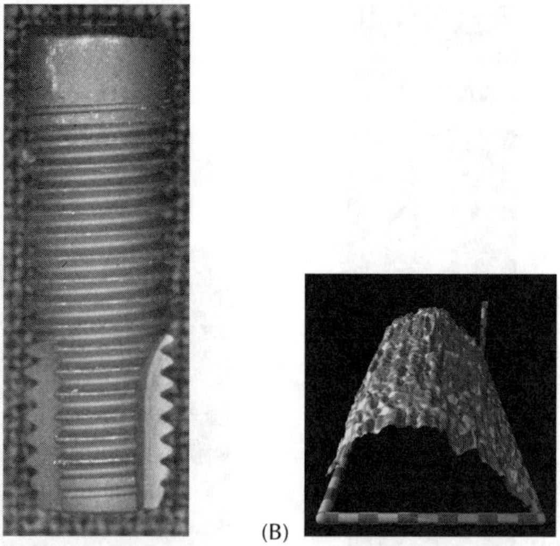

FIGURE. 1.1
(A) Astra implant. (B) Digital image showing surface roughness of Astra implant.

optics. Nine areas measuring 245 × 245 μm were measured on each implant. To separate roughness from form and waviness, a Gaussian 50-μm filter was used. Three parameters were used to describe variations in height, spatial distribution, and increased surface area compared with a flat reference plane: S_a = average height deviation, S_{cx} = average wavelength, and S_{dr} = developed surface area. The six implant types were:

1. Astra® (Astra Tech AB, Mölndal, Sweden) TiO_2 blast titanium grade 3 screws (Figure 1.1A). S_a = 1.11 μm, S_{cx} = 9.98 μm, and S_{dr} = 31%. This surface demonstrated a homogenous structure. The irregularities were equally distributed over the surface (Figure 1.1B).
2. Brånemark® (Nobel Biocare AB, Göteborg, Sweden) Mark II type titanium grade 1 screws (Figure 1.2A). S_a = 0.68 μm, S_{cx} = 8.09 μm, S_{dr} = 22%. A turned implant with visible marks from the cutting tool; an example of a surface with a clear orientation (Figure 1.2B).
3. IMZ® (Friedrichsfeld AG, Mannheim, Germany) titanium plasma-sprayed (TPS) titanium grade 2 cylinders (Figure 1.3A). S_a = 2.62 μm, S_{cx} = 16.32 μm, S_{dr} = 78%. A rough rather inhomogeneous structure and some small smooth parts were visible (Figure 1.3B).
4. ITI® (Institut Straumann AG, Waldenburg, Switzerland) hollow TPS titanium grade 4 screws and cylinders (Figure 1.4A). S_a = 2.35 μm, S_{cx} = 13.15 μm, S_{dr} = 87%. A rough rather inhomogeneous structure and some small smooth parts were visible (Figure 1.4B).

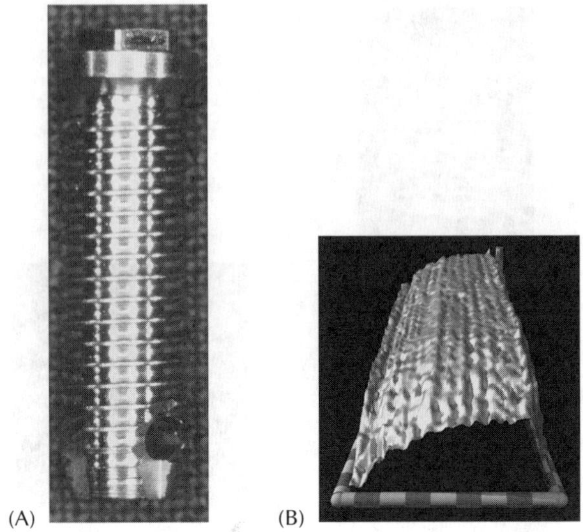

FIGURE 1.2
(A) Brånemark implant. (B) Digital image showing surface roughness of Brånemark implant.

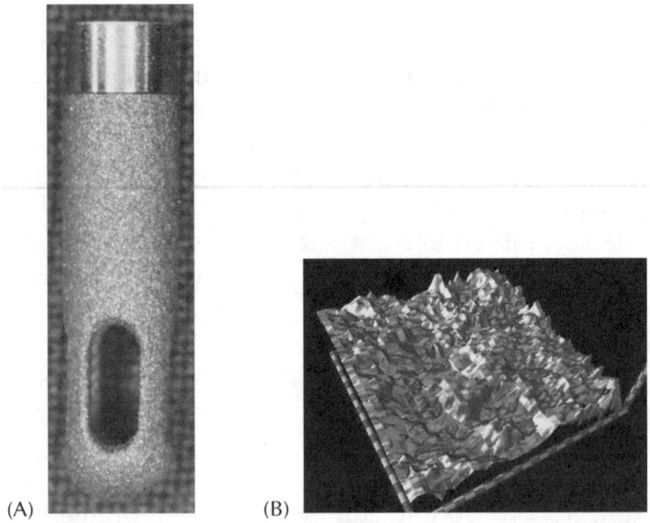

FIGURE 1.3
(A) IMZ implant. (B) Digital image showing surface roughness of IMZ implant.

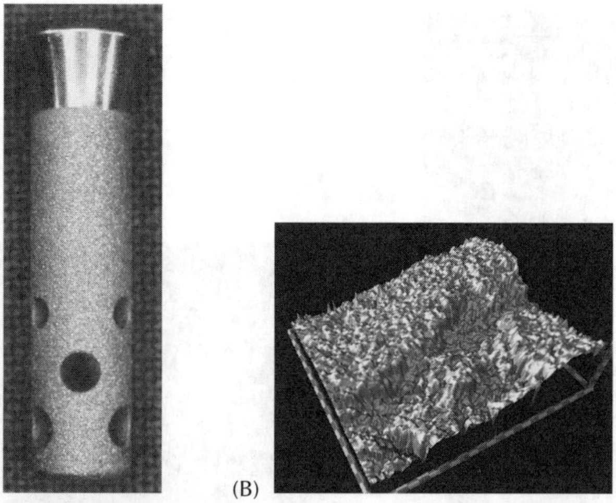

(A) (B)

FIGURE 1.4
(A) ITI implant. (B) Digital image showing surface roughness of ITI implant.

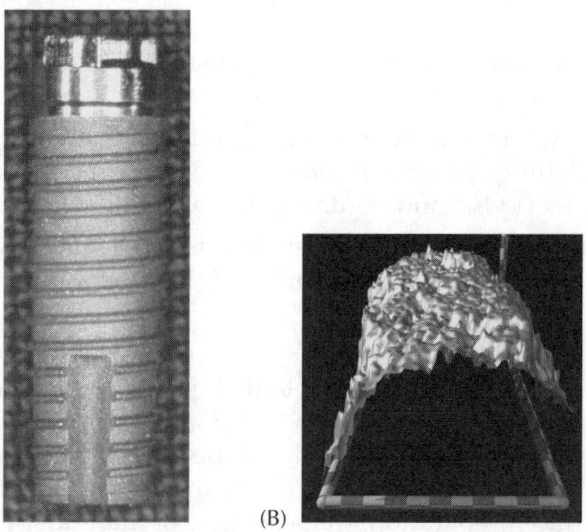

(A) (B)

FIGURE 1.5
(A) Southern implant. (B) Digital image showing surface roughness of Southern implant.

5. Southern® (Southern Implants Irene, South Africa) sand-blasted acid-etched titanium grade 4 screws (Figure 1.5A). S_a = 1.43 μm, S_{cx} = 12.18 μm, S_{dr} = 50% (Figure 1.5B).
6. Steri-Oss® (Steri-Oss, Yorba Linda, California, U.S.) HL series 3.8-mm diameter acid-etched titanium grade 4 screws (Figure 1.6A). S_a = 0.82 μm, S_{cx} = 9.29 μm, S_{dr} = 26% (Figure 1.6B).

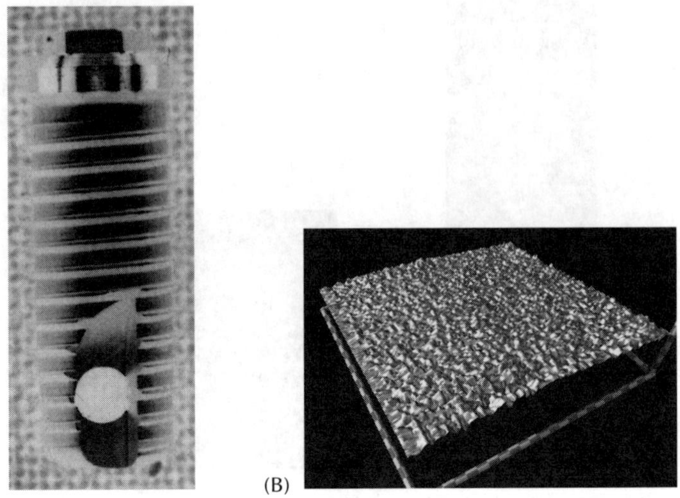

(A) (B)

FIGURE 1.6
(A) Steri-Oss implant. (B) Digital image showing surface roughness of Steri-Oss implant.

Three types of surface modifications were analyzed:

1. Surface with clear orientation of irregularities due to cutting procedure during turning (Brånemark)
2. Surface without a dominating direction (orientation), machined with techniques that remove material during manufacturing (Astra, Steri-Oss, and Southern implants)
3. Surface without a dominating direction, machined with a process that adds material to the surface (plasma-sprayed ITI and IMZ implants)

Implants were grouped according to their shapes in three main categories: screws (Brånemark, Steri-Oss, Astra and Southern implants), hollow cylinders and screws (ITI implants), and cylinders (IMZ implants). All inserted oral implants were made of machined, commercially pure titanium, but they differed in surface preparation, shape, degree of titanium purity, and modality of insertion (submerged or nonsubmerged).

In general, the final prostheses were placed 4 to 8 months after implant placement in mandibles and 7 to 10 months after placement in maxillae. However, in one trial,[44,45] mandibular overdentures were attached to the implants 6 to 12 weeks after implant placement. Cross-arch fixed prostheses were screw-retained on four to six implants.[29,30,41] Removable overdentures were retained by clip attachments to bars supported by two implants[26] or were retained by two ball attachments.[44,45] Crowns were cemented on single implants.[22]

TABLE 1.4

Patients with Failed Implants and Relative Risk Values for Included Studies

Study	Comparison	Time of Outcome (Number of Patients with Failures/Total Number of Patients per Group)	Relative Risk (95% Confidence Interval)
Kemppainen 1997[22]	Astra versus ITI	1 year (1/37 versus 0/45)	3.63 (0.15, 86.61)
Batenburg 1998[26]	Brånemark versus IMZ	1 year (1/30 versus 1/29)	0.97 (0.06, 14.74)
	Brånemark versus ITI	1 year (1/30 versus 0/29)	2.90 (0.12, 68.50)
	IMZ versus ITI	1 year (1/29 versus 0/29)	3.00 (0.13, 70.74)
Åstrand 1999[29] and Engquist 2002[30]	Astra versus Brånemark	1 yr (1/33 versus 4/33)	0.25 (0.03, 2.12)
		3 years (2/33 versus 5/33)	0.40 (0.08, 1.92)
Moberg 2001[41]	Brånemark versus ITI	1 year (1/20 versus 0/20)	3.00 (0.13, 69.52)
		3 years (2/19 versus 1/18)	1.89 (0.19, 19.13)
Tawse-Smith 2001[44]	Steri-Oss versus Southern (conventional loading)	1 year (1/12 versus 0/12)	3.00 (0.13, 67.06)
Tawse-Smith 2002[45]	Steri-Oss versus Southern (early loading)	1 year (5/12 versus 0/12)	11.00 (0.67, 179.30)

1.3 Results

A total of 957 implants (349 turned implants and 608 with roughened surfaces) were placed in 326 patients (238 mandibles and 88 maxillae) in the five trials. Astra, Brånemark, and IMZ implants were placed according to the submerged (two-stage) technique; Steri-Oss, Southern, and ITI implants were inserted according to a nonsubmerged (one-stage) protocol. In one study,[45] mandibular implants were early-loaded at 6 weeks instead of the conventional 12-week period.

During the follow-up periods considered in this review (1 and 3 years), 25 implant failures (one due to implant fracture) occurred. Thirteen of the failed implants had roughened surfaces and 12 had turned surfaces. Eighteen were early failures (10 implants had roughened surfaces) and seven were late failures (three had roughened surfaces and one fractured). Peri-implantitis (advanced marginal bone loss with signs of infection such as suppuration) affected six implants (five had roughened surfaces). Two were successfully treated; outcomes for two were uncertain; and two implants failed. No meta-analyses could be attempted. Implant failures and marginal bone level changes are presented in Tables 1.4 and 1.5, respectively.

1.3.1 Astra versus Brånemark Implants

One trial[29,30] with a parallel design compared submerged Astra versus submerged Brånemark screws in totally edentulous patients for 3 years. Thirty-

TABLE 1.5

Mean (Standard Deviation) Marginal Bone Level Changes per Patient and Mean Differences (95% Confidence Interval) between Groups

			Intervention A		Intervention B		
Study	**Comparison (A versus B)**	**Time of Outcome**	**Number of Patients**	**Mean (SD)**	**Number of Patients**	**Mean (SD)**	**Mean Difference (95% Confidence Interval)**
Kemppainen 1997[22]	Astra versus ITI	1 year	37	–0.15 (0.10)	45	–0.13 (0.09)	–0.02 (–0.06, 0.02)
Åstrand 1999[29]	Astra versus Brånemark	1 year	32	–0.26 (0.60)	33	–0.17 (0.37)	–0.09 (–0.33, 0.15)
Engquist 2002[30]		3 years	32	–0.23 (0.88)	33	–0.17 (0.44)	–0.06 (–0.40, 0.28)
Tawse-Smith 2001[44]	Steri-Oss versus Southern (conventional loading)	1 year	11	–0.07 (0.38)	12	–0.08 (0.20)	0.01 (–0.24, 0.26)
Tawse-Smith 2002[45]	Steri-Oss versus Southern (early loading)	1 year	7	–0.12 (0.15)	12	–0.12 (0.23)	0.00 (–0.17, 0.17)

three fully edentulous patients (17 maxillas and 16 mandibles) were originally included in each group. No baseline unbalances for sex, bone quantity, or length of implant used appeared in the two groups. Eight patients treated with Brånemark implants were scored as having type 4 bone quality (very soft bone) according to the Lekholm and Zarb classification[50] versus one patient in the Astra group. No withdrawals occurred during the study period. Baseline radiographs were missing for one mandible in the Astra group. According to a sample size calculation, a minimal number of 15 patients were to be included and followed in order to detect a true difference of 0.4 mm in marginal bone level changes between the tested implants with 90% power in mandibles.

Nine Brånemark implants failed in five patients (one patient lost five implants and the bridge) versus two Astra implant failures in two patients (one failure was due to implant fracture between 1- and 3-year follow-ups). Two additional Astra implants were successfully treated for peri-implantitis (suppuration combined with advanced bone loss). At patient levels no statistically significant differences for failures and marginal bone level changes between the implant systems appeared after 3 years of function.

1.3.2 Astra versus ITI Implants

One trial[22] with a parallel design compared submerged Astra versus nonsubmerged ITI hollow cylinders and screws for single tooth replacement for 1 year. Thirty-seven patients received 46 Astra implants (36 maxillary and 10 mandibular implants) and 45 patients received 56 ITI implants (34 maxillary and 22 mandibular implants; 18 hollow screws were placed in mandibular posterior areas). It was unclear whether baseline differences arose between the two groups since ITI hollow screws were placed only in posterior mandibles. No patients dropped out. One maxillary Astra implant failed to integrate (early failure). All ITI implants were successful. At patient levels we noted no statistically significant differences for failures and marginal bone level changes between the implant systems after 1 year of function.

1.3.3 Brånemark versus IMZ Implants

One trial[26] with a parallel design compared two Brånemark and two IMZ submerged implants supporting overdentures in edentulous mandibles for 1 year. Thirty patients were included in each group. It was unclear whether baseline differences appeared in the two groups. One patient in the IMZ group dropped out before the 1-year examination.

One Brånemark and one IMZ implant failed prior to the abutment connection operation. At patient levels no statistically significant difference was noted for failures after one year of function.

1.3.4 Brånemark versus ITI Implants

Two trials[26,41] with parallel designs compared submerged Brånemark and nonsubmerged ITI hollow screws in totally edentulous mandibles. One trial[26] compared two implants supporting overdentures for 1 year. Thirty patients were included in each group. It was unclear whether baseline differences occurred in the two groups. One patient of the ITI group dropped out before the 1-year examination.

One Brånemark implant failed prior to the abutment connection operation. At patient levels, no statistically significant differences appeared for failures between implant systems after 1 year of function.

One trial[41] compared implants supporting fixed bridges for 3 years. Twenty patients were included in each group. No baseline differences appeared for sex, age, or location of implant. Three patients died before the 3-year examination (one in the Brånemark group and two in the ITI group). One patient with Brånemark implants did not attend the 3-year radiographic examination.

Two Brånemark implants failed (one early failure and one for peri-implantitis between years 1 and 2). One ITI implant failed because of peri-implantitis at 2 years. However, two additional ITI implants were found affected by peri-implantitis at the 3-year examination and were under treatment. Their outcome was unknown at the time of reporting. At patient levels, no statistically significant differences for failures of the systems were noted after 3 years of function.

1.3.5 IMZ versus ITI Implants

One trial[26] with a parallel design compared two submerged IMZ cylinders and two nonsubmerged ITI hollow screws supporting overdentures in edentulous mandibles for 1 year. Thirty patients were in each group. It was unclear whether baseline differences appeared. One patient of each group dropped out before the 1-year examination. One IMZ implant failed prior to the abutment connection operation. At patient levels, no statistically significant differences were noted for failures after 1 year of function.

1.3.6 Steri-Oss versus Southern Implants

One trial[44,45] of parallel design compared nonsubmerged Steri-Oss and nonsubmerged Southern implants for the treatment of total mandibular edentulism using two unsplinted implants supporting an overdenture for 2 years. This trial comprised two additional groups for each implant system (12 subjects in each group): a control group in which mandibular implants were loaded at 12 weeks and a test group in which implants were early loaded at 6 weeks. Patients having type 4 bone were to be excluded, but none was found. There were no baseline unbalances in bone quality and quantity among the four groups. However, the Steri-Oss and Southern implants in conventionally loaded groups were longer than those in the early loaded groups. The Steri-Oss implants were described as having turned surfaces, but after analyzing the surface of an implant kindly provided by the authors, we realized that the implant surface was chemically treated.

The following information is based on the results at 1-year follow-up. No drop-out occurred at 1 year. One patient in the Steri-Oss conventionally loaded group (12 weeks) had an early implant failure, and five patients in the Steri-Oss early loaded group (6 weeks) had seven early failures. No implants were lost in the Southern groups. Most of the failed implants were placed by one surgeon who only used Steri-Oss implants. At patient levels, no statistically significant differences in failures and marginal bone level changes were noted after 1 year of function.

1.4 Discussion

In order to properly compare the effects of different implant characteristics, an ideal trial should be designed in a way that only the characteristic of interest (i.e., surface roughness, implant shape, or implant material) is different (test versus control group); all other parameters should be identical. This was not done in the RCTs we included in the present SR because the trials compared implants with combinations of different surface characteristics, shapes, dimensions, and levels of purity of titanium. The implants were placed according to different surgical protocols (submerged versus nonsubmerged). Therefore, the present systematic review presents comparisons between different implant systems and not comparisons of specific implant characteristics.

In general, high success rates were reported for all implant systems. No statistically significant differences were found when root-formed titanium implants with different surface characteristics and shapes were compared. No trial described implants made or coated with other materials.

Only one trial[29] undertook a sample size calculation for detecting a true difference in marginal bone levels of 0.4 mm, considered to be of clinical significance. However, whether the 0.4 mm difference bears any clinical significance is questionable, considering that it is very difficult to achieve valid bone loss measurements of less than 0.2 mm even in an *in vitro* situation.[51] Thus, the number of subjects included in the few available trials was likely to be too low and follow-up periods too short to detect a significant difference, if any. In other words, we cannot exclude the possibility that differences in effectiveness among various modified surfaces, materials, and shapes exist.

While it was not the aim of this review to evaluate comparisons of submerged and nonsubmerged implants, three trials[22,26,41] failed to demonstrate differences in success rates or marginal bone losses when comparing implants with different surfaces used in submerged and nonsubmerged fashions. The great majority of the implants placed in nonsubmerged mode were in mandibles, where success rates are usually higher.[18] However, if these findings are substantiated by more robust RCTs, it will be possible to reduce patient discomfort and treatment costs by using a nonsubmerged technique.

It was judged premature to make any meta-analytic comparisons with respect to clinical effectiveness of oral implants with various degrees of surface roughness by grouping different implant systems having similar degrees of surface roughness due to the limited number of patients and short follow-up periods presently available. Such comparisons will be attempted when additional data become available.

None of the trial authors characterized the implant surfaces. This is understandable because they relied on the information provided by manufacturers or published in other studies. However, after analyzing the surfaces of some implants, we realized that the surface descriptions of the Steri-Oss implants reported in two trials[44,45] did not correspond to what we actually found. In fact, the surfaces were acid-etched and not turned, as described in the articles. Such findings were indeed unexpected. In experimental research, it is recommended that authors characterize in detail the surface properties of their implants. We feel that the same recommendation should apply to clinical trials in which implant characteristics should be described in detail and possibly independently verified.

The randomization and concealment of allocation procedures were considered unclear for all trials except one,[26] despite clarifications by the authors of four trials.[22,26,29,30,44,45] These aspects of trial designing and reporting need to be improved because RCTs in which randomization and allocation concealment procedures were inadequately conducted tended to overestimate treatment effects.[10,52]

In another investigation it was found that the design, analysis, and reporting of RCTs on oral implants were generally poor.[11] This supports the determination that so many trials had to be excluded from the present review. Investigators should design studies carefully and decide to use a parallel group or a split-mouth design at the outset and not combine both designs in one study. Split-mouth studies ideally should include equal numbers of implants per patient in each group. The analysis of these studies should be "paired" and take the pairing of implants within patients into account. Another related problem is that both split-mouth and parallel group studies are analyzed at the level of the implant, not taking the clustering of implants within a patient into account. The design and analysis of these studies are usually complex and it is recommended that statisticians be involved in the initial planning stages and writing protocols for such studies. Such trials should be reported according the Consolidated Standards of Reporting Trials (CONSORT) guidelines[53] (http://www.consort-statement.org/).

The generalization of the results of the included trials to ordinary clinical conditions should be considered with extreme caution. In general, treatments were administered by experienced clinicians and the follow-up regimens were strict. It is unlikely that dentists with noncomparable experience could match similar positive results. The observation that the inclusion of a less trained surgeon might have influenced the result of one trial[45] could support this suggestion.

1.5 Conclusions

Based on the available results of RCTs, no reliable evidence supports the superiority of one type of implant surface, material, or shape over another for root-formed osseointegrated implants. No trials described implants made or coated with materials other than titanium. No statistically significant differences were observed for implant systems placed according to submerged or nonsubmerged procedures.

These conclusions are based on a few RTCs with relatively short follow-up periods and few patients, so basically we do not know whether certain implant characteristics or systems are superior to others due to the scarcity of reliable information. In order to understand whether any surface modification or material can significantly improve the effectiveness of oral implants, more well designed long-term RCTs are needed. It is recommended that such trials include sufficient numbers of patients to reveal true differences if any. Trials should also be of sufficient duration (5 years or longer). Ideally, they should investigate only one aspect, such as the effects of various degrees of surface roughness or the role of calcium–phosphate coating, thus minimizing the numerous confounding factors such as different implant shapes or clinical procedures.

Acknowledgments

We wish to thank Sylvia Bickley (Cochrane Collaboration) for her assistance with literature searching and Emma Tavender (Cochrane Collaboration) for her help with the preparation of this review. We also thank Drs. Per Åstrand, Bertil Friberg, Klaus Gotfredsen, Henny Meijer, Pentti Kemppainen, Alan Payne, Gerry Raghoebar, Mario Roccuzzo, and Andrew Tawse-Smith for providing us information on their trials. We are indebted to Drs. Alan Payne and Pentti Kemppainen for providing us with the implants used in their trials for surface roughness analyses and to Prof. Tomas Albrektsson for his critical and valuable comments and invaluable help in attempting to identify unpublished RCT data.

The financial support of the Swedish Medical Research Council (9495), Jubileumsfonden (Sweden) and the PPP Foundation (U.K.) is gratefully acknowledged. No financial support was received from industry.

References

1. Stout, K.J., Davies, E.J., and Sullivan, P.J., *Atlas of Machined Surfaces*, London, Chapman & Hall, 1990.
2. Binon, P.P., Implants and components: entering the new millennium, *Int. J. Oral Maxillofac. Implants*, 15, 76, 2000.
3. Evidence-Based Medicine Working Group, Evidence-based medicine: a new approach to teaching the practice of medicine, *J. Am. Med. Assoc.*, 268, 2420, 1992.
4. Newman, M.G., Improved clinical decision making using the evidence-based approach, *Ann. Periodont.*, 1, i, 1996.
5. Anderson, J.D., Need for evidence-based practice in prosthodontics, *J. Prosthet. Dent.*, 83, 58, 2000.
6. Guyatt, G.H., Sackett, D.L., and Cook, D.J., Users' guides to the medical literature. II. How to use an article about therapy or prevention. B. What were the results and will they help me in caring for my patients? *J. Am. Med. Assoc.*, 271, 59, 1994.
7. Colditz, G.A., Miller, J.N., and Mosteller, F., How study design affects outcomes in comparisons of therapy. I. Medical, *Stat. Med.*, 8, 441, 1989.
8. Esposito, M., Worthington, H.V., and Coulthard, P., In search of truth: the role of systematic reviews and meta-analyses for assessing the effectiveness of rehabilitation with oral implants, *Clin. Implant Dent. Rel. Res.*, 3, 62, 2001.
9. Jadad, A., *Randomized Controlled Trials: A User's Guide*, London, BMJ Publishing Group, 1998.
10. Schulz, K.F. et al., Empirical evidence of bias: dimensions of methodological quality associated with estimates of treatment effects in controlled trials, *J. Am. Med. Assoc.*, 273, 408, 1995.
11. Esposito, M. et al., Quality assessment of randomized controlled trials of oral implants, *Int. J. Oral Maxillofac. Implants*, 16, 783, 2001.
12. Clarke, M. and Oxman, A.D., *Cochrane Reviewers' Handbook 4.1*, June 2000 update. Review Manager (RevMan) (computer program), Oxford, The Cochrane Collaboration, 2000.
13. Sacks, H.S. et al., Meta-analyses of randomized controlled trials, *New Engl. J. Med.*, 316, 450, 1987.
14. Jadad, A.R. and McQuay, H.J., Meta-analyses to evaluate analgesic interventions: a systematic qualitative review of their methodology, *J. Clin. Epidemiol.*, 49, 235, 1996.
15. Glenny, A.-M. et al., The assessment of systematic reviews in the field of dentistry, *Eur. J. Oral Sci.*, submitted, 2002.
16. Moher, D. et al., Improving the quality of reports of meta-analyses of randomised controlled trials: the QUOROM statement, *Lancet*, 354, 1896, 1999.

17. Esposito, M. et al., Interventions for replacing missing teeth: different types of dental implants, protocol for a Cochrane review, Oxford, The Cochrane Library, software update, 2002.
18. Esposito, M. et al., Biological factors contributing to failures of osseointegrated oral implants. 1. Success criteria and epidemiology, *Eur. J. Oral Sci.*, 106, 527, 1998.
19. Esposito, M. et al., Differential diagnosis and treatment strategies for biologic complications and failing oral implants: a review of the literature., *Int. J. Oral Maxillofac. Implants*, 14, 473, 1999.
20. Friberg, B., Gröndahl, K., and Lekholm, U., A new self-tapping Brånemark implant: clinical and radiographic evaluation, *Int. J. Oral Maxillofac. Implants*, 7, 80, 1992.
21. Jones, J.D. et al., Clinical evaluation of hydroxyapatite-coated titanium plasma-sprayed and titanium plasma-sprayed cylinder dental implants: a preliminary report, *Oral Surg. Oral Med. Oral Pathol. Oral Radiol. Endod.*, 84, 137, 1997.
22. Kemppainen, P., Eskola, S., and Ylipaavalniemi, P., A comparative prospective clinical study of two single-tooth implants: a preliminary report of 102 implants, *J. Prosthet. Dent.*, 77, 382, 1997.
23. Manz, M.C., Radiographic assessment of peri-implant vertical bone loss: DI-CRG interim report no. 9, *J. Oral Maxillofac. Surg.*, 55 (Suppl. 5), 62, 1997.
24. Morris, H.F., Manz, M.C., and Tarolli, J.H., Success of multiple endosseous dental implant designs to second-stage surgery across study sites, *J. Oral Maxillofac. Surg.*, 55 (Suppl. 5), 76, 1997.
25. Truhlar, R.S. et al., Bone quality and implant design-related outcomes through stage II surgical uncovering of spectra-system root form implants, *J. Oral Maxillofac. Surg.*, 55 (Suppl. 5), 46, 1997.
26. Batenburg, R.H.K. et al., Mandibular overdentures supported by two Brånemark, IMZ or ITI implants: a prospective comparative preliminary study: one-year results, *Clin. Oral Implants Res.*, 9, 374, 1998.
27. Karlsson, U., Gotfredsen, K., and Olsson, C., A 2-year report on maxillary and mandibular fixed partial dentures supported by Astra Tech dental implants: a comparison of two implants with different surface textures, *Clin. Oral Implants Res.*, 9, 235, 1998.
28. Morris, H.F. and Ochi, S., Hydroxyapatite-coated implants: a case for their use, *J. Oral Maxillofac. Surg.*, 56, 1303, 1998.
29. Åstrand, P. et al., Astra Tech and Brånemark System implants: a prospective 5-year comparative study: results after one year, *Clin. Implant Dent. Rel. Res.*, 1, 17, 1999.
30. Engquist, B. et al., Marginal bone reaction to oral implants: a prospective comparative study of Astra Tech and Brånemark System implants, *Clin. Oral Implants Res.*, 13, 30, 2002.
31. Jones, J.D. et al., A 5-year comparison of hydroxyapatite-coated titanium plasma-sprayed and titanium plasma-sprayed cylinder dental implants, *Oral Surg. Oral Med. Oral Pathol. Oral Radiol. Endod.*, 87, 649, 1999.
32. Manz, M.C., Factors associated with radiographic vertical bone loss around implants placed in a clinical study, *Ann. Periodont.*, 5, 137, 2000.
33. Morris, H.F. and Ochi, S., Survival and stability (PTVs) of six implant designs from placement to 36 months, *Ann. Periodont.*, 5, 15, 2000.
34. Morris, H.F. and Ochi, S., Influence of two different approaches to reporting implant survival outcomes for five different prosthodontic applications, *Ann. Periodont.*, 5, 90, 2000.

35. Morris, H.F. and Ochi, S., Influence of research center on overall survival outcomes at each phase of treatment, *Ann. Periodont.*, 5, 129, 2000.
36. Morris, H.F., Ochi, S., and Winkler, S., Implant survival in patients with type 2 diabetes: placement to 36 months, *Ann. Periodont.*, 5, 157, 2000.
37. Truhlar, R.S., Morris, H.F., and Ochi, S., Stability of the bone-implant complex: results of longitudinal testing to 60 months with the Periotest device on endosseous dental implants, *Ann. Periodont.*, 5, 42, 2000.
38. Truhlar, R.S., Morris, H.F., and Ochi, S., Implant surface coating and bone quality-related survival outcomes through 36 months post-placement of root-form endosseous dental implants, *Ann. Periodont.*, 5, 109, 2000.
39. van Steenberghe, D. et al., A prospective split-mouth comparative study of two screw-shaped self-tapping pure titanium implant systems, *Clin. Oral Implants Res.*, 11, 202, 2000.
40. Gotfredsen, K. and Karlsson, U., A prospective 5-year study of fixed partial prostheses supported by implants with machined and TiO_2-blasted surface, *J. Prosthodont.*, 10, 2, 2001.
41. Moberg, L.E. et al., Brånemark system and ITI dental implant system for treatment of mandibular edentulism: a comparative randomized study: 3-year follow-up, *Clin. Oral Implants Res.*, 12, 450, 2001.
42. Khang, W. et al., A multi-center study comparing dual acid-etched and machined-surfaced implants in various bone qualities, *J. Periodontol.*, 72, 1384, 2001.
43. Roccuzzo, M. et al., Early loading of sandblasted and acid-etched (SLA) implants: a prospective split-mouth comparative study, *Clin. Oral Implants Res.*, 12, 572, 2001.
44. Tawse-Smith, A. et al., One-stage operative procedure using two different implant systems: a prospective study on implant overdentures in the edentulous mandible, *Clin. Implant Dent. Rel. Res.*, 3, 185, 2001.
45. Tawse-Smith, A. et al., Early loading on unsplinted implants supporting mandibular overdentures using a one-stage operative procedure with two different implant systems: a 2-year report, *Clin. Implant Dent. Rel. Res.*, 4, 33, 2002.
46. Geertman, M.E. et al., Clinical aspects of a multicenter clinical trial of implant-retained mandibular overdentures in patients with severely resorbed mandibles, *J. Prosthet. Dent.*, 75, 194, 1996.
47. Meijer, H.J. et al., Implant-retained mandibular overdentures: 6-year results of a multicenter clinical trial on three different implant systems, *J. Oral Maxillofac. Surg.*, 59, 1260, 2001.
48. Boerrigter, E.M. et al., A controlled clinical trial of implant-retained mandibular overdentures: clinical aspects, *J. Oral Rehabil.*, 24, 182, 1997.
49. Meijer, H.J. et al., A controlled clinical trial of implant-retained mandibular overdentures; 5 years' results of clinical aspects and aftercare of IMZ implants and Branemark implants, *Clin. Oral Implants Res.*, 11, 441, 2000.
50. Lekholm, U. and Zarb, G.A. Patient selection and preparation, in Brånemark, P.-I., Zarb, G.A., and Albrektsson, T., Eds., Tissue-Integrated Prostheses, Chicago, Quintessence Publishing, 1985, p. 199.
51. Benn, D.K., Estimating the validity of radiographic measurements of marginal bone height changes around osseointegrated implants, *Implant Dent.*, 1, 79, 1992.
52. Schulz, K.F., Subverting randomization in controlled trials, *J. Am. Med. Assoc.*, 274, 1456, 1995.

53. Moher, D., Schultz, K.F., and Altman, A.F., The CONSORT statement: revised recommendations for improving the quality of reports of parallel-group randomized trials, *Lancet*, 357, 1191, 2001.

Section II

Can Implant Macro Design and Micro Texturing Improve Bone Response?

2

Toward an Optimized Dental Implant Design

Stig Hansson

CONTENTS

2.1 Introduction 29
2.2 Wolff's Law and Its Implications for Dental Implant Design 30
2.3 Determining Which Parts of an Implant Should Be Provided with Retention Elements 31
2.4 Ideal Surface Roughness from a Biomechanical Angle 33
2.5 Ideal Implant Thread 34
2.6 The Implant–Abutment Interface 36
  2.6.1 Flat-to-Flat or Conical Interface 36
  2.6.2 A Conical Implant–Abutment Interface: At the Level of the Marginal Bone versus a More Coronal Location 38
2.7 Summary 39
References 40

2.1 Introduction

The primary function of dental implants is to carry loads. The loads can be quite significant and the implants are small.[1] This means that a great strain is exerted on the supporting bone which is often in limited supply and of inferior quality.[2] The desire to apply an early loading or immediate loading protocol implies an even greater strain on the bone.

All available bone is needed to resist the loads from an implant and to give support to soft tissue; a high marginal bone level is often a prerequisite for an esthetically acceptable treatment result. In spite of this, it is an accepted reality today that a substantial amount of marginal bone is lost during the first year after implant installation.[3] Can this bone loss be avoided? Does the

0-8493-1474-7/03/$0.00+$1.50

fate of the marginal bone depend on the design of the implant? Does the ability of an implant to support load also depend on implant design?

2.2 Wolff's Law and Its Implications for Dental Implant Design

In 1866, von Meyer gave a lecture on the structure of cancellous bone at the Natural Sciences Society in Zürich. Among the audience was the mathematician and founder of graphic statics, C. Culmann, who was struck by the fact that the orientation of the trabeculae bore a strong resemblance to principal stress trajectories — a mathematical concept used in solid mechanics. One of Culmann's students constructed the principal stress trajectories for a curved beam loaded in a manner expected for a human femur.[4]

The similarity of the trajectories of the trabeculae of the femur and those of the principal stresses of the curved beam was striking.[5] von Meyer concluded that the structure of cancellous bone is correlated to the magnitude and the direction of the loads to which it is exposed. The trajectories of the cancellous bone often meet at right angles and so do principal stress trajectories. Wolff expressed his conviction that the remodeling of bone as a response to the history of mechanical loading follows mathematical laws.[6] Wolff's theories about bone remodeling became known as Wolff's law. Wolff did not give a precise definition of the law. *Dorland's Illustrated Medical Dictionary* states that, "A bone, normal or abnormal, develops the structure most suited to resist the forces acting upon it."[7]

Wolff's law received widespread acceptance and a vast number of observations were interpreted as supporting it.[8] However, bone modeling and remodeling are the results of complex interactions of many different factors of which mechanical stimulation is only one. Bertram and Swartz raised serious objections against an uncritical application of Wolff's law.[9] They suggested that the adaptation of the form of bone to new functional requirements presupposes a regenerative or reparative response. Such a reparative response prevails after the installation of a dental implant.

Wolff's law implies that nature economizes on bone and tends to dispose of bone that is not optimally used. This means that in order to preserve bone tissue, a dental implant should be designed so that it induces a mechanical stimulation of the surrounding bone when loaded. However, if bone is subject to extreme stresses, it is resorbed.[10] This puts another constraint on the proper design of a dental implant. An implant should be designed not to give rise to high stress peaks in the bone when loaded. Thus we have established two operational biomechanical criteria of a good implant design which, when applied, will likely result in a favorable bone response.

A dental implant should have such a design so that, when loaded, it induces a mechanical stimulation in the surrounding bone and high stress peaks do not arise in the bone. In the search for the ultimate implant design, we can use powerful mathematical tools like the finite element method in order to meet these criteria.[11]

2.3 Determining Which Parts of an Implant Should Be Provided with Retention Elements

Dental implants are primarily anchored in bone by means of mechanical interlocking. Axial loads on the implant are transmitted to the bone via retention elements on the implant surface. The most commonly used retention elements are threads and the irregularities of rough surfaces.

Linkow and Cherchève recommended that a dental implant should have a smooth endosseous neck portion — a design principle that has been widely applied.[12] In a combined three-dimensional and axisymmetric finite element study, Hansson compared an axially loaded cylindrical implant equipped with a smooth endosseous neck portion with the same implant whose neck was equipped with retention elements (Figure 2.1).[13] The shear stress at the interface between implant and bone was calculated. At the smooth neck, it was assumed that only compressive stresses were resisted at the implant–bone interface. At implant surfaces provided with retention elements, it was assumed that shear stresses also were resisted at the interface. It follows from the assumptions that the bone outside the smooth neck did not take part in absorbing the load. This violates the first criterion of a good

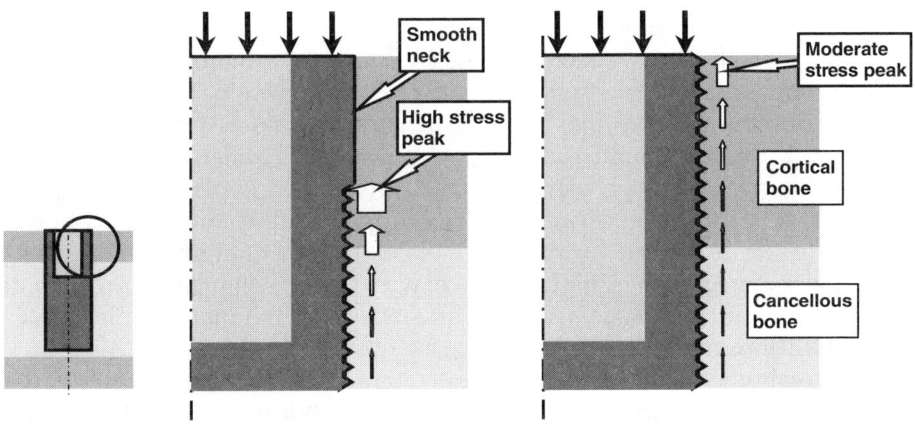

FIGURE 2.1
At the implant with a smooth endosseous neck, a high stress peak arose where the retention elements started. The peak stress at the implant where the retention elements extend to the top marginal bone was substantially lower.

dental implant design: that bone should be mechanically stimulated. Where the retention elements started at the implant with the smooth neck, a high stress peak arose in the bone. This violates the second criterion of a good dental implant design: that high stress peaks should be avoided. At the implant whose neck portion was equipped with retention elements, all the surrounding bone took part in resisting the load and the peak bone–implant interface shear stress was much reduced.

In order to investigate the generality of the results, a number of variations were made in the model. In all cases, the measure to provide the implant neck with retention elements resulted in a substantial reduction of peak interface shear stress. The results of this theoretical study unequivocally indicate that the endosseous neck portion of an implant should be equipped with retention elements. Another result of this study was that an increase in the axial stiffness of an implant results in decreased peak stresses. An increase in axial stiffness can be brought about by an increased wall thickness, for instance, by switching from a standard thread to a microthread.

In a study of loaded porous-coated dental implants provided with machined necks of two different lengths, Al-Sayyed and coworkers found that marginal bone resorption in dogs was more pronounced at the implants with the long machined necks.[14] It was suggested that the marginal bone resorption was caused by disuse atrophy in accordance with Wolff's law, i.e., due to a violation of the first criterion of a good dental implant design.

In a clinical study comprising four different screw-shaped dental implants provided with smooth necks of different lengths, Jung et al. found that the marginal bone stabilized at the level of the first thread.[15] This bone loss down to the first thread can also be interpreted as a result of insufficient mechanical stimulation of the marginal bone, i.e., due to a violation of the first criterion of a good dental implant design.

A very substantial marginal bone loss was reported around a screw-shaped titanium implant provided with a long, smooth, conical neck.[16-17] Quirynen et al. found that the marginal bone resorption progressed down to the level of the first thread around most of the implants.[16] Palmer et al., however, obtained remarkably high marginal bone levels for an implant, similar in its outer shape, whose conical neck was equipped with a microthread and a rough surface produced by means of blasting with titanium dioxide.[18] At baseline, the average marginal bone level was 0.5 mm below the upper lateral edge of the implant. Five years later, this average marginal bone level had moved 0.1 mm more coronally.

The notably favorable marginal bone conditions at this implant can be regarded as yet another confirmation that Wolff's law applies to dental implant design: a dental implant should be designed so that the surrounding bone, and especially the marginal bone, will be mechanically stimulated. It also indicates that marginal bone resorption is a phenomenon that can be avoided.

2.4 Ideal Surface Roughness from a Biomechanical Angle

Animal studies have shown that the bone–implant interface shear strength can be increased by means of a rough surface.[19-20] A rough surface will relieve the loads on retention elements of bigger dimensions. A substantial amount of research effort has been spent on trying to find the kind of surface roughness that maximizes interface shear strength. It has been the practice to characterize rough implant surfaces by means of different surface roughness parameters.[21]

While it can be assumed that an unequivocal relationship exists between the sizes and shapes of irregularities constituting a rough surface and bone response, an unequivocal relationship between a certain set of values of a certain set of surface roughness parameters and bone response cannot be postulated *a priori*. Hansson showed the absence of a clear relationship between the values of a set of surface roughness parameters and the detailed topography of a surface.[22] Consequently, surface roughness parameters are not reliable predictors of interface shear strength.

Another approach to evaluating surface roughness is to study the retention elements constituting the rough surface. The ideal surface roughness maximizes interface shear strength. Hansson and Norton developed a mathematical model for the estimation of the interface shear strength achieved by a rough implant surface.[23-24] A rough surface was conceived as consisting of pits. The model focuses on the sizes, shapes, and packing densities of these pits. It takes into account the fact that the bone tissue close to an implant surface has a reduced content of collagen and mineral and that the mineral and collagen content give bone its strength.[25-37] The gist of the model is expressed by the following formula:

$$\tau_i = f_{pe} \cdot f_{pd} \cdot \tau_b$$

where τ_i represents bone-implant interface shear strength; f_{pe} is a factor between 0 and 1, the value of which depends on the sizes and shapes of the pits constituting the rough surface (it takes into account the fact that the bone tissue immediately adjacent to the implant surface has reduced strength); f_{pd} is a factor between 0 and 1, the value of which depends on how densely packed the pits are; and τ_b is the shear strength of the surrounding bone.

From the above formula, it is evident that the theoretical maximum of the interface shear strength equals the shear strength of the surrounding bone. The model predicts that the packing density of the pits on a rough surface should be as high as possible and that up to a pit size of about 10 μm, the interface shear strength increases with increasing pit size (Figure 2.2).

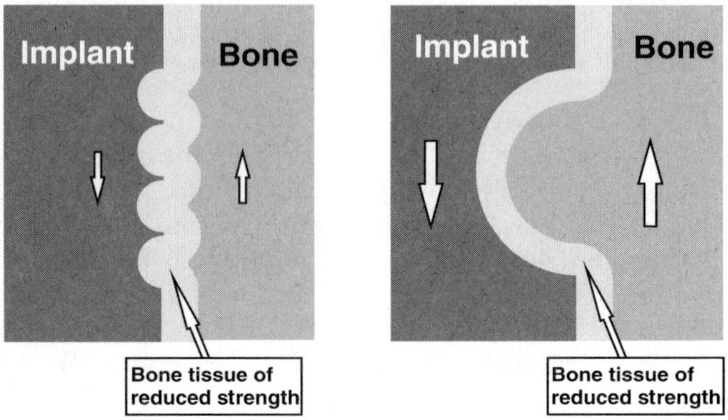

FIGURE 2.2
Left: with very small pits on the implant surface, the bone plugs protruding into the pits consist of bone tissue of reduced strength. Consequently, the interface shear strength is low. Right: with bigger pits, a substantial part of the bone plug protruding into a pit consists of bone of full strength. The interface shear strength is higher.

2.5 Ideal Implant Thread

Screw-shaped endosseous implants dominate the dental implant market today. The thread is probably the most important element of these implants. In spite of this, few scientific studies have addressed the question of thread design. Bechtol measured the holding power of vitallium bone screws with different thread profiles.[38] Variations in pull-out force for the different thread designs were within the limits of experimental error.

Knefel investigated five different thread profiles by means of photoelasticity.[39] The most favorable stress distribution was obtained for a thread profile that had sharp edges. This is remarkable because general engineering experience demonstrated theoretically and experimentally teaches that sharp edges tend to produce high stress concentrations.[40] It can be suspected that the experimental set-up was not precise enough to reveal local stress concentrations.

Albrektsson and coworkers recommended that the thread tops be rounded in order to relieve stress concentrations and predicted small stresses in the bone at interior points of the thread.[41] This is, however, a qualitative statement and no recommendation was given as to the magnitude of the radius of curvature of the thread top, nor does the implant designer find any guidance concerning the values of flank angle, thread depth, pitch, etc. in the implant literature.

It is evidently difficult to devise an experimental method that can disclose the relative benefits of small variations on a thread profile. Another possibility to evaluate different thread profiles is to approach the problem theoretically, for instance, to use the finite element method. The application of such a tool normally means that the calculations are made on an imagined physical model that deviates substantially from a typical clinical situation. The geometry and the loads are idealized. The properties of the bone, the conditions at the implant–bone interface, and the boundary conditions are also idealized. The element mesh implies yet another approximation. This means that the calculations are made on a mathematical model that differs quite a lot from a clinical situation. Consequently, we cannot expect that the calculated stresses will occur in reality. However, if we compare two different designs and in a theoretical calculation find that one design is better than the other, we often have good reason to believe that this design will become the design of choice in a real situation.[42]

Hansson and Werke investigated the effects of variations of thread profiles on the magnitude of the stress peaks in bone.[43] The study was made via finite element analysis of an infinitely long and infinitely stiff screw-shaped implant embedded in cortical bone. The implant–bone interface was assumed to resist compressive stress but not tensile or shear stress. The implant was subjected to a standard axial load per unit of implant length. With these assumptions made, the stress pattern in the bone outside the different thread turns will be identical. The hypothesis was that the thread profile that would minimize the maximum stress in the bone would be the thread profile of choice.

The profile of the thread was characterized by the depth, the top radius of curvature, the flank angle, and a straight part at the bottom of the thread. All these variables were varied and 840 different thread profiles were investigated. The profile of the thread affected the stress pattern in the bone. In all calculation examples, the maximum tensile bone stress was located outside the top of the thread. In most cases, the maximum compressive stress arose outside the point where the lower flank of the thread passed into the curved top. Bone stresses near the bottom of the thread were usually minor. These results agree well with the results of Kohn et al. who predicted stress concentrations at the thread tops and gradually decreasing bone stresses when moving toward the interior of the thread.[44]

With big values of the flank angle combined with a rather long straight part at the bottom of the thread, the maximum compressive stress was located at the flank near the thread bottom. In most cases, the peak tensile stress was more dangerous than the peak compressive stress — closer to the ultimate stress of bone.

After slight modification of the mathematical model that made it possible to analyze unsymmetrical threads, calculations were made for the thread profiles of three clinically used implants: the Brånemark implant, the ITI implant, and a recently introduced implant known as MicroThread™ (Astra Tech, Mölndal, Sweden). The MicroThread implant (Figure 2.3) is equipped with two types of thread: a microthread at the neck portion and a thread of more standard dimensions at the body portion. For the Brånemark and ITI implants, the profiles were obtained by measurements on implants. For the MicroThread implant, the nominal values of the parameters defining the

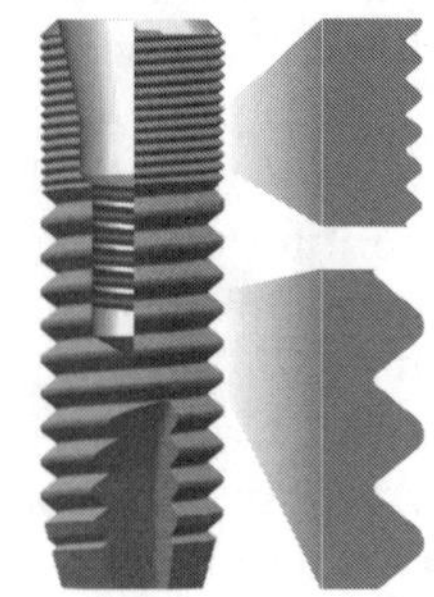

FIGURE 2.3
The MicroThread implant of Astra Tech includes a microthread and macrothread with optimized profiles. The implant also incorporates (1) retention elements at the endosseous neck portion, (2) optimized surface roughness, and (3) a conical implant–abutment interface at the level of the marginal bone.

thread were used. The peak tensile stresses in the bone resulting from the standardized load were 2.29 MPa and 2.27 MPa, respectively, for the Brånemark and ITI implant threads. For the microthread and the bigger thread of the MicroThread implant, the peak tensile stresses were substantially smaller: 1.84 MPa and 1.86 MPa, respectively. This means that the threads of the MicroThread implant performed better than the threads of the other two implants and comply with the second criterion of good implant design. A microthread has an additional merit. A switch from a standard thread to a microthread while keeping the major diameter of an implant the same will result in increased axial stiffness of the implant which in turn will bring about a reduction of the peak bone stresses.[13]

2.6 The Implant–Abutment Interface

2.6.1 Flat-to-Flat or Conical Interface

The implant and the surrounding bone can be regarded as a single structure. The load from the superstructure is transmitted to this structure by means of the abutment. In solid mechanics, Saint-Venant's principle states that a change in the distribution of the load on a structure, without change of the resultant force, alters the stresses in a region close to the area where the load is applied but not far from it.[45]

The design of the implant–abutment interface affects the way a load is applied on the implant–bone structure. For this reason, the design of the implant–abutment interface may also affect the stress pattern in the marginal bone.

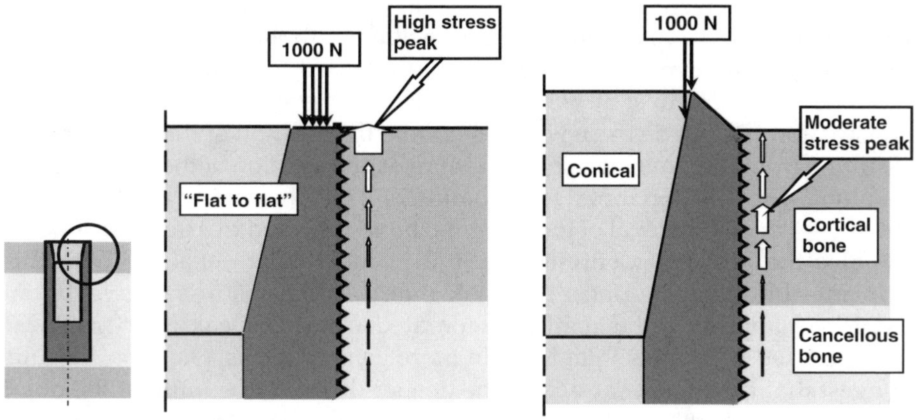

FIGURE 2.4
With the flat-to-flat implant–abutment interface, a high stress peak arose at the uppermost marginal bone. Peak stress was substantially lower for the conical interface at the level of the marginal bone and it had a more apical location.

In a finite element study, Hansson compared a conical implant–abutment interface at the level of the marginal bone with a "flat-to-flat" implant–abutment interface (Figure 2.4).[46] The implant studied was cylindrical and provided with retention elements all the way to the top. The retention elements were not modelled. The implant–bone interface was assumed to resist compressive and shear stresses but not tensile stress. For the implant with the flat-to-flat interface, a standardized axial load was applied on a flat horizontal peripheral surface on top of the implant. For the implant with the conical interface, the same axial load was applied on an inner conus in the implant.

The design of the implant–abutment interface and the points of application of the axial load had a profound effect on the stress state in the marginal bone. The peak bone–implant interface shear stress was located at the top marginal bone for the flat-to-flat implant–abutment interface. The more peripheral the location of the load, the higher the peak stress. The conical implant–abutment interface brought about a substantial decrease in the peak bone–implant interface shear stress as compared to the flat-to-flat interface. This means that the conical interface showed better compliance with the second criterion of good implant design. It also moved the peak interface shear stress further down in the bone. The further down in the inner conus the axial load was distributed, the further down in the marginal bone the peak interface shear stress settled.

An arbitrary oblique load on an implant can be divided into axial and horizontal components. Assuming an implant provided with retention elements at the endosseous neck portion, Stoiber and Mailath et al. found that the peak stresses in the bone resulting from a vertical load were located high up in the marginal bone.[47-48] The peak bone stresses resulting from a horizontal load also were located very high up. Thus the peak stresses resulting from the horizontal load component coincided with those resulting from the axial load component and are consequently added to each other.

Stoiber and Mailath et al. feared marginal bone resorption due to excessive stresses and tried to devise a way to separate the location of the peak stresses resulting from the axial load component from the location of the peak stresses resulting from the horizontal load component.[47-48] The conical implant–abutment interface at the level of the marginal bone analyzed by Hansson appears to solve the problem identified by Stoiber and Mailath et al.[46-48] With this implant–abutment interface, the peak interface shear stress caused by an axial load appears to be spatially separated from the peak interface shear stress caused by a horizontal load. In more general terms, Hansson's results suggest that the more central and the deeper down in the implant the point of application of the axial load, the more favorable the stress distribution in the marginal bone.[46]

2.6.2 A Conical Implant–Abutment Interface: At the Level of the Marginal Bone versus a More Coronal Location

Hansson found that a conical implant–abutment interface at the level of the marginal bone produced a more favorable stress distribution than a flat-to-flat interface.[46] In a finite element study, Hansson investigated whether the benefit remained if the conical interface was located more coronally.[49] Cylindrical implants provided with 0.1 mm deep microthreads extending up to the uppermost cortical bone were studied. The microthreads were modelled with finite elements.

The implant–bone interface was assumed to resist compressive stress but not tensile or shear stress. One implant was provided with a conical implant–abutment interface located at the level of the marginal bone. On another implant, the same conical interface was located 2 mm more coronally (Figure 2.5). A standard axial load was applied on the inner coni of the implants.

For the implant with the conical interface at the level of the marginal bone, moderate tensile, compressive, and von Mises stresses arose outside the uppermost thread. The peak tensile, compressive, and von Mises stresses had more apical locations. Thus the peak stresses resulting from an axial load component were spatially separated from those resulting from a horizontal load component. For the implant with the conical interface located 2 mm more coronally, the highest tensile, compressive, and von Mises stresses arose outside the uppermost thread. The peak tensile, compressive, and von Mises bone stresses were substantially higher with the latter implants. The conclusion was that the beneficial biomechanical effect of the conical interface was lost if the conical implant–abutment interface was located 2 mm more coronally.

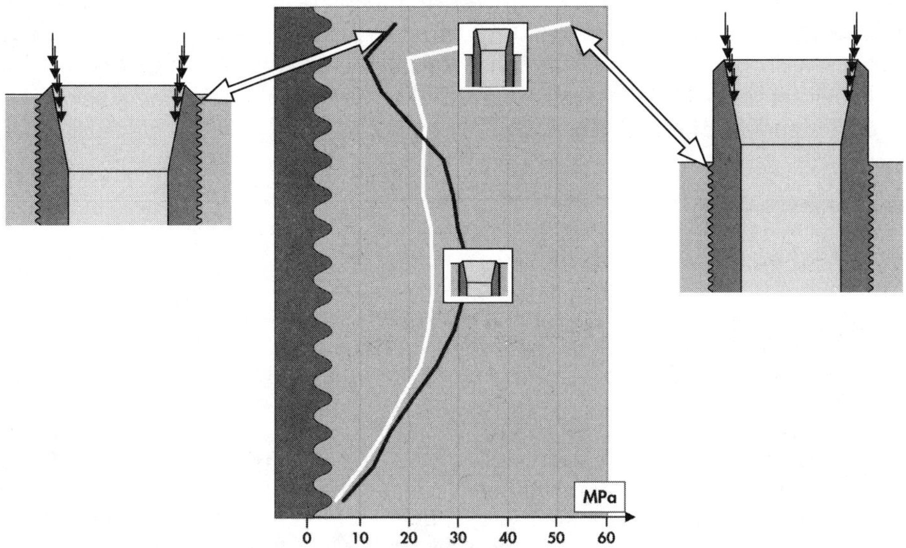

FIGURE 2.5
The peak compressive bone stresses at the different thread levels. With the conical implant–abutment interface at the level of the marginal bone, the peak stress at the uppermost thread turn was moderate. The highest stress appeared further down in the bone. With the conical interface located 2 mm more coronally, an unfavorably high stress peak arose at the uppermost thread turn.

2.7 Summary

Based on Wolff's law, two biomechanical criteria of a good dental implant design were set up. They imply that a dental implant should be designed so that, when loaded, it induces mechanical stimulation in the surrounding bone and high stress peaks are avoided. The incorporation of certain design features makes an implant comply with these criteria. An implant should be equipped with retention elements extending all the way to the uppermost marginal bone.

The retention elements should have such a design so they do not give rise to high stress concentrations. It is possible to find a thread profile that relieves stress peaks. If an implant has high axial stiffness, stress peaks are further reduced. If the outer diameter of an implant is fixed, a shallow microthread makes it possible to combine effective retention elements with high axial stiffness.

The bone–implant interface shear strength can be increased by means of a rough surface. A surface roughness consisting of densely packed pits of sufficient size and appropriate shape maximizes the interface shear strength.

Stress peaks can be further reduced by means of a suitable design of the implant–abutment interface. One such suitable design is a conical implant–abutment interface at the level of the marginal bone. The above conclusions regarding design features led to development of the Astra Tech MicroThread implant (Figure 2.3).

References

1. Brunski, J.B., Biomaterials and biomechanics in dental implant design, *Int. J. Oral Maxillofac. Implants*, 3, 85, 1988.
2. Lekholm, U. and Zarb, G., Patient selection and preparation, in *Tissue Integrated Prostheses*, Brånemark, P.-I., Zarb, G., and Albrektsson, T., Eds., Quintessence Publishing, Chicago, 1985, p. 117.
3. Tarnow, D.P., Cho, S.C., and Wallace, S.S., The effect of inter-implant distance on the height of inter-implant bone crest, *J. Periodontol.*, 71, 546, 2000.
4. Hart, R.T., Quantitative Response of Bone to Mechanical Stress, dissertation, Case Western Reserve University, Cleveland, OH, 1983.
5. von Meyer, H.V., Die Architektur der Spongiosa, *Arch. Anat. Physiol. Wissen. Med.*, 34, 615, 1867.
6. Wolff, J., *Das Gesetz der Transformation der Knochen*, A. Hirschwald, Berlin, 1892.
7. *Dorland's Illustrated Medical Dictionary*, 25th ed., W.B. Saunders, Philadelphia, 1974.
8. Treharne, R.W., Review of Wolff's law and its proposed means of operations, *Orthop. Rev.*, 10, 35, 1981.
9. Bertram, J.E.A. and Swartz, S.M., The law of bone transformation: a case of crying Wolff? *Biol. Rev. Cambridge Philosoph. Soc.*, 66, 245, 1991.
10. Frost, H.M., Skeletal structural adaptations to mechanical usage (SATMU): redefining Wolff's law: the bone modeling problem, *Anat. Rec.*, 226, 403, 1990.
11. Zienkiewicz, O.C., The finite element method in engineering science, 4th ed., McGraw-Hill, New York, 1989.
12. Linkow, L.I. and Cherchève, R., *Theories and Techniques of Oral Implantology*, C.V. Mosby, Saint Louis, 1970.
13. Hansson, S., The implant neck: smooth or provided with retention elements: a biomechanical approach, *Clin. Oral. Implants Res.*, 10, 394, 1999.
14. Al-Sayyed, A. et al., Predictable crestal bone remodelling around two porous-coated titanium alloy dental implant designs, *Clin. Oral Implants Res.*, 5, 131, 1994.
15. Jung, Y.-C., Han, C.-H., and Lee, K.-W., A 1-year radiographic evaluation of marginal bone around dental implants, *Int. J. Oral Maxillofac. Implants*, 11, 811, 1996.
16. Quirynen, M., Naert, I., and van Steenberghe, D., Fixture design and overload influence marginal bone loss and fixture success in the Brånemark system, *Clin. Oral Implants Res.*, 3, 104, 1992.
17. Engquist, B., Nilson, H., and Åstrand, P., Single-tooth replacement by osseointegrated Brånemark implants, *Clin. Oral Implants Res.*, 6, 238, 1995.
18. Palmer, R.M., Palmer, P.J., and Smith, B.J., A 5-year prospective study of Astra single tooth implants, *Clin. Oral Implants Res.*, 11, 179, 2000.

19. Carlsson, L. et al., Removal torques for polished and rough titanium implants, *Int. J. Oral Maxillofac. Implants,* 3, 21, 1988.
20. Gotfredsen, K. et al., A histomorphometric and removal torque analysis for TiO_2-blasted titanium implants, *Clin. Oral Implants Res.*, 3, 77, 1992.
21. Wennerberg, A., On Surface Roughness and Implant Incorporation, thesis, Göteborg University, Göteborg, Sweden, 1996.
22. Hansson, S., Surface roughness parameters as predictors of anchorage strength in bone: a critical analysis, *J. Biomech.,* 33, 1297, 2000.
23. Hansson, S. and Norton, M., The relation between surface roughness and interfacial shear strength for bone anchored implants, in Towards an Optimized Dental Implant and Implant Bridge Design: A Biomechanical Approach, thesis, Chalmers University of Technology, Göteborg, Sweden, 1997.
24. Hansson, S. and Norton, M., The relation between surface roughness and interfacial shear strength for bone anchored implants: a mathematical model, *J. Biomech.*, 32, 829, 1999.
25. Hansson, H.-A., Albrektsson, T., and Brånemark, P.-I., Structural aspects of the interface between tissue and titanium implants, *J. Prosth. Dent.*, 50, 108, 1983.
26. Albrektsson, T. et al., Ultrastructural analysis of the interface zone of titanium and gold implants, *Adv. Biomater.*, 4, 167, 1982.
27. Albrektsson, T., Hansson, H.-A., and Ivarsson, B., Interface analysis of titanium and zirconium bone implants, *Biomater.,* 6, 97, 1985.
28. Albrektsson, T. and Hansson, H.-A., An ultrastructural characterization of the interface between bone and sputtered titanium or stainless steel surfaces, *Biomater.,* 7, 201, 1986.
29. Linder, L. et al., Electron microscopic analysis of the bone–titanium interface, *Acta Orthop. Scand.,* 54, 45, 1983.
30. Johansson, C. et al., Ultrastructural differences of the interface zone between bone and Ti6Al4V or commercially pure titanium, *J. Biomed. Eng.*, 11, 3, 1989.
31. Johansson, C., Hansson, H.-A., and Albrektsson, T., Qualitative, interfacial study between bone and tantalum, niobium or commercially pure titanium, *Biomater.,* 11, 277, 1990.
32. Sennerby, L. et al., Structure of the bone-titanium interface in retrieved clinical oral implants, *Clin. Oral Implants Res.*, 2, 103, 1991.
33. Sennerby, L., Thomsen, P., and Ericson, L.E., Early tissue response to titanium implants inserted in rabbit cortical bone II. Ultrastructural observations, *J. Mater. Sci.: Mater. Med.*, 4, 494, 1993.
34. Young, J.Z., *The Life of Mammals*, Oxford University Press, 1957.
35. Currey, J.D., Differences in the tensile strength of bone of different histological types, *J. Anat.*, 93, 87, 1959.
36. Currey, J.D., The mechanical consequences of variation in the mineral content of bone, *J. Biomech.*, 2, 1, 1969.
37. Vose, G.P., The relation of microscopic mineralization to intrinsic bone strength, *Anat. Rec.*, 144, 31, 1962.
38. Bechtol, C.O., Internal fixation with plates and screws, in *Metals and Engineering in Bone and Joint Surgery,* Bechtol, C.O., Ferguson, A.B., and Laing, P.G., Eds., Williams & Wilkins, Baltimore, 1959.
39. Knefel, T., Dreidimensionale spannungsoptische Untersuchungen verschiedener Schraubenprofile bei zahnärztlichen Implantaten, dissertation, Ludwig Maximilians Universität, München, 1989.

40. Peterson, R.E., *Stress Concentration Design Factors*, John Wiley & Sons, New York, 1974.
41. Albrektsson, T. et al., The interface zone of inorganic implants *in vivo*: titanium implants in bone, *Ann. Biomed. Eng.*, 11, 1, 1983.
42. Meijer, H.J.A. et al., A comparison of three finite element models of an edentulous mandible provided with implants, *J. Oral Rehab.*, 20, 147, 1993.
43. Hansson, S. and Werke, M., On the role of the thread profile for bone implants, with special emphasis on dental implants, in Towards an Optimized Dental Implant and Implant Bridge Design: A Biomechanical Approach, thesis, Chalmers University of Technology, Göteborg, Sweden, 1997.
44. Kohn, D.H., Ko, C.C., and Hollister, S.J., Localized stress analysis of dental implants using homogenization theory, ASME-BED Advances in Bioengineering, Winter Annual Meeting of American Society of Mechanical Engineers, Anaheim, CA, 1992.
45. Timoshenko, S.P. and Goodier, J.N., *Theory of Elasticity*, McGraw-Hill, Singapore, 1984.
46. Hansson, S., Implant–abutment interface: biomechanical study of flat top versus conical, *Clin. Implant Dent. Rel. Res.*, 2, 33, 2000.
47. Stoiber, B., *Biomechanische Grundlagen enossaler Schraubenimplantate*, dissertation, Universitätsklinik für Zahn, Mund, und Zahnheilkunde, Wien, 1988.
48. Mailath, G. et al., Die Knochenresorption an der Eintrittstelle osseointegrierter Implantate: ein biomechanisches Phänomen: eine Finite-Element Studie, *Zeitschr. Stomatol.*, 86, 207, 1989.
49. Hansson, S., A conical implant–abutment interface at the level of the marginal bone improves the distribution of the stresses in the supporting bone: an axisymmetric finite element analysis, *Clin. Oral Implants Res.*, in press, 2003.

3

Implant Surface Design for Development and Maintenance of Osseointegration

Robert M. Pilliar

CONTENTS

3.1 Introduction 43
3.2 Implant Maintenance: Avoidance of Crestal Bone Loss 44
3.3 Sintered Porous Surfaces: Rationales of Design and Use 47
3.4 Surface Modification for Enhancing Osteoconductivity 50
3.5 Maintenance of Osseointegration and Implant Design 51
3.6 Summary 53
References 55

3.1 Introduction

It is generally accepted that a necessary requirement for success of bone interfacing endosseous dental implants (and orthopedic joint replacement implants intended for major load-bearing applications) is achievement and maintenance of rigid implant fixation to host bone (osseointegration). For all cementless implant designs including those with so-called bioactive surfaces, this results primarily through mechanical interlock of bone and biomaterial at a macroscopic or microscopic level.

An important preference of cementless implants is the ability to become osseointegrated rapidly, thereby minimizing the risks that inadvertent early forces will act on the implant and cause excessive relative displacement at the host–bone interface that would inhibit bone formation and osseointegration. The factors recognized as affecting the strength of fixation and/or the rate of osseointegration include implant topography, surface chemistry, nature of the host site (vascularity, osteogenic potential), and the stress/strain field acting on the early repair tissues that form within the

0-8493-1474-7/03/$0.00+$1.50

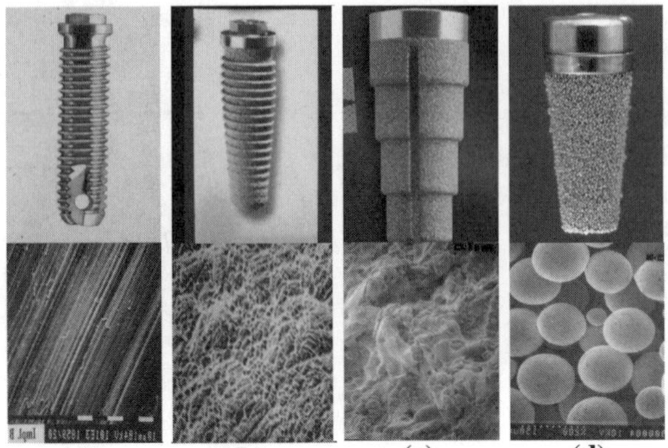

(a) (b) (c) (d)

FIGURE 3.1
Four endosseous dental implants; scanning electron micrographs showing different bone-interfacing surface preparations: (a) machined, (b) grit-blasted and acid-etched, (c) Ti plasma-sprayed, and (d) sintered porous surface.

implant–bone interface zone. The action of the stress/strain field is dependent on imposed forces and implant surface design and serves as the focus of this chapter.

Figure 3.1 shows some current designs and highlights their different surface features. Differences in osseointegration potential due to implant surface geometry appear to affect both rate of osseointegration and strength of fixation.[1-9] In terms of surface chemistry effects, calcium phosphate coatings (usually formed by plasma spraying) have been shown[10-14] to significantly affect rate of development of interface fixation (as determined by interface shear strength tests).

The matter of differentiating the effects of surface chemistry and topography remains an issue, particularly with plasma spray-coated hydroxyapatite (HA) implants that have highly irregular surfaces. In addition to the requirement for good vascularity at the implant site, mechanical strains can promote local osteogenesis, thereby contributing to implant osseointegration.[15-19] Mechanical stimulation using controlled cyclic loads has been shown to promote bone fracture healing.[20] It has also been proposed to promote osseointegration of implants.[16-18,21,22] The tissue differentiation hypothesis proposed by Carter et al.[23] suggests that low distortional and hydrostatic strains act to promote osteogenesis. Our studies appear to support this hypothesis.[17,18,22]

3.2 Implant Maintenance: Avoidance of Crestal Bone Loss

This chapter aims to identify implant design strategies shown to be beneficial for promoting more rapid implant osseointegration and ensuring long-term implant stability. While implants of virtually all designs have been reported to produce high success rates in favorable situations (mandibular location, bone density of type I or II,[24] and sufficient bone height to accomodate implants >10 mm in length), less favorable outcomes have been reported for implants placed in maxillae where shorter implant lengths are often indicated and for implants placed in posterior mandible locations in bone of low density (types III and IV).[25,26]

A review of the major causes and mechanisms of dental implant failure following the establishment of osseointegration suggests that excessive crestal bone loss is the most common root cause of failure. The resulting formation of a significant peri-implant pocket presents a site susceptible to bacterial accumulation resulting in further bone loss due to chronic local inflammation. This can progress to eventual implant loss. Alternatively, if sufficient apical implant support is maintained following substantial crestal bone loss, the resulting high bending moment acting on the implant can lead to implant fatigue failure.[27] Regardless of the mode of failure, preventing or at least limiting the extent of crestal bone loss appears to be a desirable strategy for improving the performance and long-term survival of endosseous dental implants.

Four possible causes of crestal bone loss are recognized, including local bone overload, under-stressing of peri-implant crestal bone, establishment of "biologic width," and peri-implant infection (peri-implantitis).

Mechanical overload is noted most often as the cause of crestal bone loss.[28] During normal implant function, cyclic forces are transmitted from the implant to the peri-implant bone and, depending on the design of the implant, high local stress concentrations can develop in the bone juxtaposing the coronal portion of the implant. The bone next to the tip region of machined thread elements represents a zone of especially high stress concentration. Freestanding implants that experience significant transverse force components are especially susceptible to developing unacceptably high regions of local stress in the juxtaposing bone. The shorter the implant length, the higher are these stresses. Hence, the observed high failure rates for implants smaller than 10 mm in length with sintered porous-surfaced implants representing a notable exception.[26]

Localized high stresses may cause microcracking of bone. Depending on the level and frequency of loading, bone remodeling and repair of the microcracks may occur or, alternatively, local microdamage may continue to accumulate leading to substantial loss of crestal bone. Predictions of the *absolute* magnitude of local stresses using finite element methods have been reported but are questionable because of the number of assumptions and over-simplifications that must be used with this approach. While reliable prediction of absolute bone stresses and strains is not possible, finite element analysis has proven helpful for assessing qualitatively how design changes including changes in surface features may affect local stresses and strains (resulting in *relative* increase, decrease, or no effect). Hansson[29] used this approach to suggest design improvements with threaded implants to reduce the probability of peri-implant crestal bone overloading.

A second noted cause of crestal bone loss, again stress-related, is local under-stressing of bone, also called "stress shielding." It is caused when high stiffness implant structures bear the major portions of loads and it can result in bone disuse atrophy.[30] Because the most coronal regions of virtually all currently used dental implants are prepared with smooth surface geometries (Figure 3.1), force transfer from implant to bone is poor in this region. Only compressive forces can be effectively transferred across the implant–bone interface in this region. The transfer of shear forces at the smooth coronal region can occur only as a result of friction. This transmits limited force to the apposing bone and consequent minimal mechanical stimulation of that bone. Bone loss ensues if local stresses and strains fall below a critical threshold value (~1.6 MPa[31] or 100 $\mu\varepsilon$[32]). This appears to explain the limited crestal bone loss observed around implants to a depth corresponding to the level at which bone retention elements (threads and coatings) are located.[33]

Confounding this issue, however, is the matter of biologic width that suggests a strictly physiological cause for crestal bone loss.[34] This phenomenon is claimed to result in the formation of a 1.5 to 2 mm deep layer of gingival tissue between the bone crest and the superior implant component surface (abutment–fixture junction). This suggests that, even assuming the presence of bone retention elements along the most coronal region of the implant, and hence adequate mechanical stimulation of bone along the full implant length,[31] crestal bone loss may occur as a result of the development of this soft gingival tissue layer. Follow-up studies of our earlier work on porous-surfaced implants prepared with very short (0.75 mm) smooth coronal regions placed in canine mandible sites using quantitative histological assessment suggest that biologic width establishment and possibly stress shielding[33] are responsible for the observed crestal bone loss.

Crestal bone loss may also result from local infection due to bacterial and biofilm formation at the coronal region of an implant. Surface roughness is important in this regard and is the major reason all current designs are fabricated with smooth coronal regions. Assuming that the formation of minimal biologic width is a dominant factor in peri-implant tissue response, and recognizing the general principle that the formation of a biofilm is best defended against through early development of a stable connective tissue–implant interface,[36] the design of the coronal implant surface to encourage rapid soft connective tissue attachment appears to be a worthwhile strategy. Current practice involves a smooth coronal region that has an optimal surface roughness (0.05 to 0.2 μm Ra) believed to allow a degree of gingival tissue attachment while preventing easy bacterial colonization.[37] Other studies propose the use of microgrooves and other textured surfaces to enhance soft connective tissue attachment while inhibiting epithelial growth apically.[38]

3.3 Sintered Porous Surfaces: Rationales of Design and Use

Dental implants designed with porous surfaces formed by sintering metal powders are unique by virtue of their three-dimensional interconnected porous structures (Figure 3.2).[39] If the resulting pores and interconnecting channels are of appropriate size, rapid bone ingrowth will occur, assuming appropriate conditions during tissue healing. These include the general requirements of adequate blood supply, osteogenic potential of host tissues, and limited or no movement of the implant relative to host bone.

Our studies with dogs suggest maximum relative shear displacements at the bone–porous-surface implant interface of 50 μm for acceptable bone formation and ingrowth throughout the porous structure (Figure 3.3).[40] In addition, pore size preferably should be equal to or greater than 100 μm to allow rapid bone ingrowth throughout the porous region, typically composed of two or three sintered powder layers (~0.3 mm in width).[39] Our recent studies have shown that bone formation and fixation of well stabilized porous-surfaced implants made of Ti6Al4V occur through both distance osteogenesis (appositional bone formation) and local (contact) osteogenesis. This is in contrast to plasma spray-coated designs in which bone formation within the interface zone occurs primarily by distance osteogenesis.[41] As a result, more rapid implant fixation is possible with sintered porous-surfaced designs (or presumably any design that provides a three-dimensional interconnected porous network for bone ingrowth) due to the two-front bone formation process.

Finite element analysis incorporating homogenization methods was used to model the implant surface structure (porous-surfaced or plasma-sprayed geometry) to predict local tissue strains during healing within the interface zone (including regions of the implant surface within which tissue could

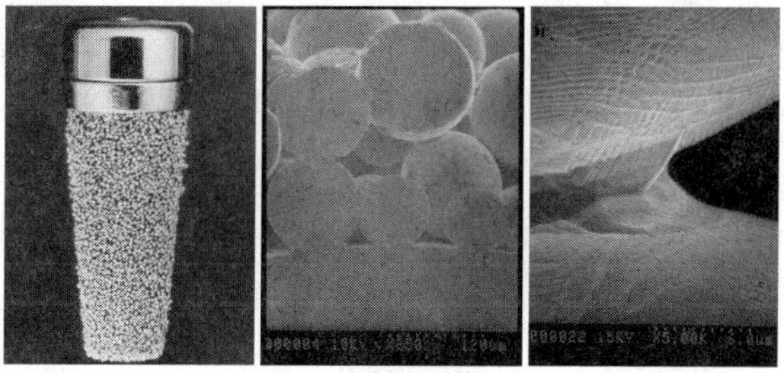

(a) (b) (c)

FIGURE 3.2
Porous-surfaced dental implant prepared by sintering Ti6Al4V powders to a Ti6Al4V machined core: (a) tapered truncated conical-shaped implant, (b) scanning electron micrograph of sinter surface–solid core junction showing particle–particle and particle–substrate sinter necks, (bar = 120 μm), (c) higher magnification scanning electron micrograph of sinter neck region showing thermal etching that develops during sintering (bar = 6 μm).

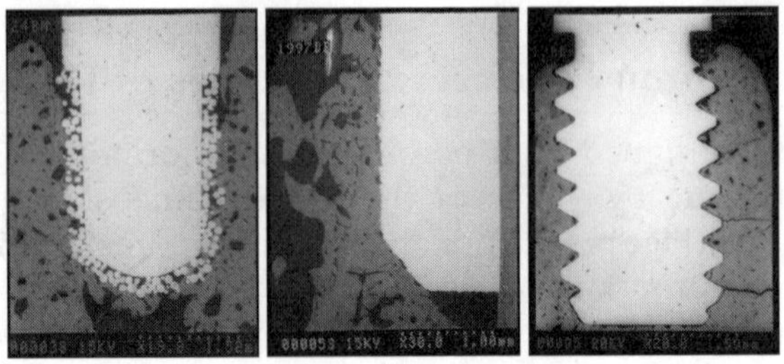

FIGURE 3.3
Back-scattered scanning electron micrographs of implants subjected to rotational displacements of 50 to 75 μm: (a) sintered porous-surfaced implant showing bone ingrowth, (b) Ti plasma spray-coated implant showing bone closely juxtaposed to the irregular plasma-sprayed coating surface, (c) machined threaded implant with bone formed within the thread region. *Note*: (b) was taken at slightly higher magnification: 30× versus approximately 20× for (a) and (c).

form). The results of the analyses indicated significant differences in local tissue strains for premineralized healing tissues juxtaposing the porous-surfaced and plasma-sprayed designs, the former resulting in more regions of lower distortional and volumetric strains.[17]

This favors osteogenesis according to the tissue differentiation hypothesis proposed by Carter and coworkers.[15] In addition, the open-pored sintered structure should also favor the ingrowth of new blood vessels compared with the close-ended surface openings of a plasma spray-coated surface. The increased vascularity may also contribute to the observed faster bone formation and fixation strength development of porous-surfaced compared with plasma spray-coated implants. Significant differences in pull-out strength and interface zone structure were only observed during the early postimplantation healing period (up to 8 days in our rabbit model studies). By 16 days, we noted no significant differences in pull-out strength or extent of bone formation in the interface zones for the two designs.[22] Recent studies using the rabbit femoral condyle model have shown that bone forms within the pores of porous-surfaced implants as early as 6 days after implantation.[42]

Relative movement at the bone–implant interface is known to inhibit the rate of osseointegration and, for excessive interface displacements, can completely prevent osseointegration. Assuming that the relative movement is limited to less than approximately 150 μm, sintered porous-surfaced implants can develop fibrous tissue anchorage of implants (a unique feature in which fibrous repair tissues can form and interdigitate throughout the three-dimensional porous network).[43] Depending on subsequent loading history, this "pseudoligamentous" attachment tissue may mineralize, remodel, and be replaced by bone through a process similar to that during callus formation and spontaneous bone fracture healing, thereby producing "delayed" osseointegration. Such a sequence of events was observed around porous-surfaced femoral hip implant components in humans.[44] For other designs, excessive early movement led to formation of a fibrous tissue capsule around the implant that was likely to thicken progressively with continued loading, leading to eventual gross implant loosening.

Due to the inhibitory effect of relative movement on bone formation within the peri-implant interface zone, absolute implant stability and a period of nonfunction are recommended as standard protocols for endosseous dental implant placement and use regardless of design in order to attain osseointegration in the shortest time. In canine studies investigating tolerable relative movement for bone ingrowth of porous-surfaced implants positioned in dog mandibular sites, we observed that in situations where relative shear displacements below 50 μm were imposed at regular intervals (30 torque-controlled loading cycles at 0.5 Hz every second day), bone formation occurred predominantly from the outer pore regions inward (greater percent bone area within the outer pores than within the pores adjoining the solid core), suggesting that appositional bone formation was dominant[22] and similar to osseointegration of plasma spray-coated designs.

Finite element analysis incorporating the critical displacement value for bone ingrowth determined in our dog studies ($\Delta_{critical}$ = 50 μm) predicted critical strain levels for (1) localized bone formation (distortional strain <3%) and (2) appositional bone formation (bone interface strain <8%;[17] see Figure 3.4. For higher levels of relative displacement (initial shear displacement >50 μm) resulting in higher tissue strains, soft tissue anchorage (pseudoligamentous attachment) was observed with porous-surfaced implants.[40,45] This response was somewhat variable with bone ingrowth occurring in some cases at initial shear displacements ~75 μm — an outcome also observed with plasma spray-coated implants (Figure 3.3b).

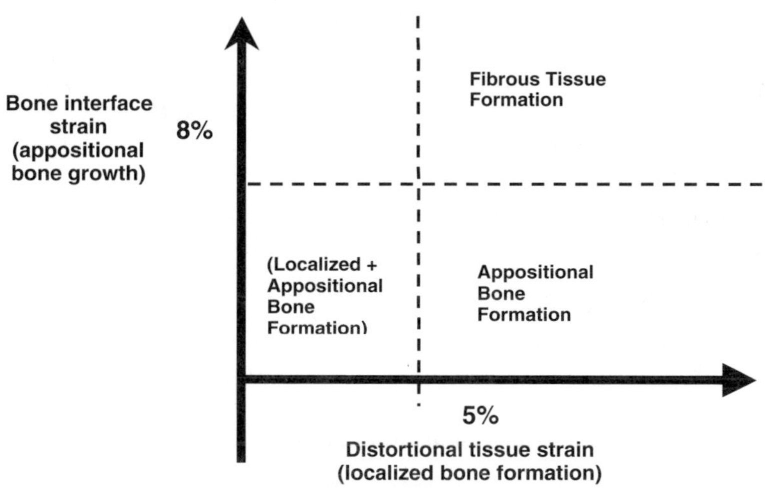

FIGURE 3.4
Summary of mechanical strain effects on peri-implant tissue formation within the implant–bone interface zone.

Machined threaded implants were also included in our canine relative micromovement effect studies (Figure 3.3c). Unlike the porous-surfaced or plasma spray-coated implants, these had no capacity for resisting imposed torques. They developed bony crypts within which they freely counter-rotated. This indicates the critical need for splinting or other means of preventing implant rotation as a result of torquing of machined threaded designs.

3.4 Surface Modification for Enhancing Osteoconductivity

Increasing the rate of bone formation along implant surfaces is an important issue, particularly for endosseous dental implants designed for immediate or early functional loading and for implants placed in low density (types III and IV) bone (typically the posterior mandible). Implant surface modifications such as acid etching in combination with grit blasting[46] and calcium phosphate coatings formed directly by plasma spraying,[47] sputtering,[48] wet chemical deposition (sol–gel),[49,50] or precipitation from solution on alkali- and heat-treated titanium substrates to form biomimetic coatings[51] have been investigated as ways to increase osteoconductivity.

Increasing osteoconductivity by these surface design strategies has been proposed to be related to the altered implant topography that results from surface modification arising from enhanced interface zone fibrin clot retention during healing.[52] Alternatively, it may be due to the formation of surfaces that, as a result of their chemical constitution, allow preferential adhesion of bioactive molecules involved in osteoblast and preosteoblast adhesion, thereby leading to accelerated bone formation. Unfortunately, as previously noted, the associated surface roughening resulting from current methods for forming calcium phosphate coatings or films and the rapid alteration of prepared smooth surfaces due to heterogeneous coating or film dissolution *in vivo* have confounded the ability to differentiate the effects of topography and surface chemistry.

The effectiveness of sintered porous-surfaced structures for promoting osteoconductivity was demonstrated by Dziedzic[53] who compared bone growth along porous-surfaced and smooth (polished) Ti6Al4V implants placed in rat tibiae. Measurements of bone contact demonstrated significant levels with porous-surfaced implants (two different pore size ranges were studied) while virtually no bone contact was observed with the smooth-surfaced samples. This experiment confirmed previous observations that suggested the osteoconductive nature of sintered porous-surfaced implants. The submicron-sized thermal etch features that develop during sintering of the Ti6Al4V powders (Figure 3.2b) may also contribute to osteoconductivity.[54]

We recently investigated the further enhancement of osteoconductivity of sintered porous-surfaced implants by adding a calcium phosphate thin film over the sintered Ti alloy structure.[42,55] A 0.5 to 1 μm thick calcium phosphate overlayer film was made by sol–gel deposition using an inorganic sol–gel solution similar to that reported by Qui et al.[56] and a process for coating porous-surfaced Ti6Al4V samples developed in our laboratory. Thin films were formed over the sintered powders. They were characterized by thin film x-ray diffraction and FTIR methods and shown to be crystalline; they consisted of hydroxyapatite and other calcium phosphate phases. Implants were placed in tibiae or femoral condyles of rabbits and left for 2 weeks (tibial implants) or 6, 9, 12, or 16 days in femoral condyle sites as described by Simmons et al.[22]

Mechanical pull-out tests (femoral condyle implants), back-scattered scanning electron microscopy, and light microscopy (for interface zone structure characterization) were used for assessment. The results indicated significantly higher interface stiffness and force for pull-out at each of the two early periods (6 and 9 days for femoral condyle implants; see Figure 3.5)[42] and more extensive implant–bone contact at 2 weeks (tibial implants) for the calcium phosphate-coated devices. Whether the enhanced osteoconductivity of this implant design represents a clinically significant improvement remains to be determined.

These studies, like others, were confounded by surface irregularities associated with the thin CaP films. Thus, the question whether topography or chemistry affects osteoconductivity remains equivocal.

3.5 Maintenance of Osseointegration and Implant Design

As noted, loss of crestal bone can result from local regions of high stress that cause microfractures or very low stress that produces bone loss via disuse atrophy. Hansson[29] proposed the introduction of retention elements along the most coronal portion of an implant as a means to promote stress transfer from implant to host bone over a greater interface area. This presumably would distribute strain energy over a greater volume of peri-implant bone and moderate high level local strains. A combined three-dimensional and axisymmetric finite element analysis was used to support this hypothesis. Unfortunately, introduction of surface retention elements along the coronal implant region also introduced structural features that increased the risks of plaque retention and peri-implantitis.

Porous-surfaced implant designs provide a more effective means of dissipating implant forces over a greater volume of bone as a result of the three-dimensional bone-implant interlock. This allows the transfer of tensile, shear, and compressive forces from implant to bone. Transverse force components acting on osseointegrated porous-surfaced implants during occlusion are transferred efficiently to bone on the downstream (by compression) and upstream (by tension) sides of the implant as well as by shear. This results in a more symmetric and uniform pattern of peri-implant bone stressing and lower peak stresses compared with machined threaded implants.

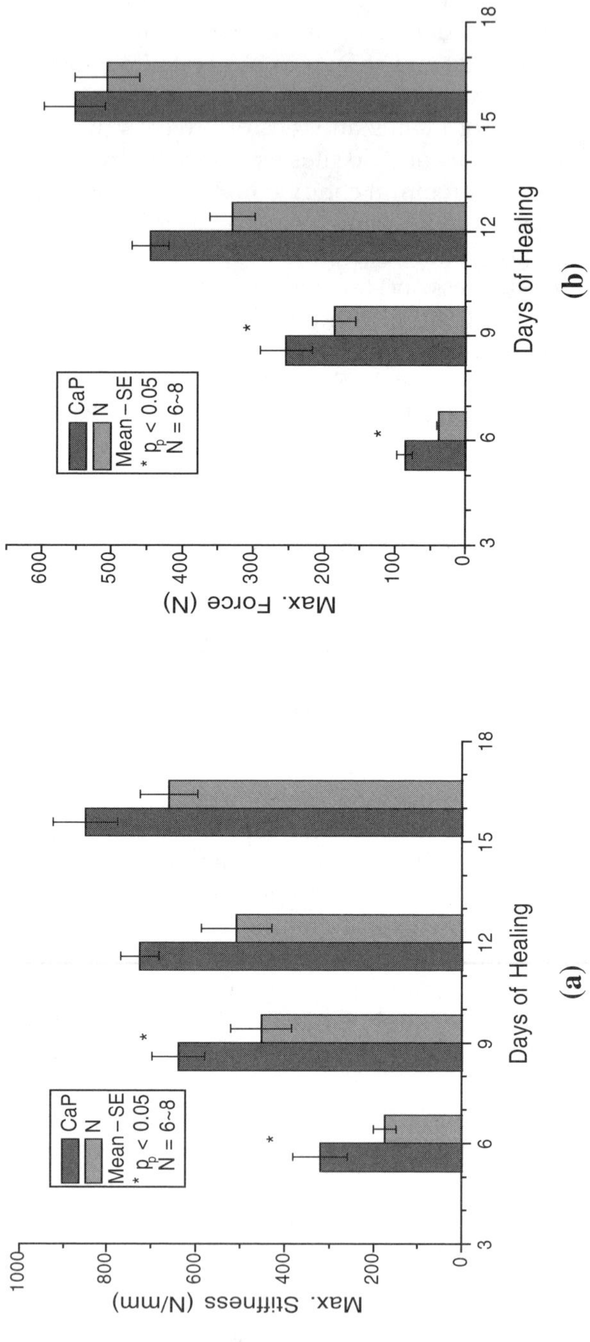

FIGURE 3.5
Mechanical pull-out test results for sol–gel Ca–P-coated versus standard porous-surfaced implants.

Finite element analyses of porous-surfaced and threaded implant designs were used to illustrate this difference.[57] Figure 3.6 shows the results of such analyses for implants acted on by a small horizontal force (2 N). In the two-dimensional finite element model, no bonding was assumed along the threaded implant surface while bonding and interface tensile force transfer was assumed with the porous-surfaced design reflecting the observed differences in bone bonding for the two designs. The model predicts a more symmetric distribution of stresses and lower *local* peak stresses in crestal bone next to the porous-surfaced implants. It also predicts lower overall stresses and strains in peri-implant crestal bone with the porous-surfaced implants.

3.6 Summary

Implant surface characteristics profoundly affect the rate of development of implant fixation through peri-implant bone formation and the stability of the fixation under long-term function. Both excessively high local strains and physiologically abnormally low bone strains can result in crestal bone loss. In addition, implant surface design has been shown to influence the peri-implant healing process; both surface chemical composition and topography appear to play roles. The extent to which one or the other of these factors is important remains to be determined.

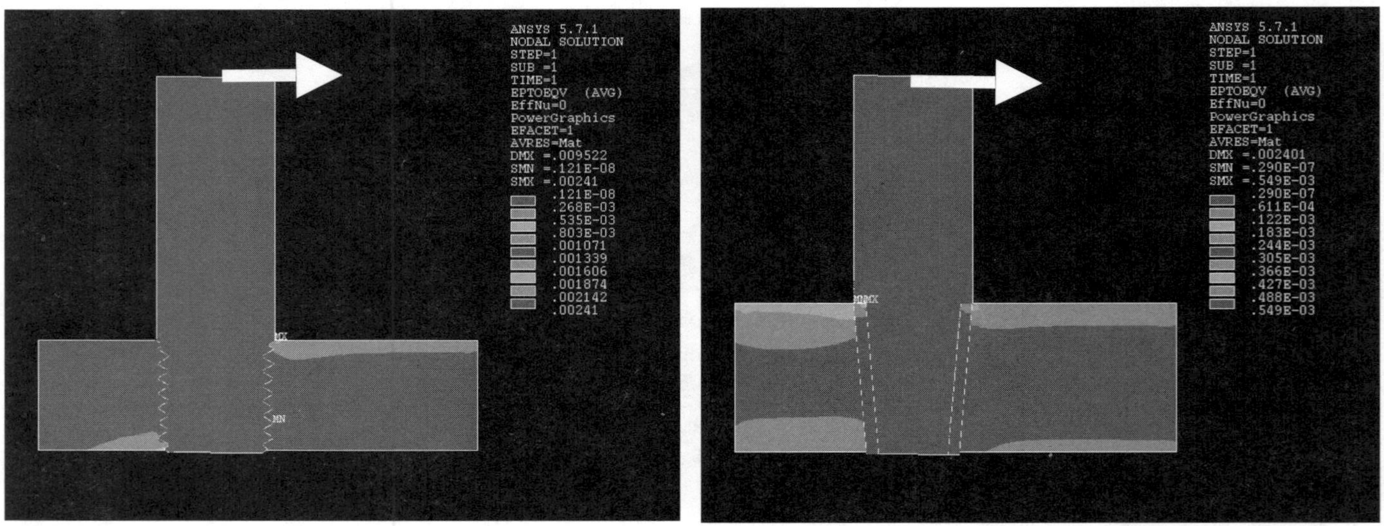

(a) (b)

FIGURE 3.6
Finite element analyses (two-dimensional model) of (a) threaded and (b) porous-surfaced implant with a horizontal force acting on the abutment (orthodontic spring, force = 2 N). The model predicts a more symmetric stress/strain distribution in crestal bone about the porous-surfaced implant (medial and distal aspects). The maximum predicted strain is approximately six times greater with the threaded design (i.e., 2410 versus 394 $\mu\varepsilon$ for the 2 N applied orthodontic force (arrow).

References

1. Pilliar, R.M., An overview of surface variability of metallic endosseous dental implants: textured and porous surface-structure designs, *Implant Dentistry,* 7, 305, 1998.
2. Albrektsson, T. et al., Osseointegrated titanium implants, *Acta Orthop. Scand.,* 52, 155, 1981.
3. Wennerberg, A., Albrektsson, T., and Lausmaa, J., Torque and histomorphometric evaluation of c.p. titanium screws blasted with 25- and 75-μm-sized particles of Al_2O_3, *J. Biomed. Mater. Res.,* 30, 251, 1996.
4. Wennerberg, A. et al., Experimental study of turned and grit-blasted screw-shaped implants with special emphasis on effects of blasting material and surface topography, *Biomaterials,* 17, 15, 1996.
5. Maniatopoulos, C., Pilliar, R.M., and Smith, D.C., Threaded versus porous-surfaced designs for implant stabilization in bone-endodontic implant model, *J. Biomed. Mater. Res.,* 20, 1309, 1986.
6. Thomas, K.A. and Cook, S.D., An evaluation of variables influencing implant fixation by direct bone apposition, *J. Biomed. Mater. Res.,* 19, 875, 1985.
7. Buser, D. et al. Removal torque values of titanium implants in the maxilla of miniature pigs, *Int. J. Oral Maxillofac. Implants,* 13, 611, 1998.
8. Klokkevold, P.R. et al., Osseointegration enhanced by chemical etching of the titanium surface: a torque removal study in the rabbit, *Clin. Oral Implants Res.,* 8, 442, 1997.
9. Cochran, D.L. and Buser, D., Bone response to sandblasted and acid-attacked titanium: experimental and clinical studies, in *Bone Engineering,* Davies, J.E., Ed., e.m. squared inc., Toronto, 2000, p. 391.
10. Jansen, J.A. et al., Histologic evaluation of the osseous adaptation to titanium and hydroxyapatite-coated titanium implants, *J. Biomed. Mater. Res.,* 25, 973, 1991.
11. Cook, S.D. et al., Torsional stability of HA-coated and grit-blasted titanium dental implants, *J. Oral Implantology,* 28, 359, 1992.
12. Thomas, K.A. et al, Effect of surface macrotexture and hydroxylapatite coating on the mechanical strengths and histological profiles of titanium implant materials, *J. Biomed. Mater. Res.,* 21, 1395, 1987.
13. Hulshoff, J.E.G. et al., Evaluation of plasma-spray and magnetron-sputter Ca–P-coated implants: an *in vivo* experiment using rabbits, *J. Biomed. Mater. Res.,* 31, 329, 1996.
14. Jansen, J.A. et al., The effect of surface roughness and calcium-phosphate coating on bone regenerative implant surfaces, in *Bone Engineering,* Davies, J.E., Ed., e.m. squared inc., Toronto, 2000, p. 345.
15. Carter, D. and Giori, N., Effect of mechanical stress on tissue differentiation in the bony implant bed, in *The Bone–Biomaterial Interface,* Davies, J.E., Ed., University of Toronto Press, Toronto, 1991, p. 367.
16. Prendergast, P.J., Huiskes, R., and Soballe, K., Biophysical stimuli on cells during tissue differentiation at implant interfaces, *J. Biomechanics,* 30, 539, 1997.
17. Simmons, C.A., Meguid, S.A., and Pilliar, R.M., Differences in osseointegration rate due to implant surface geometry can be explained by local tissue strains, *J. Orthop. Res.,* 19, 187, 2001.

18. Simmons, C.A., Meguid, S.A., and Pilliar, R.M., Mechanical regulation of localized and appositional bone formation around bone-interfacing implants, *J. Biomed. Mater. Res.*, 55, 63, 2001.
19. Pilliar, R.M., Mechanical factors and osseointegration: influence of implant design, in *Aging, Osteoporosis and Dental Implants*, Zarb, G. et al., Eds., Quintessence, Chicago, 2002, p. 35.
20. Kenwright, J. and Goodship, A.E., Controlled mechanical stimulation in the treatment of tibial fractures, *Clin. Orthop.*, 241, 36, 1989.
21. Carter, D.R., Loboa-Polefka, E.G., and Beaupre, G.S., Mechanical influences on skeletal regeneration and bone resorption, in *Bone Engineering*, Davies, J.E., Ed., e.m. squared inc., Toronto, 2000, p. 358.
22. Simmons, C.A., Valiquette, N., and Pilliar, R.M., Osseointegration of sintered porous-surfaced and plasma spray-coated implants: an animal model study of early postimplantation healing response and mechanical stability, *J. Biomed. Mater. Res.*, 47, 127, 1999.
23. Carter, D.R., Mechanical loading history and skeletal biology, *J. Biomech.*, 20, 1095, 1987.
24. Lekholm, U. and Zarb, G.A., Patient selection, in *Tissue-Integrated Prostheses: Osseointegration in Clinical Dentistry*, Brånemark, P.-I., Zarb, G.A., and Albrektsson, T., Eds., Quintessence, Chicago, 1989, p. 199.
25. Deporter, D.A. et al., A prospective human clinical trial of Endopore dental implants in restoring the partially edentulous maxilla using fixed prostheses, *Int. J. Oral Maxillofac. Implants*, 16, 527, 2001.
26. Deporter, D.A. et al., Managing the posterior mandible of partially edentulous patients with short, porous-surfaced dental implants: early data from a clinical trial, *Int. J. Oral Maxillofac. Implants*, 16, 653, 2001.
27. Morgan, M.J., James, D.F., and Pilliar, R.M., Fractures of the fixture component of an osseointegrated implant, *Int. J. Oral Maxillofac. Implants*, 8, 409, 1993.
28. Quirynen, M., Naaert, I., and Steenberghe, D., Fixture design and overload influence marginal bone loss and fixture success in the Branemark system, *Clin. Oral Implants Res.*, 3, 104, 1992.
29. Hansson, S., The implant neck: smooth or provided with retention elements, *Clin. Oral Implants Res.*, 10, 394, 1999.
30. Pilliar, R.M. et al., Dental implant design: effect on bone remodeling, *J. Biomed. Mater. Res.*, 25, 467, 1991.
31. Vaillancourt, H., Pilliar, R.M., and McCammond, D., Finite element analysis of bone remodeling around porous-coated dental implants, *J. Appl. Biomater.*, 6, 267, 1995.
32. Roberts, W.E., Fundamental principles of bone physiology, metabolism and loading, in *Osseointegration in Oral Rehabilitation*, Naert, I., van Steenberghe, D., and Worthington, P., Eds., Quintessence, London, 1993, p. 157.
33. Al-Sayyed, A. et al., Predictable bone remodeling around two porous-coated titanium alloy dental implant designs, *Clin. Oral Implants Res.*, 5, 31, 1994.
34. Abrahamsson, I. et al., The peri-implant hard and soft tissues at different implant systems: a comparative study in the dog, *Clin. Oral Implants Res.*, 7, 212, 1996.
35. Deporter, D.A. et al., A histometric assessment of bone and peri-implant mucosal tissue contact around sintered porous-surfaced dental implants in dogs, submitted, 2002.

36. Gristina, A.G. and Naylor, P.T., Implant-associated infection, in *Biomaterials Science: An Introduction to Materials in Medicine,* Ratner, B.D. et al., Eds., Academic Press, San Diego, 1996, p. 205.
37. Quirynen, M. et al., An *in vivo* study on the influence of the surface roughness of implants on the microbiology of supra- and subgingival plaque, *J. Dent. Res.,* 72, 1304, 1993.
38. Brunette, D.M. and Chehroudi, B., The effects of the surface topography of micromachined titanium substrata on cell behavior *in vitro* and *in vivo, J. Biomech. Eng.,* 121, 49, 1999.
39. Pilliar, R.M., Porous-surface metallic implants for orthopedic applications, *J. Biomed. Mater. Res.,* 21[A1], 1, 1987.
40. Pilliar, R.M., Deporter, D.A., and Watson, P.A., Tissue-implant interface: micromovement effects, in *Material in Clinical Applications,* Vincenzini, P., Ed., Techna, Faenza, Italy, 569, 1995.
41. Simmons, C.A. and Pilliar, R.M., A biomechanical study of early tissue formation around bone-interfacing implants: the effect of implant surface geometry, in *Bone Engineering,* Davies, J.E., Ed., e.m. squared inc., Toronto, 2000, p. 369.
42. Gan, L. et al., Sol–gel-formed calcium phosphate porous-surfaced implants: film formation and short-term *in vivo* studies, presented at Canadian Biomaterials Society Annual Meeting, Toronto, June 2002.
43. Pilliar, R.M. et al. Radiographic and morphologic studies of load-bearing porous surface-structured implants, *Clin. Orthop.,* 156, 249, 1981.
44. Engh, C.A. and Bobyn, J.D., *Biological Fixation in Total Hip Arthroplasty,* Slack Inc., Thorofare, NJ, 1985, chap. 6.
45. Pilliar, R.M., Lee, J.M., and Davies, J.E., Interface zone: factors influencing its structure for cementless implants, in *Biological, Material, and Mechanical Considerations of Joint Replacement,* Morrey, B.F., Ed., Raven Press, New York, 1993, p. 225.
46. Cochran, D.L. et al., Bone response to loaded and unloaded titanium implants with sandblasted and acid-etched surface: a histometric study in the canine mandible, *J. Biomed. Mater. Res.,* 40, 1, 1998.
47. Klein, C.P.A.T. et al., Calcium phosphate plasma-sprayed coatings and their stability: an *in vivo* study, *J. Biomed. Mater. Res.,* 28, 909, 1994.
48. Jansen, J.A. et al., Application of magnetron sputtering for producing ceramic coatings on implant materials, *Clin. Oral Implants Res.,* 4, 28, 1993.
49. Langstaff, S. et al., Thin film phosphate based bioactive substrates, *Mat. Res. Soc. Symp. Proc.,* 87, 414, 1996.
50. Montenero, A. et al., Sol–gel derived hydroxyapatite coatings on titanium substrate, *J. Mater. Sci.,* 35, 2791, 2000.
51. Kokubo, T. et al., Spontaneous formation of bone apatite layer on chemically treated titanium metals, *J. Am. Ceram. Soc.,* 79, 1127, 1996.
52. Davies, J.E. and Hosseini, M.M., Histodynamics of endosseous wound healing, in *Bone Engineering,* Davies, J.E., Ed., e.m. squared inc., Toronto, 2000, p. 1.
53. Dziedzic, D.M., Effects of Implant Surface Topography on Osteoconduction, M.Sc. thesis, University of Toronto, Toronto, Canada, 1995.
54. Pilliar, R.M., Davies, J.E., and Smith, D.C., The bone–biomaterial interface for load-bearing implants, *MRS Bulletin,* 16, 55, 1991.
55. Nguyen, H. et al., Osteoconduction of calcium phosphate thin films on porous implants in rabbit tibiae, *J. Dent. Res.,* 76, 282, (Abstr. 2151), 1997.

56. Qui, Q. et al., Bone growth on sol–gel calcium phosphate thin films *in vitro*, *Cells Mat.*, 3, 351, 1993.
57. Genady, S., personal communication, 2002.

4

Bone Response to Surface Roughness: Measurements and Results from Experimental and Clinical Studies

Ann Wennerberg and Tomas Albrektsson

CONTENTS

4.1 Introduction 60
4.2 Surface Roughness 60
4.2.1 Measurement and Evaluation 60
4.2.1.1 Methods 60
4.2.1.2 How to Measure and Evaluate Surface Topography of Oral Implants 61
4.2.2 Surface Roughness and Experimental Results 63
4.2.2.1 Experimental Studies of Surface Roughness and Bone Fixation 64
4.2.3 Surface Roughness and Clinical Results of Studies of Commercially Available Implants Prepared with Different Techniques 65
4.2.3.1 Blasted Surface 65
4.2.3.2 Blasted and Acid-Etched Surface 66
4.2.3.3 Acid-Etched Surface 67
4.2.3.4 Hydroxyapatite-Coated Surface 68
4.2.3.5 Oxidized Surfaces 68
4.2.3.6 Titanium Plasma-Sprayed Surface 68
4.2.3.7 Turned Surface 69
References 69

0-8493-1474-7/03/$0.00+$1.50

4.1 Introduction

Turned titanium implant surfaces have been shown to function well in dental practice for decades.[1-4] However, based mainly on experimental studies, several manufacturers abandoned turned surfaces for surface-enlarged implants. The alleged clinical reason is the possibility of loading surface modified implants sooner than generally recommended for turned implants. Better stability caused by greater contact area and a fibrin clot-retentive surface that may trigger bone healing are arguments used in promoting surface-modified implants. Examples of methods used to alter the surface topographies of commercial implants are grit blasting, titanium plasma spraying, chemical surface coating, and etching (used alone or in combinations). Other methods designed to alter surface topography can be found in various *in vitro*[5-6] and *in vivo*[7-9] studies.

In general, experimental studies have shown firmer bone fixations with roughened surfaces.[10-11] The different surface alteration methods produced different heights of individual surface irregularities and different spatial dimensions. Increases in height often, but not always, demonstrated increases in wavelength. However, whether the variation in height or wavelength is most important for improving implant incorporation by bone tissue is still unknown. A careful topographical characterization is necessary for a reliable interpretation of the role of implant surface roughness for bone incorporation. We also need further knowledge of equipment that measures arbitrary designs and different surfaces and interpretation of measurements.

4.2 Surface Roughness

4.2.1 Measurement and Evaluation

4.2.1.1 Methods

Surface topography relates to the degree of roughness of the surface and the orientations of surface irregularities. Surface roughness exists in two principal planes: at a right angle to the surface and in the plane of the surface.[12] For a careful topographical characterization, it is necessary to use measuring methods that provide numerical and visual data for height and spatial variation of the surface irregularities.

Today three major groups of instruments supply such data: (1) mechanical contact stylus instruments, (2) optical instruments, and (3) scanning probe microscopy (SPM). Each method has its own area of application. Only the optical methods are appropriate for threaded oral implants.[13] Among the optical instruments, confocal laser scanning profilometers and interferometers are recommended. The horizontal resolution of optical instruments is dependent on the wavelength of light and can hardly be better than 0.3 μm. However, vertical resolution can be as good as 0.05 nm. Typical maximal measuring area is a few square millimeters and maximal vertical range is several millimeters. If excellent resolution can be maintained, the vertical range is limited to approximately 100 μm. Instruments are rapidly improving and better vertical resolution and measuring range are to be expected.

4.2.1.2 How to Measure and Evaluate Surface Topography of Oral Implants

Parts of threaded implants, for example, the top area, flank, or valley, generally have different degrees of roughness (Figure 4.1) due to the manufacturing process, particularly fabricating the screws. The tops will usually be the roughest parts.[13] Assuming all parts of an implant are of equal importance with respect to bone incorporation, measurements should be taken from the top, flank, and valley areas. The number of required measurements depends on the homogeneity of the surface structure and must be decided at the start of every new study. A stable and small value of the standard deviation could serve as an indication.[14]

Nine measurements (three tops, three flanks, and three valleys) on each implant and three implants for every surface modification appeared sufficient for a reliable interpretation of threaded oral implant surface roughness.[15] Three-dimensional measurements are more reliable than two-dimensional measurements due to considerably increased data. Generally measurements should be as large as possible in view of resolution and vertical measuring ability of the chosen instrument. They are also dependent on the size of the surface to be evaluated. For oral implants, an area from 150 × 150 μm to 350 × 350 μm is a realistic size. The sampling distance is of importance for the parameter calculation. Too great a distance will result in

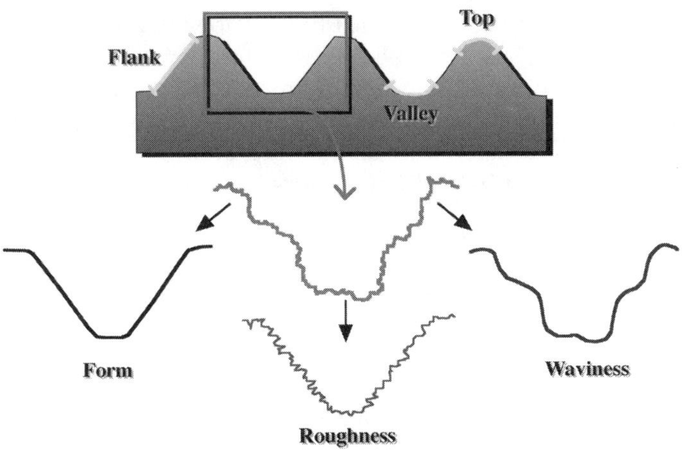

FIGURE 4.1
Top: flank, valley, and top of a threaded oral implant. Bottom: form, waviness, and roughness.

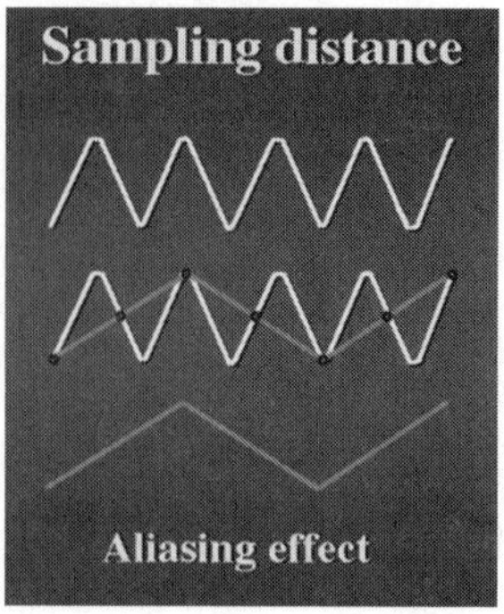

FIGURE 4.2
Too much distance between measuring points will result in a loss of information and an artificial increase of wavelength.

a loss of important frequency components and the surface profile will appear smoother than it actually is because of the so-called aliasing effect (Figure 4.2). Independent measuring method undercuts are impossible to measure. Surfaces with large numbers of undercuts will appear to have shorter wavelengths than are actually the case (Figure 4.3).

Surface topography consists of form, waviness, and roughness (Figure 4.1). Surface roughness parameters are defined after form and waviness are removed.[16] A digital filter is used to separate these components. The roughness is related to the finest irregularities with the spatial frequencies within the measurement; waviness relates to medium spatial frequencies; and form to the lowest spatial frequencies. The point at which roughness becomes waviness has not been defined and must be decided before evaluation because the size of the filter is based on this decision. The numerical values depend on the filter and filter size chosen.

A Gaussian filter is recommended for three-dimensional measurements.[17] A number of parameters can numerically describe the appearance of surface roughness. A parameter should be sensitive to a specific surface characteristic. In most cases, several parameters are needed for a careful characterization. Surface roughness parameters are often separated into three groups, depending on the characteristics of the surface they quantify: amplitude, spatial distribution, and hybrid parameters.

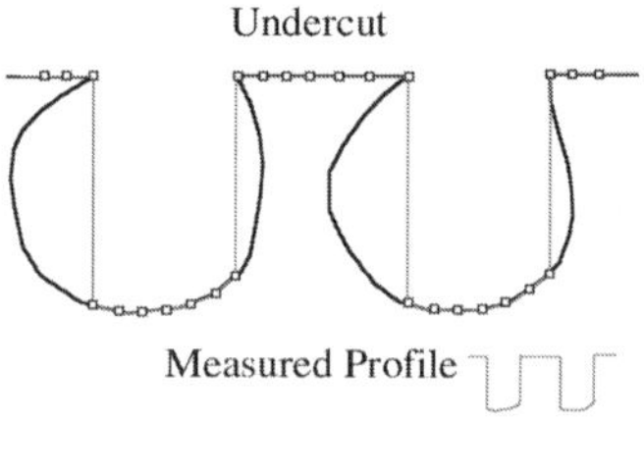

FIGURE 4.3
Undercuts cannot be measured; a loss of spatial information will occur.

Stout and coworkers[17] recommended a primary set of 13 parameters, perhaps too many parameters for oral implants, but at least one parameter from each of the three groups should be included in a careful topographical evaluation.

Amplitude parameters are solely height descriptive. Examples are R_a, R_q, R_z, and R_t for two-dimensional measurements (profiles). S_a, S_q, S_z, and S_t are corresponding parameters for three-dimensional measurements (surfaces).

Spacing parameters describe the spacing between irregularities. Examples are S_m and S (two-dimensional) and S_{cx}, $S_{cy,}$ S_{al}, and S_{ds} (three-dimensional). The two-dimensional S_m parameter is the average value of the length of the center line section containing a profile peak and adjacent valley. It should cross the center line, in contrast to the S parameter that represents mean spacing of adjacent local peaks.

Hybrid parameters include information about height and spatial distribution, for example, the parameters $S_{\Delta q}$ and S_{dr} describe shape, i.e., if an irregularity has a pointed or rounded curvature ($S_{\Delta q}$) and the developed surface area ratio (S_{dr}) is the ratio between a 3D measurement and a 2D, i.e., the ratio between a rough area and a totally flat reference plane.

A clear description of the parameters used is necessary. Information should be provided about measuring equipment, numbers of measurements, lengths and areas of measurement, and types of filters. Otherwise, the stated parameter value will be impossible to interpret and provide very little value to other researchers.

4.2.2 Surface Roughness and Experimental Results

Surface structures equal in all directions with respect to height and spatial deviations are designated isotropic (Figure 4.4). Techniques for producing such surfaces on which the irregularities are randomly oriented include abrasive blasting, plasma spraying, etching, and oxidizing. Other machining processes, such as turning and milling, produce surfaces with distinct and

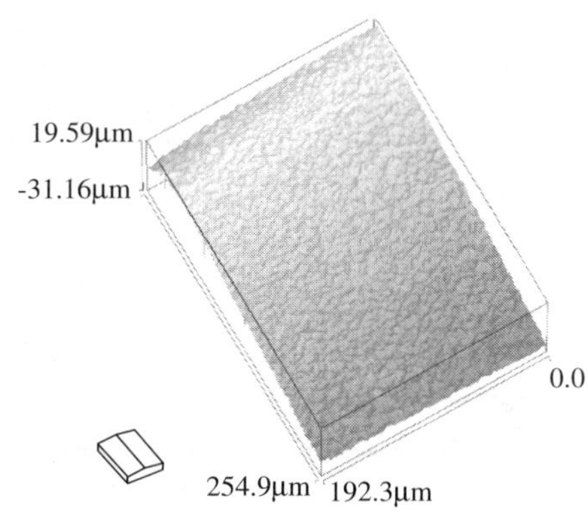

FIGURE 4.4
An oxidized implant surface; a surface structure without a dominating direction.

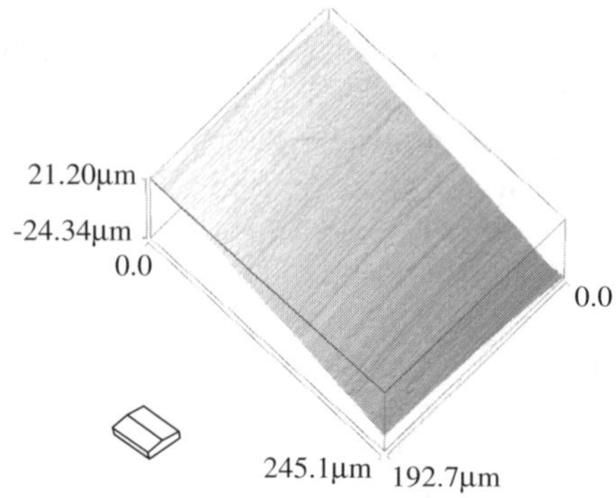

FIGURE 4.5
A turned implant surface; a surface structure with a dominating direction. Marks from the cutting procedure are clearly visible.

dominant directions, i.e., anisotropic surfaces. Several oral implants have been machined with isoptropic or anisotropic surfaces (Figure 4.5).

4.2.2.1 Experimental Studies of Surface Roughness and Bone Fixation

Several experimental studies *in vivo* reported better bone fixation for surface-enlarged implants compared with turned or polished implants.[10,15,18-19] Some studies revealed positive correlations of increasing surface roughness and implant incorporation,[11,20-22] while others found no such correlation.[23] A study published in 1991 by Buser et al.[24] pointed to the possibility of an optimal degree of surface roughness. A series of studies was designed with the intent of investigating whether an optimum level of surface roughness exists.

The surface structures on screw-shaped turned implants were altered by using blasting materials of different particle sizes. Turned implants were used as controls. Every implant had a diameter of 3.75 mm and a pitch height of 0.6 mm. The blasting material was TiO_2 or Al_2O_3 and the median sizes of the particles were 25 μm, 75 μm, and 250 μm, respectively. The implants were cleaned in an ultrasonic bath and the surface topography of each device was well characterized by an optical confocal profilometer using the same record described above.

The major finding was that a surface with an S_a value of 1.45 μm, S_{cx} value of 11 μm, and an S_{dr} ratio of 1.50 resulted in the firmest bone fixation. The evaluation methods used were peak removal torque and calculation of the amount of bone in contact with the implant surface. This series of studies was published in a number of international journals in the 1990s.[25-30] A control study using implants prepared with two different surface roughness levels, i.e., each screw was its own control, confirmed the findings.[31]

It may be speculated that rabbit bone reacts differently from human bone in response to various surface modifications. A study in human jaw bones[19] was carried out to compare turned and TiO_2 blasted microimplants histomorphometrically after healing periods of 4 (mandible) to 6 (maxillae) months. Significantly more bone was in contact with the blasted implant surface than with the turned one. The conclusion was that human bone and rabbit bone reacted similarly.

An interesting finding in the study by Ivanoff and coworkers[19] was that the S_a values were very similar for the turned and the blasted microimplants if the parameter mean value was calculated from measurements undertaken from tops, valleys, and flanks. If, on the other hand, only measurements from the flank areas were considered, parameter values obtained corresponded well with results achieved in previous studies investigating surfaces machined in the same manner. This finding indicates that a topographical evaluation should be undertaken in every new study and that one cannot rely on earlier investigations to reliably monitor surface roughness. Furthermore, the results may be interpreted as if the isotropy of a surface were the most important topographical property for implant incorporation in bone. In a thesis by Hallgren-Höstner,[32] the importance of isotropy versus anisotropy and checkered surface patterns was investigated. The blasted isotropic surface was found preferable in terms of bone fixation related to these surface modifications. Increasing the average wavelength from 10 μm to about 40 μm did not improve implant incorporation. Waviness seemed to be less important than roughness.

4.2.3 Surface Roughness and Clinical Results of Studies of Commercially Available Implants Prepared with Different Techniques

All values that follow were measured by a confocal laser scanning profilometer, the TopScan 3D™ (Heidelberg Instruments, Heidelberg, Germany). The diameter of the helium-neon laser beam is approximately 1 μm. All measurements had sizes of 250 × 250 μm. Nine measurements were taken from each implant (three tops, three valleys, and three flanks). Three implants from each manufacturer were measured. A Gaussian filter (50 × 50 μm) was used to separate roughness from errors of form and waviness.

4.2.3.1 Blasted Surface

The Tioblast™ (Astratech AB, Mölndal, Sweden) is surface blasted with TiO_2 particles. The blasting procedure results in an isotropic surface. The implants had an average height deviation (S_a) of 1.07 μm, an average wavelength (S_{cx}) of 10.11 μm, and an increased surface area (S_{dr}) of 29%.

Tioblast is today one of the best documented implant systems with several short- and medium-time follow-up studies. Furthermore, there are three published clinical reports that span more than 5 years.[33–34,36b] Palmer et al.[33] in a prospective paper, report results of 15 implants. Of these, one became a drop-out for unknown reasons. In total, 14 implants were followed for 5 years with no losses, and the implants showed a maintained bone height.

Norton[34] summarizes the up to 7-year outcome of 27 implants. However, of those only 14 implants were available for review, and, therefore, the best survival rate over the 4- to 7-year period was 95.6% and the worst case (assuming that all drop-outs are failures) survival rate was as low as 60.8%. Bone height figures were not available for 4 to 7 years. However, in a separate study, Norton[35] reported on the same material when followed for up to 4 years and then reported on maintained bone heights. This surface must be described as well-documented from a clinical perspective, but still too few implants have been included in the referred studies in relation to the recommended minimum figures for a proper success report.[36] However, enough implants were included in a study published by Godfredsen and Karlsson,[36b] in which 133 Astra implants, turned and Tioblast were followed-up for 5 years. The survival rate after 5 years was 95.1% for the turned surface and 100% for the TiO_2 blasted surface. Marginal bone resorption was 0.21 mm and 0.51 mm, respectively.

4.2.3.2 Blasted and Acid-Etched Surface

The surface of the SLA™ (Institute Straumann AG, Waldenburg, Switzerland) is first blasted with large size particles and then acid etched. The surface modification resulted in a structure that includes high frequency and medium frequency wavelengths. The implants had average height deviations of 1.42 μm, average wavelengths of 16.60 μm, and increased surface area of 33%.

From a long-term clinical perspective, no publications covered this implant type. Rocuzzo et al.[37] published a prospective, short-term, split-mouth study of 68 SLA and 68 titanium plasma sprayed (TPS) implants of the same design. At 1-year follow up, they noted no implant losses. The accumulated bone height levels showed mean marginal bone losses of 0.65 mm and 0.77 mm for SLA and TPS implants, respectively. In a multicenter study published in 2002,[38] SLA implants were evaluated in a prospective study; 138 implants were followed up for 2 years and 326 implants were followed up for 1 year. Inclusion criteria included adequate oral hygiene and adequate bone volume to harbor the implant. Exclusion criteria were moderate or heavy smoking, severe bruxism, and other conditions. No data were published on bone height levels, making it impossible to evaluate implant success according to the Albrektsson and Zarb[36] criteria. However, only six implants were unaccounted for and only three failed, pointing to good 2-year clinical results for the SLA implant.

The Southern implant™ (Irene, South Africa) is another implant machined with a blasted and etched surface. The average height deviation is very similar to that for the SLA implant. The Southern implant had a more dense structure; average wavelength was several microns shorter than the SLA. This resulted in a greater enlarged surface compared to the SLA results. S_a was 1.43 μm, S_{cx} was 12.18 μm, and S_{dr} value was 50% for the Southern implant.

Steri-Oss machined implants and surface roughened Southern implants were compared in a randomized study of mandibular overdentures.[39] Inclusion called for edentulous patients with minimal bone stock of 13 to 15 mm; exclusion criteria included bruxism or any history of smoking. The study was claimed to compare two types of implants of different surface roughnesses although no actual evaluation of roughness was published. Furthermore, the two tested implant systems differed in design although both were threaded screws. Forty-eight implants of both types were tested for a follow-up of 2 years. Eight Steri-Oss implants failed. All were inserted by the same surgeon. None of the Southern implants failed, but four implants were considered as only surviving. Drop-out patients had Steri-Oss (two) and Southern (four) implants. The four Southern implants were the same ones considered as "only surviving."

When tested at our laboratories, the Steri-Oss™ surface described as machined was in fact acid etched with a roughness (S_a) of 0.8 μm. The Southern implant had S_a roughness of 1.4 μm. Whether the higher failure rate of Steri-Oss™ implants is coincidental, dependent on differences in roughness or design between the two tested implants, or based on implantation by the same surgeon is unknown.

4.2.3.3 Acid-Etched Surface

The surface of the Osseotite™ (Implant Innovations, Palm Beach Gardens, FL) is etched in a two-step procedure, resulting in an isotropic surface with high frequency irregularities. The measured implants had an average height deviation of 0.94 μm, an average wavelength of 11.68 μm, and an increased surface area of 20%.

We were unable to find any long-term clinical reports of this implant. However, Testori et al.[40] published a prospective multicenter clinical study in a 4-year report. This was a well performed study of 485 implants of which 219 were mandibular and 266 maxillary; 73% of the implants were placed in posterior locations, 39 implants (7.4%) were drop-outs, and 6 failed. Bone height measurements indicated steady state conditions. The cumulative success rate (CSR) was reported as 98.7% at an average of 52 months (loading time 43 months), but this high figure may in part relate to the fact that smokers, bruxers, and clenchers were in the exclusion group.

In another study published by Testori et al.,[41] Osseotite™ microtextured, acid-etched implants were evaluated in a prospective multicenter study of 282 mandibular and 123 maxillary implants placed in posterior parts of the jaws. Exclusion criteria included active periodontal infection and static or dynamic bruxism. Smoking was not an exclusion criterion. No data were published on bone height levels; the authors only reported survival rates. Of the placed implants, 206 were followed up for a full 3 years. Nine implants failed and 16 were unaccounted for. The cumulative survival rate was 97.7% at 3 years of follow up.

Other papers on results of this implant [42-43] span much shorter follow-up times and are clearly less impressive from a design point of view.

4.2.3.4 Hydroxyapatite-Coated Surface

The coating procedure of the Steri-Oss™ Replace system (Nobel Biocare, Yorba Linda, CA) alters the surface chemistry and the topography. In general this machining method gives a rather rough and isotropic surface. The Steri-Oss HA coated implants had an average height deviation of 1.68 μm, an average wavelength of 13.74 μm, and an increased surface area of 55%.

From a clinical perspective, numerous short- and intermediate-term reports cited acceptable clinical results with HA-coated Calcitec™ implants (Sulzer Medica, now known as Centerpulse Dental, Carlsbad, CA) but no investigations with acceptable 5-year clinical data have been found in the literature.[44]

4.2.3.5 Oxidized Surfaces

The surface of the TiUnite™ (Nobel Biocare AB, Göteborg, Sweden) is oxidized in a manner that increases the thickness of the oxidized layer in the apical direction. The process results in an isotropic surface characterized by craterous structures. The implants had an average height deviation of 1.08 μm, an average wavelength of 10.98 μm, and an increased surface area of 37%.

From a clinical view, we found only one relatively long-term follow-up of oxidized implants.[45] However, the reported oxidized implant probably differed in design and surface characteristics compared to the TiUnite. The paper reports the outcomes of implants of 339 Ticer oxidized screws (32 were lost to follow-up) and 30 cylinders (one was lost to follow-up). The precise times of follow-ups for individual implants and the precise localizations of the implants were insufficiently described. Inclusion criteria were not adequately reported, particularly with respect to whether patients were consecutive. The frequency of patient recall, parameters examined at the recalls, and bone height measurements were not reported. Because of these shortcomings, it was difficult to interpret this paper and compare the results with those found in other publications.

4.2.3.6 Titanium Plasma-Sprayed Surface

The Steri-Oss™ Replace system (Nobel Biocare, Yorba Linda, CA) had the roughest implant surface among those measured. The implants had an average height deviation of 3.86 μm, an average wavelength of 19.55 μm, and an increased surface area of 134%. No long-term follow-up studies have been published.

The Bonefit™ (Institute Straumann AG, Waldenburg, Switzerland) has a smoother surface than the Steri-Oss™ implant, although it is still rough compared with devices produced by other machining methods. The surface of the implants was found to have an average height deviation of 2.35 μm, an average wavelength of 13.15 μm, and an increased surface area of 87%.

Buser et al.[46] reported good long-term survival results for plasma-sprayed Bonefit implants. Their fine study evaluated 488 implants for survival at 5 years or more. Of the total of 2359 implants (most followed up for less than 5 years), only 127 (5.4%) drop-outs were registered. Implant subgroups showed slightly better results for screw-type implants than for hollow cylinder types. Mandibular implants showed an overall survival rate of 95% compared to 87% for maxillary implants. The only major criticism of this paper is the absence of bone height measurement, making it impossible to evaluate the implants for success. In another fine paper, Merickse-Stern et al.[47] reported a survival rate of 84.6% for cylindrical plasma-sprayed implants after a mean observation period of 14 years.

4.2.3.7 Turned Surface

Cutting marks from the machining process that produces the MK III™ (Nobel Biocare, Göteborg, Sweden) resulted in an oriented anisotropic surface. The implants had an average height deviation of 0.71 μm, an average wavelength of 9.84 μm, and an increased surface area of 19%. The MK III implants had rougher surfaces compared to the turned coronal parts of the Osseotite™ implant. The average height deviation for Osseotite™ coronal part was 0.53 μm, average wavelength was 8.6 μm, and the developed surface area was 15%.

The turned Brånemark implant was, by far, the best documented implant.[3] The literature contains several long-term reports showing good clinical results.[2] However, experimental studies clearly indicate that significantly more bone is found around HA-coated, intermediary roughened or oxidized implants compared to turned implants[15] and it has been suggested that these newer surfaces should be preferred over turned implants. Claims that turned implants do not function well in poor bone have proven untrue. The only positively documented long-term cases of good clinical results in poor bone were reported with turned implants.[48-49] Comparative studies with split-jaw designs with turned and intermediary roughened implants have failed to definitively prove the automatic superiority of roughened surfaces.[50-52]

References

1. Albrektsson, T. and Sennerby, L., State of the art in oral implants, *J. Clin. Paradontol.*, 18, 474, 1991.
2. Roos, J., Sennerby, L., and Albrektsson, T., An update on the clinical documentation on currently used bone-anchored endosseous implants, *Clin. Update*, 24, 194, 1997.

3. Eckert, S. et al., Validation of dental implant systems through a review of the literature supplied by system manufacturers, *J. Prosth. Dent.*, 77, 271, 1997.
4. Arvidsson, K. et al., Five-year prospective follow-up report of the AstraTech dental implant system in the treatment of edentulous mandibles, *Clin. Oral Implant Res.*, 9, 225, 1998.
5. Chehroudi, B. et al., The role of connective tissue in inhibiting epithelial downgrowth on titanium-coated percutaneous implant, *J. Biomed. Mater. Res.*, 26, 493, 1992.
6. Chehroudi, B., McDonnell, D., and Brunette, D.M., The effects of micromachined surfaces on formation of bone-like tissue on subcutaneous implants as assessed by radiography and computer image processing, *J. Biomed. Mater. Res.*, 34, 279, 1997.
7. Hallgren, C. et al., The importance of surface texture for bone integration of screw-shaped implants: an *in vivo* study of implants patterned by photolithography, *J. Biomed. Mater. Res.*, 57, 485, 2001.
8. Li, J. et al., Surface-dimpled commercially pure titanium implant and bone ingrowth, *Biomaterials*, 18, 691, 1997.
9. Sul, Y.T. et al., Oxidized implants and their influence on the bone response, *J. Mater. Sci. Mater. Med.*, 12, 1025, 2001.
10. Feighan, J.E. et al., The influence of surface blasting on the incorporation of titanium alloy implants in a rabbit intramedullary model, *J. Bone Joint Surg.*, 77-A, 1380, 1995.
11. Gotfredsen, K., Berglundh, T., and Lindhe, J., Anchorage of titanium implants with different surface characteristics: an experimental study in rabbits, *Clin. Implant Dent. Relat. Res.*, 2, 120, 2000.
12. Thomas, T., *Rough Surfaces*, 2nd ed., Imperial Collage Press, London, 1999.
13. Wennerberg, A. and Albrektsson, T., Suggested guidelines for the topographic evaluation of implant surfaces, *Int. J. Oral Maxillofac. Implants*, 15, 331, 2000.
14. Bennett, J.M. and Mattsson, L., *Introduction to Surface Roughness and Scattering*, 1st ed., Optical Society of America, Washington, D.C., 1989.
15. Wennerberg, A., On Surface Roughness and Implant Incorporation, Ph.D. thesis, Göteborg University, Göteborg, Sweden, 1996.
16. British Institution, Assessment of surface texture: methods and instrumentation: general information and guidance, BS 1134, London, 1988.
17. Stout, K.J. et al., The development of methods for the characterisation of roughness in three dimensions, Commission of the European Communities, Birmingham, 1993.
18. Lazzara, R.J. et al., A human histologic analysis of Osseotite and machined surfaces using implants with two opposing surfaces, *Int. J. Periodon. Restorative Dent.*, 19, 117, 1999.
19. Ivanoff, C.J. et al., Histologic evaluation of the bone integration of TiO_2 blasted and turned titanium microimplants in humans, *Clin. Oral Implant. Res.*, 12, 128, 2001.
20. Hahn, H. and Palich, W., Preliminary evaluation of porous metal surfaced titanium for orthopedic implants, *J. Biomed. Mater. Res.*, 4, 571, 1970.
21. Robertson, D.M., St. Pierre, L., and Chahal, R., Preliminary oberservations of bone ingrowth into porous materials, *J. Biomed. Mater. Res.*, 10, 335, 1976.
22. Carlsson, L. et al., Removal torques for polished and rough titanium implants, *Int. J. Oral Maxillofac. Implants.*, 3, 21, 1988.
23. Vercaigne, S. et al., Bone healing capacity of titanium plasma-sprayed and hydroxylapatite-coated oral implants, *Clin. Oral Implant Res.*, 9, 261, 1998.

24. Buser, D. et al., Influence of surface characteristics on bone integration of titanium implants: a histomorphometric study in miniature, *J. Biomed. Mater. Res.*, 25, 889, 1991.
25. Wennerberg, A. et al., A histomorphometric and removal torque study of screw-shaped titanium implants with three different surface topographies, *Clin. Oral Implant Res.*, 6, 24, 1995.
26. Wennerberg, A., Albrektsson, T., and Andersson, B., An animal study of c.p. titanium screws with different surface topographies, *J. Mater. Sci. Mater. Med.*, 6, 302, 1995.
27. Wennerberg, A. et al., Experimental study of turned and grit-blasted screw-shaped implants with special emphasis on effects of blasting material and surface topography, *Biomaterials*, 17, 15, 1996
28. Wennerberg, A., Albrektsson, T., and Andersson, B., Bone tissue response to commercially pure titanium implants blasted with fine and coarse particles of aluminum oxide, *Int. J. Oral Maxillofac. Implants*, 11, 38, 1996.
29. Wennerberg, A., Albrektsson, T., and Lausmaa, J., Torque and histomorphometric evaluation of c.p. titanium screws blasted with 25- and 75-micron-sized particles of Al_2O_3, *J. Biomed. Mater. Res.*, 30, 251, 1996.
30. Wennerberg, A. et al., A 1-year follow-up of implants of differing surface roughness placed in rabbit bone, *Int. J. Oral Maxillofac. Implants*, 12, 486, 1997.
31. Wennerberg, A. et al., A histomorphometric evaluation of screw-shaped implants each prepared with two surface roughnesses, *Clin. Oral Implant Res.*, 9, 11, 1998.
32. Hallgren-Höstner, C., On the Bone Response to Different Implant Textures: A Three-Dimensional Analysis of Roughness, Wavelength and Surface Patterns of Experimental Implants, Ph.D. thesis, Göteborg University, Göteborg, Sweden, 2001.
33. Palmer, R.M., Palmer, P.J., and Smith, B.J., A 5-year prospective study of Astra single tooth implants, *Clin. Oral Implant Res.*, 11, 179, 2000.
34. Norton, M.R., A 4–7 year follow-up on the biological and mechanical stability of single tooth implants, *Clin. Implant Dent. Relat. Res.*, 3, 214, 2001.
35. Norton, M.R., Marginal bone levels at single tooth implants with a conical fixture design: the influence of surface macro- and microtexture, *Clin. Oral Implant Res.*, 9, 91, 1998.
36. Albrektsson, T. et al., The long-term efficacy of currently used dental implants: a review and proposed criteria of success, *Int. J. Oral Maxillofac. Implants*, 1, 11, 1986.

36b. Gotfredsen, K. and Karlsson, U., A prospective 5-year study of fixed partial prostheses supported implants with machined and TiO_2-blasted surface, *J. Prosthodont.*, 10, 1, 2–7, 2001.

37. Roccuzzo, M. et al., Early loading of sandblasted and acid-etched (SLA) implants: a prospective split-mouth comparative study, *Clin. Oral Implant Res.*, 12, 572, 2001.
38. Cochran, D.L. et al., The use of reduced healing times on ITI implants with a sandblasted and acid-etched (SLA) surface: early results from clinical trials on ITI SLA implants, *Clin. Oral Implant Res.*, 13, 144, 2002.
39. Tawse-Smith, A. et al., Early loading of unsplinted implants supporting mandibular overdentures using a one-stage operative procedure with two different implant systems: a 2-year report, *Clinical Implant Dent. Rel. Res.*, 4, 33, 2002.
40. Testori, T. et al., A prospective multicenter clinical study of the Osseotite implant: four-year interim report, *Int. J. Oral Maxillofac. Implants*, 16, 193, 2001.

41. Testori, T. et al., A multicenter prospective evaluation of 2-months loaded Osseotite implants placed in the posterior jaws: 3-year follow up results, *Clin. Oral Implant Res.*, 13, 154, 2002.
42. Sullivan, D., Sherwood, R., and Mai, T., Preliminary results of a multicenter study evaluating a chemically enhanced surface for machined commercially pure titanium implants, *J. Prosth. Dent.*, 78, 379, 1997.
43. Lazzara, R. et al., A prospective multicenter study evaluating loading of Osseotite implants two months after placement: one-year results, *J. Esth. Dentistry*, 10, 280, 1998.
44. Albrektsson, T., Hydroxyapatite-coated implants: a case against their use, *J. Oral Maxillofac. Surg.*, 56, 1312, 1998.
45. Graf, H.L. et al., Klinisches Verhalten des ZL-duraplant-Implantatsystems mit Ticer Oberfläche: Prospektive Studie Mitteilung 1: Überlebensraten, *Z. Zahnärtzl Implant.*, 17, 124, 2001.
46. Buser, D. et al., Long-term evaluation of non-submerged ITI implants. Part 1: 8-year life table analysis of a prospective multicenter study with 2359 implants, *Clin. Oral Implant Res.*, 8, 161, 1997.
47. Merickse-Stern, R. et al., Long-term evaluation of submerged hollow cylinder implants: clinical and radiographic results, *Clin. Oral Implant Res.*, 12, 252, 2001.
48. Friberg, B., On Bone Quality and Implant Stability Measurements, Ph.D. thesis, University of Göteborg, Göteborg, Sweden, 1999.
49. Bahat, O., Brånemark system implants in the posterior maxilla: clinical study of 660 implants followed for 5 to 12 years, *Int. J. Oral Maxillofac. Implants*, 15, 646, 2001.
50. Lindhe, J., Prospective clinical trials on implant therapy in the partially edentulous dentition using the Astra Tech dental implant system, in *Transactions of Workshops, 13th European Conference on Biomaterials*, European Society for Biomaterialsm 1997, p. 9.
51. Karlsson, U., Gotfredsen, K., and Olsson, C., A 2-year report on maxillary and mandibular fixed partial dentures supported by Astra Tech dental implants: a comparison of two implants with different surface textures, *Clin. Oral Implants Res.*, 9, 235, 1998.
52. Åstrand, P. et al., Astra Tech and Brånemark implants: a prospective 5-year comparative study: results after one year, *Clin. Implant Dent. Relat. Res.*, 1, 17, 1999.

5

From Microroughness to Resorbable Bioactive Coatings

Serge Szmukler-Moncler, Peter Zeggel, Daniel Perrin, Jean-Pierre Bernard, and Hans-Georg Neumann

CONTENTS

5.1 Introduction 74
  5.1.1 Choosing a Surface that Meets Early and Immediate Loading Requirements 75
5.2 Materials and Methods 77
  5.2.1 First *In Vivo* Study: Testing the Safety of the Coating 77
    5.2.1.1 The Animal Model 77
    5.2.1.2 Implants 77
    5.2.1.3 Histology Processing and Histomorphometric Analysis 78
    5.2.1.4 Results 78
  5.2.2 Second *In Vivo* Study: Testing Efficacy of the Coating 78
    5.2.2.1 Animal Model 80
    5.2.2.2 Implants 80
    5.2.2.3 Histology Processing and Histomorphometric Analysis 81
    5.2.2.4 Statistical Analysis 81
    5.2.2.5 Results 81
  5.2.3 Third *In Vivo* Study: Testing Efficacy of the Coating 82
    5.2.3.1 Animal Model 82
    5.2.3.2 Implants 82
    5.2.3.3 Histology Processing and Histomorphometric Analysis 86
    5.2.3.4 Statistical Analysis 86
    5.2.3.5 Results 86
  5.2.4 Results of Human Biopsies Following Immediate Loading Protocol 86
    5.2.4.1 Immediate Loading Model 87

0-8493-1474-7/03/$0.00+$1.50

5.2.4.2 Implants....87
5.2.4.3 Histology Processing and Histomorphometric Analysis....87
5.2.4.4 Results....87
5.2.5 Coating Characterization....87
5.3 Discussion....88
References....96

5.1 Introduction

Considerable scientific evidence indicates that surface state modulates the bone response to implant placement. The last decade can be described as the "surface quest" decade, because most manufacturers left standard machined surface production to introduce modified surfaces as shown in Table 5.1. The trend in dental implantology is to reduce the time between implant placement and loading through early or immediate loading protocols. Implementation of a new optimized implant surface should follow these trends and enhance the predictability of both types of protocols. Ideally, the same implant surface should suit both purposes optimally.

The requirements for a predictable early and immediate loading are distinct. The early loading approach requires a safe loading before 3 to 4 months of healing in the mandible and 5 to 6 months in the maxilla. A surface that responds to these requirements should, therefore, foster healing at the bone–implant interface. Conversely, the immediate loading approach

TABLE 5.1

Main Surface Treatments, Brand Names, and Manufacturers

Treatment Type	With	Brand Name and Manufacturer
Machined		Mark II–IV, Nobel Biocare; Clones
Sandblasted	Al_2O_3	EVL, SERF; STI, Idhe; Ankylos
	TiO_2	Tioblast, Astra
	TCP + acid	RBM, Lifecore; SBM, Paragon; BioHorizon
Plasma sprayed	Ti atmospheric (APS)	ITI-TPS, Straumann
	Ti vacuum (VPS)	Pitt-Easy, Oraltronics
	HA	MTX, Sulzer, Calcitec; Friatec
Etched	Acid	Osseotite, 3i; ETK, Eutoteknika
	Sandblasting and etching	DPS, Friatec; ITI-SLA, Straumann, Promote, Camlog; Ha-Ti
Anodic oxidation	Thick TiO_2	TiUnit, Nobel Biocare
Electrochemical deposition	Resorbable CaP	FBR, Oraltronics

Note: TCP = tricalcium phosphate; APS = atmospheric plasma spraying; VPS = vacuum plasma spraying.

requires the highest tolerance to micromotion during the bone healing period. A surface that concomitantly meets both requirements would most suitably take into account the trends in implantology.

This chapter describes the rationale that led to the development of a surface aimed to address early and immediate loading requirements. It also provides related histological data.

5.1.1 Choosing a Surface that Meets Early and Immediate Loading Requirements

Based on the literature, a machined surface can be considered a basic non-optimized surface. An implant surface can be roughened and provides a bioinert surface in contact with bone. The aim then is to introduce roughness and undercuts at the implant surface into which bone might grow and create a mechanical interlock.

Various roughening methods exist, including sandblasting with alumina, titanium oxide, or resorbable tricalcium phosphate particles and titanium plasma spraying. The most recent technique is chemical etching with or without prior sandblasting. Surfaces can be changed also by implementing bioactive coatings; however, the biologic principle that stays behind is interaction between bone and the surface to stimulate bone growth directly from the implant surface. The literature is replete with studies comparing several surface treatments in various animal models. A survey of the literature comparing implant surfaces shows a definite trend.

When roughened bioinert and bioactive surfaces are compared, it appears clear that bioactive surfaces increase bone–implant contacts (BICs), particularly during the first weeks of healing.[1-4] Buser et al.[1] measured six distinct surfaces 3 and 6 weeks after implantation. The electropolished surfaces were the smoothest. The roughest were the titanium plasma-sprayed surfaces or those with bioactive HA coatings. Although rougher surfaces tended to provide more bone at the interface, the highest BIC was always achieved by the bioactive HA plasma-sprayed surface. Similarly, when the bone–implant interface strength is compared mechanically for textured bioinert and bioactive surfaces by torque or push-out, the bioactive coatings appear to induce greater mechanical resistance.

For example, Wong et al.[5] compared push-out data of a bioactive HA coating and several roughened surfaces, among them textured sandblasted and etched (SLA) surfaces after 3 months of implantation in the knees of mini-pigs. The HA-coated implant required 841 N for push-out; the SLA interface was broken after the application of only 389 N. To review details of these studies, readers are referred to Larsson et al.[4] It appears that bioactive HA coatings best meet the requirements for safe early loading, i.e., a surface that leads to the highest bone-to-implant contact, the shortest healing after implant insertion, and/or the highest implant anchorage at the shortest time as evidenced by removal torque or push-out methods.

The requirement for submitting an optimized surface to immediate loading is intended to increase tolerance to micromotion. A survey of the literature shows that bioactive coatings provide higher tolerance to micromotion than bioinert surfaces.[6] The work of Søballe et al.[7] serves as an example. They compared TPS-coated and HA–TPS-coated surfaces in a controlled micromotion model. A device implanted in dog knees allowed 150 μm of micromotion to a cylindrical implant. At each gait, the coated cylinders were moved up and down by that amount of micromovement. After 12 weeks, the HA-coated cylinders were osseointegrated while the bioinert TPS-coated implants displayed fibrous integration. The tolerated threshold of micromotion was higher for the HA-coated surface; thus the HA-coated surface seems more suitable for the purpose of immediate loading.

The HA-coated surface seems to meet adequately the requirements for enhanced predictability of the early and immediate loading protocols. However, several concerns[8-11] may challenge the short-term achievements:

1. HA coatings may flake.[12,13]
2. HA-coated titanium interface strength may decrease subsequently to functional loading[14] and the coating may delaminate from its substrate over the long term.
3. The dissolution extent of the coating is unpredictable.[1,10,15-17]
4. Little is known about the maintenance of osseointegration in case of total dissolution of the plasma-sprayed HA-coating.[10]
5. HA coatings may induce dramatic bone loss if contaminated by dental plaque.[8,11,18]
6. Third-body wear in orthopedic applications has been described.[16,19]

In order to avoid the drawbacks of HA plasma-sprayed coatings, some manufacturers proposed specific post-treatments aimed to increase coating crystallinity[20,21] in the hope of achieving safer long-term behavior. However, since no long-term data are available, the concern about long-term use cannot be completely alleviated. A number of trials aimed to eradicate the mid- and long-term risks of HA plasma-sprayed implants by means of a fully resorbable bioactive coating.[6,22-26] Such a resorbable coating should combine the initial advantages of CaP coatings and obliterate the mid- or long-term concerns for coating stability, deleterious inflammatory responses, and third-body wear.

Formulation of a resorbable bioactive coating should include a given bioactive material, a given structural phase, and a given morphology. This second generation of bioactive coatings should display simultaneously (1) enough lability to be completely dissolved during the first months following implantation and (2) adequate dissolution kinetics capable of initiating the cascade of events that leads to bioactivity before vanishing. In addition, the heavy release of Ca and PO_4 ions during the dissolution phase should not interfere with the ongoing osseointegration process.[6,22,23] This is of outmost importance because plasma-sprayed CaP coatings have been documented to impede bone apposition at dissolving areas[29-35] and to attract macrophages and multinucleated cells.[16,21,34,35]

The following section addresses the issues of early and immediate loading and summarizes experimental data gathered on a novel resorbable bioactive coating obtained by electrochemical deposition and known by a number of trade names.*

5.2 Materials and Methods

5.2.1 First *In Vivo* Study: Testing the Safety of the Coating

Because the literature shows that the dissolution of HA-coatings may interfere with bone apposition,[27,31-35] the first step was to investigate whether a similar result would occur for this resorbable coating since a massive release of Ca and PO_4 ions in the environment was expected during the healing phase.

5.2.1.1 The Animal Model

A female farmer Land Race pig model was used as described by Perrin et al.[36] The adult animals were about 14 months old. After a month of quarantine, the premolars were extracted to allow 90 to 100 mm of area for implant placement. The maxilla is specially suitable for this purpose because of its spongy bone quality. This model offers the opportunity of placing 8 to 10 implants per hemimaxilla, and is particularly suitable for screening studies because a large number of test implants can be investigated in one animal. Furthermore, at experiment completion, the animals are not sacrificed. Implants and the surrounding bones are retrieved through segmental osteotomy. The first experimentation evaluating this coating was a pilot study involving a single animal. It was dedicated to screening the safety of this fully resorbable bioactive coating.[22]

5.2.1.2 Implants

ITI TPS-coated hollow-screw implants including the necks (Figure 5.1) were coated with the resorbable BONIT–FBR coating. Three implants were inserted in the mandible and three in the maxilla. Implants were left to heal for 12 weeks in a submerged way and retrieved through segmental osteotomy.

---

* The coating is a proprietary process of DOT GmbH, Rostock, Germany. It is named BONIT® by DOT GmbH, FBR® by Oraltronics GmbH, Bremen, Germany, and μCaP® by Aesculap AG, Tütlingen, Germany.

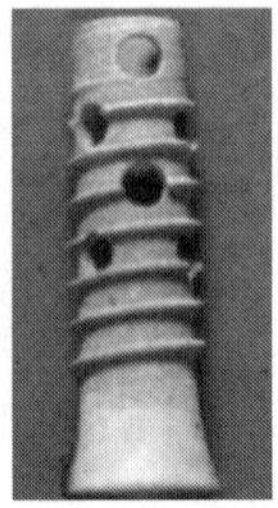

FIGURE 5.1
ITI TPS-coated hollow-screw covered by BONIT–FBR coating. The implant neck was also coated in this experiment.

5.2.1.3 Histology Processing and Histomorphometric Analysis

After retrieval, the blocks were washed in a saline solution and immediately fixed in 10% formalin and processed for histology. They were dehydrated in an ascending series of alcohol rinses and embedded in glycol-methacrylate resin (Technovit 7200 VLC, Kulzer, Germany). After polymerization, the specimens were sectioned mesiodistally at about 150 μm and then ground to 30 to 50 μm. They were stained with toluidine blue and basic fuchsin. Histomorphometry was performed under a light microscope coupled with a color image analyzing system (Samba, Allocate, France).

5.2.1.4 Results

Healing was uneventful and all implants osseointegrated. Examination with the naked eye indicated the coating at the neck level seemed to have vanished from all implants. In the mandible, the most distal implant had to be removed for a surgical reason; a reverse torque of 160 Ncm was required to unscrew it. In the mandible, cortical bone apposition was found; Histomorphometry was not performed because of the small number of implants. In the maxilla, type IV bone with very loose trabeculae was found. Thin trabecules of bone were found along the implant surface (Figure 5.2), particularly between the implant threads, leading to 60 ± 3.6% of bone apposition. The coating was completely resorbed, as confirmed via scanning electron microscopy (Figure 5.3).

The internal core of the hollow screw was also covered with similar thin bone trabecules. It is noteworthy that no deleterious bone response was observed similar to that described for resorbing areas of plasma-sprayed HA coatings.[29-35] Macrophages and multinucleated cells were not found at the interface as described for studies of plasma-sprayed HA coatings.[21,28,35]

5.2.2 Second *In Vivo* Study: Testing Efficacy of the Coating

The first pilot study showed that the resorbable coating was completely dissolved in the mandible and the maxilla after 12 weeks of healing, without

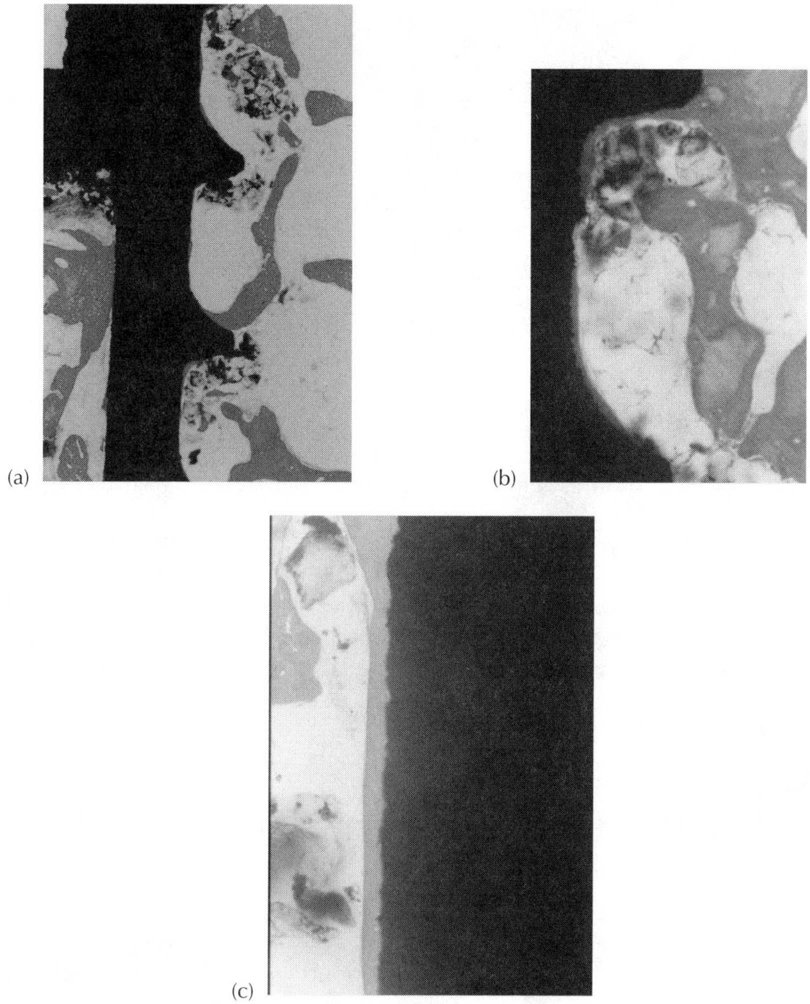

FIGURE 5.2
Bone apposition at the BONIT–FBR coated ITI implants after 12 weeks of healing. (a) Low magnification of the bone–implant interface. Thin trabecules of bone run along the implant surface, particularly between the threads. Note the very loose trabecular bone. Original mag × 5. (b) Higher magnification of the bone–implant interface. At this magnification (original mag × 25), the bone trabecules are clearly identified. No coating remnant was found. Remainder of the polishing paper was encrusted in the embedding material and is a preparation artefact. (c) Bone–implant interface at the hollow part of the implant. Note the continuous thin bone trabecule running along the hollow part that is completely covered by the resorbable coating because of the wet electrochemical deposition method. Original mag × 25.

inducing any unexpected bone reactions. However, demonstration of its efficacy against a bioinert osteophilic surface like the well documented titanium plasma-sprayed surface (TPS) was warranted. In addition, the question of the time required for the entire dissolution of the BONIT–FBR coating was raised. Therefore, evaluation of the coating after a shorter period of 6

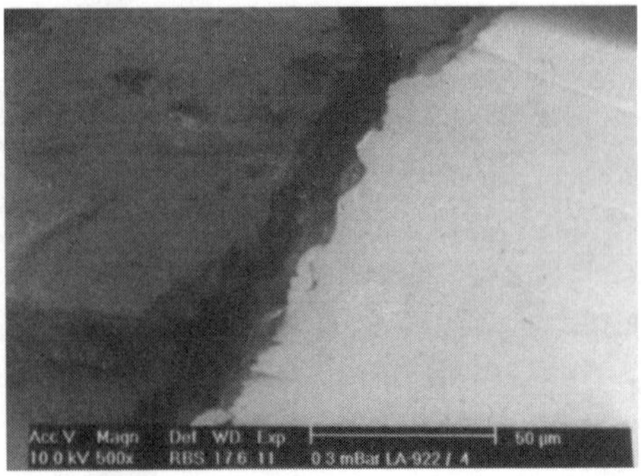

FIGURE 5.3
Scanning electron micrograph of the interface. No coating rests were found at the interface. Bone (dark) on the left side has separated from the implant surface (right) because of shrinkage during preparation. Shrinkage led to cohesive fracture of the bone. Usually in HA-coated implants, shrinkage leads to fracture at the coating–metal interface. Original mag × 500.

weeks was considered relevant because this duration corresponds to the present practice of reducing healing periods in implant dentistry.[37-38]

In this second pilot study,[26] two hypotheses were tested: (1) after 6 weeks of healing, the coating would increase the percentage of bone–implant contact (BIC) when compared to control implants and (2) the coating would undergo homogeneous partial resorption.

5.2.2.1 Animal Model

The same Land Race pig model as in the previous study was used.

5.2.2.2 Implants

The two-stage Pitt-Easy Bio-Oss® implant system (Oraltronics GmbH, Bremen, Germany) was used (Figure 5.4). Implants 4.9 mm × 8 mm roughened

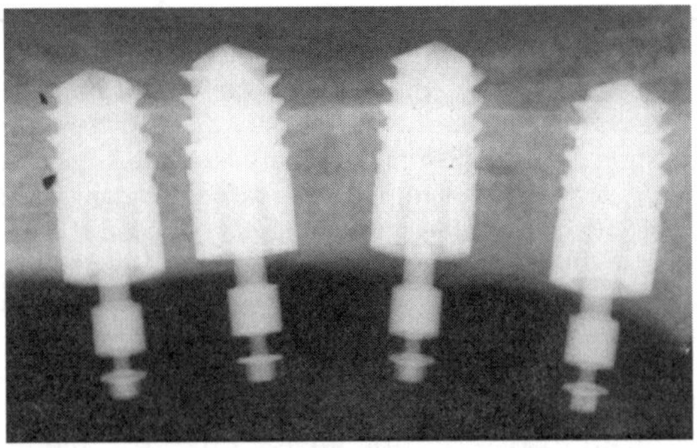

FIGURE 5.4
Radiograph of the FBR-coated Pitt-Easy implants placed for 6 weeks. Control and test implants were inserted alternately.

by titanium plasma spraying (TPS) served as control implants. The TPS surfaces of the Pitt-Easy Bio-Oss test implants were further coated with a 15- to 20-μm BONIT–FBR layer. Sample size was n = 8 for both groups.

The implants were inserted in the maxillae; the test and control implants were inserted alternately, eight implants in each hemimaxilla (four for the test and four for the control groups). On one side, the most distal implant belonged to the test group and was followed by a control implant. On the contralateral side, a control implant was inserted most distally followed by a test implant. Implants were placed flush with bone level and each received a cover screw. They were left to heal in a submerged way for 6 weeks and retrieved by segmental osteotomy.

5.2.2.3 Histology Processing and Histomorphometric Analysis

Immediately after retrieval, each hemimaxilla block section was cut in two pieces to allow better fixation. The blocks were indexed, washed in saline solution, fixed in 10% formalin, and processed for histology. They were dehydrated in an ascending series of alcohol rinses and embedded in glycol-methacrylate resin (Technovit 7200 VLC, Kulzer, Germany). After polymerization, the specimens were sectioned mesiodistally at about 150 μm and then ground to 30 to 50 μm. They were stained with toluidine blue and basic fuchsin. The von Kossa staining was used in some sections to delineate the calcified tissue borders. Histomorphometric measurements were performed by the eye-grid method.

5.2.2.4 Statistical Analysis

To evaluate the histomorphometric results, the Wilcoxon rank test for non-parametrical data was used at the confidence level of $\alpha = 5\%$.

5.2.2.5 Results

All implants osseointegrated within 6 weeks. One implant in the control group showed inflammation and was not included in the analysis. Histomorphometric measurements of direct bone apposition were 73.0 ± 6.2% for the BONIT–FBR group and 49.8 ± 16.4% for the control TPS group (Figure 5.5). The difference in bone apposition was statistically significant ($p = 0.009$) and confirmed the first hypothesis of this study.

Extensive bone apposition was found, primarily between the threads at the spongy level. More bone contacted the internal part of the screw when compared to the TPS surface (Figure 5.6). The bioactive coating had a pronounced osteoconductive effect in the spongy bone (Figure 5.7). In one test implant, bone was lacking around the apical third. Nevertheless, new bone trabecules were found in contact with the implant surface (Figure 5.8). It seems that the BONIT–FBR coating had the ability to conduct bone apposition since it was replaced by bone.

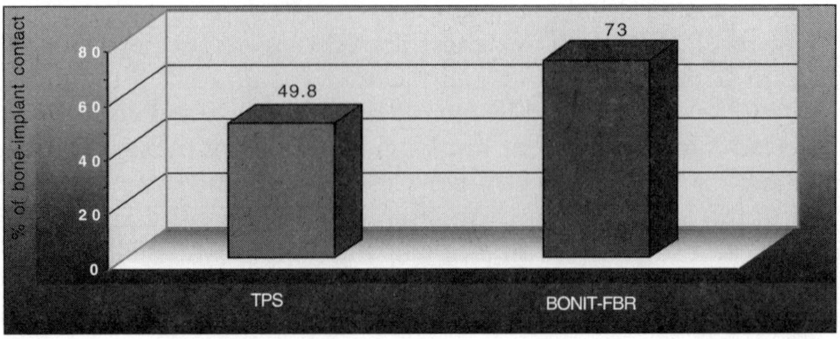

FIGURE 5.5
BICs at the TPS control implants and the BONIT–FBR coated implants after 6 weeks of implantation.

The bioactive BONIT–FBR layer was fully resorbed. In two sections only, minute spots with the rest of the coating were found, indicating a resorption rate of >99%. Macrophages or multinuclear cells around the coated implants were not observed at the interface or at a distance. At the circumscribed coating remnant, direct bone apposition was found. In one spot, bone was growing inside the coating at the expense of the coating (Figure 5.9). These results disprove the second hypothesis that a partial homogeneous dissolution occurred after 6 weeks of healing.

5.2.3 Third *In Vivo* Study: Testing Efficacy of the Coating

Evaluation of the first two pilot studies showed that the bioactive coating was completely resorbed within a 6- to 12-week period. The coating proved safe and bioactive when compared to an osteophilic TPS bioinert surface. Since this resorbing coating was aimed at replacing plasma-sprayed HA coatings, testing was warranted to verify whether tolerance to micromotion under immediate loading conditions was at least as good for the BONIT–FBR coating as for plasma-sprayed HA coatings.

5.2.3.1 Animal Model

The pig model described above did not suit the purpose of an immediate loading study because pigs are not amenable to easy and regular hygiene programs. Therefore, the beagle dog model was used as in a previous immediate loading study involving the mandible.[25,26] Three male beagles were selected for this immediate loading study.[23]

5.2.3.2 Implants

ITI TPS-coated implants 4.1 mm × 6 mm (Figure 5.10) were used (Straumann AG, Waldenburg, Switzerland). Implants were divided into a test group and

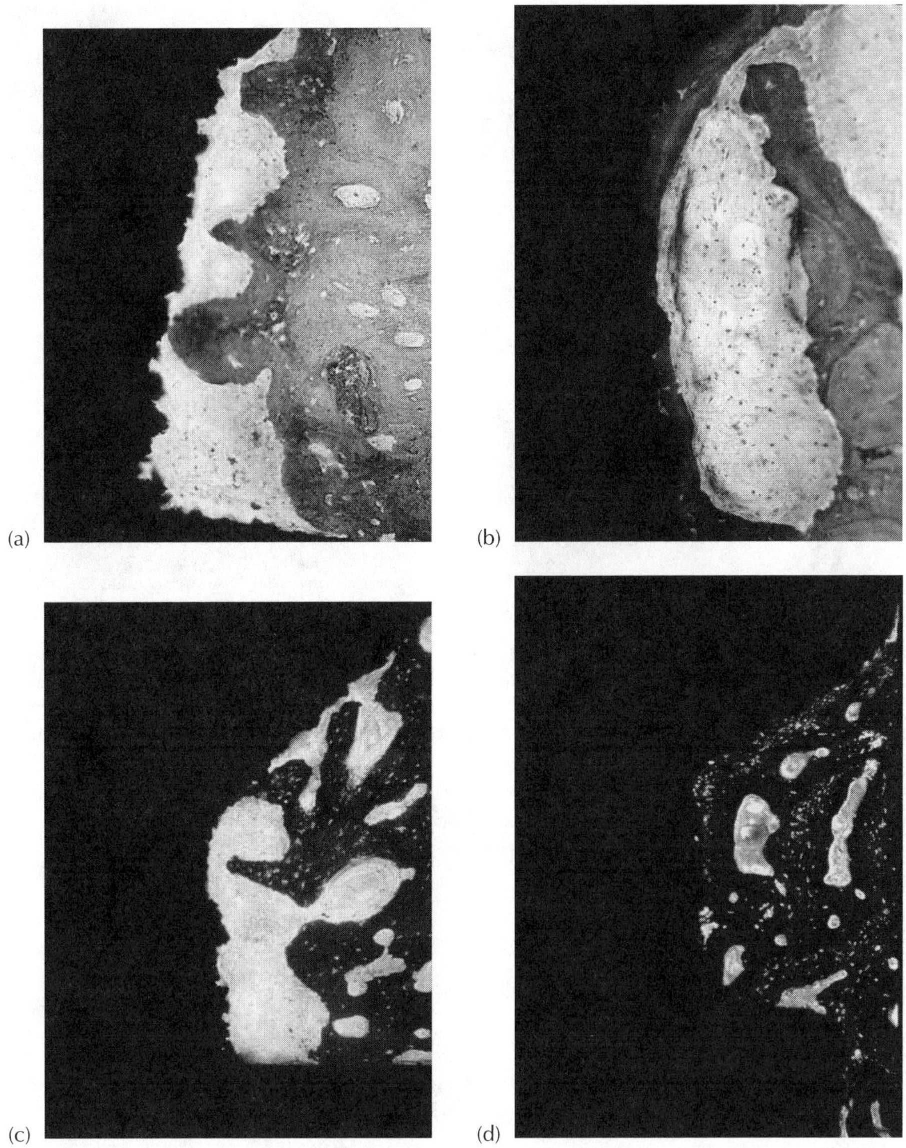

FIGURE 5.6
Bone–implant interface. (a) Interface at TPS-coated control implants. Bone growth is centripetal in the direction of the implant surface. Toluidine blue staining. (b) Interface at BONIT-FBR-coated test implants. (*Source (a) and (b):* Zeggel, P., *Int. Mag. Oral Implantology*, 1, 52–57, 2000. With permission.) Note the good bone coverage of the implant surface; bone growth is centrifugal and centripetal, providing two mineralization fronts. Toluidine blue staining. (c) Interface at TPS-coated control implant. Bone growth contacts the implant surface. Von Kossa staining. (d) Interface at BONIT-FBR-coated test implant. Note woven bone filling the core thread level. Von Kossa staining.

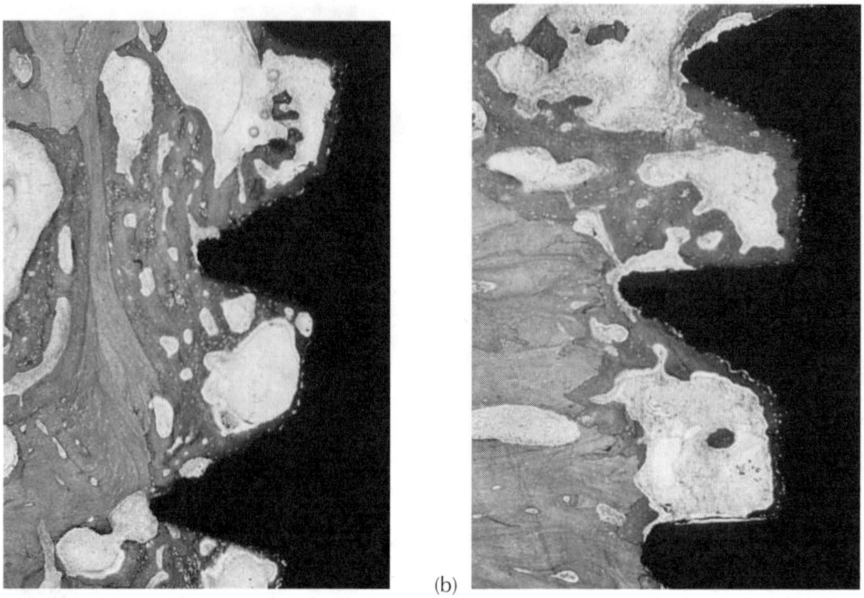

(a) (b)

FIGURE 5.7
Bioconductive effect of BONIT–FBR coating. (a) Overview of bone–implant interface. Bone covers the entire surface even when remote from the pristine bone. New bone is deeper stained than old bone. Toluidine blue staining. (b) Interface view at higher magnification. The same conductive effect is found. New bone is deeper stained than old bone. Toluidine blue staining.

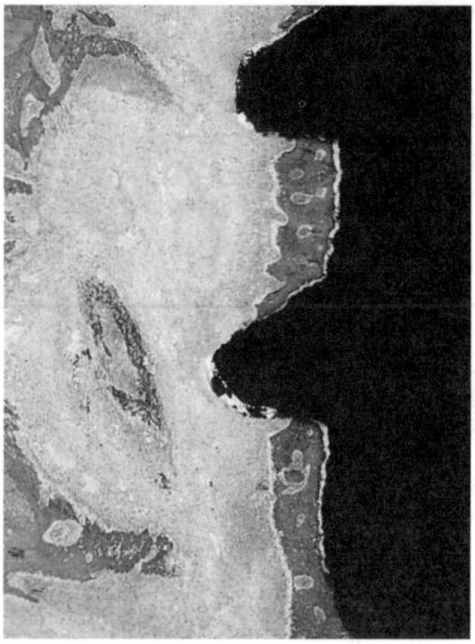

FIGURE 5.8
Bone–implant interface at the apical third of an implant. This BONIT–FBR-coated implant was devoid of surrounding bone at this level. Nonetheless, bone covered the implant surface without bone at the implant vicinity. Toluidine blue staining.

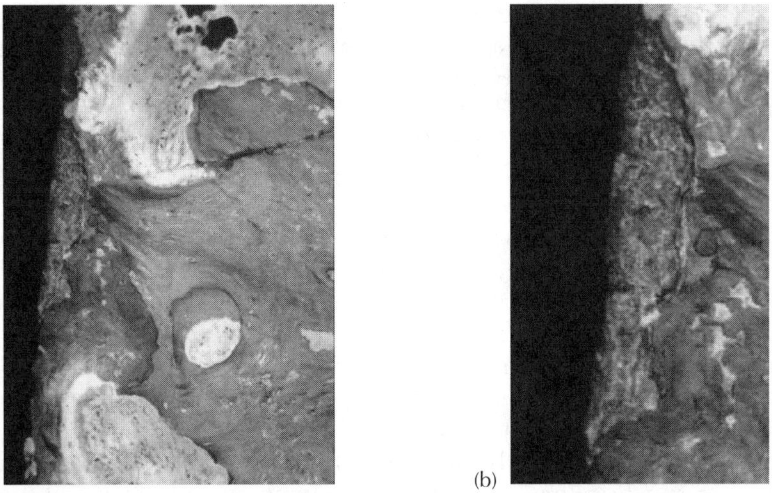

(a) (b)

FIGURE 5.9
Spot with remnant coating. (a) A minute spot was found with a coating rest. Note that new bone is in contact with the coating; the old bone (less stained) is at a distance. Toluidine blue–von Kossa staining. (b) Higher magnification of the remnant coating. In the middle of the coating, bone (stained in brown) is growing at the expense of the coating. Toluidine blue–von Kossa staining.

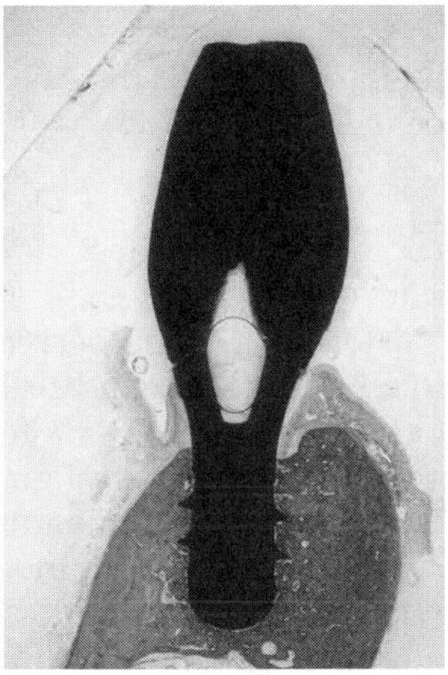

FIGURE 5.10
Overview of a BONIT–FBR coated implant immediately loaded for 7 months in the beagle mandible. Note the short implant and high crown/implant ratio (13/6) and type I dense bone quality. Paragon staining. (*Source:* Zeggel, P., *Int. Mag. Oral Implantology,* 1, 52–57, 2000. With permission.)

two control groups (positive and negative). The negative control group was treated with TPS roughened as standard implants. The positive control group was TPS treated and then HA plasma-sprayed (CAM BV, Leiden, Netherlands). The test group was TPS treated and subjected to further coating with a 15- to 20-μm BONIT–FBR layer. Sample size was seven or eight implants.

The test and control implants were inserted alternately in the mandibles. Implants were placed as to avoid any contact with any adjacent tooth or implant. The rough surface was left flush with the bone level. The abutments were screwed in the implants, then preformed metallic crowns 10 mm high were seated on the abutments. Occlusion in the molar area was adapted to achieve slight under-occlusion as recorded with a 0.2-mm paper. After finalization of the occlusion, the crowns were cemented per-operatively and excess cement was removed completely. Finally, the flaps were sutured around all implants. The dogs were fed soft diets during the first week corresponding to soft tissue healing, then hard food was provided. Implants remained in function for 7 months. The animals were euthanized by overdoses of pentothal and the implants were retrieved *en bloc.*

5.2.3.3 Histology Processing and Histomorphometric Analysis

Samples were fixed and processed for histology as previously described. Thin sections were obtained according to the vestibulo-lingual direction. They were stained with toluidine blue and basic fuchsin and histomorphometrical analysis was performed using the eye grid method as previously mentioned.

5.2.3.4 Statistical Analysis

To evaluate the histomorphometric results, the ANOVA pairwise comparison was used at the confidence level of $\alpha = 5\%$.

5.2.3.5 Results

Soft tissue healing was uneventful. During the loading period, one HA-coated implant was lost. Histologically, the peri-implant hard tissues were found to be dense bones in all dogs (Figure 5.10). The BIC was 56.4 ± 10.6% for the TPS-coated control group, 61.0 ± 26.4% for the HA-coated control group, and 64.6 ± 7.6% for the BONIT–FBR test group. These BIC data were not statistically different. No BONIT–FBR remnants were observed. The HA coating was fragmented and particles were found away from the interface, embedded into bone. The deleterious effect at the locally resorbing plasma-sprayed HA coating was found as previously described in the literature.

5.2.4 Results of Human Biopsies Following Immediate Loading Protocol

Based on the results of the above *in vivo* studies, the question remained whether the same dissolution window found in the pig model would be found on human biopsy. In addition, documenting the bone apposition levels for immediately loaded implants was an interesting project. Massei et al.[39] provided answers to both issues.

5.2.4.1 Immediate Loading Model

Patients undergoing implant therapy according to an immediate loading protocol were asked to participate in this study. Each patient was proposed to receive an added implant to be retrieved after 8 to 12 weeks of function. After signing informed consents, the patients joined the study. Massei et al.[39] reported on the first three patients who volunteered for this protocol.

5.2.4.2 Implants

FBR-coated two-stage Pitt-Easy implants 3.25 or 3.75 mm × 8 mm were used (Oraltronics GmbH, Bremen, Germany). Each of three patients (31 to 67 years old) received an added implant in the wise molar tooth region (WHO 38 or 48) loaded 1 to 3 days after implant placement. The implants were retrieved after 8, 10, and 12 weeks of function. The loading protocol involved (1) slight under-occlusion of the acrylic crowns during the first 4 weeks, (2) a punctiform occlusion between the fourth and eighth week gained by adding acrylic material, and (3) full occlusal loading after the eighth week achieved by adding more acrylic material.

5.2.4.3 Histology Processing and Histomorphometric Analysis

The three samples were trephined, fixed, and processed for histology as previously described. The thin sections were stained with toluidine blue and basic fuchsin and histomorphometry was performed as previously described.

5.2.4.4 Results

Healing was uneventful. All three immediately loaded implants were clinically stable and were osseointegrated. BICs varied from 54.4 to 70.1%. The biopsies showed that the bone quality was type II (cortical and normal trabecular bone) and type III (cortical and loose trabecular bone). At the spongy level and particularly between the threads, continuous bone apposition was observed similar to apposition observed for *in vivo* experiments; the coating bioactivity was confirmed. At the 8- and 12-week biopsies, the coating was completely dissolved. The 12-week samples showed mature lamellar bone arranged parallel to the thread surface.

5.2.5 Coating Characterization

The BONIT coating was obtained by electrochemical deposition following a proprietary process (DOT GmbH, Rostock, Germany). Figure 5.11 shows the

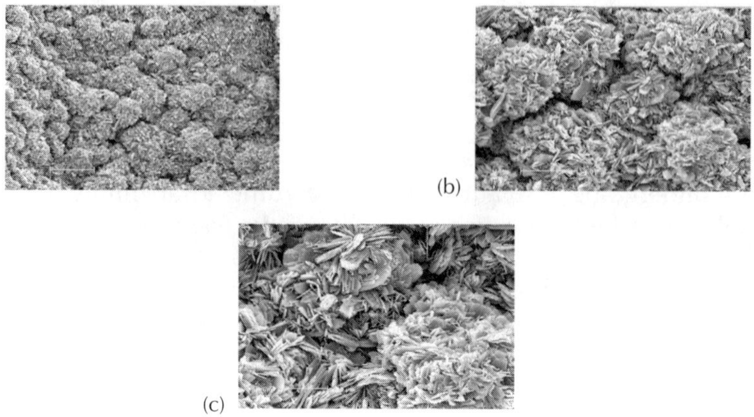

FIGURE 5.11
Scanning electron micrograph of FBR-coated Pitt-Easy implant. (a) General view of the coating (× 200). (b) Higher magnification (× 500) of the coating. Its porosity is seen and can explain the specific capillarity effect observed in Figures 5.12 and 5.13. (c) Detail of coating. The porosity and morphology are seen. The plates are 10 to 20 μm long. If torn off, they would dissolve rapidly in the environment, without requiring the activation of phagocytizing cells.

coating deposited on top of a VTPS coating at various magnifications. This coating consists mainly of brushite; the Ca:P ratio is 1.1 ± 0.1. This means that a limited amount of an added phase, probably an amorphous HA, was codeposited. The brushite plates were 10 to 20 μm long. They started growing perpendicularly to the roughened titanium surface and covered each undercut even at the submicroscopic level because of the wet no-line-of-sight process. This 15- to 20-μm thick coating was highly porous and presented a very high capillarity effect as shown in Figure 5.12.

5.3 Discussion

Plasma-sprayed bioactive coatings are in disrepute in the orthopedic and dental fields due to drawbacks peculiar to the deposition process. In the plasma-spraying method, the starting HA powder undergoes a rapid and dramatic temperature elevation followed by a rapid air quenching. This alters the structure and the solubility properties of the final coating material when compared to the starting powder. It results in an inhomogeneous coating made of a mixture of crystalline and amorphous structures of distinct calcium phases[40,41] and leads to unpredictable dissolution patterns when inserted in bone.[1,10,13,33,42]

Furthermore, the biologic properties of the plasma-sprayed HA coatings may differ dramatically according to coating manufacturer even if they meet the FDA recommendations.[33] Because young patients are treated more fre-

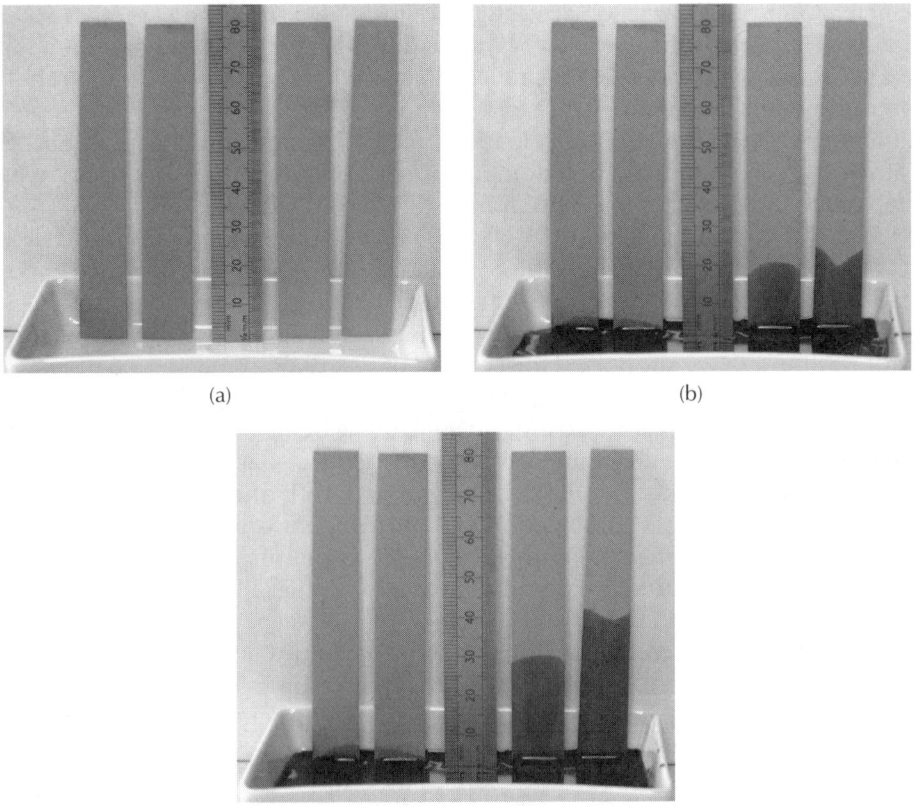

(a) (b) (c)

FIGURE 5.12
Comparative capillarity of the TPS and the BONIT–FBR coatings. (a) Before the start of the experiment, the TPS-coated strips are on the left side of the graduated rule; the TPS-BONIT–FBR-coated strips are on the right side. (b) The capillarity observed after 10 seconds. Note the difference between the TPS- and the BONIT–FBR-coated strips. (c) Capillarity observed after 45 seconds. At the BONIT–FBR coated implants, the colored water was drawn 32 to 40 mm, whereas at the TPS-coated strips, it was drawn only 2 to 3 mm. Between 10 and 45 seconds, the level dramatically increased at the BONIT–FBR-coated strips whereas it did not change at the TPS-coated strips.

quently with orthopedic and dental implants, the life expectancy of a bioactive coating must in fact cover a span of many tens of years. Little is known about the long-term behavior of bioactive coatings. Several authors suggested that *in vivo* loaded conditions alter the adhesion and biologic characteristics of HA plasma-sprayed coatings.[10,13,14] Some post-treatments have been tried to improve their adherence or homogenize the plasma-sprayed coating structures[20,21,43] but their efficiency in long-term weight-bearing or loaded applications has not been proven.

A way to eradicate every concern about the mid- and long-term performance of a bioactive coating would be to use resorbable bioactive materials.

Such materials have been investigated in the past decade.[31,32,44] Maxian et al.[33,34] reported on a poorly crystalline HA plasma-sprayed coating made of 60% crystalline HA that was mostly resorbed within 12 weeks in a rabbit femur model. The coating used by Maxian et al.[31] was tested in a dog experiment involving immediately loaded dental implants in the mandible.[25] However, after 6 months of loading, evidence of only partial resorption was reported; the complete resorption intended was never reached.

Physical vapor deposition (PVD) also has been used to obtain resorbable CaP coatings.[44] Unfortunately, this method produces thin HA coatings in the 0.5- to 5-μm range only. We tried similar coatings 1 μm and 5 μm thick without reaching the achievements of the plasma-sprayed HA coating control.[27] Although we supported the concept of resorbable bioactive coatings,[6,25] we sought thicker resorbable coatings in the 10- to 30-μm range without necessarily using HA as a coating substance. The BONIT–FBR coating mainly made of brushite and obtained by electrochemical deposition represented an alternative to both the plasma-sprayed and PVD thin HA coatings. The BONIT–FBR coating is produced by a room temperature process that allows for a complete coverage of complex shapes and porous surfaces and should permit additional stuffing with other active molecules like antibiotics[45] and/or growth factors.[46]

Brushite belongs to the calcium phosphate family and is a precursor of HA.[47,48] It was observed in the early external calluses of fractured human long bones[49] using selected area diffraction (SAD) before it was known to be involved in biologic calcifications occurring under acidic conditions.[47,49,50] Wen et al.[49] suggested that the reason greater amounts of brushite were not found during bone healing by x-ray diffraction analysis was because of its rapid transformation into HA. Indeed, in contrast to HA, brushite is more stable at pH <4 and less stable at physiological pH.[47] Cui et al.,[51] using SAD, found for the first time a consistent number of brushite particles in the external periosteal calluses of repaired femoral fractures in children. They speculated that the reason children heal faster might be related to the presence of brushite particles that serve as ion reservoirs for bone matrix mineralization.[49] Subsequently, they argued that the brushite mineral phase should be considered a component in designing implant materials for bone regeneration and repair.[51]

Villareal et al.[52] reported on a specific biologic activity for the brushite phase *in vitro*. They found that albumin absorption on brushite was five times higher than on HA. They also measured for osteoblast cells in culture on pellets, higher protein production, and higher alkaline phosphatase (ALP)-specific activity for brushite when compared to HA. Brushite has been considered an ion reservoir of Ca and PO_4[47,49,53] and this can explain its positive effect on the osteoblastic population and its performance with the BONIT–FBR coating determined by Liefeith et al.[54]

Brushite seems to convert into HA when immersed in various aqueous solutions. According to Kumar et al.,[48] the process seems to start as soon as 6 hours and may be complete at 48 hours. However, Liefeith et al.[54] measured a gradual transformation of the Ca:P ratio of the BONIT coating in a cell culture testing environment. The starting Ca:P ratio was 1.06; after 7 days it increased to 1.40, and reached 1.62 after 14 days of culture.

The biologic activity of brushite in contact with mineralized tissues has been under focus for several years as a bone cement application.[55-58] Brushite-based bone cements were introduced to challenge HA-based bone cements because of their higher dissolution, thus warranting a faster bony substitution. Several *in vivo* studies documented the ability of brushite bone cements to resorb and be replaced by bone.[55-58] Brushite coatings were investigated for orthopedic applications; however, they were converted into HA before *in vivo* testing.[48,61]

A limited number of brushite-coated implants were tested in a rabbit femur model[61] and compared with uncoated porous (bioinert) implants. The bioactive coatings (HA and brushite) induced more bone apposition and higher push-out strength than uncoated implants.

Extrapolation from the present studies to other electrochemically deposited brushite coatings should be undertaken cautiously because the plasma-sprayed process and variation of the deposition parameters (tension, current, time, and electrolyte composition) can play key roles in the coating morphology in terms of grain size, plate size, and porosity, that in turn can greatly affect the solubility and bioreactivity of the coating. Kumar et al.[48] described an electrochemically deposited brushite coating with a surface topography that included volcano-like structures and an amorphous-like phase enriched in potassium. The BONIT–FBR morphology shown in Figure 5.11 is devoid of this typical feature due to H bubbling at the metal–Ca–P interface. This confirms that the electrochemical deposition parameters are distinct. Similarly, the coating obtained by Redepenning et al.[61] was brushite with a Ca:P ratio slightly <1, whereas the BONIT layer was mainly brushite and included an amorphous structure that led to a Ca:P ratio of 1.1 ± 0.1 instead of 1.0.

Because the literature indicates that dissolution of plasma-sprayed HA coatings may impede direct bone apposition,[29-35] the first step was to determine whether a similar feature would be found for the BONIT–FBR coating,[22] because it leads to a massive release of Ca and PO_4 ions into the environment during the healing phase. This feature was not found at 6 weeks,[24] 12 weeks,[22,62] 24 weeks,[62] or 7 months of healing,[23] whether pig, dog, or sheep models were considered. In addition, Massei et al.[39] confirmed the absence of this undesirable feature in three biopsies from human mandibles.

Another consistent discrepancy with plasma-sprayed HA coatings was the absence of cellular reaction to the dissolution process of the resorbable BONIT–FBR coating. Dissolution of plasma-sprayed HA coatings often showed coating removal activity mediated by macrophages and multinucleated cells,[21,28,34,35] including HA particles present within macrophages.[21] Such an activity was not observed at any milestone (3, 6, 8, and 10 weeks and 3, 6, and 7 months) in any animal model (pig, dog, or sheep) or in humans for the BONIT–FBR coating.[22-24,39,62] The reasons for this difference may relate to the distinct dissolution patterns. Plasma-sprayed HA coatings appear to undergo first a physicochemical dissolution of the amorphous phase followed by the release of dense crystalline particles that are less soluble.[63,64] These particles require the activation of phagocytizing cells to clear them from the interface and dissolve them intracellularly. Conversely, considering the structure and morphology of the BONIT–FBR coating, a distinct dissolution pattern may take place. Brushite is more soluble than HA. It dissolves rapidly in elemental ions and does not require the involvement of phagocytizing cells. In case of torn-away particles and particles released from the coating, the thin brushite plates are more prone to dissolution than the dense particles of HA and their removal from the interface would not require the activation of phagocytizing cells.

Based on thermodynamics, brushite is one the most soluble CaP phases[47] and might be considered too soluble to allow bone substitution. It was not clear whether the dissolution kinetics and thickness of the brushite phase were adapted to gain bioactivity properties similar to those of plasma-sprayed HA coatings. The dissolution kinetics measured in an acidic Sörensen glycin solution at 37°C differed from the kinetics of a 50 μm plasma-sprayed HA coating and the 15-μm BONIT coating. Complete dissolution of the BONIT–FBR coating was obtained after 90 seconds while 240 minutes were required to dissolve the HA coating.[65] Thin radio-frequency deposited amorphous HA coatings of 0.5 μm were found to be effective when compared to a machined titanium control surface.[44] However, PVD-deposited 1-μm and 5-μm thick HA coatings could not compare with the HA plasma-sprayed coatings in an immediate loading model in dogs.[25] The BIC at the plasma-sprayed HA coating was 67.4 ± 8.3% — statistically different from the 47.5 ± 10.3% and 49.0 ± 5.9%, respectively, obtained for the 1-μm and 5-μm HA coatings.[25] Therefore, it seems that the release of a minimal number of Ca and PO_4 ions is necessary before initiation of the cascade of events that leads to bioactivity equivalent to that obtained for plasma-sprayed HA coatings.

In cell culture with human fetal osteoblasts (hFOB), the BONIT–FBR coating showed a bioactive effect when compared to a bioinert TPS surface; its proliferation rate was higher and the osteoblasts were completely spread.[54] Bioactivity was confirmed *in vivo* in the pig model since the BONIT–FBR coating enhanced the BIC from 49.8 ± 16.4% to 73.0 ± 6.2% (+ 23%). Interestingly, the standard deviation at the bioactive coating was much lower than those observed at the TPS implants. A characteristic finding at the coated implants was the consistent new bone apposition formed between the threads at the spongy bone level in the form of continuous bone trabecules of variable thickness, according to the environing bone quality.

The pristine bone was removed during the drilling process and nonetheless new bone was found as soon as 6 weeks after implant placement. The bioconductive property of the coating, particularly at the between-thread level, was consistently found in the animal model and was further confirmed in all three human biopsies. In one instance, bone was missing around the apical part of an implant; nevertheless trabecules of bone were found at the surfaces of BONIT–FBR-coated implants. The bioactivity pattern of bone growth from the surfaces of coated implants was verified in animal and human samples.

Weber et al.[25] reported a statistically significant difference between HA-coated (67.4 ± 8.3%) and TPS (39.1 ± 9.6%) implants submitted to an immediate loading protocol and left to function for 6 months. In a similar experiment after 7 months, no statistically significant difference was found among the plasma-sprayed HA coating, the BONIT–FBR coating, and the TPS control implants as described.[23] The reason for the distinct results probably lies in the bone quality encountered. In the first study,[25] implants were placed in types II and III bone quality, whereas in the second study, the implants were placed in dense bones of type I.[23] It is well known that the added value of a bioactive coating is maximized in spongy bone,[10,66,67] while in a cortical bone environment, enhanced BIC is not seen.[67,68] Therefore, the use of the BONIT-FBR coating is expected to be most relevant in suboptimal situations involving spongy bone applications, when bone healing stimulation is requested or short healing is a goal.

It should be stressed that although most experimental studies were performed with dental implants, the results might be transposable with good reliability to orthopedic implants, as suggested by Cook et al.[69] who compared femoral and mandibular animal models for the evaluation of HA-coated implants. They concluded that the similarity of the mandibular and femoral transcortical models allowed both types of data to be used by dental or orthopedic implant designers. They added that since similar results were obtained by both methods, the results provided a degree of validation of the results previously reported for each model. In addition, the data obtained with the acetabulum cup model in sheep[62] strengthened this assumption.

The resorption process seems to initiate rapidly. After 17 days in cell culture, the original coating was partially degraded. It was no longer continuous and the remaining coating was only 4 to 5 μm thick as compared to the initial 15 to 20 μm. Reprecipitated round particles were seen on the surface displaying a Ca:P ratio of 1.62, including elements from the medium (Na, K, and S).

After 28 days of culture, the original bioactive coating completely disappeared.[54] *In vivo*, a coated acetabulum cup retrieved after 3 weeks from a sheep showed that the coating was partially degraded; it was able to induce bone ingrowth in the deeper layers of the TPS coating.[62] After 6 weeks in the pig maxilla, the coating was over 99% dissolved. Only 2 minute spots were undergoing dissolution; in one spot, bone was seen growing from the middle of the remaining coating as revealed by toluidine blue–von Kossa staining. At later periods, i.e., after 3 months and 7 months, no coating remnants could be found. From these animal data, a dissolution window of 6 to 12 weeks was assessed.[24] Human biopsies obtained from immediately loaded commercially available FBR-coated implants (Oraltronics GmbH, Bremen, Germany) after 8, 10, and 12 weeks[39] confirmed the validity of this resorption window. They also confirmed the remarkable bone conduction between the implant threads observed earlier in the pig model.[22,24] More generally, these histological data also suggest that once osseointegration is achieved, the bioactive coating is no longer required.

It should be stressed that the use of fully resorbable coatings renders irrelevant the issue of addressing the interfacial adherence of the coating on its substrate in the long-term[70] or under fatigue tests as performed for plasma-spayed coatings.[71] An important characteristic of resorbable coating is the ability to withstand the insertion phase under shear or pressure. Zeggel[72] reported a shear resistance of 11 to 25.3 MPa with the stud-pull test. The result is in the same range as those for plasma-sprayed HA coatings. Interestingly, if the coating would tear off locally, e.g., at the tips of threads during insertion, the morphology of the coating (entangled plates, not dense particles as with plasma-sprayed coating) and the wet electrochemical deposition method (no line-of-sight; plates growing directly from the surface even at the submicronic level) would still allow the coating to remain, at least in the valleys of the TPS-coated tips, and provide a certain level of bioactivity.

In addition, in the worst case scenario, i.e., when very tight insertion is performed in dense bone, only the coatings at the tips of the threads would tear off, leaving most of the implant surface still coated, especially at the between-thread level. It is important to accelerate the apposition of new bone at the core thread level because the drilling sequence removes pristine bone and leaves a gap to be filled between the adjacent bone and the implant surface. Accelerated new bone formation at this level entails the earliest move from primary stability, obtained by the macrogeometry of the threads and usually provided by the tips of the threads, to secondary stability achieved by micromechanical anchorage (long-lasting osseointegration) between the titanium-textured surface (e.g., TPS) and the newly formed bone along the majority of the implant surface.

A pronounced capillarity effect was found for the BONIT–FBR coating. Figure 5.12 shows the striking difference in capillarity between two TPS and two BONIT–FBR coated titanium strips. The colored water was drawn 30 to 42 mm in height at the BONIT–FBR strips, whereas TPS wettability was limited to a maximum of 2 to 3 mm. In the clinic, an unprecedented capillarity effect with blood (Figure 5.13) was also described by several authors.[73-75] This was probably due to the porosity exhibited by this coating as shown in Figure 5.11.

This property might explain the remarkable bone conduction found in the animal and human samples, especially at sites remote from the original old bone or placed in loose trabecular bone of type IV. Davies and colleagues[77-78] theorized on the capacity of the bioinert textured Osseotite titanium surface to allow for the attachment of collagen fibers, on its capacity to facilitate migration of osteoblastic cells up to the implant surface, and on its capacity to aggregate platelets and release growth factors at the implant surface. It stands to reason that these properties are even more applicable in the case of this three-dimensional open bioactive structure and they explain the histological findings.

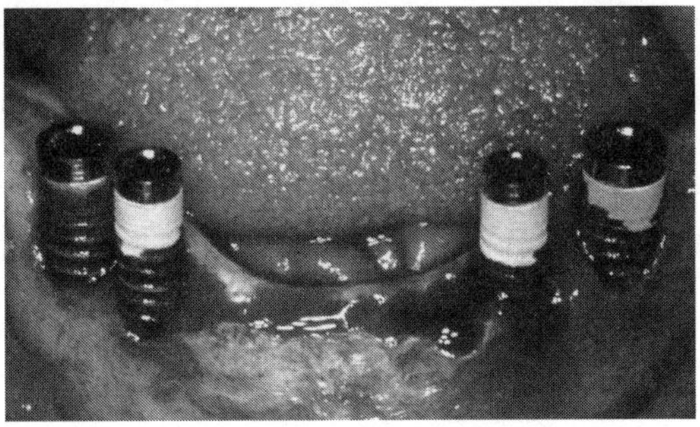

FIGURE 5.13
Blood capillarity observed at four FBR-coated Pitt-Easy implants inserted in the mandible of an edentulous patient. (*Source:* Böttcher, R., *Dent. Implantol. Paradontol.*, 4, 306–312, 2000. With permission.)

To take full advantage of this resorbable coating, blood should be first come in contact with the coating and be absorbed in depth via the capillarity effect. Contact with a cooling solution or saliva should be therefore avoided.[24,73,76] Clinically, more attention should be dedicated during surgery to avoid the absorption of saliva or any fluids other than blood. This explains why insertion of FBR-coated implants should be performed without the aid of a cooling solution. Malchiodi et al.,[76] in an immediate loading prospective clinical study on FBR-coated implants, reported eight failures during the first 2 months. Two could be attributed to biomechanical reasons while the remaining six related to inflammation complications. During the learning curves of the 11 centers involved in this clinical trial, it is possible that insufficient attention was paid to bringing the coating first in contact with blood and avoiding the absorption of other fluids.

Clinical studies with the FBR-coated Pitt-Easy dental implants are ongoing. The first results confirmed that halving the standard healing period in the mandible (6 to 8 weeks instead of 3 to 4 months) and in the maxilla (10 to 14 weeks instead of 24 to 32 weeks) was highly predictable. A 2-year life-table analysis based on 159 implants inserted in 56 patients showed a cumulative success rate of 98.11%.[73] Similarly, an immediate loading study involving 156 implants mostly (73.1%) placed in the posterior regions to support short-span bridges in 62 patients is in progress. Malchiodi et al.[76] reported on eight failed implants of 156 after at least 6 months of follow-up, corresponding to a cumulative success rate of 94.87% despite the demanding mechanical conditions and the learning curves of the practitioners with the various immediate loading indications and the FBR coating.

Glauser et al.[73] reported a noteworthy cumulative success rate of 85.8% for immediately loaded machined Brånemark MK IV implants for similar indications. Eighteen of 127 implants (14.2%) were lost in 10 patients of 41 (24.4%). In the maxilla, the cumulative success rate was 80.3%; in the mandible, the rate was 94.1%. The immediately loaded FBR-coated Pitt-Easy implants performed better. Only eight of 156 implants (5.1%) were lost in six of 62 patients (9.7%). In addition, only two of 82 implants (2.4%) failed in the maxilla, providing a better prognosis than implants in the mandible.

Furthermore, the results from 11 separate centers with various degrees of experience with immediate loading protocols involved in the FBR-coated implants clinical trial compared well with results from a single experienced center.[79] This makes the results of the immediate loading study with FBR-coated implants promising in terms of enhancing the predictability of immediate loading protocols by means of this fully resorbable bioactive coating.

In conclusion, the above *in vivo* and human histologic data are well correlated. They indicate that the BONIT–FBR coating is bioactive, osteoconductive, and resorbable within 3 months. The data suggest that bioactive coatings do not have to remain after osseointegration is achieved. The use of second generation members of this coating family is expected to be most relevant in the short term, particularly for spongy bone applications where bone healing stimulation is desirable. Implementing this coating on dental implants allowed a predictable decrease of the duration of implant therapy and enhanced the predictability of immediate loading protocols. The fully resorbable second generation coating should be able to replace the first generation of plasma-sprayed HA coatings to achieve an enhanced bone response.

Further studies are warranted to confirm these histological and clinical results and to gain a better understanding of the dissolution and substitution processes of this fully resorbable bioactive coating.

References

1. Buser, D. et al., Influence of surface characteristics on bone integration of titanium implants: a histomorphometric study in miniature pigs, *J. Biomed. Mater. Res.*, 25, 889, 1991.
2. Godfredsen, K. et al., Anchorage of TiO_2-blasted, HA-coated and machined implants: an experimental study with rabbits, *J. Biomed. Mater. Res.*, 29, 1223, 1995.
3. Vercaigne, S. et al., Bone healing capacity of titanium plasma-sprayed and hydroxylapatite-coated oral implants, *Clin. Oral Implants Res.*, 9, 261, 1998.
4. Larsson, C. et al., The titanium-bone interface *in vivo*, in *Titanium in Medicine*, Brunette, S.M. et al., Eds., Springer, Berlin, 2001, p. 587.
5. Wong, M. et al., Effect of surface topology on the osseointegration of implant materials in trabecular bone, *J. Biomed. Mater. Res.*, 29, 1567, 1995.
6. Szmukler-Moncler, S., Reingewirtz, Y., and Weber, H.P., Bone response to early loading: the effect of surface state, in *Biological Mechanisms of Tooth Movement and Craniofacial Adaptation*, Davidovitch, Z. and Norton, L.A., Eds., Harvard Society for the Advancement of Orthodontics, Boston, 1996, p. 611.
7. Søballe, K. et al., The effects of osteoporosis, bone deficiency, bone grafting and micromotion on fixation of porous-coated hydroxyapatite-coated implants, in *Hydroxyapatite Coatings in Orthopaedic Surgery*, Geesink, R.G.T. and Manley, M.T, Eds., Raven Press, New York, 1993, p. 107.

8. Johnson, B.W., HA-coated dental implants: long term consequences, *Calif. Dent. Assoc. J.,30,* 33, 1992.
9. Wheeler, S.L., Eight-year clinical retrospective study of titanium plasma-sprayed and hydroxyapatite-coated cylinder implants, *Int. J. Oral Maxillofac. Implants,* 11, 340, 1996.
10. Caullier, H. et al., Histological and histomorphometrical evaluation of the application of screw designed calcium phosphate (Ca-P)-coated implants in the cancellous maxillary bone of the goat, *J. Biomed. Mater. Res.,* 35, 19, 1997.
11. Ong, J.L. and Chan, D.C., Hydroxyapatites and their use as coatings in dental implants: a review, *Crit. Rev. Biomed. Eng.,* 28, 667, 2000.
12. Liao, H., Fartash, B., and Li, J., Stability of HA-coatings on titanium oral implants (IMZ): Two retrieved cases, *Clin. Oral Implants Res.,* 8, 68, 1997.
13. Rohrer, M.D. et al., Postmortem histologic evaluation of mandibular titanium and maxillary HA-coated implants from one patient, *Int. J. Oral Maxillofac. Implants,* 14, 579, 1999.
14. Kangasniemi, I.M.O. et al., *In vitro* testing of fluoroapatite and HA plasma-sprayed coatings, *J. Biomed. Mater. Res.,* 28, 563, 1994
15. Dhert, W.J.A. et al., A histological and histomorphometrical investigation of fluoroapatite, magnesium whitlockite and hydroxyapatite plasma-sprayed coatings in goats, *J. Biomed. Mater. Res.,* 27, 127, 1993.
16. Bauer, T.W., Severe osteolysis after third-body wear due to HA particles from acetabular cup coating, *J. Joint Bone Surg., Br.,* 80, 745, 1998.
17. Iamoni, F. et al., Histomorphometric analysis of a half-hydroxyapatite-coated implant in humans: a pilot study, *Int. J. Oral Maxillofacial Implants,* 14, 729, 1999.
18. Golec, T.S. and Krauser, J.T., Long-term perspective studies on hydroxyapatite- coated endosteal and subperiosteal implants, *Dent. Clin. N. Amer.,* 36, 39, 1992.
19. Bloebaum, R.D. etpal., Analysis of particles in acetabular components from patients with osteolysis, *Clin. Orthopaed.,* 338, 109, 1997.
20. Burgess, A.V. et al., Highly crystalline MP-1 hydroxyapatite coating. I: *In vitro* characterization and comparison to other plasma-sprayed hydroxyapatite coatings, *Clin. Oral Implants Res.,* 10, 245, 1999.
21. Burgess, A.V. et al., Highly crystalline MP-1 hydroxyapatite coating. II: *In vivo* performance on endosseous root implants in dogs, *Clin. Oral Implants Res.,* 10, 245, 1999b.
22. Szmukler-Moncler, S. et al., Evaluation of a soluble calcium phosphate coating obtained by electrochemical deposition: a pilot study in the pig maxillae, in *Biological Mechanisms of Tooth Eruption, Reabsorption and Implant Replacement,* Davidovitch, Z. and Mah, J., Eds., Harvard Society for the Advancement of Orthodontics, Boston, 1998, p. 481.
23. Szmukler-Moncler, S. et al., Immediate loading of single crowns retained by short implants: a histologic study with various surfaces in the canine mandible, *Clin. Oral Implants Res.,* 11, 373, 2000.
24. Szmukler-Moncler, S. et al., Evaluation of BONIT,® a fully resorbable calcium phosphate (CaP) coating obtained by electrochemical deposition, after 6 weeks of healing: a pilot study in the pig maxillae, in *Key Engineering Materials,* Trans Tech Publications, Zurich, 2001, 192-195, 395.
25. Weber, H.P. et al., Clinical and histomorphometric analysis of osseointegration of immediately loaded freestanding implants in dogs, *Clin. Oral Implants. Res.,* 8, 434, 1997.

26. Corso, M. et al., Clinical and radiographic evaluation of early loaded free-standing dental implants with various coatings in beagle dogs, *J. Prosth. Dent.*, 82, 428, 1999.
27. Klein, C.P.A.T. et al., Plasma-sprayed coatings of TTCP, HA, α-TCP on titanium alloys: an interface study, *J. Biomed. Mater. Res.*, 25, 53, 1991.
28. Klein, C.P.A.T. et al., A new saw technique improves preparation of bone sections for light and electron microscopy, *J. Appl. Biomater.*, 5, 369, 1994.
29. Klein, C.P.A.T. et al., Calcium phosphate plasma-sprayed coatings and their stability: an *in vivo* study, *J. Biomed. Mater. Res.*, 28, 909, 1994.
30. Gottlander, M. and Albrektsson, T., Histomorphometric studies of hydroxyapatite-coated and uncoated CP titanium threaded implants in bone, *Int. J. Oral Maxillofac. Implants*, 6, 399, 1991.
31. Maxian, S.H., Zawadski, J.P., and Dunn, M.G., Mechanical and histological evaluation of amorphous calcium phosphate and poorly crystallized hydroxyapatite coatings on titanium implants, *J. Biomed. Mater. Res.*, 27, 717, 1993.
32. Maxian, S.H., Zawadski, J.P., and Dunn, M.G., Effect of Ca/P coating resorption and surgical fit on the bone/implant interface, *J. Biomed. Mater. Res.*, 28, 1311, 1994.
33. Dalton, J.E. and Cook, S.D., *In vivo* mechanical and histological characteristics of HA-coated implants vary with coating vendor, *J. Biomed. Mater. Res.*, 29, 239, 1995.
34. Gottlander, M., Johansson, C., and Albrektsson, T., Short- and long-term animal studies with a plasma-sprayed calcium phosphate-coated implant, *Clin. Oral Implants Res.*, 8, 345, 1997.
35. Karabuda, C. et al., Histologic and histomorphometric comparison of immediately placed HA-coated and titanium plasma-sprayed implants: a pilot study in dogs, *Int. J. Oral Maxillofac. Implants*, 14, 510, 1999.
36. Perrin, D. et al., Bone response to alteration of surface topography and surface composition of sandblasted and acid etched (SLA) implants, *Clin. Oral Implant Res.*, 13, 465, 2002.
37. Szmukler-Moncler, S. et al., Timing of loading and effect of micro-motion on bone-implant interface: a review of experimental literature, *J. Biomed. Mater. Res. Appl. Biomater.*, 43, 192, 1998.
38. Szmukler-Moncler, S. et al., Considerations preliminary to the application of early and immediate loading protocols in implant dentistry, *Clin. Oral Implants Res.*, 12, 12, 2000.
39. Massei, G. et al., Immediately-loaded FBR-coated Pitt-Easy Bio-Oss implants: a histologic evaluation in 3 patients after 8–12 weeks of function, *Clin. Oral Implants Res.*, 12, 409, 2001.
40. Weng, J. et al., Further studies on the plasma-sprayed amorphous phase in hydroxyapatite coatings and its desamorphisation, *Biomaterials*, 14, 578, 1993.
41. Cheang, P. and Khor, K.A., Addressing processing problems associated with plasma spraying of hydroxyapatite, *Biomaterials*, 17, 537, 1996.
42. Cune, M. etpal., Clinical retrospective evaluation of FA/HA coated (Biocomp) dental implants: results after 1 year, *Clin. Oral Implants Res.*, 7, 345, 1996.
43. Filliagi, M.J., Pilliar, R.M., and Coombs, N.A., Post-plasma-spraying heat treatment of the HA coating/Ti-6Al-4V implant system, *J. Biomed. Mater. Res.*, 27, 191, 1993.
44, Cooley, D.R. et al., The advantages of coated titanium implants prepared by radio-frequency sputtering from hydroxyapatite, *J. Prosth. Dent.*, 67, 93, 1992.

45. Gautier, H., Daculsi, G., and Merle, C., Association of vancomycin and calcium phosphate by dynamic compaction: *inpvitro* characterization and microbiological activity, *Biomaterials*, 22, 2481, 2001.
46. Gauthier, O. et al., Human growth hormone locally released in bone sites by calcium-phosphate biomaterials stimulate ceramic bone substitution without systemic effects: a rabbit study, *J. Bone Mineral Res.*, 13, 739, 1998.
47. Johnsson, M.S. and Nancollas, G.H., The role of brushite and octacalcium phosphate in apatite formation, *Crit. Rev. Oral Biol. Med.*, 3, 61, 1992.
48. Kumar, M., Darathy, H., and Riley, C., Electrodeposition of brushite coatings and their transformation to hydroxyapatite in aqueous solutions, *J. Biomed. Mater. Res.*, 45, 302, 1999.
49. Wen, H.B. et al., Microstructural investigation of the early external callus after diaphyseal fractures of human long bones, *J. Struct. Biol.*, 114, 115, 1995.
50. Hesse, A. and Heimbach, D., Causes of phosphate stone formation and the importance of methalaxis by urinary acidification: a review, *World J. Urol.*, 17, 308, 1999.
51. Cui, F.Z. et al., Microstructure of external periosteal callus of repaired femoral fractures in children, *J. Struct. Biol.*, 117, 204, 1996.
52. Villareal, D.R., Sogal, A., and Ong, J.L., Protein adsorption and osteoblast response to different calcium phosphate surfaces, *J. Oral Implantol.*, 24, 67, 1998.
53. Roufosse, A.H. et al., Identification of brushite in newly deposited bone mineral from embryonic chicken, *J. Ultrastruct.*, 68, 235, 1979.
54. Liefheith, K. et al., Electrochemical deposited CaP coating on TPS substrates. *Proc. 2nd Int. Tissue Culture Meeting*, Davos, Switzerland, June 2000.
55. Mirtchi, A., Lemaitre, J., and Terao, N., Calcium phosphate cements: study of α-tricalcium phosphate-monocalcium phosphate system, *Biomaterials*, 10, 475, 1989.
56. Muntig, E., Mirtschi, A., and Lemaitre, J., Bone repair of defects filled with a phospho-calcic hydraulic cement: an *in vivo* study, *J. Mater. Sci. Biomater. Med.*, 4, 337, 1993.
57. Bohner, M., Calcium orthophosphate in medicine: from ceramics to calcium phosphate cements, *Injury*, 31, 37, 2000.
58. Frayssinet, P. et al., Short-term implantation effects of DCDP-based calcium phosphate cement, *Biomaterials*, 19, 971, 1998.
59. Constantz, B.R. et al., Histological, chemical, and crystallographic analysis of four calcium phosphate cements in different rabbit osseous sites, *J. Biomed. Mater. Res.*, 43, 451, 1998.
60. Redepenning, J. and McIsaac, J.P., Electrocrystallisation of brushite coatings on prosthetic alloys, *Chem. Mater. Commun.*, 2, 625, 1990.
61. Redepenning, J. et al., Characterization of electrolytically prepared brushite and hydroxyapatite on orthopaedic implants, *J. Biomed. Mater. Res.*, 30, 287, 1996.
62. Schreiner, U., Evers, J., and Scheller, G., Der Effekt einer löslichen Calcium-phosphat-Beschichtung auf die Osteointegration einer Hüftpfanne. Ergebnisse eines Schaafs-Modells, *Zeit. Orthopäd.*, S160, 139, 2001.
63. Clemens, J.A.M. et al., Healing of gaps around calcium phosphate-coated implants in trabecular bone of the goat, *J. Biomed. Mater. Res.*, 36, 55, 1997.
64. Gross, K.A. et al., *In vitro* changes of HA coatings, *Int. J. Oral Maxillofac. Implants*, 12, 589, 1997.

65. Hildebrand, G., Liefeith, K., and Neumann, H.G., Quantitative Analyse des Degradationverhaltens verschiedener Ca/P Schichten in simulierter Körperflussigkeit, *Medizintechnik Workshop*, Tübingen, Germany, May 1998.
66. Saadoun, A.P. and LeGall, M.L., Clinical results and guidelines on Steri-Oss endosseous implants, *Int. J. Periodontol. Restor. Dent.*, 12, 487, 1992.
67. Janssen, J.A. and van der Waerden, J.P.C.M., Histologic investigation of the biologic behavior of different hydroxyapatite plasma-sprayed coatings in rabbits, *J. Biomed. Mater. Res.* 27, 603, 1993.
68. Oonishi, H. et al., The effect of hydroxyapatite coating on bone growth into porous titanium alloys implants, *J. Bone Joint Surg.*, 71B, 213, 1989.
69. Cook, S.D. et al., A comparison of femoral and mandibular animals models for the evaluation of HA-coated implants, *J. Oral Implantol.*, 18, 359, 1992.
70. Ogiso, M., Yamashita, Y., and Mastumoto, T., The process of physical weakening and dissolution of the HA-coated implant in bone and soft tissue, *J. Dent. Res.*, 77, 1426, 1998.
71. Kummer, F.J. and Jaffe, W.L., Stability of a cyclically loaded hydroxyapatite coating: effect of substrate material, surface preparation, and testing environment, *J. Appl. Biomater.*, 3, 211, 1992.
72. Zeggel, P., Bioactive calcium phosphate coatings for dental implants: a summarizing characterization of BONIT–FBR, *Int. Mag. Oral Implantol.*, 1, 52, 2000.
73. Böttcher, R. et al., Shortened healing periods for FBR-coated Pitt-Easy Bio-Oss implants: preliminary results from a prospective multi-center study in private practices, *Clin. Oral Implants Res.*, 12, 395, 2001.
74. Böttcher, R., Fast Bone Regeneration (FBR®) ein Anwenderbericht, *Dent. Implantol. Parodontol.*, 4, 306, 2000.
75. Semmler, R., Doppelbeschichtung beschleunigt Knochenreaktion, *Implantol. J.*, 5, 22, 2001.
76. Malchiodi, L. et al., Immediate loading of FBR-coated Pitt-Easy Bio-Oss implants: preliminary results from a prospective multi-center study, *Clin. Oral Implants Res.*, 12, 408, 2001.
77. Davies, J.E., Mechanisms of endosseous integration, *Int. J. Prosthodont.*, 11, 391, 1998.
78. Park, J.Y., Gemmel, C.H., and Davies, J.E., Platelet interactions with titanium: modulation of platelet activity by surface topography, *Biomaterials*, 22, 2671, 2001.
79. Glauser, R. et al., Immediate loading of Brånemark implants in all oral regions: preliminary results of a prospective clinical study, *Clin. Oral Implants Res.*, 11, 389, 2000.

Section III

Cell and Tissue Reactions to Biomaterials

6

Improving the Bio-Implant Interface by Controlling Cell Behavior Using Surface Topography

Donald M. Brunette, Ali Khakbaznejad, Masanori Takekawa, Mitsuru Shimonishi, Hiroshi Murakami, Marco Wieland, Babak Chehroudi, Jeannette Glass-Brudzinski, and Marcus Textor

CONTENTS

6.1 Introduction 103
6.2 Strategy in Selecting Potential Experimental Systems 104
6.3 Cell Responses to Topography 105
6.4 Cell Population Density 107
6.5 Role of Extracellular Matrix 108
  6.5.1 High Population Density Cultures 108
  6.5.2 Formulation of Bone Nodules in Culture 110
  6.5.3 Exogenously Added Collagen 110
6.6 Cell Responses to Surfaces Produced by Industrial Processes 113
  6.6.1 Osteoblast Migration on Rough and Machined-Like Surfaces 114
  6.6.2 Resistance of Tissue Equivalent/Ti Interface to Cell-Generated Forces 114
6.7 Cell Selection in an *In Vivo* Model 117
6.8 Conclusions 118
Acknowledgment 118
References 119

6.1 Introduction

Commercially available implant systems vary widely in their surface topographies[1] and manufacturers vigorously promote the benefits of the

0-8493-1474-7/03/$0.00+$1.50

topographies employed on their devices. The question of what constitutes the best topography has not been definitively answered, in part because tests comparing implant systems that differ only in topography are rare. In contrast to differences in clinical opinion on the most desirable surface, there is widespread agreement that topography is an important and powerful modulator of cell behavior and thus an important factor in implant performance.

This review will largely concern itself with titanium surfaces, but it should be noted that topography and chemistry can interact to produce effects that are greater than can be achieved by either factor independently.[2] The advantage of using topography to control cell behavior is that it is a somewhat abiding influence. Unlike some other approaches that influence tissue response such as the use of chemical coatings or release of growth factors that will be present only transiently, topographical features in the range of the size of a cell can exert their influence more or less indefinitely. This chapter deals with issues of design of studies to explore how topography can be modified to improve the bio-implant interface.

6.2 Strategy in Selecting Potential Experimental Systems

The options and tradeoffs in experimental systems faced by the investigator hoping to improve the bio-implant interface are shown in Figure 6.1. Extant choices range from the reductionist approach of molecular biology to the complex clinical situations encountered in true experiments in humans. Between the extremes are approaches of cell and tissue culture and animal models of varying complexity. Associated with the gradient from the reductionist to the clinical approaches are other gradients associated with the strengths and weaknesses of the various approaches.

Most agree that true experiments in humans are required to establish the effectiveness of a surface. While high in relevance, the approach of true experimentation in humans has drawbacks in that such experiments are slow and expensive, and consequently not well suited to screening large numbers of surfaces. Indeed, conclusions based on the Cochrane approach of systematic review have yet to yield unequivocal conclusions about the relative merits of various systems (see Esposito, Chapter 1, this volume). Conversely simple *in vitro* tests are rapid and relatively inexpensive, but can be low in relevance.

The conclusions of such studies are framed often in well-hedged phrases of the form, "surface X influences process Y that may play a role in…." The conventional wisdom in the pharmaceutical industry is that drug discovery can be thought of as a funnel-shaped selective process in which large numbers of compounds are screened with high throughput assays of relatively high specificity, such as effects on drug metabolizing enzyme systems. Candidate drugs that perform poorly on such tests are winnowed away. The best

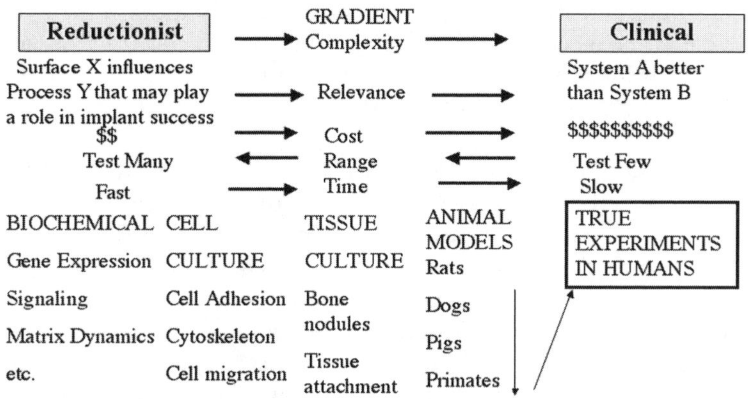

FIGURE 6.1
Outline of experimental strategies for improvement of the bio-implant interface. This chapter argues that high cell population density, tissue equivalent approaches, and simple animal models have received less attention than they merit.

suited few are tested more extensively in animal models and the best of these selected for clinical trials. For optimizing topography, however, there are a number of reasons why the wide funnel approach may not be optimal. Chief among the reasons, in our view, is that the responses of cells to topography are not specific, that is, many diverse responses and interactions are involved so that the response on any single test may not predict overall performance.

6.3 Cell Responses to Topography

Abundant literature on cell responses to surface topography is available. Research on the topic that began with Harrison's observations of cells moving on fibers[3] now spans almost a century. A variety of phenomena have been reported, but four cell behaviors may be of particular relevance to the implant interface:

1. Contact guidance, the phenomenon whereby oriented surface features, such as grooves, direct cell locomotion.[4]
2. Cell selection, the process whereby surface topographic features, such as roughness, lead to the preferential accumulation of certain cell populations. For example, macrophages prefer rough surfaces in contrast to fibroblasts that prefer smooth surfaces.[5]
3. Cell differentiation; in some instances the differentiation of cells is influenced by the topography of the surfaces with which they are in contact. For example, bone nodule production is increased on Ti surfaces with deep grooves.[2]

4. Cell-mediated matrix organization; classically associated with the so-called two-center effect of Weiss,[6] in which cell traction acts on extracellular matrix to produce tracts of cells and fibers between two or more centers of attachment.

If one examines any of these responses in detail, however, it quickly becomes evident that several biochemical or biophysical processes are involved. As a well studied example, consider surfaces containing multiple grooves. In studying the effects of such surfaces and other topographies, the most precise means of producing surfaces has been microfabrication, a set of techniques originally developed for the microelectronics industry and introduced into cell biological studies by Brunette et al.[7,8] A number of laboratories, including those of Brunette, Curtis, and Jansen, are currently active in this area and some of their approaches and findings are reviewed in recent publications.[9-11] For purposes of uniformity of comparison, not to mention convenience, examples will focus on data taken from the Brunette lab where the types of surfaces examined are more or less similar among studies on various cell populations. In brief, microfabricated grooved Ti-coated substrata have been found to affect:

1. Cell adhesion[12]
2. Direction, persistence, and speed of locomotion (fibroblasts) and direction of locomotion (but not speed) of epithelial cells[13]
3. Cytoskeletal organization (fibroblasts,[14] osteoblasts,[15] and epithelium[16])
4. Extracellular matrix organization of collagen[15] and fibronectin[17]
5. Gene expression of fibronectin[18] and matrix metalloproteinase[19]

Thus, if one considers a simple substrate such as a grooved surface, the complex mixtures of processes produced often interact with each other. The interactions are illustrated in Figure 6.2. Grooved surfaces have been found to affect all the processes listed in the diagram. For example, as cells are oriented by the grooves, they in turn orient the extracellular matrix by their tractional forces and migration.[17] The extracellular matrix would also be altered relative to what occurs on smooth surfaces by changes in gene expression and secretion of fibronectin[18] and matrix metalloproteinase.[19]

The existence of a modified matrix might well be expected to modify cell adhesion. As cells multiply, the phenomenon of contact inhibition of movement would also be expected to alter cell orientation and the distribution of cell tractional forces. On occasion, one effect may dominate all the others. For example, a material that cannot support cell attachment would not normally be considered a good candidate for an implant to be integrated with adjacent tissue. The plurality of responses often makes it difficult to predict which of the many possible effects of topography will significantly alter the bio-implant interface and thus implant performance.

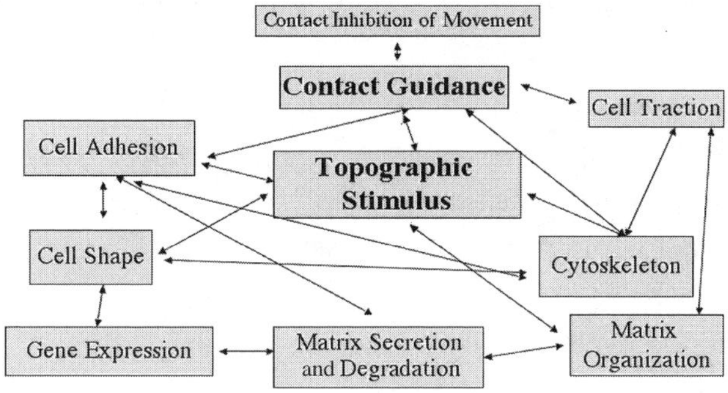

FIGURE 6.2
Processes altered (in comparison to smooth surfaces) when cells are cultured on a grooved Ti surface. The topographic stimulus has many effects; topography is a powerful modulator of cell behavior, but not necessarily a specific one.

In short, although topography is a very powerful modulator of cell behavior, it is not necessarily a very specific one and the effects are complex. Although such microfabricated surfaces used in simple cell culture are very good models for understanding certain processes, such as the control of cell locomotion, they are not necessarily good at predicting what happens when surfaces are implanted *in vivo*. One approach to making the predictions more certain is to alter conditions so that *in vivo* conditions are mimicked more closely and the effects of possible interactions incorporated into the model system. A particularly important difference between simple cell cultures and tissues *in vivo* is cell population density.

6.4 Cell Population Density

Typically, studies in cell culture investigating the effects of surfaces on such processes as cell locomotion are conducted under conditions of low cell population density. The goal of *in vitro* studies is usually to understand the underlying mechanisms of cell behavior, and it is generally preferable to employ low cell population densities because the complications introduced by cell interactions are avoided. However, such interactions may be important in determining implant performance. Cell population density is in fact one of the most important modulators of cell physiology and early tissue culturists were often careful to account for cell population density effects in their interpretations of data. The following examples have been selected to show the wide range of processes influenced by cell population density:

1. Amount and type of collagen produced[20,21]
2. Casein secretion[22]
3. Cell migration (contact inhibition of movement)[23]

4. Cell proliferation (contact inhibition of growth)[24]
5. Sensitivity to drugs[25]
6. "Spontaneous" transformation[26]
7. Estrogen receptors[27]
8. Erythropoietin production[28]
9. Response to epidermal growth factor[29]
10. Na–K pump[30]
11. Vitamin D effects on calcium accumulation[31]
12. Vitamin B_{12} requirements[32]

Since the studies on this list use populations as diverse as tendon fibroblasts, mammary epithelium, and various transformed cell lines, it is clear that cell population density may be expected *a priori* to be an important factor to be controlled in almost any cell culture study. A second conclusion is that cell population density effects may be involved in studies where cell populations interact, as such studies typically take place under conditions of high population density. Finally, if one wishes to predict behavior on implant surfaces at the high population densities found in tissues, it would appear to be useful to test the effects of surface topography on cell behavior under conditions of high cell population density.

6.5 Role of Extracellular Matrix

Many cell biological studies directed at improving our understanding of the bio-implant interface ignore a basic tenet of connective tissue organization: that a tissue comprises cells and extracellular substance. Generally speaking, there are two approaches to studying the role of the extracellular matrix on cell behavioral response to topography. The first is simply allowing the cells to grow to high population densities and fortify the medium, if necessary, with components that promote collagen production. This is the approach often used for *in vitro* studies of bone formation where the culture period is prolonged and ascorbic acid added on a regular basis. The second approach is to add the extracellular matrix exogenously. This approach is used in many of the systems, sometimes called tissue equivalents,[33] in which cells at high population density are incorporated into a collagen gel. Examples of these approaches appear below.

6.5.1 High Population Density Cultures

Figure 6.3 shows the orientation of newborn rat osteoblasts cultured on a 10-μm grooved surface as a function of time in culture up to day 21. Under

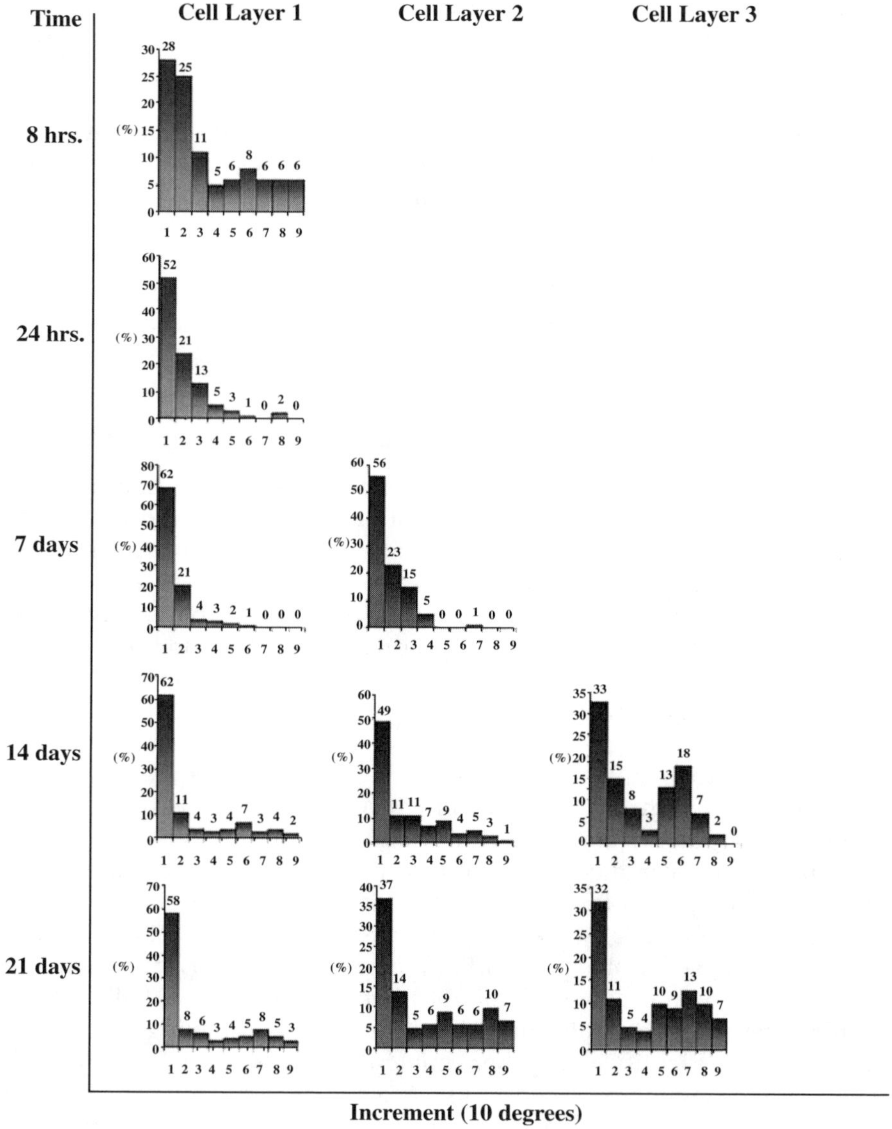

FIGURE 6.3
Orientation of osteoblasts growing on a grooved surface in which the grooves are 10 μm deep and 42 μm wide with a pitch (groove + ridge) of 47 μm. Each plot represents the orientation of cells in a layer; the percent cells in each 10-degree increment is plotted. Initially, a single cell layer is found. On day 7, a second layer is noted. By day 14, a third layer appears. Cells within the first two layers are largely oriented with the grooves. The third cell layer has a significant proportion of cells oriented at an angle (~60 degrees) with the groove.

the conditions of the experiment, the cells formed a monolayer initially; by day 7, a second layer of cells formed on the grooved surface. One week later, a third cell layer could be observed. It is noteworthy that the first two cell layers, both of which can be accommodated within the topographic features of the grooves, show marked alignment with the grooves. The third cell layer is more mixed; a significant proportion of the cells is oriented at an oblique angle to the grooves and the first layers.

This phenomenon of the overlaying of sheets of cells with differing orientations has been called *orthogonal multilayering* by Elsdale and Foley[34] for the special case in which the most common angle of the first layer to the second is 90 degrees. With osteoblasts on this grooved surface, many cells in the third cell layer were oriented at a roughly 60-degree angle to the cells of the lower layers. Thus, the net effect is that the topography of the surface can influence the orientation of cells at some distance from the surface, and this effect would not be seen in low population density cultures.

6.5.2 Formulation of Bone Nodules in Culture

For osteoblasts derived from rat newborn calvaria, the formation of bone-like nodules is promoted by conditions that promote collagen formation (in particular, ascorbic acid addition) and an exogenous source of organic phosphate. Under these conditions, bone formation on grooved surfaces increases with the depth of feature. Moreover, the effect depends on the surface chemistry of the substratum; HA surfaces produce more bone nodules than Ti surfaces and the effects of topography and chemistry are synergistic.[2]

A greater increase in nodule production brought about by HA was observed in the deepest grooves. Because bone *in vivo* can consist of orthogonally layered sheets, it was of interest to examine the orientation of cells in these nodules. On a grooved surface in which the osteoblasts were stained with propidium iodide (PI) and optically sectioned by confocal microscopy (Figure 6.4), cells near the bottom of a forming nodule are oriented with grooves and subsequent layers do not exhibit this tendency.

To obtain more details, some nodules were processed for histology and sectioned. As expected, the cells within the grooves were oriented with the grooves. The uppermost layer of cells, however, formed a capsule-like structure at almost right angles to the cells in the grooves. Staining by the von Kossa method to identify areas where mineralization occurred revealed that the bulk of the staining occurred in the area between the two orthogonally arranged cell layers. It is currently unknown whether cell orientation *per se* influences the process of mineralization or whether other factors affected by position in the multilayer, such as nutrient supply, play a role.

6.5.3 Exogenously Added Collagen

Figure 6.5 shows an example of the second approach, namely examining the influence of exogenously added matrix. The methodology is described by Glass-Brudzinski et al.[35] The interaction of fibroblasts with the matrix was manipulated as follows. In the control group, fibroblasts were added to the grooved Ti substratum and the only collagen in the system was that synthe-

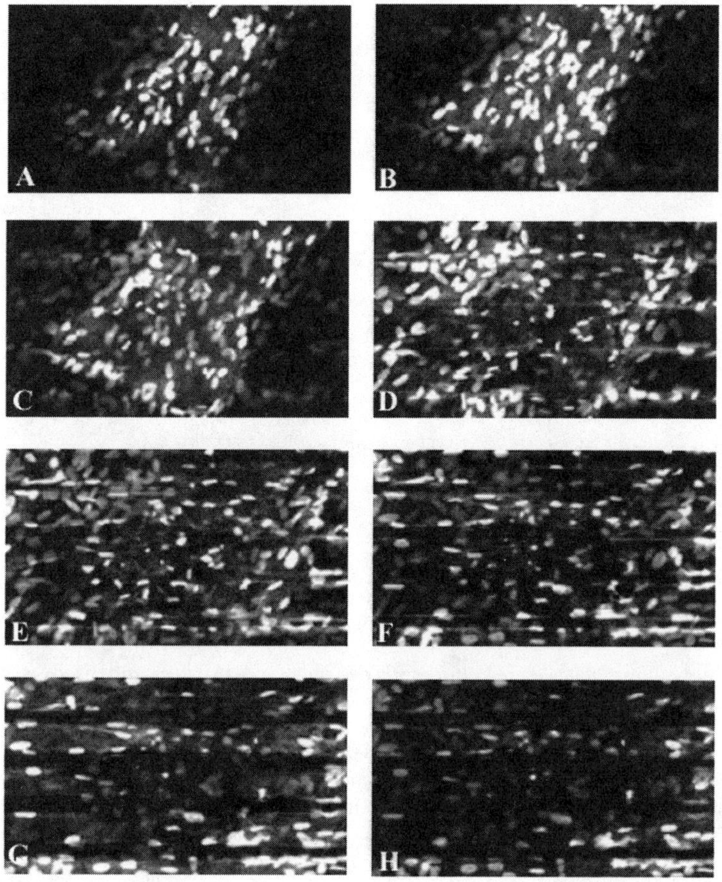

FIGURE 6.4
Optical sections through a forming bone-like nodule in which the nuclei have been stained with propidium iodide. The osteoblasts were cultured on a grooved Ti surface on which the grooves were 10 μm deep and 42 μm wide with a pitch (groove + ridge) of 47 μm. The cells found in the optical sections closest to the grooved surface (G and H) are generally oriented with the grooves, but orientation is progressively lost so that the cells at the upper surface of the nodule are oriented at an angle to the grooves.

sized and secreted by the cells. In the second group, called the cell–gel group, the fibroblasts were cultured on a grooved substratum and the culture was subsequently overlaid with a collagen gel. Finally, in the third group designated the gel group, fibroblasts were mixed with the collagen and medium and the gelling mixture added to the substratum.

At various times, the cultures were fixed and stained with PI and cell orientation assessed by means of confocal microscopy. The confocal microscope enabled optical sections to be produced so that the orientation of cells in different zones at or above the surface could be measured.

In light of the observation of Cooper et al.[36] that the relative binding of fibroblasts to titanium is five to ten times lower than binding to type 1

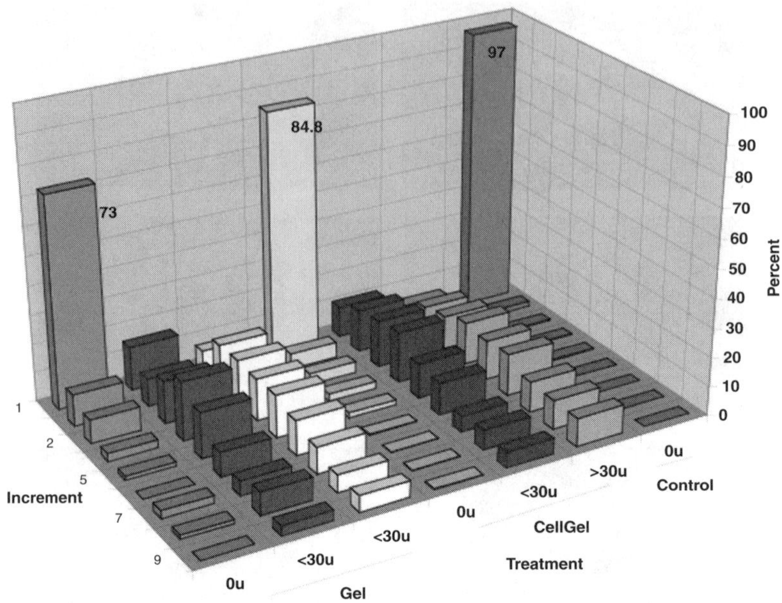

FIGURE 6.5
Human gingival fibroblasts were cultured for two weeks on a surface with grooves 30 μm deep and 35 μm wide with a pitch (groove + ridge) of 175 μm Ti surface under three conditions: (1) control (no collagen gel added), (2) cell–gel in which cells cultured on the surface were overlaid with a collagen gel, and (3) cells were added to the gel before placement on the Ti surface. Cells were subsequently stained with propidium iodide and optical sections were taken at the level of the surface (0 μm), less than 30 μm above the surface, and greater than 30 μm above the surface. The distribution of orientation of cells (expressed as percent of cells) is given for each of the 10-degree increments between 0 and 90 degrees. Cells leave the surface for the gel under the cell-gel condition, but conversely leave the gel for the Ti surface (gel condition). Orientation with the grooves is found for all conditions at the level of the surface, but is less pronounced under the gel and cell–gel conditions.

collagen gels, the first question of interest was the distribution of cells between the gel and the titanium substrata. The results showed that cells were found on the surface for all groups. This indicates that some fibroblasts remained on the surface even though adhesive opportunities were available in the collagen gel. In fact, some cells originally on the surface (i.e., in the cell–gel condition) did migrate into the gel. Many cells remained on the Ti and remained oriented with the grooves, although their alignment was reduced in comparison with the control (i.e., no gel) culture. Similarly, in the gel condition thought to mimic what happens when tissues interact with the implant surface *in vivo*, some fibroblasts, initially located in the collagen gel migrated to the Ti surface and became aligned with the grooves although once again they were less well aligned than the cells in the control and cell–gel conditions.

Overall, these results show that collagen alters fibroblast interaction with the surface. Moreover, the order in which the cells encounter the collagen affects cell orientation and the number of cells on the surface. Such findings may be relevant considerations when alternative courses of action are possible with respect to the order in which cells and matrix contact the surface. For example, in some situations, it may be possible to place cells on an implant before insertion. This approach was employed by Boyko et al.[37] who implanted tooth roots with attached periodontal ligament cells in dogs and observed the formation of periodontal ligament-like structures with cells having the appropriate orientations — a result that did not occur if the roots were simply reimplanted.

6.6 Cell Responses to Surfaces Produced by Industrial Processes

In contrast to the microfabricated surfaces used in studies of cell behavior, the surfaces used in clinical trials are typically those produced by the industrial techniques of implant manufacturers. As a general rule there is less flexibility in surface feature design on such surfaces, but they are eminently more practical and in some instances have been characterized thoroughly.[1,38] Since industrially produced surfaces have been implanted in humans, they represent the most feasible approach to comparing effects on cell behavior in model systems to actual implant performance. Two of the more widely used surfaces in implantology are machined surfaces characterized by small parallel grooves and rough surfaces such as the SLA surface of the Straumann-ITI implant system.

Davies[39] speculated that one advantage of the rough surfaces is that they may bind or entangle fibrin fibers and thus provide pathways by which the cells adjacent to the implant can migrate to the implant surface. Another possibility is that the cells, once on the surface, may be involved in mechanical integration of the device with adjacent connective tissue through a mechanism known as the two-center effect. In brief, the two-center effect was so named by Weiss[6] who observed that a cellular bridge formed between two explants when they were placed in a plasma clot gel.

Subsequent investigation by Harris and coworkers[40-42] demonstrated that the basis for this effect was that the cells exerted a tractional force on the fibers that acted to align them and that more cells subsequently became aligned as a result of the fiber orientation. They demonstrated that ligament-like structures can be formed under suitable conditions *in vitro* as a result of cell traction. Since the direction of cell traction is determined by cell orientation and cell orientation can be controlled by topography, the possibility arises of using implant topography to produce desired connective tissue organization adjacent to implant surfaces. Questions of interest in addressing this possibility are (1) the orientation and migratory behavior of cells on the surfaces, (2) how the attachment to the surfaces survives the tractional forces generated by the cells, and (3) the orientation of extracellular matrix in relation to the surface.

6.6.1 Osteoblast Migration on Rough and Machined-Like Surfaces

Figure 6.6 illustrates osteoblast migration on machined-like and rough SLA surfaces in a series of frames extracted from a time-lapse movie in which the cells were labeled with a molecular dye and images captured using a CCD camera capable of forming images under conditions of low light. Incubation conditions were similar to those used by Damji et al.[13] It is evident that the osteoblasts exhibit contact guidance on the grooves made by the machining process. In contrast, the direction of migration of osteoblasts on the SLA surface appears to be more or less random. Nevertheless, it can be seen that the cells enter pits formed by blasting and in some instances appear to be trapped in them at least for short periods.

The motion and orientation of cells on the SLA surface have a component in what might be considered the Z direction relative to an XY plane that parallels the implant surface. There is thus the potential to orient cell tractional forces so that components of the cell-generated forces are directed perpendicular to the implant surface. Moreover, the cells are in positions in which they may be mechanically interlocked with the surface. Such a micromechanical linkage has the potential to stabilize the bio-implant interface.

6.6.2 Resistance of Tissue Equivalent/Ti Interface to Cell-Generated Forces

Tranquillo et al.[33] emphasized that mixtures of collagen gels and embedded cells that have the capability of contraction may be considered as tissue equivalents. In their seminal *Nature* paper on cell traction, Harris et al.[43] noted that "collagenous structures such as tendons, ligaments ... need not be laid down by direct secretion of collagen fibers into their eventual arrangement. Instead. fibroblast traction can rearrange and repack collagen into these patterns even beginning from a totally random meshwork."

Stopack and Harris[40] demonstrated that small heterogeneities in cell distributions can be magnified by positive mechanical feedback so that even the formation of complex tissue arrangements can be explained through the action of tractional forces (reviewed by Harris[42]). Tractional forces have been shown to produce the two-center effect, in which bridges of aligned cells and fibers formed between two tissue explants cultured in plasma or collagen gels. As the structural geometry of extracellular matrix is largely controlled by directed cellular activity, control of cell orientation at fixed sites on an implant should enable control of soft connective tissue organization and the promotion of tissue integration.

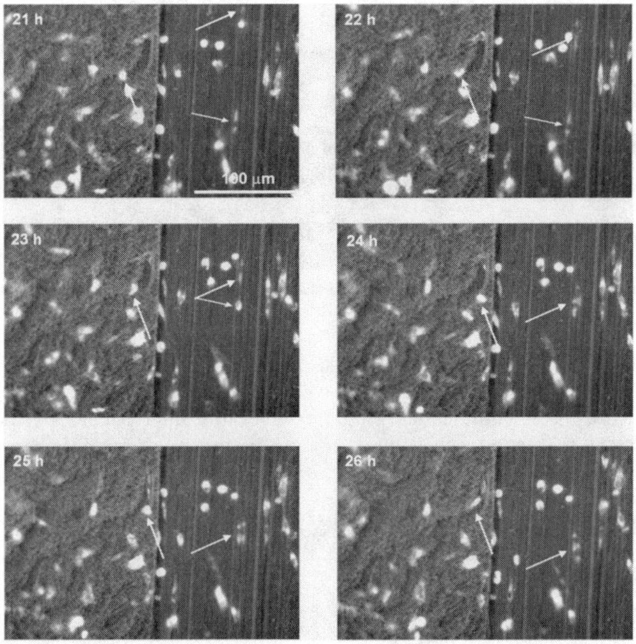

FIGURE 6.6
Time-lapse sequence of osteoblasts stained with CellTracker® Orange on machined-like and SLA surfaces after 21 to 26 hours of culture. Cells were stained and then observed using epifluorescence optics as they migrated on Ti-coated surfaces replicated in epoxy from SLA (right) and machined-like Ti surfaces (left). The digital images of the cells were overlaid on the digital image of a scanning electron micrograph of the precise areas to be examined so that the interaction of the cells with local topographic features could be determined. On the SLA surface, the cells did not move in any preferred direction; the cells exhibited interaction with the pits formed by blasting occasionally entering these pits (arrow on left sides of frames). On the machined-like surface, the cells exhibited contact guidance, that is, they followed the grooves on the surface (arrows on right side, of frames).

Inoue et al.[44] have shown that surface topography of Ti or Ti alloy surfaces can lead to the production of a two-center-like effect *in vitro* when the surfaces are placed on a lawn of fibroblasts, and that the orientation of the cells is influenced by surface topography. The model developed by Takekawa at the Faculty of Dentistry at the University of British Columbia was adapted from the work of Harris and coworkers. It consists of Ti surfaces mounted on an epoxy block and embedded in collagen gel — a fibroblast tissue equivalent (Figure 6.7). Tractional forces develop within the gel over time and can displace the tissue equivalent from the surface. The time at which this occurs, however, depends on the surface. Figure 6.8 shows a smooth surface in which the interface is disrupted after 64 hours. In contrast, the SLA surface is still attached to the tissue equivalent at the same time of culture.

The orientation of cells on the surface was examined by PI staining and confocal microscopy. As predicted from time-lapse studies, some of the fibro-

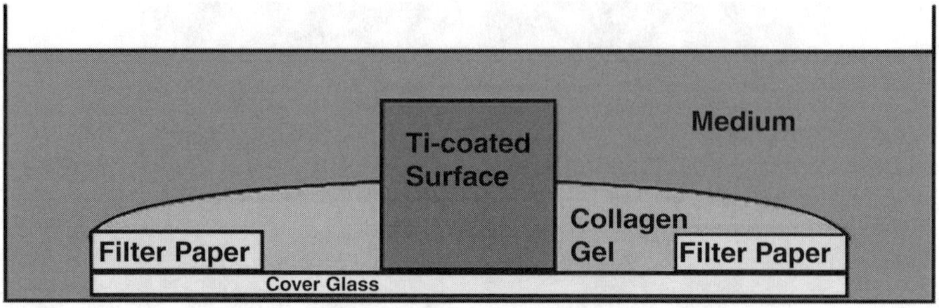

FIGURE 6.7
Culture system used to investigate ability of surfaces to resist cell generated forces. Surface is mounted on an epoxy block and placed in a collagen gel–human gingival fibroblast mixture, sometimes called a tissue equivalent. The gel extends to a filter paper ring that anchors the gel–cell mixture, so that when cells contract the gel, it is removed from the surface.

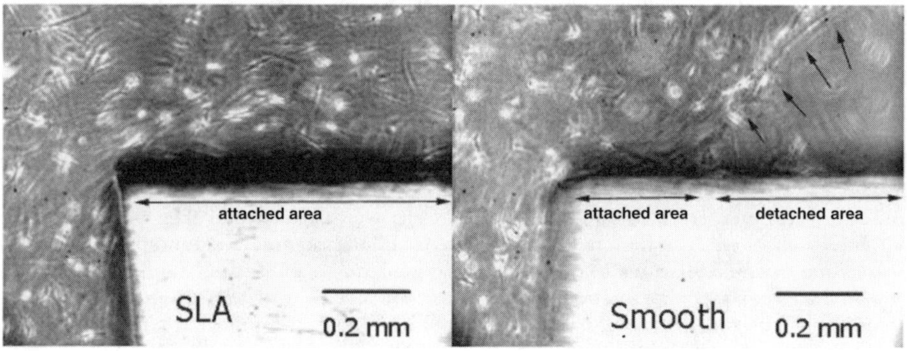

FIGURE 6.8
Phase contrast micrographs of surfaces (SLA and smooth) embedded in gel after 64 hours of culture. For the SLA figure, the epoxy block is at a slight angle to the surface of the culture slide, resulting in a black band. In some instances, the cells are oriented obliquely to the Ti surface. On the smooth surface, the gel has contracted from the Ti surface.

blasts had vertical or oblique orientations relative to the SLA surface but cells on the smooth surface were parallel to the surface. This vertical orientation of the fibroblasts on the SLA surface may prolong survival by disrupting the formation of the contractile ring of fibroblasts with cells oriented parallel to the Ti surface, as described by Glass-Brudzinski et al.[35] The survival of attachment to the SLA and smooth Ti was compared using the Mantel–Cox log rank approach and found to be statistically different ($p = <0.005$) with the SLA surfaces supporting tissue-equivalent attachment for a longer time. It is clear that more work with this model system is required to sort out the roles of cells and collagen entrapment with the surface in producing this effect.

6.7 Cell Selection in an *In Vivo* Model

Cell selection provides another example of the complexity of applying the principles of cell behavior to predicting events *in vivo*. By analogy to the work of Rich and Harris[45] who demonstrated that fibroblasts prefer rough surfaces, Brunette[46] speculated that one would expect rough Ti implant surfaces to attract cells of the monocyte series. Brunette reasoned that since monocytes can form osteoclasts, an accumulation of cells from the monocytic family might be detrimental to the performance of the implant because bone loss might be stimulated. It has subsequently become clear that rough surfaces can be very successful clinically so Brunette's worries were to an extent unfounded.

The question thus arises whether rough Ti implant surfaces attract macrophages *in vivo* as was observed for other rough surfaces. Accordingly, we implanted surfaces of varying roughness subcutaneously in rats. We found that macrophage-like cells, as assessed by morphology, were present on rough SLA surfaces in strikingly greater numbers (Figure 6.9) than on smooth surfaces or grooved microfabricated surfaces in which each facet of the groove was smooth. Moreover, the SLA surfaces were associated with a higher frequency of bone formation than the smooth or grooved surfaces.

Thus, in this model, the mere presence of macrophages on an implant surface is not necessarily detrimental and it is possible that the products of

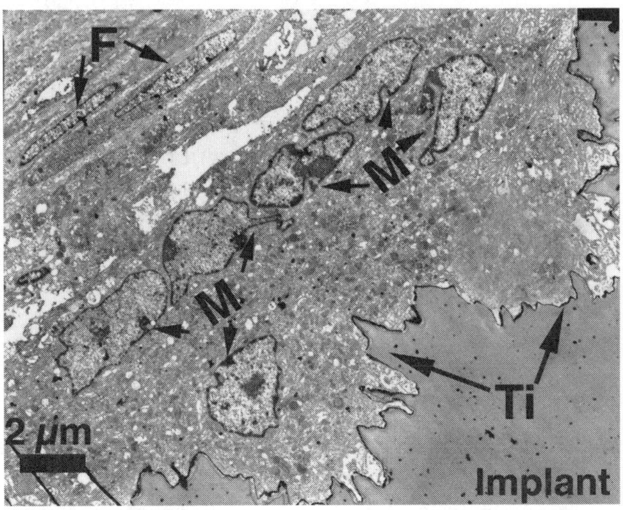

FIGURE 6.9
Transmission electron micrograph of cells in the vicinity of a Ti-coated epoxy replica of an SLA surface implanted subcutaneously in a rat for 2 weeks. M = macrophage-like cells; F = fibroblasts. Details of production of the replica are given in Wieland, M. et al.[49]

macrophages on these surfaces may exert positive effects on bone formation. Another factor is the potential for interaction between the macrophages and connective tissue cells. McKee and Nanci[47] suggested that an osteopontin coating may be involved in selectively activating the cellular mechanisms required for macrophage attachment, signal transduction, and phagocytosis. In their recent review on macrophage interactions with material surfaces, Thomsen and Gretzer[48] concluded that additional experimental models with different degrees of experimental complexity are required.

One approach would be the systematic investigation of macrophage responses to the topography of industrial and microfabricated Ti surfaces and the correlation of those responses with bone formation. The rat subcutaneous model has several advantages for such a study including relatively low cost that allows the use of sufficient animals for appropriate statistical analysis, availability of immunological reagents, uniformity of animals, rapid responses, and experimental convenience. Other models are also being investigated, but it appears likely that the most successful approaches will enable complex cell–cell and cell–material interactions to occur and be assessed.

6.8 Conclusions

Topography is a powerful modulator of cell behavior but not necessarily a specific one. Based on the plurality of responses to topographic stimuli and the possibility of cell interactions, simple cell culture systems may be limited in their ability to predict responses. Thus, the approach of using models in which cell interactions occur has merit.

Examples where this approach led to promising insights include tissue-equivalent collagen gels, the role of cell orientation in interface stability, high population density osteoblast cultures, the possible role of cell orientation in bone formation, and rodent *in vivo* models in which cell selection, in particular macrophage accumulation on rough surfaces, could be demonstrated.

In some instances, these models provide information that correlates with implant performance and allow questions to be posed about cell interactions and cell selection. In other situations, they test possibilities that cannot be realistically tested in simpler systems.

Acknowledgment

These studies were supported by the Canadian Institutes of Health Research.

References

1. Wennerberg, A., Albrektsson, T., and Andersson, B., Design and surface characteristics of 13 commercially available oral implant systems, *Int. J. Oral Maxillofac. Implants*, 8, 622, 1993.
2. Perizzolo, D., Lacefield, W.R., and Brunette, D.M., Interaction between topography and coating in the formation of bone nodules in culture for hydroxyapatite- and titanium-coated micromachined surfaces, *J. Biomed. Mater. Res.*, 56, 494, 2001.
3. Harrison, R.G., The reaction of embryonic cells to solid structures, *J. Exp. Zool.*, 17, 521, 1914.
4. Weiss, P. and Taylor, A., Fish scale as substratum for uniform orientation of cells *in vitro*, *Anat. Rec.*, 124, 381, 1956.
5. Rich, A. and Harris, A.K., Anomalous preferences of cultured macrophages for hydrophobic and roughened substrata, *J. Cell. Sci.*, 50, 1, 1981.
6. Weiss, P., "Attraction fields" between growing tissue cultures, *Science*, 115, 293, 1952.
7. Brunette, D.M, Kenner, G.S., and Gould T.R., Grooved titanium surfaces orient growth and migration of cells from human gingival, *J. Dent. Res.*, 62, 1045, 1983.
8. Brunette, D.M., Fibroblasts on micromachined substrata orient hierarchically to grooves of different dimensions, *Exp. Cell Res.*, 164, 11, 1986.
9. Brunette, D.M., Principles of cell behaviour on titanium surfaces and their application to implanted devices, in *Titanium in Medicine*, Brunette, D.M. et al., Eds., Springer-Verlag, Heidelberg, 2001, p. 485.
10. Curtis, A.S. and Wilkinson, C.D., Reactions of cells to topography, *J. Biomater. Sci. Polym. Ed.*, 9, 1313, 1998.
11. Wallboomers, X.F. and Jansen, J.A., Cell and tissue behavior on micro-grooved surfaces, *Odontology*, 89, 2 ,2001.
12. Chehroudi, B., Gould, T.R.L., and Brunette, D.M., Effects of a grooved titanium-coated implant surface on epithelial cell behaviour *in vitro* and *in vivo*, *J. Biomed. Mater. Res.*, 23, 1067, 1989.
13. Damji, A., Weston, L., and Brunette, D.M., Directed confrontations between fibroblasts and epithelial cells on micromachined grooved substrata, *Exp. Cell Res.*, 228, 114, 1996.
14. Oakley, C. and Brunette, D.M., The sequence of alignment of microtubules, focal contacts, and actin filaments in fibroblasts spreading on smooth and grooved titanium substrata, *J. Cell Sci.*, 106, 343, 1993.
15. Qu, J., Chehroudi, B., and Brunette, D.M., The use of micromachined surfaces to investigate the cell behavioural factors essential to osseointegration, *Oral Dis.*, 2, 102, 1996.
16. Oakley, C. and Brunette, D.M., The response of single, pairs, and clusters of epithelial cells to substratum topography, *Biochem. Cell Biol.*, 73, 473, 1995.
17. Abiko, Y. and Brunette, D.M., Immunohistochemical investigation of tracks left by the migration of fibroblasts on titanium surfaces, *Cells Mater.*, 3, 161, 1993.
18. Chou, L. et al., Effects of titanium on transcription and post-transcriptional regulation of fibronectin in human fibroblasts, *J. Biomed. Mater. Res.*, 31, 209, 1996.

19. Chou, L. et al., Effects of surface composition and topography on 72-kDa gelatinase gene expression and secretion, *J. Biomed. Mater. Res.*, 39, 437, 1998.
20. Schwarz, R.I. and Bissel, M.J., Dependence of the differentiated state on the cellular environment: modulation of collagen synthesis in tendon cells, *Proc. Natl. Acad. Sci. U.S.A.*, 74, 4453, 1977.
21. Trombley, L., Absher, M., and Kelley, J., Lung cell population density determines the ratio of type III to type I collagen, *Am. Rev. Respir. Dis.*, 123, 694, 1981.
22. Talhouck, R.S., Neiswander, R.L., and Shanbacher, F.L., *In vitro* culture of cryopreserved bovine mammary cells on collagen gels: synthesis and secretion of casein and lactoferrin, *Tissue Cell*, 22, 583, 1990.
23. Abercrombie, M. and Heaysman, J.E.M., Observations on the social behaviour of cells in tissue culture. I. Speed of movement of chick heart fibroblasts in relation to their mutual contacts, *Exp. Cell Res.*, 5, 111, 953.
24. Stoker, M., Contact and short-range interactions affecting growth of animal cells in culture, *Curr. Topics Dev. Biol.*, 2, 107, 1967.
25. Olive, P.L. and Durand, R.E., Drug and radiation resistance in spheroids: cell contact and kinetics, *Cancer Metastasis Rev.*, 13, 121, 1994.
26. Rubin, H., Cellular epigenetics: effects of passage history on competence of cells for "spontaneous" formation, *Proc. Natl. Acad. Sci. U.S.A.*, 90, 10715, 1993.
27. Shull, J.D. and Pennington, K.L., Changes in population density elicit quantitative and qualitative changes in the estrogen receptor in intact GH4C1 pituitary tumor cells, *J. Steroid Biochem. Mol. Biol.*, 44, 53, 1993.
28. Hagiwara, M., Chen, I.L., and Fisher, J.W., Erythropietin production in long-term cultures of human renal carcinoma cells: the role of cell population density, *Exp. Cell Res.*, 154, 619, 1984.
29. Blay, J. and Brown, K.D., Contradistinctive growth responses of cultured rat intestinal cells to epidermal growth factor depending on cell population density, *J. Cell Physiol.*, 129, 343, 1986.
30. Tenang, E.M. and McCaldin, B., The influence of virus transformation and cell population density on some membrane properties of mouse fibroblasts in culture, *Biochem. Med. Metab. Biol.*, 38, 338, 1987.
31. Kim, Y.S. et al., Cell density-dependent vitamin D effects on calcium accumulation in rat osteogenic sarcoma cells (ROS 17/2), *Calcif. Tissue Int.*, 41, 218, 1987.
32. Matsuya, Y. and Yamane, I., Population-dependent requirements of vitamin B_{21} and metabolically related substances of several mouse cell types in serum-free, albumin-fortified medium, *Cell Struct. Funct.*, 11, 9, 1986.
33. Tranquillo, R.T., Durrani, M.A., and Moon, A.G., Tissue engineering science: consequences of cell traction force, *Cytotechnology*, 10, 225, 1992.
34. Elsdale, T. and Foley, R., Morphogenetic aspects of multilayering in Petri dish cultures of human fetal lung fibroblasts, *J. Cell Biol.*, 41, 298, 1969.
35. Glass-Brudzinski, J., Perizzolo, D., and Brunette, D.M., Effects of substratum surface topography in the organization of cells and collagen fibers in collagen gel cultures, *J. Biomed. Mater. Res.*, in press, 2002.
36. Cooper, L.F., A role for surface topography in creating and maintaining bone at titanium endosseous implants, *J. Prosthet. Dent.*, 84, 522, 2000.
37. Boyko, G.A., Melcher, A.H., and Brunette, D.M., Formation of new periodontal ligament by periodontal ligament cells implanted *in vivo* after culture *in vitro*: a preliminary study of transplanted roots in the dog, *J. Periodont. Res.*, 16, 73, 1981.

38. Wieland, M. et al., Wavelength-dependent roughness: a quantitative approach to characterizing the topography of rough titanium surfaces, *Int. J. Oral Maxillofac. Implants,* 16, 163, 2001.
39. Davies, J.E., Mechanisms of endosseous integration, *Int. J. Prosthodont.*, 11, 391, 1998.
40. Harris, A.K., Stopack, D., and Wild, P., Fibroblast traction as a mechanism for collagen morphogenesis, *Nature*, 290, 249, 1981.
41. Stopack, D. and Harris, A.K., Connective tissue morphogenesis by fibroblast traction. 1. Tissue culture observations, *Dev. Biol.*, 90, 383, 1982.
42. Harris, A.K., Physical forces and pattern formation in limb development, in *Developmental Patterning of the Vertebrate Limb*, Hinchcliffe, J.R. et al., Eds., Plenum Press, New York, 1991, p. 203.
43. Harris, A.K., Stopack, D., and Wild, P., Fibroblast traction as a mechanism for collagen morphogenesis, *Nature*, 290, 249, 1981.
44. Inoue, T. et al., Effect of the surface geometry of smooth and porous-coated titanium alloy on the orientation of fibroblasts *in vitro*, *J. Biomed. Mater. Res.*, 21, 107, 1987.
45. Rich, A. and Harris, A.K., Anomalous preferences of cultured macrophages for hydrophobic and roughened substrata, *J. Cell Sci.*, 50, 1, 1981.
46. Brunette, D.M., The effects of implant surface topography on the behavior of cells, *Int. J. Oral Maxillofac. Implants*, 3, 231, 1988.
47. McKee, M.D. and Nanci, A., Osteopontin at mineralized tissue interfaces in bone, teeth and osseointegrated implants: ultrastructural distribution and implications for mineralized tissue formation, turnover and repair, *Microscopy Res. Tech.*, 33, 141, 1996.
48. Thomsen, P. and Gretzer, C., Macrophage interactions with modified material surfaces, *Curr. Opin. Solid State Mater. Sci.*, 5, 163, 2001.
49. Wieland, M. et al., Use of Ti-coated replicas to investigate the effects on fibroblast shape of surfaces with varying roughness and constant chemical composition, *J. Biomed. Mater. Res.*, 60, 2002.

7

Osteoblast Response to Pure Titanium and Titanium Alloy

Michael L. Paine and Jennifer C. Wong

CONTENTS

7.1 Introduction 123
7.2 Titanium Dioxide: Dental Implant or Orthopedic Interface to Bone 124
 7.2.1 Osteoblast Phenotype Related to Titanium Substrata: Morphology and Integrin Expression 126
 7.2.2 Bone Morphogenetic Proteins 129
 7.2.3 Enamel Matrix-Derived Proteins as Osteopromoters 131
 7.2.4 Local and Systemic Delivery of Microbiologicals at Time of Implant Placement to Improve Success Rates 132
 7.2.5 DNA Microarrays: Possible Experimental Protocol to Identify Important Cellular Responses and Molecular Pathways of Osteoblasts Exposed to Dental Implant Interface 133
7.3 Proteomics as the Future 137
7.4 Conclusions 137
Acknowledgments 138
References 138

7.1 Introduction

Commercially pure titanium (c.p. Ti) and titanium alloy (Ti-6Al-4V) are highly regarded as skeletal biomaterials because of their good biocompatibility. Commercially pure titanium resists corrosion because of its outer oxide layer, and shares this characteristic with Ti-6Al-4V. Commercially pure titanium is used to fabricate endosseous dental implants and coat devices con-

0-8493-1474-7/03/$0.00+$1.50

structed of titanium alloy. Although c.p. Ti is not a strong enough material to be used in orthopedic devices, the addition of aluminum (Al) and vanadium (V) creates an alloy (Ti-6Al-4V) with significantly greater strength. This improved strength, together with its low elastic modulus and excellent biocompatibility, makes Ti-6Al-4V a preferred orthopedic material.

Attempts have been made in recent years to define the biological responses occurring at the metallic osseous interfaces of c.p. Ti and Ti-6Al-4V. To improve on long-term bonding and survival or hasten short-term bonding of metals to the living skeleton, a detailed understanding of the composition of the interfacial zones and the timing of its genetic construction is required. Initial and early cellular reactions observed at the time of placement of the implanted device may explain differences detected in the interfacial zones between similar and dissimilar metals.

This chapter reviews some of the current literature discussing the cellular and genetic responses of osteoblasts at the implant interfacial zone. Discussion is limited to c.p. Ti and Ti-6Al-4V metals, and covers both *in vitro* and *in vivo* studies. This chapter concludes by suggesting that a well-executed *in vitro* experimental design using bone cells and DNA microarrays may add to the relevant information needed by prosthetic manufacturers to improve both the short- and long-term physical properties of osseointegration.

7.2 Titanium Dioxide: Dental Implant or Orthopedic Interface to Bone

Titanium dioxide (TiO_2) is a solid with a melting point of 1855°C. TiO_2 is polymorphous — it exists in multiple modifications or crystal structures. The following crystal structures have been recognized for TiO_2: rutile (tetragonal), anatase or octahedrite (tetragonal), and brookite (orthorhombic).[1] However, two additional oxides have been described recently. One is an orthorhombic structure in which titanium is seven-coordinated to oxygen.[2] The other is a cotunnite-structured oxide in which titanium is nine-coordinated to oxygen.[3] TiO_2 also exists in an amorphous state.

Two other notable forms of titanium oxides are ilmenite ($FeTiO_3$) and perovskite ($CaTiO_3$).[1] Technically and commercially, only the anatase and rutile forms are of significance. Rutile has a density of 4.23 g/ml, anatase has a density of 3.90 g/ml, and brookite has a density of 4.13 g/ml. This density difference is explained by different crystal structures. Geometry dictates that the rutile modification is more closely packed than the anatase crystal.

The most important commercial application of TiO_2 is as a pigment for providing brightness, whiteness, and opacity to such products such as paints and coatings, plastics, papers, inks, fibers, foods, and cosmetics (e.g., DuPont White Pigment and Mineral Products, Wilmington, DE). TiO_2 is by far the most widely used white pigment in the world. Both the anatase and rutile crystal structures (as powders) are used in the manufacture of white pigments. TiO_2 must be developed to an ideal particle size in order to realize its optical properties. Normally, the particle size is one half the wavelength of visible light or about 0.3 μ. The property that gives this white powder its unmatched performance is its high refractive index (only diamonds have a higher refractive index than TiO_2). The refractive index is a measure of the ability to bend light and from this we attain opacity. Only magnesium oxide is whiter than TiO_2, but the refractive index of magnesium oxide is much lower. This means that much more magnesium oxide is required in a product to achieve opacity; hence, for practical purposes, TiO_2 is preferred. TiO_2 is usually associated with iron, either as ilmenite or leuxocene ores and the ores are the principal raw materials used in manufacturing TiO_2 pigment. TiO_2 is also readily mined in one of the purest forms, rutile beach sand.

Regarding the surface oxide layer on c.p. Ti dental implant systems, spectroscopic studies suggest that the oxide is amorphous and its thickness is approximately 2 to 17 nm. Generally speaking, the thinnest oxide layers on dental implants, say, less than 10 nm, are amorphous, morphologically homogeneous, and have essentially no contrast in transmission electron microscopy (TEM) images. As the oxide thickness is increased up to 40 nm, a texture corresponding to the grain structure of the oxidized metal becomes gradually more visible. At the same time, the oxide becomes increasingly more crystalline.[4]

It is believed that properties of oxide films covering titanium implant surfaces are of crucial importance for successful osseointegration, in particular at compromised bone sites. Various chemical treatments of c.p. Ti and Ti-6Al-4V are employed by implant manufacturers in attempts to influence the biological response to implants at the time of placement and improve and hasten osseointegration.

For example, anodic oxides have been prepared on c.p. Ti by galvanostatic mode in acetic acid (CH_3COOH)[4] to achieve oxide layers with the following characteristics: (1) oxide layer thickness ranging from 200 to 1000 nm with barrier and porous structure dominating the surface morphology; (2) pore sizes approximately 8 μm in diameter; and (3) porosity in the range of 12.7 to 24.4%. The crystal structures of the titanium oxides present were amorphous, anatase, and mixtures of anatase and rutile. The chemical surface compositions consisted mainly of TiO_2. These experimental oxide layers were compared to the native (thermal) oxides on turned implants (controls) which were amorphous, 17 nm thick, and had chemical compositions of TiO_2.[4]

This chapter does not set out to describe the oxide layer characteristics of dental implants or orthopedic devices. However, it is important to recognize that the biological responses to titanium implants occur on amorphous, anatase, or rutile TiO_2, rather than on the metal itself. No doubt considerable industry effort is directed at altering the oxide surface chemistry and physical characteristics of implant devices in attempts to improve the success rates and longevity of implants. The success of implants also includes the immediate biological events that occur at the time of implant placement.

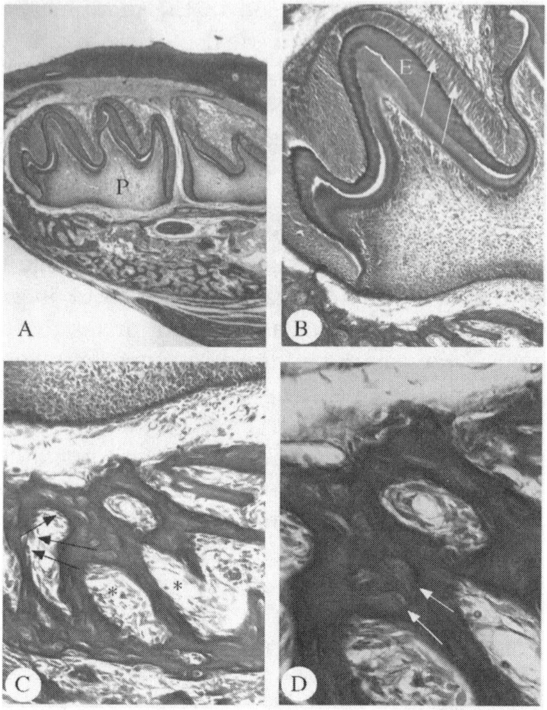

FIGURE 7.1
(See color insert following Page 272.) The developing cancellous bone from the mandible of a 5-day postnatal mouse. Tissue prepared by Mallory–Heidenhain stain. Panels A and B show dental pulp (P) and enamel (E) of a first molar. Arrows point to osteoblasts in panel C and to osteocytes in panel D. Bone marrow is identified by asterisks. Panels B, C, and D are magnified 10, 20, and 40×, respectively.

7.2.1 Osteoblast Phenotype Related to Titanium Substrata: Morphology and Integrin Expression

Osseointegration is characterized by direct apposition of bone matrix and osteoblasts (Figure 7.1) to the implant surface without intervening soft or fibrous tissue. Dental implants typically fail to achieve total osseointegration but, based on criteria used to judge implant success, even a sparse amount of bone-to-implant contact may result in a clinically successful implant.[5]

A number of *in vitro* studies have addressed the nature of the cellular and molecular events occurring at the bone–metal interface. These studies focused mainly on cell adhesion and morphology, DNA synthesis, integrin expression, and synthesis of various proteins including collagen and alkaline phosphatase.[6,7] It is assumed that a better understanding of each of these phenotypic events may ultimately result in the development of a perfect implant material with ideal surface properties that can be positioned in bone under conditions that favor complete osseointegration.

Cell lines of osteoblast lineage can provide a rapidly proliferating and differentiating system for testing biomaterials *in vitro*. A study by Hendrich and colleagues investigated the effect of standard orthopedic implant materials on osteoblast proliferation and differentiation using a human osteoblast cell culture system.[8] The human fetal osteoblast cell line hFOB1 · 19[9] was cultured on polystyrene (control), c.p. Ti, stainless steel, and cobalt–chrome–molybdenum. Lower cell numbers and delayed proliferation were noted on stainless steel and cobalt–chrome–molybdenum compared to c.p. Ti and polystyrene substrates. Higher levels of alkaline phosphatase and osteocalcin were measured on c.p. Ti than on stainless steel or cobalt–chrome–molybdenum. This increase in the levels of alkaline phosphatase and osteocalcin is an indication of osteoblast differentiation.[10] No differences in collagen type I production were noted in this study.[8]

Integrins are heterodimeric cell adhesion proteins connecting extracellular matrices (ECMs) to the cytoskeleton and transmitting signals in both directions. They thus mediate cell adhesion to the ECM. Integrins are also involved in many biological processes such as growth, differentiation, migration, and cell death.[11] Integrins constitute a family of transmembrane proteins and eukaryotic cells contain at least 16 α and 8 β integrin subunits. Different combinations of the α and β subunits dimerize to form at least 22 different receptors with distinct but overlapping ECM protein specificity.[12]

Of the known integrin heterodimers, ten contain the nearly ubiquitously expressed β1 integrin subunit. Heterodimers of the β1 integrin subfamily bind ECM components such as fibronectin (α3, α4, α5, α8, and αv), collagen (α1 and α2), and laminins (α1, α2, α3, α6, α7, and α9).[11] The major underlying theme of scientific discovery related to the integrins involves cell adhesion and subsequent modifications during development, wound healing, metastasis, and angiogenesis. Perhaps the most studied integrins relate to the fibronectin receptors present on mammalian fibroblasts. Fibronectin receptors were initially identified as plasma membrane glycoproteins that bound to fibronectin affinity columns and could be eluded by peptides containing Arg–Gly–Asp (or RGD) amino acid sequences. This RGD string is present in fibronectin and is responsible for cell binding. Simply put, integrin fibronectin receptors function as transmembrane linkers to mediate interactions between the actin cytoskeleton and fibronectin of the ECM.

Integrins can also function as activators of intracellular signaling machinery.[13] The cytoplasmic domain of β1 integrin can interact with cytoskeletal proteins such as α-actinin and talin or with signaling molecules such as focal adhesion kinase (FAK) and integrin-linked kinase (ILK).[11] One of the many signaling mechanisms triggered by the β1 integrins is the mitogen-activated protein (MAP) kinase cascade.[14] Under cell culture conditions using 3T3 or REF52 fibroblasts, activation of MAP kinases depends on integrin engagement with the ECM, that is, MAP kinases are activated only when cells adhere to substrata coated with integrin ligands.[14] Intracellular signals can change the affinity of integrins for their extracellular ligands.[15] Therefore, integrins allow bidirectional transfer of information through cell membranes.

Because the biologic fixation of orthopedic implants depends on optimal cell interactions at the interface, investigators have examined whether integrins are involved in the attachment of osteoblasts to implant materials. In a study by Sinha and Tuan,[16] immunohistochemistry was used to examine the expression of integrins in primary human osteoblasts cultured on polystyrene and on rough and polished disks of orthopedic alloys Ti-6Al-4V and cobalt–chrome–molybdenum. Their results demonstrated the level of complexity of expression profiles that exist among the different integrin subunits.[16] Integrin subunits $\alpha 2$, $\alpha 3$, $\alpha 4$, $\alpha 5$, αv, $\alpha 6$, $\beta 1$, and $\beta 3$ were expressed by the osteoblasts cultured on polystyrene coated with various ECM molecules; $\alpha 5$ and $\alpha 6$ were notably absent in cells attached to the alloys. Also, the presence or absence of $\alpha 3$ and $\beta 3$ varied depending on the metal surface type. The nature of the metal alloy appeared to influence the expression of particular integrins. Thus the ability of cells to adhere to and receive messages from the extracellular matrix may be influenced by the substratum.

Unfortunately, the study by Sinha and Tuan[16] and similar studies suffer from their inability to assign a definitive molecular activity at the metal interface with absolute certainty. For example, human $\beta 1$ integrin subunit can be expressed in four different (alternatively spliced) variants that differ in their cytoplasmic domains.[17] Protein isoforms generally exist to perform different biological functions. Alternative splicing resulting in multiple protein isoforms offers another level of complexity when studying gene activities.

A second problem related to but independent of the first complication is the quality of the antibody used. The study by Sinha and Tuan[16] used multiple antibodies to the same antigen and these authors note that they achieved varied results. Explanations offered included technique and equipment, method of fixation and permeabilization, antibody specificity and titer, immunostaining conditions (temperature and humidity), species cross-reactivity (most commercial antibodies are raised in rabbit hosts), and finally the time of the cells in culture prior to experimentation. The authors acknowledged that antibodies to the same antigen purchased from different sources produced conflicting data. A particular problem is species cross-reactivity when investigating multiple proteins belonging to a genetically related family.

Recently, the intracellular signaling pathway for osteoblast adhesion to Ti-6Al-4V was investigated and compared to integrin-mediated adhesion to fibronectin.[7] Primary osteoblasts from fetal rat calvaria were plated onto Ti-6Al-4V, fibronectin, and poly-L-lysine (control) and the levels of focal adhesion kinase (FAK), mitogen-activated protein kinase (MAP kinase), and the c-fos and c-jun AP-1 transcription factors were compared. At a molecular level, it appeared that osteoblast adhesion to Ti-6Al-4V implants was similar to adhesion to fibronectin. Osteoblast adhesion to Ti-6Al-4V also led to osteoblast proliferation. This study provided some evidence for the biocompatibility of Ti-6Al-4V at a molecular level.[7]

7.2.2 Bone Morphogenetic Proteins

Substantial progress has been made in the area of *in vivo* bone morphogenetic protein (BMP) research as it relates to clinical uses. BMPs are members of the transforming growth factor beta (TGF-β) superfamily of secreted signaling molecules that have important functions in many biological contexts.[18,19] Several BMP receptors have been cloned and characterized and, in addition, the intracellular signal transduction and transcriptional factors associating with BMP receptors are being investigated.

BMPs bind to specific serine and threonine kinase receptors that transduce the signal to the nucleus through Smad proteins.[20] Intracellular signaling cascades triggered by BMPs, which eventually activate Smad transcription factors, ultimately regulate expression of specific target genes. Nuclear cofactors that cooperate with the Smads in regulating specific target genes depending on the cellular context have also been identified.[18,20]

BMPs are well established agents for inducing orthotopic and ectopic bone formation, but their clinical usefulness may be limited by a short *in vivo* half-life and low specific activity.[21] This can be partly addressed with the use of moldable carriers. When implanted locally to animals with appropriate carriers (such as collagen), recombinant human BMP-2 (rhBMP-2) reproduces ectopic bone-forming activity.[19,22] *In vitro*, rhBMP-2 is shown to induce differentiation of mesenchymal stem cells into osteoblast and chondroblast cells and prevent the former cells from differentiating into cell types other than the latter cells.[22] Clinical applications for rhBMP-2 in which suitable biocompatible, biodegradable, and nonimmunogenic carriers are employed to correct large bony defects are being developed.[22] Experimentally significant bone formation can be produced in multiple animal models such as rodents and nonhuman primates.[22] Such preclinical studies show that bone induced by rhBMP-2 seems to behave morphologically and mechanically like normal bone. Clinical trials are underway to determine its usefulness in the orthopedic, oral, and maxillofacial fields.[22]

Another study investigated the combined effects of BMP-2 and TGF-β. BMPs have the ability to induce ectopic bone, while TGF-β stimulates proliferation of osteoblasts and chondrocytes and production of extracellular matrix. A morphometric study in mice revealed that the quantity of newly formed bone induced by a combination of rhBMP-2 and TGF-β could be greater than by use of rhBMP-2 alone.[23]

Gene therapy is an alternative route for exploiting the bone-inductive activities of BMPs. Investigators examined the osteogenic activity of an adenovirus containing BMP-7 cDNA under control of the CMV promoter (AdCMV-BMP-7).[24] Adenovirus vectors have been shown to readily infect a wide variety of cell types *in vitro* including osteoblasts, fibroblasts, and myoblasts. Using this vector, high levels of BMP-7 can be generated in the monkey kidney cell line COS7.[24] Transduction of murine myoblast cells with AdCMV-BMP-7 suppresses the muscle phenotype and induces *in vitro* osteoblast differentiation. AdCMV-BMP-7 with a bovine bone-

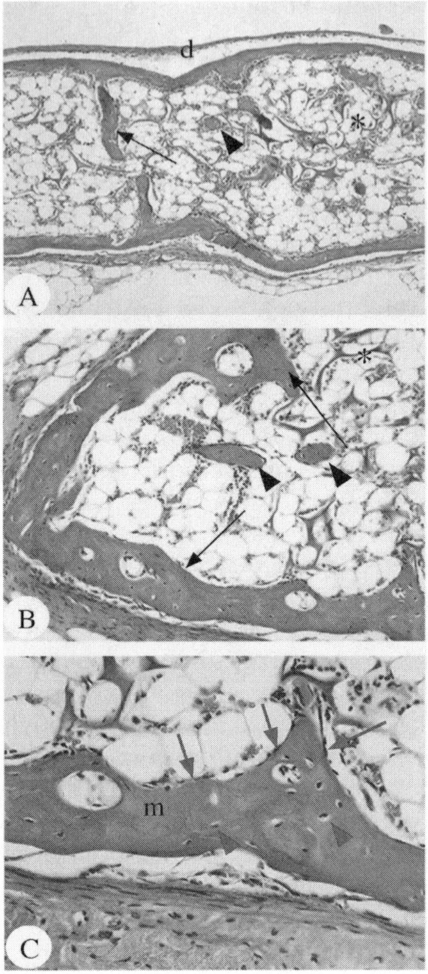

FIGURE 7.2
(See color insert.) Panels A and B: Newly formed cancellous bone (black arrows), ossicles (black arrowheads), and marrow cavities (asterisks) are formed after subcutaneous implantation of the adenovirus vector AdCMV-BMP-7 with a bovine bone-derived collagen carrier. Panel A also shows dermis (d). Panel C: bone matrix (m), osteoblasts (arrows), and osteocytes (arrowheads) are shown. Panels A, B, and C are magnified 10, 20, and 40×, respectively.

derived collagen carrier was implanted into mouse muscles and dermal pouches, and ossicles containing cortical and trabecular bone resulted (Figure 7.2).[24]

These cited studies using recombinant forms of BMP-2 and BMP-7 demonstrate the current discussion of the use of biologically active molecules to repair or induce bone in areas void of bone. It is conceivable that similar, molecular-based applications may be developed in the future to improve success rates of implants placed in immediate extraction sites. Immediate extraction sites often present void of contact bone or with the coronal portion of the implant remaining exposed due to the tooth root architecture.

7.2.3 Enamel Matrix-Derived Proteins as Osteopromoters

Enamel matrix-derived proteins (EMDPs) have been available commercially for dental treatment in Europe since 1995 and in the U.S. since 1997 (see *Journal of Clinical Periodontology*, Vol. 9, Part 2, 1997). Biora AB of Malmö, Sweden markets such a product registered under the name Emdogain®. Emdogain is a porcine-derived enamel matrix product and its principal component is the enamel matrix protein amelogenin. Emdogain has been marketed primarily to treat periodontal lesions by regenerating the affected periodontal ligament[25] but suggestions in the literature indicate that this product can also hasten the processes of wound healing.[26]

Embryonic enamel matrix proteins may be involved in the formation of cellular and acellular cementum during development of the periodontal attachment apparatus, suggesting that these proteins might be used clinically to promote periodontal regeneration.[27] Schwartz and colleagues analyzed the effects of Emdogain on osteoblast cells and found that it can influence cell proliferation and differentiation depending on the cell maturation stage.[28] The following methodologies were used to measure these parameters: (1) proliferation (cell number and [3H]-thymidine incorporation); (2) differentiation (alkaline phosphatase and osteocalcin production); and (3) matrix synthesis ([35S]-sulfate incorporation and percentage of collagen production).

Emdogain stimulates proliferation of preosteoblasts, but has no effect on differentiation; in osteoblast-like (MG63) cells, it inhibits proliferation and stimulates differentiation. In normal human osteoblast cells, it increases proliferation and differentiation.[28] Collagen production and proteoglycan sulfation were not affected by Emdogain, but both cellular activities increased in the presence of other growth factors like BMP-2 or TGF-β. These studies suggest that Emdogain may work as a growth factor but, if that is the case, its mechanism of action is different from those of BMP-2 and TGF-β. It has also been shown that Emdogain prolongs the growth of primary cultures of mouse calvaria osteoblasts.[29] EMDPs enhanced collagen-I, interleukin-6, and prostaglandin G/H synthase-2 expression, but did not stimulate the expression of osteocalcin and IGF-I.

To determine the effects of Emdogain on bone regeneration in rat femurs after drill-hole injury, defects in bone were filled with either Emdogain or its carrier, propylene glycol alginate (PGA).[30] Early formation of trabecular bone (days 4 through 7) occurred in the medullary cavities at cylindrical bone defects for both study groups; cuboidal osteoblasts were clearly observed as were many multinucleated giant cells indicating active bone remodeling. No significant differences were noted between the PGA- and Emdogain-applied groups with respect to calcium and phosphate ratios or mass at day 7. However, at day 7, the bone volume fractions of newly formed bone trabeculae were significantly higher in the Emdogain-applied group than in the PGA-applied controls, but this difference was no longer apparent 28 days postoperatively. The authors concluded that Emdogain possesses an osteopromotive effect (rather than an osteoinductive effect) on bone and medullary regeneration during healing of injured long bones.[30] This conclusion was also reached in a study by Boyan and colleagues who, to further understand the effect of Emdogain on bone formation, attempted to induce *de novo* bone formation in nude mouse calf muscle.[31]

To date, no clinical studies addressing the use of Emdogain to improve clinical parameters of osseointegration during the healing process after dental implant placement have been published, although the issue seems like a logical clinical study. If Emdogain has osteopromotive potential, its use with dental implants may be indicated to quicken osseointegration to allow for shorter treatment periods.

7.2.4 Local and Systemic Delivery of Microbiologicals at Time of Implant Placement to Improve Success Rates

Clinically, the success or failure of a dental implant is based on simple criteria: whether the implant osseointegrates and whether it can be restored into a functional dental unit. Degrees of osseointegration are generally not taken into account in human clinical studies, because of the difficulty in obtaining biopsy materials from the numbers of patients needed to draw scientifically valid conclusions. The literature does, however, include a number of case reports on human biopsies and postmortem studies that addressed relative amounts of bone (percent volume) and bone-to-implant contacts adjacent to implants.[32,33]

In one study, 30 c.p. Ti implants (Nobelpharma) were retrieved from 17 patients (despite remaining clinically stable). The authors measured approximately 84% direct bone-to-implant contact and approximately 80% average surface bone area in individual threads, as evaluated in a computerized morphometric system at the light microscopic level.[33]

Animal experimentation is addressing ways to improve the degree of osseointegration as measured by bone quantity at the bone-to-implant interface. Ti-6Al-4V implants were placed in the tibiae of Sprague-Dawley rats to determine whether prior treatment (of the implant) with fibroblast growth factor-1 (FGF-1) enhanced healing and bone response.[34] Animals were injected with a radiopharmaceutical imaging agent, technetium-99m-methylene diphosphonate (Tc-99m-MDP), which concentrates in bone in areas of higher osteoblastic activity. A histomorphometric analysis was carried out 2 weeks after implant placement and samples treated with FGF-1 demonstrated significantly greater amounts of bone (percent volume) and bone-to-implant contact adjacent to implants when compared to controls. Images of Tc-99m-MDP supported these findings by demonstrating a significantly greater uptake of Tc-99m-MDP adjacent to FGF-1-treated implants. Thus, this study showed that FGF-1 could increase bone production around implants in a rat model.[34]

Intermittent systemic administration of parathyroid hormone (PTH) increases bone formation by stimulating osteoblastic activity. Skripitz and Aspenberg addressed the question of how systemic PTH (1-34) administration influences the bony fixation of stainless steel screws over time.[35] Stainless steel screws were implanted in the tibiae of rats injected three times a week with a physiologic dose (60 μg/kg) of human PTH (1-34). The treatments lasted 1, 2, and 4 weeks, after which the animals were euthanized. Pull-out strength was used to measure the degree of fixation. At 2 and 4 weeks, PTH-treated animals showed significant increases in pull-out strength that reflects the mechanical properties of the bone within the screw threads. PTH also increased the fraction of metal surface having contact with bone without an intervening soft tissue layer. These results suggest that intermittent PTH treatment can enhance early implant fixation by enhancing the density of the surrounding bone and by increasing the implant-to-bone contact.[35]

7.2.5 DNA Microarrays: Possible Experimental Protocol to Identify Important Cellular Responses and Molecular Pathways of Osteoblasts Exposed to Dental Implant Interface

Numerous variables related to osseointegration determine the short- and long-term clinical success of dental implant treatments (Figure 7.3). One such variable is the bone cell response to a titanium-based metal or metal oxide surface. A greater understanding of the molecular interplay of osteoblasts and metal surface chemistry is needed to improve implant design. Also, a better knowledge of osteoblast gene up- and down-regulation may shed light on molecular pathways initiated during the early stages of osseointegration. This may lead to routine local and/or systemic delivery of biological molecules at the time of implant placement.

The study proposed here would address this aspect of implant and cell biology. DNA microarray analysis could be used to distinguish cell activities present in cultured osteoblasts contacting either c.p. Ti or Ti-6Al-4V and compared to osteoblasts cultured on an artificial collagen or fibronectin extracellular matrix. A working hypothesis for this experiment would be that phenotypic differences will be noted for osteoblasts in contact with the metal oxide surface. Such differences, as measured by the various parameters associated with osseointegration, may ultimately contribute to the different degrees of success or failure of implants. It is anticipated that the more clinically important molecular activities will be present for both c.p. Ti and Ti-6Al-4V, and absent for the cells grown on a collagen or fibronectin matrix.

Thus this protocol is aimed at identifying the key molecules and molecular signaling pathways involved in the very early stages of osseointegration. It is envisioned that particular molecules such as cytokines, growth factors, and/or bone-morphogenes may be up-regulated when osteoblasts are in

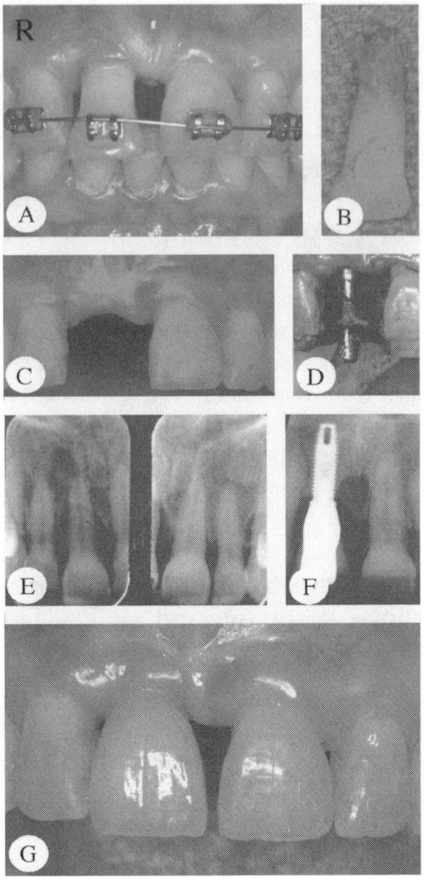

FIGURE 7.3
Clinical implant case of the maxillary right central incisor. The patient underwent orthodontic extrusion (A) prior to extraction. The tooth was stabilized in its final position for approximately 6 months prior to a nontraumatic extraction (B). Soft tissue healing 2 months after extraction (C). At the time of implant placement, a surgical guide was used (D). Radiographs were made prior to treatment (E) and after treatment was completed (F). Final clinical appearance of the patient (G).

direct contact with titanium or titanium alloy. Poor integration or failure of integration may be related to the inactivation of these particular proteins. If a certain molecule is essential to initial integration events, for example, a BMP (BMP-2 or BMP-7), it may be possible to engineer or coat implant surfaces with these molecules. Alternatively, a patient could be treated with locally delivered BMP-2 prior to implant placement. This treatment might hasten and/or improve bone adaptation to metal surfaces.

Microarrays entail the isolation, quantitation, and analysis of messenger RNAs from each sample. Microarrays can presently screen the entire human genome (for example, Affymetrix, Inc., Santa Clara, CA). A Medline and PubMed search performed indicated that the proposed project is indeed novel. The most similar project found was in part supported by Astra Tech AB and published by Mustafa and colleagues.[10] It used osteoblast cells grown on titanium discs to look at cell attachment (by scanning electron microscopy), proliferation ([3H]-thymidine uptake), and differentiation (osteocalcin synthesis and alkaline phosphatase activity). The work we propose would be more broadly based in that it would screen approximately 40,000 gene responses rather than only two. Microarrays are extremely powerful initial screening tools. Genes shown to be up- or down-regulated would subsequently become the foci of further investigations. The significance of this work would be the potential to rewrite current protocols of implant placement to specifically address the immediate molecular response to a bone–metal interface.

The choice of collagen and fibronectin as control substrate molecules is based on the following. The total skeletal mass consists of two components: (1) an organic unmineralized matrix that includes mainly type 1 collagen and comprises about one third of total bone weight and (2) the inorganic mineral phase of bone that constitutes about two thirds of the skeleton and is mainly composed of hydroxyapatite crystals (the main form of bone mineral).[36] The presence of the osteoblasts and the collagen extracellular matrix, however, precedes any mineral component of bone. Type I collagen can be used as a control substrate for these experiments.

Commercially pure human type I collagen can be purchased from Sigma-Aldrich Co. (St. Louis, MO, Catalogue #C5483). In solution (in sodium acetate buffer or weak acid), collagen can be applied to tissue culture plates, washed and dried, and then used as a substrate for cell growth. Fibronectin is an adhesion glycoprotein of ECM. Multiple domains of fibronectin show binding affinities to collagen, fibrin, heparin, and specific membrane receptors. The most notable domain, Arg–Gly–Asp (RGD), is recognized by integrins and mediates cell adhesion. Fibronectin is involved in widespread interactions and functions such as cell migration, cytoskeletal assembly, tyrosine phosphorylation, and metastasis. Human-derived fibronectin (Sigma-Aldrich, Catalogue #F2006) can be dissolved in 0.05M Tris buffered saline and applied to culture plasticware.

Human osteoblast cell line hFOB1.19 is well studied and can be purchased from the American Type Culture Collection (ATCC, Manassas, VA) for experiments.[9] This cell line was established by transfection of limb tissue obtained from a spontaneous miscarriage with the temperature-sensitive expression vector pUCSVtsA58 and the neomycin resistance expression vector pSV2-neo. Clones were selected in the presence of 0.6 mg/ml G418. Cells grown at a permissive temperature of 33.5°C exhibit rapid cell division. Little or no cell division occurs at a restrictive temperature of 39.5°C.

The cells have the ability to differentiate into mature osteoblasts expressing the normal osteoblast phenotype. At the restrictive temperatures, cell division is slowed, differentiation increases, and a more mature osteoblast phenotype is produced. The cells thus provide a homogenous, rapidly proliferating model system for studying normal human osteoblast differentiation, osteoblast physiology, hormonal, growth factor, and other cytokine effects on osteoblast function and differentiation. The recommended medium for hFOB1.19 cells is a 1:1 mixture of Ham's F12 medium and Dulbecco's modified Eagle's medium with 2.5 mM L-glutamine and 0.3 mg/ml G418 and 10% fetal bovine serum. Cells should be maintained at a temperature of 34°C.

Commercially pure titanium and Ti-6Al-4V discs must be prepared for this study. To extract the the quantities of mRNA needed for the microarray experiment two 3 × 10-cm tissue culture dishes are required for each experiment. The internal dimensions of the dishes are approximately 83 mm, so metal discs approximately 1 mm thick and 10 to 80 mm in diameter would be required. It is apparent from the literature that c.p. Ti or Ti-6Al-4V discs of many dimensions can be prepared from multiple sources including implant companies. For example, 16-mm Ti-6Al-4V discs were prepared by Biomet, Inc. (Warsaw, IN) for a study by Sinha and Tuan[16]; 22-mm Ti-6Al-4V discs by Zimmer (Warsaw, IN) for a study by Krause and colleagues[7]; 10 mm in diameter and 2.5 mm thick c.p. Ti discs were prepared by Astra Tech (Mölndal, Sweden) for a study by Nishio and colleagues[37]; and 15-mm c.p. Ti and Ti-6Al-4V discs of 1 mm thickness by Titanium International (Melbourne, Australia) for a study by Zreiqat and Howlett.[38]

The advantage of a larger disc (for example, 80 mm) would be that all cells grown in the culture dish would be in intimate contact with metal, which in turn would allow for the rapid removal of all the cells from culture and followed by rapid mRNA purification. Speed of cell manipulation is required to ensure a highly purified and nondegraded RNA result. A source for c.p.Ti and Ti-6Al-4V discs will have to be identified, and a dental implant manufacturer is preferred. Ideally, the metals will have to be machined with surface finishes similar to those of dental implants. In addition, if special chemical modifications are employed to create surface oxides with characteristics unique to an implant system, the same chemical treatments would be needed for the metal discs.

The final stage of this experimental protocol would be the DNA microarray analysis. The GeneChip® Human Genome U133 set is the most recent edition of DNA microarrays offered by Affymetrix, Inc. (as of February 2002). This two-chip set comprises 39,000 unique gene transcripts from the approximately 33,000 genes that create the human genome. This is the most comprehensive microarray coverage of human gene sequence information made available to the public domain to date. Protocols for microarray analysis vary. Affymetrix presently requests that approximately 20 μg of high quality total RNA for each experiment be purified and sent to its laboratories for analysis. This approach minimizes errors in experimental protocols and data interpretation, by allowing highly trained individuals to carry out RNA–DNA hybridization using very specialized and expensive equipment. Data from the chip analysis is returned to the investigator, along with computer software to aid in the interpretation of results. Gene microanalysis is an initial screening to identify differences in gene expression between experiment and control samples, and it is anticipated that data will provide many clues to gene activities that occur during osseointegration. Clearly, confirmation of findings will be needed by alternative genetic methodologies such as Northern and Western analysis or *in vivo* experimental protocols.

7.3 Proteomics as the Future

It is clear that array-based protein technologies will be essential for modern biological research, molecular diagnostics, and therapeutic development. Such technologies have the potential of providing functional analysis of perhaps tens of thousands of proteins simultaneously. Just as DNA microarray methods have established themselves over recent years, protein array-based methods are becoming prevalent within proteomics research. Novel protein biochips are under development in academic laboratories and biotechnology companies.[39-41]

Several complementary tools are available for proteome analysis including two-dimensional protein electrophoresis and mass spectrometry. Emerging technologies for proteome analysis include spotted-array-based methods and microfluidic devices.[40] Clearly some key limitations exist related to analysis of the generated data, and new computer software will be required to fully integrate proteomic information with information obtained from DNA sequences, open-reading frames, and mRNA expression profiles.

7.4 Conclusions

Available data suggest that biomaterial compositions and biomolecules influence the initial events of osseointegration, such as osteoblastic cell adhesion and spreading. Molecules such as the integrins coordinate intracellular molecular responses to the extracellular environment. These responses include signal transduction cascades that ultimately regulate cellular activities (such as gene transcription and translation, tissue morphogenesis, differentiation, and growth). In a study by Shah and colleagues, osteoblast cells grown on a Ti-6Al-4V substrate showed a more highly organized cytoskeletal network when compared to a cobalt–chrome–molydbenum alloy.[42]

Such differences in cytoskeletal arrangement suggest that different substrates elicit different molecular responses. Understanding how different substrates (or implant biomaterials) affect osteoblast morphologies, cellular properties, and molecular activities should ultimately provide important information that can be used to improve implant design, biocompatibility, and ultimately clinical success.

Acknowledgments

The authors would like to thank the organizers of the workshop on "Improving Bio-Implant Interface Interactions," and in particular, we would like to thank Siv Jamtøya and Drs. Jan Eirik Ellingsen and Staale Petter Lyngstadaas. We would also like to thank Astra Tech AB for financial and moral support and the National Institutes of Health for the academic freedom offered through its sponsored research programs. Michael Paine is grateful for grant DE13404 from the National Institute for Dental and Craniofacial Research.

We would like to also thank Pablo Bringas Jr. and Drs. Paul Krebsbach, Wen Luo, Kian Kar, and Michelle Ikoma for supplying all the images used to create the figures. The clinical case illustrated was a patient treated with a Nobelpharma implant at the Advanced Specialty Clinics of the University of Southern California by Drs. Kar and Ikoma under the supervision of Drs. Hessam Nowzari and Winston Chee. Finally, we would like to thank Caroline Paine for the many hours spent proofreading this manuscript. References 43 through 48 were included in the discussion but have not been cited in the text of this manuscript.

References

1. Budavari, S., *The Merck Index: An Encyclopedia of Chemicals, Drugs and Biologicals.*, 13th ed., Merck & Co., Inc., Whitehouse Station, NJ, 2001.
2. Dubrovinskaia, N.A. et al., Experimental and theoretical identification of a new high-pressure TiO_2 polymorph., *Phys. Rev. Lett.*, 87, 275501, 2001.
3. Dubrovinsky, L.S. et al., Materials science: the hardest known oxide, *Nature*, 410, 653, 2001.
4. Sul, Y.T. et al., Characteristics of the surface oxides on turned and electrochemically oxidized pure titanium implants up to dielectric breakdown: oxide thickness, micropore configurations, surface roughness, crystal structure and chemical composition, *Biomaterials*, 23, 491, 2002.
5. Lindhe, J., *Clinical Periodontology and Implant Dentistry*, 3rd ed., Munksgaard, Copenhagen, 1998.
6. Gronowicz, G. and McCarthy, M.B., Response of human osteoblasts to implant materials: integrin-mediated adhesion, *J. Orthop. Res.*, 14, 878, 1996.
7. Krause, A., Cowles, E.A., and Gronowicz, G., Integrin-mediated signaling in osteoblasts on titanium implant materials, *J. Biomed. Mater. Res.*, 52, 738, 2000.
8. Hendrich, C. et al., Testing of skeletal implant surfaces with human fetal osteoblasts, *Clin. Orthop.*, 394, 278, 2002.
9. Harris, S.A. et al., Development and characterization of a conditionally immortalized human fetal osteoblastic cell line, *J. Bone Miner. Res.*, 10, 178, 1995.
10. Mustafa, K. et al., Determining optimal surface roughness of $TiO_{(2)}$ blasted titanium implant material for attachment, proliferation and differentiation of cells derived from human mandibular alveolar bone, *Clin. Oral Implants. Res.*, 12, 515, 2001.

11. Brakebusch, C. et al., Genetic analysis of beta1 integrin function: confirmed, new and revised roles for a crucial family of cell adhesion molecules, *J. Cell Sci.*, 110, 2895, 1997.
12. Giancotti, F.G. and Ruoslahti, E., Integrin signaling, *Science*, 285, 1028, 1999.
13. Eliceiri, B.P., Integrin and growth receptor cross-talk, *Circ. Res.*, 89, 1104, 2001.
14. Chen, Q. et al., Integrin-mediated cell adhesion activates mitogen-activated protein kinases, *J. Biol. Chem.*, 269, 26602, 1994.
15. Schwartz, M.A., Schaller, M.D., and Ginsberg, M.H., Integrins: emerging paradigms of signal transduction, *Annu. Rev. Cell Dev. Biol.*, 11, 549, 1995.
16. Sinha, R.K. and Tuan, R.S., Regulation of human osteoblast integrin expression by orthopedic implant materials, *Bone*, 18, 451, 1996.
17. Zhidkova, N.I., Belkin, A.M., and Mayne, R., Novel isoform of beta-1 integrin expressed in skeletal and cardiac muscle, *Biochem. Biophys. Res. Commun.*, 214, 279, 1995.
18. von Bubnoff, A. and Cho, K.W., Intracellular BMP signaling regulation in vertebrates: pathway or network? *Dev. Biol.*, 239, 1, 2001.
19. Hollinger, J.O. et al., Therapeutic potential of bone morphogenetic proteins, *Expert. Opin. Investig. Drugs*, 10, 1677, 2001.
20. Kloos, D.U., Choi, C., and Wingender, E., The TGF-β–Smad network: introducing bioinformatic tools, *Trends Genet.*, 18, 96, 2002.
21. Uludag, H. et al., Characterization of rhBMP-2 pharmacokinetics implanted with biomaterial carriers in the rat ectopic model, *J. Biomed. Mater. Res.*, 46, 193, 1999.
22. Takahashi, K., Bone morphogenetic protein (BMP): from basic studies to clinical approaches, *Nippon Yakurig. Zasshi*, 116, 232, 2000.
23. Si, X., Jin, Y., and Yang, L., Induction of new bone by ceramic bovine bone with recombinant human bone morphogenetic protein 2 and transforming growth factor beta, *Int. J. Oral Maxillofac. Surg.*, 27, 310, 1998.
24. Franceschi, R.T. et al., Gene therapy for bone formation: *in vitro* and *in vivo* osteogenic activity of an adenovirus expressing BMP7, *J. Cell Biochem.*, 78, 476, 2000.
25. Heijl, L. et al., Enamel matrix derivative (EMDOGAIN) in the treatment of intrabony periodontal defects, *J. Clin. Periodontol.*, 9, 705, 1997.
26. Wennstrom, J.L. and Lindhe, J., Some effects of enamel matrix proteins on wound healing in the dento-gingival region, *J. Clin. Periodontol.*, 29, 9, 2002.
27. Gestrelius, S., Lyngstadaas, S.P., and Hammarstrom, L., Emdogain: periodontal regeneration based on biomimicry, *Clin. Oral Investig.*, 4, 120, 2000.
28. Schwartz, Z. et al., Porcine fetal enamel matrix derivative stimulates proliferation but not differentiation of preosteoblastic 2T9 cells, inhibits proliferation and stimulates differentiation of osteoblast-like MG63 cells, and increases proliferation and differentiation of normal human osteoblast NHOst cells, *J. Periodontol.*, 71, 1287, 2000.
29. Jiang, J. et al., Effects of enamel matrix derivative on gene expression of primary osteoblasts, *Oral Surg. Oral Med. Oral Pathol. Oral Radiol. Endodontol.*, 91, 95, 2001.
30. Kawana, F. et al., Porcine enamel matrix derivative enhances trabecular bone regeneration during wound healing of injured rat femur, *Anat. Rec.*, 264, 438, 2001.
31. Boyan, B.D. et al., Porcine fetal enamel matrix derivative enhances bone formation induced by demineralized freeze dried bone allograft *in vivo*, *J. Periodontol.*, 71, 1278, 2000.

32. Nystrom, E., Kahnberg, K.E., and Albrektsson, T., Treatment of the severely resorbed maxillae with bone graft and titanium implants: histologic review of autopsy specimens, *Int. J. Oral Maxillofac. Implants,* 8, 167, 1993.
33. Albrektsson, T. et al., Histologic investigations on 33 retrieved Nobelpharma implants, *Clin. Mater.,* 12, 1, 1993.
34. McCracken, M., Lemons, J.E., and Zinn, K., Analysis of Ti-6Al-4V implants placed with fibroblast growth factor 1 in rat tibiae, *Int. J. Oral Maxillofac. Implants,* 16, 495, 2001.
35. Skripitz, R. and Aspenberg, P., Early effect of parathyroid hormone (1-34) on implant fixation, *Clin. Orthop.,* 392, 427, 2001.
36. Green, J., The physicochemical structure of bone: cellular and noncellular elements, *Miner. Electrolyte Metab.,* 20, 7, 1994.
37. Nishio, K. et al., The effect of alkali- and heat-treated titanium and apatite-formed titanium on osteoblastic differentiation of bone marrow cells, *J. Biomed. Mater. Res.,* 52, 652, 2000.
38. Zreiqat, H. and Howlett, C.R., Titanium substrata composition influences osteoblastic phenotype: *in vitro* study, *J. Biomed. Mater. Res.,* 47, 360, 1999.
39. Lee, K.H., Proteomics: a technology-driven and technology-limited discovery science, *Trends Biotechnol.,* 19, 217, 2001.
40. Ezzell, C., Proteins rule, *Sci. Amer.,* April 2002, p. 40.
41. O'Donovan, C., Apweiler, R., and Bairoch, A., The human proteomics initiative (HPI), *Trends Biotechnol.,* 19, 178, 2001.
42. Shah, A.K. et al., High-resolution morphometric analysis of human osteoblastic cell adhesion on clinically relevant orthopedic alloys, *Bone,* 24, 499, 1999.
43. Shaama, F.A. et al., Titanium and stainless steel modify cytokine production in human osteoblasts, *J. Bone Min. Res.,* 11(S1), 167, 1996.
44. Cochran, D.L. et al., Evaluation of recombinant human bone morphogenetic protein-2 in oral applications including the use of endosseous implants: 3-year results of a pilot study in humans, *J. Periodontol.,* 71, 1241, 2000.
45. Fiorellini, J. P. et al., Effect on bone healing of bone morphogenetic protein placed in combination with endosseous implants: a pilot study in beagle dogs, *Int. J. Periodont. Res. Dent.,* 21, 41, 2001.
46. Skripitz, R. and Aspenberg, P., Implant fixation enhanced by intermittent treatment with parathyroid hormone, *J. Bone Joint Surg. Br.,* 83, 347, 2001.
47. Cummings, C.A. and Relman, D.A., Using DNA microarrays to study host-microbe interactions, *Emerg. Infect. Dis.,* 6, 513, 2000.
48. Fang, Y., Frutos, A.G., and Lahiri, J., Membrane protein microarrays, *J. Am. Chem. Soc.,* 124, 2394, 2002.

8

Biomedical Implant Surface Topography and Its Effects on Osteoblast Differentiation In Vitro*

Clark M. Stanford, Galen Schneider, Hiran Perinpanayagam, John C. Keller, and Ronald Midura

CONTENTS

8.1 Introduction 141
8.2 Methods and Materials 146
  8.2.1 *In Vitro* Assay 147
  8.2.2 RNA Extraction, Quantitation, and PCR 147
  8.2.3 Quantitative RT-PCR for Changes in Cbfa-1 and BSP Expression 148
  8.2.4 Quantitative Atomic Absorption Assay for Calcium 149
  8.2.5 Alkaline Phosphatase Assay 149
  8.2.6 Cell Expression (Matrix Product Production) 150
8.3 Results and Discussion 150
8.4 Summary 157
Acknowledgments 158
References 158

8.1 Introduction

The introduction of a dental implant into a prepared osteotomy initiates a cascade of wound healing events that under favorable conditions results in a mature haversian osseous interface. Since the commercial introduction of

* The information in this chapter was presented in part at the Improving Bio-Implant Interface Reactions Workshop, April 2002, University of Oslo, Norway.

0-8493-1474-7/03/$0.00+$1.50

machined surface dental implants, various empirical clinical approaches have been advocated to assure a consistent osseous interface. These approaches included surgical approaches to implant placement, loading protocols, postoperative care, and indications for prosthetic reconstruction (e.g., occlusal schemes to assure bone adaptation).

The relatively smooth surfaces characterized by machined surface implants achieved lower success rates in the posterior parts of the maxilla.[1] The goal of a number of current strategies is to provide enhanced osseous stability through microsurface-mediated events. These strategies can be divided into those that attempt to enhance the in-migration of new bone (osteoconduction) through changes in surface topography (surface roughness), biological means of manipulating the types of cells that grow onto the surface, and strategies to utilize the implant as a vehicle for local delivery of a bioactive coating (adhesion matrix or growth factor such as a bone morphogenetic protein or BMP) that may achieve osteoinduction of new bone differentiation along the implant surface.

Dental implants typically have one of three major types of macroretentive features to provide initial or primary stability during placement. These features include screw threads (tapped or self-tapping), solid body press-fit designs, and sintered bead technologies. These design features should allow bone to react to favorable compressive loading forces with adaptive modeling and remodeling responses.[2,3] Therefore, screw thread designs have been adapted to achieve compressive loading of the surrounding cortical or cancellous bone. Certain implant designs (ITI/Straumann, Institut Straumann AG, Waldenburg, Switzerland) use 15-degree cutting thread profiles that create mostly compressive versus shear interfacial stress.

Another common feature is the use of thread profiles having rounded tips (purported to reduce the shear forces at the tips). These thread designs appear to maintain bone in the compressive zone beneath the thread profile.[4-6] With the intent to improve initial bone stability, various implant designs also incorporate dual (or more) cutting thread profiles (with or without screw-based press-fits). Two sets of threads are cut at different locations in the osteotomy (across from each other) upon placement as a means to reduce initial stripping and thus improve primary implant stability (Mark III and Mark IV™, Nobel Biocare, Göteborg, Sweden). Still other thread designs (Microthread™, Astra Tech AB, Mölndal, Sweden) focus on reducing surrounding shear forces by reducing the height of the thread profile (reducing the contribution of any one thread) and increasing the number of threads per unit area of the implant surface.[7,8] This provides the added benefit of increasing the strength of the implant body by doubling the wall thickness of the implant body.[9]

Finally, orthopedic prostheses (femoral stems, pelvic acetabular caps, knee prostheses, etc.) have used various sintering technologies to create a mesh or structure of sintered beads as a surface for bone to grow into. The application of this technology to dentistry involved attempts to improve the success rates of short implants (<10 mm in length), which are associated with the highest failure rates.[1] At the University of Toronto, sintered bead technology led to the development of one commercially available implant system (Endopore™ Innova Corp., Toronto, Canada) that shows favorable clinical results (93 to 100% relative success after 3 to 5 years) with short implants (7.7 mm) even in the posterior maxilla.[10-19]

Various studies have also addressed the issue of surface roughness through various means of grit blasting followed by a surface etching or coating procedure. The techniques include titanium plasma spray (TPS),[20] abrasion (TiO_2 blasting or use of soluble abrasives), combinations of blasting and etching (e.g., Al_2O_3 with H_2SO_4/HCl),[20] thin apatite coatings,[21] or sintered beads.[16] Commercially available roughened devices using large grit-blasted and acid-etched surfaces (ITI/Straumann's SLA surfaces) have shown both laboratory and clinical evidence of elevated success rates in the area of the posterior maxilla.[20,22-25] The SLA surface is one example of a commercially available surface technology developed from animal studies (mini-pigs) using a range of surface topographies including electropolished commercially pure (c.p.) Ti, a range of roughened c.p. Ti surfaces, and a calcium phosphate-coated surface. This study revealed that a large grit-blasted surface cleaned with an acid-etching procedure achieved bone contact (50 to 60%) equivalent to the calcium phosphate-coated surface and was able to do so without the need for a soluble coating.[20]

Wong et al. looked at press-fit implants in trabecular bone sites in the minipig model over 12 weeks and characterized a near-linear increase in mechanical strength of the interface as a function of increasing roughness.[26] The role of the roughened surface is complex because the actual strength of bone contact against the titanium oxide surface is quite low (4 MPa or less) — weak enough that without surface topography (e.g., electropolished surfaces), little bone contact occurs.[27] Clinically, the combination of large grit-blasted and etched surfaces (ITI/Straumann's SLA surface) in a one-stage surgical procedure resulted in longer than 10-year cumulative survival rates of 96.2% (30.5% in the maxilla).[28]

An alternative commercially surface-etched implant design uses a combination of HCl and H_2SO_4 to create surface topography (Osseotite™, Implant Innovations, Palm Beach Gardens, FL). This alternative roughened surface appeared to have enhanced biomechanical strength in animal studies.[29] Data appear to favorably support elevated success rates in conventional two-stage protocols (delayed and early loading, e.g., 2 months after placement).[30-32] The continued application of a roughened surface topography appears to have become the current state of the art with new or modified products reflecting this increased interest.

The current clinical interest in surface technology begs the question whether true biological responses can be measured with these roughened surfaces as functions of individual cellular responses. In other words, are the favorable clinical responses simply a function of greater bone contact or can specific surface technologies influence the number of bone formative cells (osteoconduction), the type of cells present (osteoinduction), or the amount of bone cell expression and matrix elaboration per cell (osteopromotion)? Various studies have tried to address these issues using a variety of *in vitro* systems. For instance, the expression of matrix-related proteins such as alkaline phosphatase and type I collagen was enhanced on SLA surfaces.[33] The mechanism by which topography influences osteoblast expression may be mediated by the protein kinase A and PLA_2 signal transduction pathway.[34] The topography also influences subsequent expression of osteoblast-mediated cytokines and growth factors.

Most surface topographical features created on grit-blasted surfaces,* whether etched or not, may act as surface reservoirs on the ventral sides of the cells. This reservoir concept implies that matrix is secreted and assembled on the ventral side of a cell and that implant topography may have a primary effect on matrix structure. The changes in matrix structure would, in turn, influence cell adhesion, shape, and other factors leading to altered gene expression in the adherent osteoblastic cell layer on the implant surface. When relatively immature osteosarcoma cells (MG-63) are grown on roughened surfaces, increases in transforming growth factor-beta (TGF-β) and interleukin-1-beta (IL-1β) expression are observed.[35] These responses are prostaglandin-mediated and lead to decreased proliferation on rougher c.p. Ti surfaces along with increases in markers for differentiation (alkaline phosphatase activity and osteocalcin).[35]

Similar responses have also been described with primary cells derived from rat calvarial cells.[36,37] Interestingly, many of these features are seen to act through a phospholipase A2 pathway leading to a surface roughness-mediated increase in the expression of specific prostaglandins (e.g., PGE_2).[38] This suggests that osteoblasts have the capability to directly respond to cell shape changes induced by growth on roughened surfaces and/or the matrix deposited and oriented on roughened surfaces.[34]

As is typical in biomedical science, the story is rather more complex. Recent evidence indicates that the reduction in cell growth (and the corresponding increase in elaboration of an extracellular matrix) appears to occur through integrin-mediated signaling modulated by various hormones or cytokines.[34,36,39-41] Hormone-based modulation of cell response (e.g., with Vitamin D) to surface topography appears to elicit cross-talk activation of protein kinase A (PKA) and protein kinase C (PKC) major signal transduction pathways that converge on a central proliferation-controlling pathway for cell growth: the mitogen-activated protein (MAP) kinase pathway.[38] These *in vitro* studies emphasize how cell shape may influence cell interactions with implant surfaces and serve to highlight the complex interaction that connects how cells attach to a surface, transduce a signal, and then mediate and maintain a differentiated pathway.[39,42-45]

The ability to form an extracellular matrix that can undergo regulated mineralization is the ultimate phenotypic expression of osteogenic tissue. The maturation of this matrix and subsequent mineralization lead to its

* Most surface topographical features are less than 10 μm in diameter — a dimension that allows only cell processes to penetrate.

structural strength. Two patterns of mineral deposition on an extracellular matrix have been described. One is matrix vesicle-mediated mineral initiation and the second is heterogeneous nucleation of mineral crystals on a collagen scaffold. Both processes probably involve a role for Ca^{++} and collagen-binding noncollagenous glycoproteins.[46] Attention has been focused on a bone-specific glycoprotein known as bone sialoprotein (BSP), which nucleates hydroxyapatite formation *in vitro* and is localized at sites of early mineral formation in rat bone.[47-49]

Following the healing of the fibrin clot around an implant, a rapidly formed unorganized bone tissue is formed that is referred to histologically as "woven" bone. Relative to mature lamellar bone, woven bone is characterized by a higher cellularity, high content of BSP, lower levels of osteocalcin, and a less organized collagenous extracellular matrix. The ability of woven bone to form an intimate contact with a dental implant surface is modulated in part by the combination of matrix vesicle and collagen-mediated mineralization resulting in a mechanically stable matrix interface.[50]

When osteoblast cells interact with the matrix-coated implant surface, the resultant adhesion, migration, and differentiation events are modulated by surface topographical cues through changes in the assembled serum and mesenchymal-derived matrix components. A cell culture model capable of eliciting and biologically regulating the initiation of mineralization is a useful tool for understanding the role of surface topographical cues in altering states of differentiation and matrix expression in woven bone. The rat osteoblastic cell line UMR 106.01 BSP was isolated from an induced transplantable osteosarcoma and shares a number of phenotypic properties with osteoblasts. The similarities include morphological appearance,[51-53] responsiveness to calciotropic agents such as parathyroid hormone (PTH)[51,53-55] and 1,25-$(OH)_2$ vitamin D_3,[56] and a relatively high level of expression of cell surface alkaline phosphatase activity.[53,55]

Additionally, UMR cells synthesize several matrix proteins expressed by normal osteoblasts including type I collagen,[57] proteoglycans,[58,59] and BSP.[60] UMR cells are distinguished from primary osteoblasts by their relatively high expression level of the H-*ras* oncogene thought to induce the transformed states of these cells.[61] When transplanted into a host animal, UMR cells can form bone mineral trabeculae in ectopic sites demonstrating osteogenic properties.[52] The UMR cells also deposit a bioapatitic mineral into the culture environment upon exposure to organophosphates in a dose- and time-dependent fashion.[46] In studies evaluating the role of PTH, the biomineralization phenotype was shown to be reversibly inhibited at physiological doses of PTH. This effect was mediated in part through the PKA pathway.[62]

Within the body, the integration of an implant involves the recruitment of multipotential mesenchymal stem cells and their differentiation into mature osteoblasts.[63-67] The differentiation pathway of osteoblasts is marked by a number of extracellar matrix (ECM)-mediated events. These events signal both the pathway of differentiation within the maturing matrix and the way the matrix elicits signals within the matrix.[41,68,69] Ultimately, these signaling events lead to specific molecular events that act either in a permissive or inductive manner. Two specific transcription factors lead to the differentiation and maintenance of the osteoblast phenotype. These are core binding factor-1 (Cbfa-1)/RUNX2* and the recently described osterix (Osx).[70] Their expression appears necessary for the proper spatial and temporal development and maintenance of bone.

The formation of a mineralized matrix during osteogenesis and bone remodeling, cranio-facial development, osseous wound healing following surgery, and during integration of a dental implants involves the recruitment of multipotential mesenchymal stem cells and their progressive differentiation into osteoblasts.[67,72] The RUNX2/Cbfa-1 transcription factor is found in cells of osteoblast lineage and hypertrophic cartilage. It is regulated by growth factors such as BMP-7 and vitamin D, and binds to the osteoblast-specific *cis*-acting element (OSE2) promoter of the osteocalcin, BSP, and type I collagen genes.[71] The fatal homozygous cbfa1-deficient mutant mice (-/-) lack skeletons resulting from the failure to replace cartilage anlagen with bone.[73,74]

The heterozygous (+/-) state results in a condition similar to the human disease of cleidocranial dysplasia (malformed skeleton, supernumerary teeth, etc.). Cbfa-1 also functions postnatally by regulating the expression of bone extracellular matrix protein genes that encode for BSP, osteopontin, osteocalcin, and collagen-I.[75,76] Cbfa-1 plays an essential role in osteogenesis, osteoblast matrix formation, chondrocyte differentiation, and bone resorption by osteoclasts[77] and could therefore be a downstream target of integrin extracellular matrix adhesion-mediated signaling pathways.

Understanding the role of matrix-regulating factors and evaluating alteration in mineralization of the synthesized matrix may provide clues to normal bone healing and turnover and also how these processes occur around alloplastic materials placed into the body for prosthetic or reparative procedures.

The purpose of this chapter is to review recent *in vitro* work in the area of cell-mediated biomineralization as a model for woven bone formation and the impact of implant surface microtopography on alteration in osteoblast gene expression.

8.2 Methods and Materials

The studies reviewed in this chapter utilized an *in vitro* model in which a high density cell culture (or micromass) approach was used to maintain or elicit a differentiated phenotype in mammalian mesenchymal cellular studies.[78-85] For the purposes of laboratory studies of surface topography, disks of grade 2 unalloyed commercially pure titanium (ASTM F67) 15 mm in

* Cbfa-1 is a member of the Runt-related transcription factor family, RUNX2 (AML3/cbfa-1/PEBP2αB) and has recently been designated as RUNX2 by the Human Genome Organization's nomenclature committee.

diameter × 4 mm were machined and prepared to fit into standard 24-well sterile tissue culture plates.[78] Various laboratory titanium surface topographies were created for these studies. These included a machined surface topography (MS; acid-passivated 600-grit machine-surfaced c.p. Ti) and a surface polished with 1 micron diamond paste according to standard metallurgical methods for production of mirror-like surfaces.[78,86] A surface of c.p. passivated Ti grit-blasted with 50 micron Al_2O_3 particles was also included. These surfaces were used in a number of cell attachment and matrix expression studies.[86-89] Preparation and cleaning of the surfaces were performed as described.[36,78] As a reference control, cultures were also grown on standard tissue culture plastic.

8.2.1 *In Vitro* Assay

UMR 106.01 BSP cells were grown, passaged, and maintained in Eagle's minimum essential medium (EMEM) supplemented with nonessential amino acids, HEPES (20 mM, pH 7.2), fetal bovine serum (10%), and penicillin/streptomycin (25 μg per ml) as described.[46] In selective experiments, nonmineralizing subclones of the parental UMR BSP cell line, *UMR-UI* cells, were used as negative controls for mineralization.[41] Cultures of UMR 106.01 BSP cells (5000 cells per mm^2) were grown on prepared titanium surfaces for 72 hours prior to cell isolation and analysis. Replicates of each surface were evaluated (5 samples per trial) and each trial was repeated three times.

Cultures were plated and exogenous organophosphate added at 48 hours to induce mineralization. Control cultures on each surface were grown without the addition of exogenous phosphate. Outcome assessment was evaluated using multiplex polymerase chain reaction (PCR) and quantitative realtime PCR techniques.[90] Where appropriate, statistical analysis was performed with parametric ANOVA with a *post hoc* Tukey's multiple comparison analysis. Statistical significance was assumed at $\alpha = 0.05$.

8.2.2 RNA Extraction, Quantitation, and PCR

Total cell RNA was extracted separately from each culture using the RNeasy Mini Kit (Qiagen, Valencia, CA), according to manufacturer instructions. Briefly, the growth media were removed and the cultures rinsed in PBS. The cells were then resuspended in lysis buffer and homogenized by passage through a QIA shredder column. The homogenized lysate was then applied to the RNeasy column, rinsed repeatedly with a series of buffers, and eluted into RNase-free deionized water. The RNA extracts were stored at –20°C.

Aliquots of the RNA extracts were diluted in deionized water and measured for absorbance at 260 and 280 nm in a Lambda 20 Spectrophotometer (Perkin Elmer, Wellesley, MA). RNA concentration was then determined from the absorbance at 260 nm and RNA purity estimated from the ratio between the absorbances at 260 and 280 nm.

RUNX2/Cbfa-1 transcripts in the RNA extracts were detected with PCR amplification using Cbfa-1-specific primers.[91] The forward primer was designed to the first 22 bases at the 5′ terminus of the first exon in the Cbfa-1 gene.[92,93] The reverse primer was designed to 20 base pairs (bps) spanning the junction of exons 3 and 4. This primer pair generated a 655-bp amplicon from mouse and human osteoblast cell lines. They are calculated to generate a 688-bp product in rat osteoblasts due to a predicted 33-bp insert (11 amino acids) in the rat Cbfa-1 sequence.

To serve as a positive control for the RT-PCR reactions, the PCR amplification was also performed with glyceraldehyde 3-phosphate dehydrogenase (GAPDH)-specific primers designed to generate a 345-bp amplicon from exons 7 and 8 of the rat sequence. To ensure that the PCR products were from mRNA-generated cDNA, and not genomic DNA, both primer pairs were designed to span separate exons.

8.2.3 Quantitative RT-PCR for Changes in Cbfa-1 and BSP Expression

Real-time PCR primers and probes were designed with Primer Express software (Perkin Elmer) from 294 bps of known rat sequence that corresponded to exons 1 and 2 of the Cbfa-1 gene.[93] See Table 8.1. The Cbfa-1 primers were designed to span the junction of exons 1 and 2 and generate an 80-bp PCR product. The probe was designed to overlay the exon junction. The DNA probe was then modified with the 5′-reporter dye FAM (6-carboxyfluorescein) and the 3′-quencher dye TAMRA (6-carboxy-N,N,N′,N′-tetramethylrhodamine).

The TaqMan Ribosomal RNA Control Reagents Kit (Perkin Elmer) was used to detect 18S ribosomal RNA as an endogenous control. The proprietary primer and probe sequences are reportedly conserved in a diverse group of eukaryotes, including humans, mice, and rats. The TaqMan probe was modified with the 5′-reporter dye VIC and the 3′-quencher dye TAMRA.

RNA extracts from triplicate samples of each surface were analyzed (each in triplicate) by real-time RT-PCR with the TaqMan Gold RT-PCR Kit (Perkin Elmer), according to manufacturer instructions (DNA Core Facility, University of Iowa). The RNA was reverse transcribed into cDNA with random hexamers and recombinant Moloney murine leukemia virus reverse transcriptase (RT) at 48°C for 30 minutes. The RT reactions were performed in a GeneAmp PCR System 2400 (Perkin Elmer).

The Cbfa-1 target and the endogenous rRNA control were amplified by multiplex PCR with AmpliTaq Gold DNA polymerase. The thermal cycling

TABLE 8.1

PCR Primer Sequences

Cbfa1 (688bp)	5′-ATGCTTCATTCGCCTCACAAAC-3′	5′-CTACAACCTTGAAGGCCACG-3′
BSP (766bp)	5′-ATAGAAGAATCAAAGCAGAGG-3′	5′-GCAGTGTTGTACTCGTTGCC-3′
GAPDH (345bp)	5′-AGATCCACAACGGATACATT-3′	5′-TCCCTCAAGATTGTCAGCAA-3′

parameters were 50°C for 2 minutes to activate AmpErase UNG and 95°C for 10 minutes to activate AmpliTaq Gold DNA polymerase, followed by 40 cycles of 95°C for 15 seconds and 60°C for 1 minute. The real-time PCR reactions were performed in 96-well optical reaction plates (Perkin Elmer) in an ABI Prism 7700 sequence detection system (Perkin Elmer).

During the PCR reactions, the associated TaqMan probes were cleaved by DNA polymerase 5′ nuclease activity which released the 5′-reporter dye (FAM or VIC) from the effects of the 3′-quencher dye (TAMRA). Amplification of the PCR reactions during each cycle caused an increase in reporter dye release. This increase in fluorescence intensity from FAM (Cbfa-1) and VIC (rRNA) was then measured by the ABI Prism 7700.

From the real-time RT-PCR data, a logarithmic plot of the increase in fluorescence intensity versus cycle number was analyzed to determine the linear range of amplification. Within this range, a threshold level above background fluorescence emission was chosen. The fractional cycle number (Ct) at which the fluorescence intensity reached this threshold within the linear range of amplification was calculated for each dye (FAM and VIC) in each reaction tube. These data were used to calculate the relative steady state levels of Cbfa-1 mRNA in the original extracts by the *Comparative Method of Relative Quantitation in Multiplex Reactions* approach (ABI Prism 7700, User Bulletin 2, Perkin Elmer). In each reaction tube, Cbfa-1 levels were normalized to 18S rRNA by calculating ΔCt, where ΔCt = (FAM)Ct – (VIC)Ct. A constant was then subtracted to yield ΔΔCt, where ΔΔCt = ΔCt – k (k was adjusted to approximate the lowest ΔCt value). The relative levels of Cbfa-1 were then calculated as $2^{(-\Delta\Delta Ct)}$.

8.2.4 Quantitative Atomic Absorption Assay for Calcium

After exposure to the respective conditions, cultures were washed twice with saline followed by extraction of cell layer mineral with a 24-hour exposure to 0.6 N HCl in 0.02 M PBS (Ca^{++}- and Mg^{++}-free). Aliquots of extracted cell layer or media (50 µl) were added to a solution of 2.5% w/v lanthanum oxide in 25% v/v HCl followed by atomic absorption analysis of calcium content using a Perkin Elmer 2380 atomic absorption spectrophotometer optimized to 422.7 nm, slit width = 0.7 nm. The atomic absorption lamp (0.125 nmol per mL detection limit) was optimized with a calcium standard curve (2.5 to 1200 nmol per mL) using serial dilutions of calcium atomic absorption standard (Sigma Chemical Co., St. Louis, MO). Values were then normalized to total DNA content.

8.2.5 Alkaline Phosphatase Assay

Alkaline phosphatase, while not bone-specific, serves as a useful marker for mineralization-related activity. Enzyme activity was obtained from sonicated membrane preparations derived from cells cultured to 72 hours using the method described.[78]

8.2.6 Cell Expression (Matrix Product Production)

Distribution of matrix components within cultures was localized using an indirect immunolabeling protocol.[94] Monoclonal antibodies for BSP [WVID1(9C5)] and a negative control antibody (*Drosophila* even-skipped protein 3C10) were obtained through the University of Iowa's Developmental Studies Hybridoma Bank. Antigen location was determined by secondary labeling with 1:300 dilution FITC goat antimouse IgG. Following preparation of slides, planar images were collected on a BioRad confocal microscope. Digital image analysis was then performed using NIH Image Alpha-9 shareware.

8.3 Results and Discussion

UMR 106.01 BSP cells exhibit an unusual property of rapid mineralization within the *in vitro* environment. For instance, when either monolayer or high density (micromass) cultures were exposed to organophosphate, a rapid formation of bioapatitic mineral occurred (Figure 8.1).[46]

When studies were performed using a 48-hour growth period with standard growth medium followed by a change in medium and addition of an organophosphate (phospho-ser, phospho-thr, or β-glycerophosphate), a dose-dependent increase in atomic absorption-detectable calcium levels was

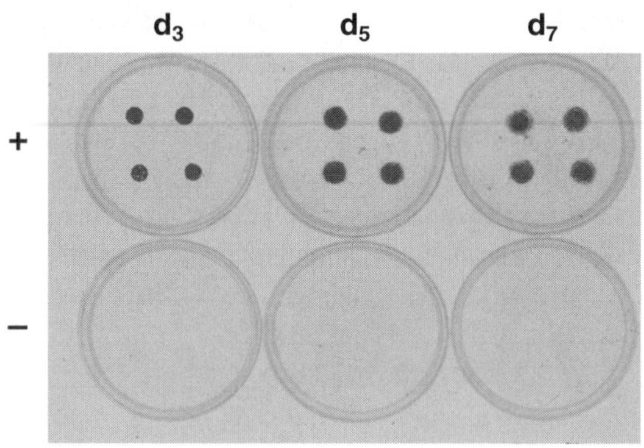

FIGURE 8.1
UMR 106.01 BSP micromass cultures (5000 cells/mm^2) grown for 3, 5, or 7 days prior to 24-hour exposure to an organophosphate (5 mM β-glycerophosphate). Cultures (EMEM + 10% serum + ascorbate) were grown on tissue culture plastic and stained with alizarin red S.

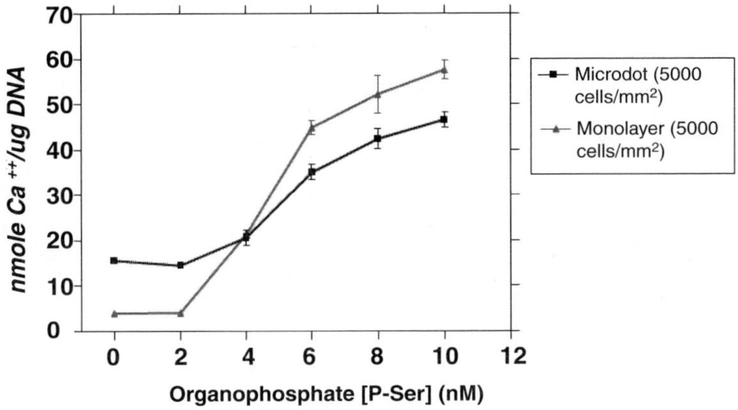

FIGURE 8.2
Dose-dependent increase in bioapatitic mineral as a function of organophosphate addition. Cultures (n = 12) were measured with atomic absorption for calcium content at 24 hours following addition of phospho-ser.

observed (Figure 8.2). Mineral formation occurred rapidly with a half maximal formation by 12 hours following the addition of organophosphate (Figure 8.3).[46] In this culture model, mineralization is initiated with the release of inorganic phosphate (tightly regulated phosphate concentration with an ED_{50} ~4 to 5 mM). Calcium content and release affect the amount of total bioapatitic mineral formed per unit of time rather than initiating the process.[3,45,46] The mineral was positive to alizarin red S stain.

Atomic absorption analysis and x-ray diffraction studies demonstrated the presence of a bioapatitic phase. One very important aspect of this culture model is that the initiation of apparent mineralization is very sensitive to

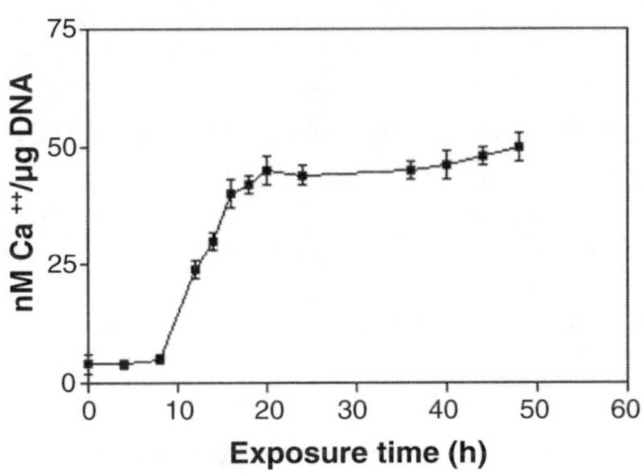

FIGURE 8.3
Calcium content increased over the first 24 hours following addition of the organophosphate.

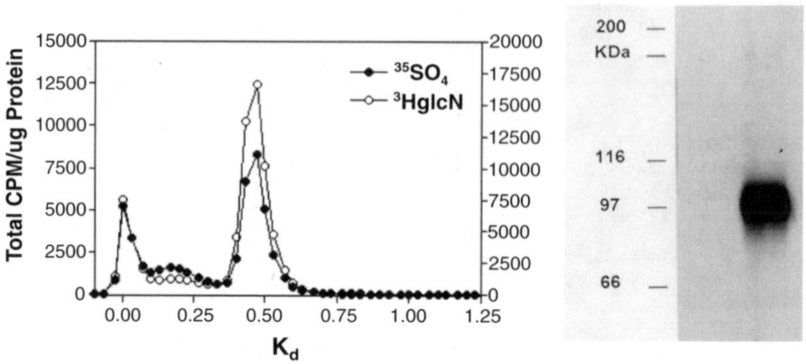

FIGURE 8.4
Bone sialoprotein is highly expressed in UMR cultures. Metabolic labeling with $^{35}SO_4$/^{3}H glucosamine was performed for 24 hours followed by extraction, batch anion exchange with Q-Sepharose, and the bound fraction chromatographically separated on a Superose-6 FPLC column. The middle peak (K_d = 0.5) provides a single band upon Western blotting with the monoclonal antibodies to BSP (Wv1D1, Hybridoma Studies Bank, University of Iowa).

both the dose and presence of organophosphate. The mineralization response is very sensitive to inhibitors of alkaline phosphatase (dose-dependent decrease with levamisole) and this mineralization response is probably related to an overexpression of BSP by this cell line (Figure 8.4). The culture model is limited in its application to studies that deal only with hormonal, cytokine, or cellular transduction processes that are essentially matrix-dependent because the responses occur prior to the elaboration of an extensive extracellular matrix. The expression appears to be mediated through the deposit of matrix vesicles into the pericellular environment.[46] The culture model acts as one approach to understanding how cell shape can be altered upon adhesion to topographically enhanced surfaces and how the direct adhesion events can alter short-term phenotypic outcomes (an important one is control of the initiation steps leading to biomineralization).

In order to study the effect of surface topography on cell expression, three different laboratory-based titanium surface topographies were used for a range of studies (Figure 8.5).[45,78,86] For instance, smooth-surfaced topographies are created with metallurgical polishing and 1-μm diamond paste creates a mirror-like surface with surface topographical features on the order of Ra = 6.3 nm and Rms (Rq) = 11.35 nm using atomic force microscopy (AFM).

A machined implant surface configuration was prepared by polishing with 600-grit Al_2O_3 papers, followed by thorough cleaning and nitric acid passivation.[78] This process produced a relatively rougher surface with uniform parallel surface topographical features defined as Ra = 160.8 nm and Rms (Rq) = 189.6 nm. A relatively rough surface topography was prepared by grit blasting a grade 2 c.p. Ti surface (Al_2O_3, 50 μm) under standard time and air pressure conditions. The surfaces were then cleaned and acid passi-

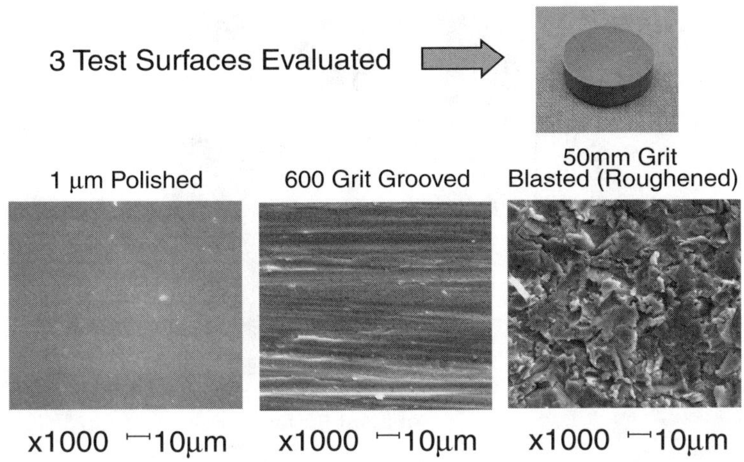

FIGURE 8.5
Scanning electron microscopy of three titanium test surfaces: a 1-µm highly polished surface, a parallel grooved surface created by polishing with 600-grit metallurgical papers, and a grit-blasted surface created with 50-µm diameter Al_2O_3. All surfaces were prepared, nitric acid passivated, and sterilized. (*Source:* Stanford, C.M. et al., *J. Dent. Res.*, 73, 1061, 1994. With permission.)

vated following ASTM standards. Topographical features measured had a peak height of Ra = 236.9 nm and Rms (Rq) = 295.4 nm.

When cell cultures are plated on the titanium surfaces and mineralization is assessed at 24 hours, the grit-blasted surfaces elicit a higher level of alizarin red S staining (a surrogate marker for calcium precipitation) relative to the 600-grit machined implant surface (Figure 8.6). These observations suggest that surface topography may influence one aspect of mineralization. In order to assess this possibility, a study of bone matrix expression was performed.

Bone matrix consists of a collagenous scaffold interlaced with noncollagenous proteins that may influence mineral formation.[40,41,46,67,95–98] One of these glycoproteins, bone sialoprotein (BSP), initiates hydroxyapatite nucleation when the protein is bound to a solid-phase agarose gel system.[48,99] Further, the presence of BSP has been localized specifically within mineralized tissues and osteoid matrix.[49,100,101] At the ultrastructural level, BSP has been localized within the early mineral accretions deposited in osteoids and near the basal surfaces of osteoblasts.[49]

UMR 106.01 BSP cells produce relatively large amounts of BSP *in vitro*.[60] Studies demonstrated that the culture model secretes BSP into the media phase at low cell densities and appears to localize the calcium-binding protein to a layer immediately above the culture surface or within the first layers of cells. Studies with the culture model have shown that the cells can detect surface cues (probably through changes in cell shape and cell

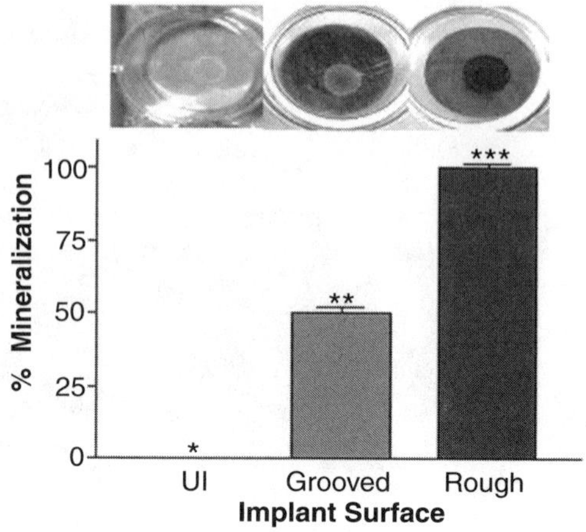

FIGURE 8.6
Osteoblasts plated at high density on grit-blasted surfaces elicited greater (p = <0.001) mineralization than the 600-grit grooved surfaces as shown by alizarin red S staining.

adhesion), resulting in greater levels of steady-state messages for BSP (Figures 8.7 and 8.8) and enhanced deposition in the cell layer (Figure 8.9) in a pattern similar to that observed in a nontransformed mandibular bovine osteoblast culture model.[40,94,102]

Since BSP expression (steady-state message and protein level) appears responsive to topographical cues, studies were performed to determine whether cellular differentiation was also influenced by surface topography.

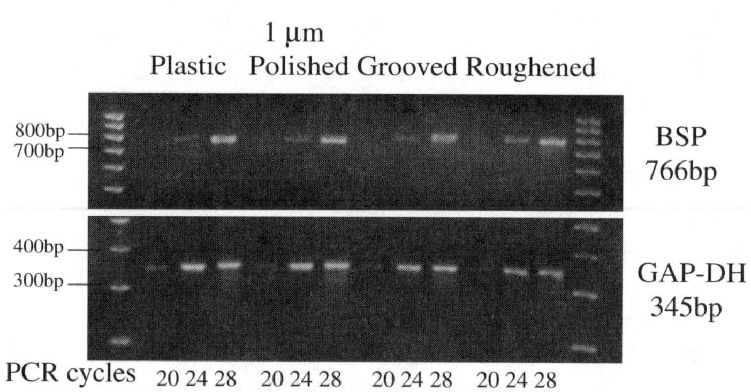

FIGURE 8.7
Primers for RT-PCR to bone sialoprotein (BSP) and glyceraldehyde 3-phosphate dehydrogenase (GAPDH) were used to demonstrate single-band amplicon product on *in vitro* laboratory surfaces consisting of tissue culture plastic or c.p. Ti disks polished to a mirror-smooth surface (1 μm polished), grooved in a pattern similar to a machined surface (600 g), or roughened using a 50-μm diameter Al_2O_3 grit-blasting procedure. Osteoblast micromass cultures were grown (5000 cells per mm^2) for 72 hours prior to RNA extraction and cDNA synthesis.

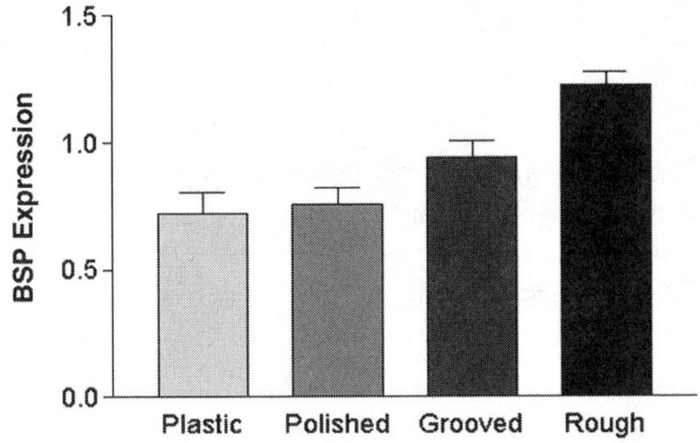

FIGURE 8.8
Steady-state mRNA for BSP was quantified by digital imaging of ethidium bromide staining. Steady-state message for bone sialoprotein was elevated in micromass cultures (5000 cells per mm^2) as compared to the housekeeping gene GAPDH when osteoblast cultures were grown on the c.p. Ti surface.

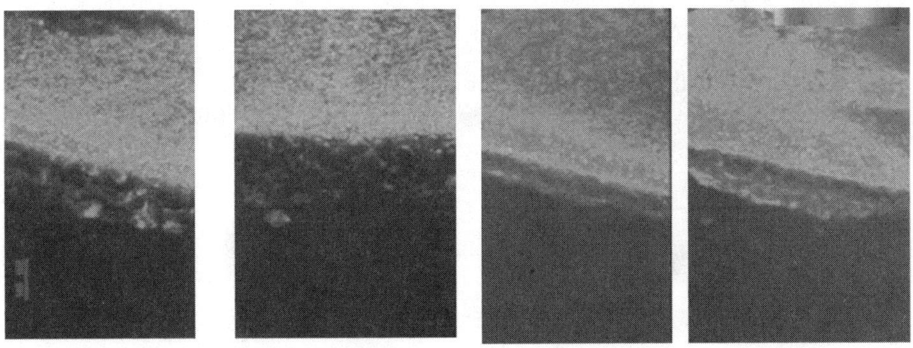

FIGURE 8.9
(See color insert.) Immunofluorescent labeling for bone sialoprotein (BSP). Cultures were grown for 72 hours and frozen-embedded. Embedded cultures were removed and cytosectioned. Sections were then labeled with a primary monoclonal antibody to BSP followed by secondary labeling with 1/300 FITC goat antimouse IgG. Cultures were grown on tissue culture plastic (TCP) or on the prepared c.p. Ti surfaces. BSP labeling occurred within a region of the micromass culture above the layer of cells directly in contact with the substratum.

In the past few years, significant strides have been made in understanding specific transcription factors that influence the differentiation cascade leading to the osteoblast pathway and the transcription factor expression needed to maintain the differentiated state.[71,103-109] Members of the RUNX2 family (AML3, Cbfa-1, and PEBP2αB) express an osteoblast- and hypertrophic chondrocyte-specific transcription factor that binds to the OSE-2 specific regions of target genes (e.g., osteocalcin, BSP, and osteopontin), leading to enhanced downstream promoter activity of the bone-related gene product.

An additional transcription factor (OSX) reported by Crombrugghe's group at M.D. Anderson Cancer Center helped to clarify the distinct role of RUNX2 in the osteoblast and chondrocyte pathways.[70] It appears that both RUNX2 and OSX expression (acting apparently downstream of RUNX2) are necessary for expression of type I collagen, BSP, and osteocalcin. The lack of expression of OSX appears to lead to the chondrogenic pathway.[70]

One aspect of RUNX2 expression has been the observation of different isoforms characterized by different groups.[110-113] This observation adds an additional layer of complexity since it suggests that RUNX2 regulation may be regulated at both the transcriptional and post-translational levels (by phosphorylation) and by means of proteolysis,[110] and implies a complex hierarchy of control over the osteoblast differentiation pathway.

Our laboratory evaluated the upstream RUNX2 N-terminal isoform (isoform 1 with 5′ side within exon 1) and a downstream isoform (isoform 3 with 5′ side within exon 3, a region within the conserved *runt* DNA-binding domain) based on the work of Xiao et al. (Figure 8.10).[91,93,102] The N-terminal isoform (isoform 1) demonstrates levels of expression associated with biomineralization in the UMR culture model (Figure 8.11).[91]

Elevated levels of mineralization are associated with higher levels of N-terminal isoform expression, whereas isoform 3 demonstrates no difference

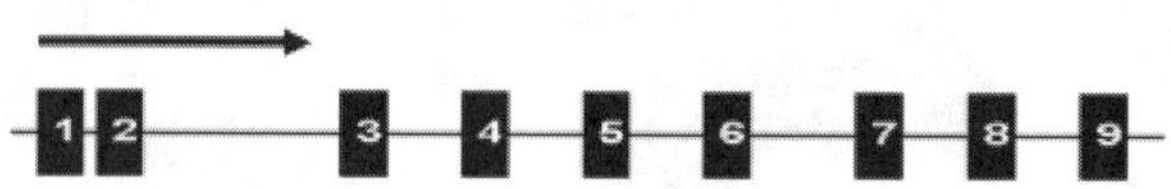

1 ATGCTTCATTCGCCTCACAAACAACCACAGAACCACAAGTGCGGTGCAAA

51 CTTTCTCCAGGAGGACAGCAAGGGGGCCCTGGTGTTTAAATGGTTAATCT

101 CTGCAGGTCACTACCAGCCACCGAGACCAACCGAGTCAGTGAGTGCTCTG

Forward Primer

Exon 1

151 AGCACAGTCCATGCAGTAATATTTAAGGCTGCAAGCAGTATTTACAACAG

TaqMan Probe **Reverse Primer**

201 AGGGCACAAGTTCTATCTGGAAAAAAAAGGAGGGACTATGGCGTCAAACA

Exon 2

251 GCCTCTTCAGTGCAGTGACACCGTGTCAGCAAAACTTCTTTTGG------

FIGURE 8.10

For the purpose of detecting different forms of RUNX2/cbfa-1 in the culture model, two sets of real-time PCR primers were made. Isoform 1 5′ primer started in exon 1, whereas the 5′ primer of isoform 3 started in exon 3.

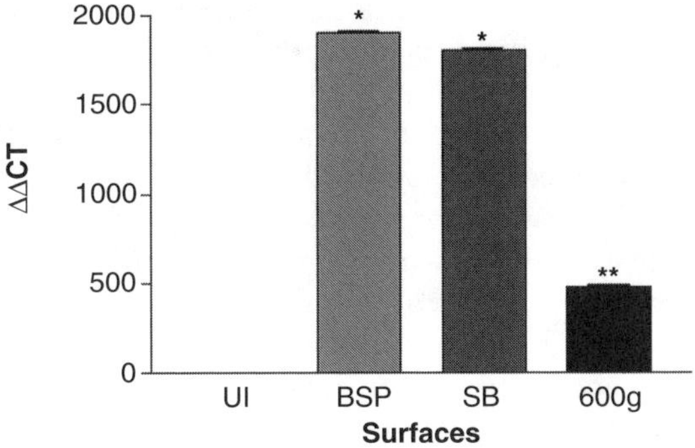

FIGURE 8.11
Expression of RUNX2/cbfa-1 isoform 1 in UMR 106.01 BSP micromass cultures (5000 cells per mm^2) was elevated on the grit-blasted surface (SB) relative to the machined (600 g) surface.

with organophosphate exposure. One interpretation for altered Cbfa-1 expression as a function of surface roughness may be changes in cell shape and subsequent alteration in the assembly of focal adhesion complexes.[39] Xiao et al. (1998) suggested osteoblasts utilize the collagen integrin receptor α-2 integrin subunit as an important component in regulating the association of the RUNX2 gene product binding to the osteocalcin and BSP promotor elements (OSE2).[114] Interestingly, recent data also suggest that assembly of focal adhesions and subsequent activation of focal adhesion kinase (FAK) may also play an important role in the processes leading to mineralization.[94]

8.4 Summary

The ability to utilize *in vitro* approaches is an important means to evaluate how cells interact with topographical surfaces. Given the wide variety of culture models (and outcomes obtained), it is important to understand the limitations and advantages each model provides. For instance, comparing the UMR model to normal osteoblastic cultures involves a number of important distinctions. First, the timeframe of mineral formation is shorter in UMR cultures than in primary cultures. This difference is best explained by the UMR system's lack of the extended proliferative and differentiation stages exhibited by primary culture systems. UMR cells manifest a fully differentiated phenotype and appear constitutively competent to produce apatitic mineral when they reach a confluent state *in vitro*.

Second, UMR cells produce apatitic mineral without necessarily establishing the *in vitro* nodules of multicellularity characteristic of primary-derived cells.[115] In primary osteoblastic culture systems, nodule formation typically represents the clonal proliferation of osteogenic cells from a heterogeneous population of primary cells. The lack of a requisite nodular morphology for mineralization in UMR cultures is likely the result of the uniform expression of a mature osteoblast-like phenotype in this cell line. However, UMR cells require a confluent state to generate a substantial calcification response implying a role for cell–cell contact in the mineralization process.

The biomedical interest in implant surfaces and the role they play in regulating osteoblast differentiation are important to the clinical predictability of developing new, innovative material surfaces. Utilizing screening assays with stable osteoblast culture lines is useful, especially as a model to define molecular events that alter gene expression and possible differentiation pathways of maturing mesenchymal cells that occur on the biomaterial surface.

Acknowledgments

The authors would like to thank Rebecca Zaharias, Kevin Holtman, Matt Clegg, and Chad Schwitters for their dedicated and hard work. These studies were supported by the U.S. National Institutes of Health (P30-DE10126–09, K1600175–14, and P60-DE13076), the Roy J. Carver Charitable Trust, and the ITI Foundation for the Promotion of Oral Implantology, Switzerland (209/2001).

References

1. Lindh, T. et al., A meta-analysis of implants in partial edentulism, *Clin Oral Implants Res.*, 9, 80, 1998.
2. Stanford, C.M., Biomechanical and functional behavior of implants, *Adv. Dent. Res.*, 13, 88, 1999.
3. Stanford, C.M. and Brand, R.A., Toward an understanding of implant occlusion and strain adaptive bone modeling and remodeling, *J. Prosth. Dent.*, 81, 553, 1999.
4. Schroeder, A. et al., The reactions of bone, connective tissue, and epithelium to endosteal implants with titanium-sprayed surfaces, *J. Maxillofac. Surg.*, 9, 15, 1981.
5. Schroeder, A. and Buser, D.A., ITI system: basic and clinical procedures, *Shigaku Odontol.*, 77 (spec.), 1267, 1989.
6. Schroeder, A. et al., *Oral Implantology Basics: ITI Hollow Cylinder System*, 2nd ed., Thieme, New York, 1996.
7. Hansson, S. and Norton, M., The relation between surface roughness and interfacial shear strength for bone-anchored implants: a mathematical model, *J. Biomech.*, 32, 829, 1999.
8. Hansson, S., The implant neck: smooth or provided with retention elements: a biomechanical approach, *Clin. Oral Implants Res.*, 10, 394, 1999.

9. Binon, P.P., Implants and components: entering the new millennium, *Int. J. Oral Maxillofac. Implants*, 15, 76, 2000.
10. Deporter, D.A. et al., A clinical and radiographic assessment of a porous-surfaced, titanium alloy dental implant system in dogs, *J. Dent. Res.*, 65, 1071, 1986.
11. Deporter, D.A. et al., A histological assessment of the initial healing response adjacent to porous-surfaced, titanium alloy dental implants in dogs, *J. Dent. Res.*, 65, 1064, 1986.
12. Lowenberg, B.F. et al., Migration, attachment, and orientation of human gingival fibroblasts to root slices, naked and porous-surfaced titanium alloy discs, and Zircalloy 2 discs *in vitro*, *J. Dent. Res.*, 66, 1000, 1987.
13. Deporter, D.A. et al., A histological comparison in the dog of porous-coated vs. threaded dental implants, *J. Dent. Res.*, 69, 1138, 1990.
14. Pilliar, R.M., Dental implants: materials and design, *J. Assoc. Dent. Can.*, 56, 857, 1990.
15. Pilliar, R.M. et al., Dental implant design: effect on bone remodeling, *J. Biomed. Mater. Res.*, 25, 467, 1991.
16. Deporter, D.A. et al., A prospective clinical study in humans of an endosseous dental implant partially covered with a powder-sintered porous coating: 3- to 4-year results, *Int. J. Oral Maxillofac. Implants*, 11, 87, 1996.
17. Vaillancourt, H., Pilliar, R.M., and McCammond, D., Factors affecting crestal bone loss with dental implants partially covered with a porous coating: a finite element analysis, *Int. J. Oral Maxillofac. Implants*, 11, 351, 1996.
18. Pilliar, R.M., Overview of surface variability of metallic endosseous dental implants: textured and porous surface-structured designs, *Implant Dent.*, 7, 305, 1998.
19. Pilliar, R.M. et al., The endopore implant-enhanced osseointegration with a sintered porous-surfaced design, *Oral Health*, 88, 61, 1998.
20. Buser, D. et al., Influence of surface characteristics on bone integration of titanium implants: a histomorphometric study in miniature pigs [comments], *J. Biomed. Mater. Res.*, 25, 889, 1991.
21. Vercaigne, S. et al., Histomorphometrical and mechanical evaluation of titanium plasma-spray-coated implants placed in the cortical bone of goats, *J. Biomed. Mater. Res.*, 41, 41, 1998.
22. Buser, D. et al., Tissue integration of one-stage implants: three-year results of a prospective longitudinal study with hollow cylinder and hollow screw implants, *Quintessence Int.*, 25, 679, 1994.
23. Buser, D. et al., Long-term stability of osseointegrated implants in bone regenerated with the membrane technique: 5-year results of a prospective study with 12 implants, *Clin. Oral Implants Res.*, 7, 175, 1996.
24. Buser, D., Belser, U.C., and Lang, N.P., The original one-stage dental implant system and its clinical application, *Periodontology*, 17, 106, 2000.
25. Cochran, D.L., A comparison of endosseous dental implant surfaces, *J. Periodontol.*, 70, 1523, 1999.
26. Wong, M. et al., Effect of surface topology on the osseointegration of implant materials in trabecular bone, *J. Biomed. Mater. Res.*, 29, 1567, 1995.
27. Brunski, J.B., Puleo, D.A., and Nanci, A., Biomaterials and biomechanics of oral and maxillofacial implants: current status and future developments, *Int. J. Oral Maxillofac. Implants*, 15, 15, 2000.

28. Buser, D. et al., Clinical experience with one-stage, non-submerged dental implants, *Adv. Dent. Res.*, 13, 153, 1999.
29. Klokkevold, P.R. et al., Osseointegration enhanced by chemical etching of the titanium surface: a torque removal study in the rabbit, *Clin. Oral Implants Res.*, 8, 442, 1997.
30. Lazzara, R.J. et al., A human histologic analysis of osseotite and machined surfaces using implants with two opposing surfaces, *Int. J. Periodont. Restor. Dent.*, 19, 117, 1999.
31. Lazzara, R.J. et al., A prospective multicenter study evaluating loading of osseotite implants two months after placement: one-year results, *J. Esthet. Dent.*, 10, 280, 1998.
32. Grunder, U. et al., Evaluating the clinical performance of the Osseotite implant: defining prosthetic predictability, *Compend. Contin. Educ. Dent.*, 20, 628, 1999.
33. Davies, J.E., Mechanisms of endosseous integration, *Int. J. Prosthodont.*, 11, 391, 1998.
34. Boyan, B.D. et al., Surface roughness mediates its effects on osteoblasts via protein kinase A and phospholipase A2, *Biomaterials,* 20, 2305, 1999.
35. Batzer, R. et al., Prostaglandins mediate the effects of titanium surface roughness on MG63 osteoblast-like cells and alter cell responsiveness to 1-α-25-(OH)2D3, *J. Biomed. Mater. Res.*, 41, 489, 1998.
36. Lohmann, C.H. et al., Surface roughness modulates the response of MG63 osteoblast-like cells to 1,25-(OH)(2)D(3) through regulation of phospholipase A(2) activity and activation of protein kinase A, *J. Biomed. Mater. Res.*, 47, 139, 1999.
37. Lohmann, C.H. et al., Maturation state determines the response of osteogenic cells to surface roughness and 1,25-dihydroxyvitamin D3, *J. Bone Miner. Res.*, 15, 1169, 2000.
38. Schwartz, Z. et al., Osteoblast response to titanium surface roughness and 1 alpha dihydroxy Vitamin D is mediated through the mitogen activated protein (MAP) kinase pathway, *J. Biomed. Mater. Res.*, 56, 417, 2001.
39. Schneider, G. and Burridge, K., Formation of focal adhesions by osteoblasts adhering to different substrata, *Exp. Cell Res.*, 214, 264, 1994.
40. Schneider, G.B., Whitson, S.W., and Cooper, L.F., Restricted and coordinated expression of beta3-integrin and bone sialoprotein during cultured osteoblast differentiation, *Bone,* 24, 321, 1999.
41. Schneider, G.B., Zaharias, R., and Stanford, C., Osteoblast integrin adhesion and signaling regulate mineralization, *J. Dent. Res.*, 80, 1540, 2001.
42. Cooper, L.F. et al., Generalizations regarding the process and phenomenon of osseointegration. II. *In vitro* studies, *Int. J. Oral Maxillofac. Implants,* 13, 163, 1998.
43. Masuda, T. et al., Generalizations regarding the process and phenomenon of osseointegration. I. *In vivo* studies, *Int. J. Oral Maxillofac. Implants,* 13, 17, 1998.
44. Cooper, L.F. et al., Formation of mineralizing osteoblast cultures on machined, titanium oxide grit-blasted, and plasma-sprayed titanium surfaces, *Int. J. Oral Maxillofac. Implants,* 14, 37, 1999.
45. Stanford, C.M., Solursh, M., and Keller, J.C., Significant role of adhesion properties of primary osteoblast-like cells in early adhesion events for chondroitin sulfate and dermatan sulfate surface molecules, *J. Biomed. Mater. Res.*, 47, 345, 1999.
46. Stanford, C.M. et al., Rapidly forming apatitic mineral in an osteoblastic cell line (UMR 106–01 BSP), *J. Biol. Chem.*, 270, 9420, 1995.

47. Hunter, G.K., Kyle, C.L., and Goldberg, H.A., Modulation of crystal formation by bone phosphoproteins: structural specificity of the osteopontin-mediated inhibition of hydroxyapatite formation, *Biochem. J.*, 300, 723, 1994.
48. Hunter, G.K. and Goldberg, H.A., Nucleation of hydroxyapatite by bone sialoprotein, *Proc. Natl. Acad. Sci. U.S.A.*, 90, 8562, 1993.
49. Bianco, P. et al., Localization of bone sialoprotein (BSP) to Golgi and post-Golgi secretory structures in osteoblasts and to discrete sites in early bone matrix, *J. Histochem. Cytochem.*, 41, 193, 1993.
50. Boyan, B.D. et al., Mechanisms involved in osteoblast response to implant surface morphology, *Annu. Rev. Mater. Res.*, 31, 357, 2001.
51. Underwood, J.C. et al., Structural and functional correlations in parathyroid hormone responsive transplantable osteogenic sarcomas, *Eur. J. Cancer (Oxford)*, 15, 1151, 1979.
52. Martin, T.J. et al., Metabolic properties of hormonally responsive osteogenic sarcoma cells, *Clin. Orthopaed. Rel. Res.*, 140, 247, 1979.
53. Partridge, N.C. et al., Morphological and biochemical characterization of four clonal osteogenic sarcoma cell lines of rat origin, *Cancer Res.*, 43, 4308, 1983.
54. Partridge, N.C. et al., Activation of adenosine 3′,5′-monophosphate-dependent protein kinase in normal and malignant bone cells by parathyroid hormone, prostaglandin E2, and prostacyclin, *Endocrinology*, 108, 220, 1981.
55. Partridge, N.C. et al., Functional properties of hormonally responsive cultured normal and malignant rat osteoblastic cells, *Endocrinology*, 108, 213, 1981.
56. Forrest, S.M. et al., Characterization of an osteoblast-like clonal cell line which responds to both parathyroid hormone and calcitonin, *Calcified Tiss. Int.*, 37, 51, 1985.
57. Partridge, N.C. et al., Parathyroid hormone inhibits collagen synthesis at both ribonucleic acid and protein levels in rat osteogenic sarcoma cells, *Molec. Endocrinol.*, 3, 232, 1989.
58. McQuillan, D.J. et al., Plasma-membrane-intercalated heparan sulphate proteoglycans in an osteogenic cell line (UMR 106–01 BSP), *Biochem. J.*, 285, 25, 1992.
59. McQuillan, D.J. et al., Proteoglycans synthesized by an osteoblast-like cell line (UMR 106–01), *Biochem. J.*, 277, 199, 1991.
60. Midura, R.J. et al., A rat osteogenic cell line (UMR 106–01) synthesizes a highly sulfated form of bone sialoprotein, *J. Biol. Chem.*, 265, 5285, 1990.
61. Scott, D.K. et al., Parathyroid hormone induces transcription of collagenase in rat osteoblastic cells by a mechanism using cyclic adenosine 3′,5′-monophosphate and requiring protein synthesis, *Molec. Endocrinol.*, 6, 2153, 1992.
62. Wang, A.M. et al., Reversible suppression of *in vitro* biomineralization by activation of protein kinase A, *J. Biol. Chem.*, 275, 11082, 2000.
63. Cooper, L.F. et al., Incipient analysis of mesenchymal stem-cell-derived osteogenesis, *J. Dent. Res.*, 80, 314, 2001.
64. Bianco, P. and Robey, P.G., Stem cells in tissue engineering, *Nature*, 414, 118, 2001.
65. Bianco, P. et al., Bone marrow stromal stem cells: nature, biology, and potential applications, *Stem Cells*, 19, 180, 2001.
66. Mustafa, K. et al., Effects of titanium surfaces blasted with TiO_2 particles on the initial attachment of cells derived from human mandibular bone: a scanning electron microscopic and histomorphometric analysis, *Clin. Oral Implants Res.*, 11, 116, 2000.

67. Aubin, J. E. et al., Osteoblast and chondroblast differentiation, *Bone,* 17, 77S, 1995.
68. Juliano, R.L. and Haskill, S., Signal transduction from the extracellular matrix, *J. Cell Biol.,* 120, 577, 1993.
69. Brand, R.A. and Stanford, C.M., How connective tissues temporally process mechanical stimuli, *Med. Hypotheses,* 42, 99, 1994.
70. Nakashima, K. et al., The novel zinc finger-containing transcription factor Osterix is required for osteoblast differentiation and bone formation, *Cell,* 108, 17, 2002.
71. Ducy, P., Cbfa1: a molecular switch in osteoblast biology, *Dev. Dynamics,* 219, 461, 2000.
72. Stein, G.S., Lian, J.B., and Owen, T.A., Relationship of cell growth to the regulation of tissue-specific gene expression during osteoblast differentiation, *FASEB J.,* 4, 3111, 1990.
73. Otto, F. et al., Cbfa1, a candidate gene for cleidocranial dysplasia syndrome, is essential for osteoblast differentiation and bone development, *Cell,* 89, 765, 1997.
74. Komori, T. et al., Targeted disruption of Cbfa1 results in a complete lack of bone formation owing to maturational arrest of osteoblasts, *Cell,* 89, 755, 1997.
75. Harada, H. et al., Cbfa1 isoforms exert functional differences in osteoblast differentiation, *J. Biol. Chem.,* 274, 6972, 1999.
76. Ducy, P. et al., A Cbfa1-dependent genetic pathway controls bone formation beyond embryonic development, *Genes Dev.,* 13, 1025, 1999.
77. Hoshi, K., Komori, T., and Ozawa, H., Morphological characterization of skeletal cells in Cbfa1-deficient mice, *Bone,* 25, 639, 1999.
78. Stanford, C.M., Keller, J.C., and Solursh, M., Bone cell expression on titanium surfaces is altered by sterilization treatments, *J. Dent. Res.,* 73, 1061, 1994.
79. Daniels, K., Reiter, R., and Solursh, M., Micromass cultures of limb and other mesenchyme, *Methods Cell Biol.,* 51, 237, 1996.
80. Solursh, M. et al., Osteogenic protein-1 is required for mammalian eye development, *Biochem. Biophys. Res. Commun.,* 218, 438, 1996.
81. Chen, Y. et al., Comparative study of Msx-1 expression in early normal and vitamin A-deficient avian embryos, *J. Exp. Zool.,* 272, 299, 1995.
82. Schramm, C.A., Reiter, R.S., and Solursh, M., Role for short-range interactions in the formation of cartilage and muscle masses in transfilter micromass cultures, *Dev. Biol.,* 163, 467, 1994.
83. Geduspan, J.S., Padanilam, B.J., and Solursh, M., Mesonephros derived IGF I in early limb development, *Progr. Clin. Biol. Res.,* 383B, 673, 1993.
84. Sonn, J.K. and Solursh, M., Activity of protein kinase C during the differentiation of chick limb bud mesenchymal cells, *Differentiation,* 53, 155, 1993.
85. Archer, C.W. et al., Myogenic potential of chick limb bud mesenchyme in micromass culture, *Anat. Embryol.,* 185, 299, 1992.
86. Swart, K.M. et al., Short-term plasma-cleaning treatments enhance *in vitro* osteoblast attachment to titanium, *J. Oral Implantol.,* 18, 130, 1992.
87. Bowers, K.T. et al., Optimization of surface micromorphology for enhanced osteoblast responses *in vitro, Int. J. Oral Maxillofac. Implants,* 7, 302, 1992.
88. Michaels, C.M., Keller, J.C., and Stanford, C.M., *In vitro* periodontal ligament fibroblast attachment to plasma-cleaned titanium surfaces, *J. Oral Implantol.,* 17, 132, 1991.

89. Stanford, C.M. and Keller, J.C., The concept of osseointegration and bone matrix expression, *Crit. Rev. Oral Biol. Med.*, 2, 83, 1991.
90. Holtman, K., Quantitative RT-PCR of estrogen receptor alpha and beta from human alveolar bone cells, *J. Dent. Res.*, 80, 273, 2001.
91. Perinpanayagam, H. et al., The N-terminal Isoform of cbfa-1 is overexpressed in rapidly mineralizing UMR106–01 osteoblasts., *J. Dent. Res.*, 81, 504, 2002.
92. Xiao, Z.S. et al., Cbfa1 isoform overexpression upregulates osteocalcin gene expression in non-osteoblastic and pre-osteoblastic cells, *J. Cell. Biochem.*, 74, 596, 1999.
93. Xiao, Z.S. et al., Genomic structure and isoform expression of the mouse, rat and human Cbfa1/Osf2 transcription factor, *Gene*, 214, 187, 1998.
94. Zaharias, R. and Schneider, G.B., FAK expression differs between mineralizing and non-mineralizing osteoblasts., *J. Dent. Res.*, 81, A-361, 2002.
95. Cooper, L.F. et al., Spatiotemporal assessment of fetal bovine osteoblast culture differentiation indicates a role for BSP in promoting differentiation, *J. Bone Miner. Res.*, 13, 620, 1998.
96. Midura, R.J. and Hascall, V.C., Bone sialoprotein: a mucin in disguise, *Glycobiology*, 6, 677, 1996.
97. Riminucci, M. et al., The anatomy of bone sialoprotein immunoreactive sites in bone as revealed by combined ultrastructural histochemistry and immunohistochemistry, *Calcified Tiss. Int.*, 57, 277, 1995.
98. Pinero, G.J. et al., Bone matrix proteins in osteogenesis and remodelling in the neonatal rat mandible as studied by immunolocalization of osteopontin, bone sialoprotein, alpha 2HS-glycoprotein and alkaline phosphatase, *Arch. Oral Biol.*, 40, 145, 1995.
99. Hunter, G.K. and Goldberg, H.A., Modulation of crystal formation by bone phosphoproteins: role of glutamic acid-rich sequences in the nucleation of hydroxyapatite by bone sialoprotein, *Biochem. J.*, 302, 175, 1994.
100. Bianco, P. et al., Bone sialoprotein (BSP) secretion and osteoblast differentiation: relationship to bromodeoxyuridine incorporation, alkaline phosphatase, and matrix deposition, *J. Histochem. Cytochem.*, 41, 183, 1993.
101. Bianco, P. et al., Expression of bone sialoprotein (BSP) in developing human tissues, *Calcified Tiss. Int.*, 49, 421, 1991.
102. Schwitters, C. et al., Bone sialoprotein expression in UMR106–01BSP osteoblasts increases *in vitro* on roughened surfaces, *J. Dent. Res.*, 81, A-439, 2002.
103. Franceschi, R.T., The developmental control of osteoblast-specific gene expression: role of specific transcription factors and the extracellular matrix environment, *Crit. Rev. Oral Biol. Med.*, 10, 40, 1999.
104. Karsenty, G. et al., Cbfa1 as a regulator of osteoblast differentiation and function, *Bone*, 25, 107, 1999.
105. Shapiro, I.M., Discovery: Osf2/Cbfa1, a master gene of bone formation, *Clin. Orthodont. Res.*, 2, 42, 1999.
106. Gao, Y.H. et al., Potential role of cbfa1, an essential transcriptional factor for osteoblast differentiation, in osteoclastogenesis: regulation of mRNA expression of osteoclast differentiation factor (ODF), *Biochem. Biophys. Res. Commun.*, 252, 697, 1998.
107. Komori, T. and Kishimoto, T., Cbfa1 in bone development, *Curr. Opin. Genet. Dev.*, 8, 494, 1998.

108. Zeng, C. et al., Intranuclear targeting of AML/CBFalpha regulatory factors to nuclear matrix-associated transcriptional domains, *Proc. Natl. Acad. Sci. U.S.A.*, 95, 1585, 1998.
109. Banerjee, C. et al., *Runt* homology domain proteins in osteoblast differentiation: aml3/cbfa1 is a major component of a bone-specific complex, *J. Cell. Biochem.*, 66, 1, 1997.
110. Banerjee, C. et al., Differential regulation of the two principal Runx2/Cbfa1 n-terminal isoforms in response to bone morphogenetic protein-2 during development of the osteoblast phenotype, *Endocrinology*, 142, 4026, 2001.
111. Javed, A. et al., *Runt* homology domain transcription factors (Runx, Cbfa, and AML) mediate repression of the bone sialoprotein promoter: evidence for promoter context-dependent activity of Cbfa proteins, *Mol. Cell. Biol.*, 21, 2891, 2001.
112. Gilbert, L. et al., Expression of the osteoblast differentiation factor RUNX2 (Cbfa1/AML3/Pebp2alpha A) is inhibited by tumor necrosis factor-alpha, *J. Biol. Chem.*, 277, 2695, 2002.
113. Zaidi, S.K. et al., A specific targeting signal directs Runx2/Cbfa1 to subnuclear domains and contributes to transactivation of the osteocalcin gene, *J. Cell Sci.*, 114, 3093, 2001.
114. Xiao, G. et al., Role of the alpha2-integrin in osteoblast-specific gene expression and activation of the Osf2 transcription factor, *J. Biol. Chem.*, 273, 32988, 1998.
115. Beresford, J.N., Graves, S.E., and Smoothy, C.A., Formation of mineralized nodules by bone derived cells *in vitro*: a model of bone formation? *Am. J. Med. Genet.*, 45, 163, 1993.

9

Cellular Interactions at Commercially Pure Titanium Implants

Lyndon F. Cooper

CONTENTS

9.1 Introduction 165
9.2 Cellular Diversity and Osseointegration 166
9.3 Understanding Biological Conditioning of the Endosseous Implant Surface 167
9.4 Osteoinduction Is a Function of the Implant–Resident Cell Population 169
9.5 Early Responses to Osteoinductive Signals 175
9.6 Potential Specialization of Bone Formation at Implants 178
9.7 Summary 178
References 179

9.1 Introduction

The progression of dentistry beyond restorative care to include regenerative therapy has been promoted by successes involving tooth root replacement using endosseous dental implants. This success of commercially pure (c.p.) titanium endosseous implants in support of dental prostheses is now well documented. There is growing consensus that uncoated, threaded c.p. titanium implants can provide survival rates greater than 95% when used to support anterior single tooth restorations[1] or mandibular prostheses supported by four to five parasymphyseal implants.[2] Clinical successes notwithstanding, we confront the absence of significant data to guide future efforts to apply endosseous implant use in the more challenging environments of low density bone and high stress situations such as single implant replacements for molar teeth.

0-8493-1474-7/03/$0.00+$1.50

A generalized view of endosseous implant success is formulated on existing data and historical reference. Foremost in this vision is the role of bone volume and, most importantly, bone density. In particular, there is a broadly based conceptualization of endosseous implant success in relationship to the quality and quantity of the interfacial bone dimension and bone volume that forms shortly following surgical implant placement.[3]

While an acceptable minimum implant to bone interfacial dimension has not yet been defined, recent clinical investigations indicate that a remarkably small quantity of bone actually exists after months of healing at a machined c.p. titanium endosseous implant and that surface topographic enhancement of the implant surface leads to improvements that are less than 100% (Table 9.1). Control of bone formation and maintenance at the endosseous implant interface is considered a key factor in assuring the immediate and long-term success of the endosseous dental implant.[4,5]

The physiological basis for the resultant bone-to-implant interface involves bone formation and the processes that underlie the maintenance of existing bone at the implant surface following initial bone healing.[4] Bone formation is dependent on the regulation of osteoblastic cells derived from host tissues and influenced by osteoinductive signals, osteogenetic stimuli, and osteoconductive mechanisms.[10] In addition to the aforementioned *in vivo* data, a large number of *in vitro* studies considers the influence of the endosseous implant on the natures and activities of various cultured osteoblastic cells.

It is the aim of this chapter to focus on cells other than differentiating osteoprogenitors and osteoblastic tumor cell lines in an effort to better understand the process of osseointegration and the relationship of implant surface parameters and clinical procedures to the formation of the implant–bone interface.

9.2 Cellular Diversity and Osseointegration

The term *integration* is used in the social arena to describe the interaction of different groups of individuals among a resident population. When the process of wound healing and bone formation is considered at the cellular level, *integration* is also a relevant term (beyond its typical connotation) in that different groups of distinct cell types must interact to achieve the goal of bone formation. It is clear from a long list of studies focusing on osteoblast interactions with implant surfaces[11,12] that few other cell types have been considered significant to the process of osseointegration.

The main question addressed is, "What can be learned about osseointegration from other cells involved in the process?" To identify the role of cells other than osteoblasts, a temporal model for cellular interactions with a c.p. titanium endosseous implant must be available. Additionally, four assump-

TABLE 9.1

Clinical Evidence of Commercially Pure (c.p.) Titanium Topography Effects on Bone-to-Implant Interface

		Bone-to-Implant Contact	
Authors	**Duration of Healing (Average)**	**Machined c.p. Titanium Implant**	**Modified c.p. Titanium Implant**
Ivanoff et al.[6]	6.3 months	9%	37% (TiOBlast)[a]
Trisi et al.[7]	12 months	7%	77% (grit-blasted)[b]
Lazarra et al.[8]	6 months	34%	73% (Osseotite)[c]

[a] P = 0.0001.
[b] P = <0.05.
[c] P = 0.0129.

tions can be stipulated for the following discussion of cellular interactions with endosseous implants.

Assumption 1 — The placement of the endosseous implant into a blood- and extracellular fluid-filled space forever changes the molecular nature of the implant surface by subjecting it to a set of biological conditioning events.

Assumption 2 — The endosseous implant surface interacts with cells resident in a fibrin blood clot that are primarily responsible for the deposition of growth factors, cytokines, chemokines, and extracellular matrix proteins that subsequently direct the induction, recruitment, and motility of osteoprogenitor cells at the implanted foreign surface.

Assumption 3 — Bone formation is provided through the induction of bone marrow-derived mesenchymal stem cells along the osteoblastic lineage. This inductive process may require or may be modulated by nonmesenchymal cells including circulating cells of the immune system.

Assumption 4 — In this chapter, the initial processes of bone formation will be considered without additional consideration of the mechanical influences on cell activity during osteogenesis or on the processes of modeling and remodeling of this formed bone for a lifetime thereafter. A new mechanical environment is established by creation of the osteotomy, the placement of an endosseous implant, and the physical properties of the endosseous implant, and it may be further affected by the inflammatory status that can influence bone formation or resorption.

9.3 Understanding Biological Conditioning of the Endosseous Implant Surface

The placement of endosseous implants results in extravasation of blood, hemostasis, and fibrin blood clot formation at the bone–implant interface. In a rat model of osseointegration, the molecular and cellular events occur-

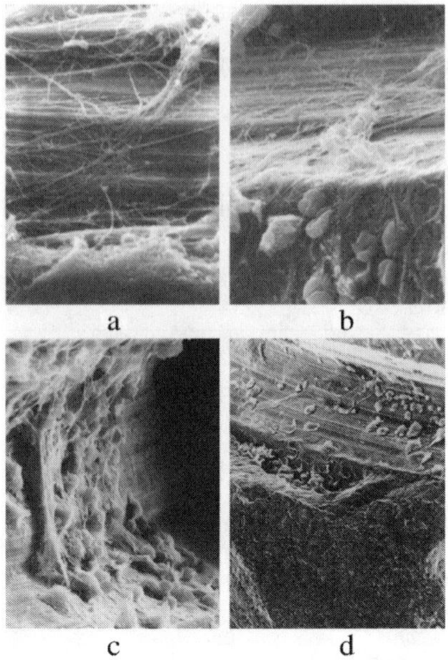

FIGURE 9.1
Cell and matrix interactions at c.p. titanium implants. (a) Surface of a machined c.p. titanium implant removed 2 days following placement in the rat tibia reveals adsorption of a fibrin network. (b) Alternative view of a machined c.p. titanium implant removed 2 days following placement reveals platelets and red blood cells present on the implant surface covered by a fibrin network. (c) Surface of a machined c.p. titanium implant removed 7 days following placement reveals complete replacement of the fibrin network by an amorphous protein layer and cell proliferation within a cell-associated matrix. (d) In other locations, single cells are adherent to the surface. Only some cells are spread. The original fibrin matrix is absent.

ring at the endosseous implant interface were evaluated at the morphological level[13] (Figure 9.1).

The interpretations from this and several similar investigations are that (1) fibrin clots form directly upon c.p. titanium implant surfaces; (2) a fibrin clot is a residence for red blood cells and platelets enriched with many growth factors and cytokines necessary for robust osteogenesis, but lacking in osteoinductive cytokines; (3) early fibrinolysis at the surface is temporally congruent with monocyte attachment and elaboration of a cell- and plasma-derived extracellular matrix adherent to the implant surface; and (4) morphological evidence suggests that surface topographies of c.p. titanium implants alter the nature of this early implant–tissue interface.

Davies et al. suggested that implant surface topography could affect the physical interaction of the implant with the fibrin clot network and the activation of included platelets.[14] Increasing surface roughness indeed leads to greater physical retention of this fibrin clot on the implant surface.[15] The cells resident in this fibrin network are likely contributors of inductive and chemotactic signals that support osseointegration.

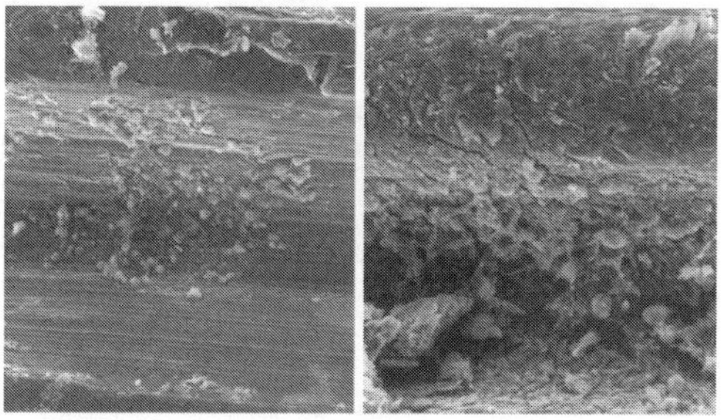

a b

FIGURE 9.2
Implant surface-dependent nature of cell and molecule adhesion to endosseous implants. (a) Adherent and spreading cells on the surface of a machined c.p. titanium implant removed 5 days after placement. (b) Adherent and spreading cells on the surface of a TiO_2-grit-blasted c.p. titanium implant removed 5 days after placement. Note the relative density and spreading of cells on the topographically enhanced implant surface.

Evaluation of both machined and titanium dioxide (TiO_2) grit-blasted implants removed from rat tibiae 2 days following placement suggests that (1) both surfaces serve as substrates for the fibrin clot, and (2) the TiO_2 grit-blasted surface retains more of the biologically contributed interface upon removal (Figure 9.2). It can be acknowledged that implant removal is not part of the normal healing process, yet this interfacial evaluation demonstrates the contribution of the fibrin clot to a process of biologically conditioning this artificial interface. This simple morphologic assessment illustrates that potentially significant macromolecular mechanical interactions may be influenced by implant surface topography (or chemistry). The presence of varying numbers of platelets, red blood cells, and monocytes further suggests that important surface-dependent variations in early cell–implant interactions may also occur within this fibrin matrix. Much is still to be learned about the incipient events that condition the implant within its biologic context.

9.4 Osteoinduction Is a Function of the Implant–Resident Cell Population

Implantation of c.p. titanium materials to ectopic sites does not result in bone formation and thus c.p. titanium is not osteoinductive. Osteoblastic adhesion to an endosseous implant surface alone does not render the osteoblast capable of osteoinduction, but micrographs of osseointegrated endosseous implants indicate that within the medullary bone, new bone forms preferentially at the endosseous surface to yield the clinically significant implant–bone interface. This implies that either the osteoblastic models available are not representative or that other molecules or cells adherent to the implant surface are osteoinductive.

Blood and serum lack osteoinductive molecules, although other important osteogenic factors are present.[16] While platelets are efficient in delivering many important growth factors, they do not contain bone morphogenetic proteins (BMPs). By exclusion, it may be deduced that other resident cells at or adherent to the implant surface might provide osteoinductive signals.

The resident cell population at the endosseous implant surface during the first days following placement includes platelets, red blood cells, and monocytes. Monocytes are typically resident among the populations of cells in blood clots. Their extravasation and differentiation along the macrophage lineage is important in wound healing.

Mice lacking macrophage chemotactic protein-1 (MCP-1) display delayed cutaneous wound healing.[17] Although a general role for macrophages in the process of osseointegration has been proposed based on evidence of macrophage adhesion to endosseous implant surfaces,[18] a specific role for macrophages remains to be defined. Evidence for their population of the implant surface is provided in numerous published micrographs of successful endosseous implants.

Molecular evidence that monocytes populate the endosseous implant can be obtained by accessing the cellular components of the implant–tissue interface by retrieval of the dental implant by a prefixation fracture method.[13] The 1.5-mm implants in rat tibae were removed 1 to 7 days following surgical placement, rinsed in ice cold PBS, and then placed into a cell lysis buffer for RNA extraction. From each implant, total RNA was precipitated and used to program reverse transcription polymerase chain reactions (PCRs) that included primer pairs specific for the monocyte/macrophage-specific extracellular receptor CD14.

In Figure 9.3, the ethidium-bromide stained, transilluminated gel results demonstrate that among the transient population of cells adherent to c.p. titanium endosseous implants, CD14-producing cells (monocytes/macrophages) are present. The time course of events further indicates that CD14 expression is present in cells adherent to the surface at days 3 and 5 following implantation. Expression of this monocyte/macrophage marker precedes BSP expression and osteocalcin expression. One interpretation of this molecular information is that monocytes/macrophages are among the early resident cells at endosseous c.p. titanium implants.

The possible wound-healing role for implant adherent monocytes was suggested by this temporal relationship and also by the important role of macrophages in directing dermal wound healing.[19] If monocytes/macrophages contribute to induction of bone formation at endosseous dental implants, then they should produce osteoinductive cytokines including BMPs.

To address the possibility that monocytes/macrophages produce BMPs, accepted cell culture models of monocytes/macrophages were examined. The expression of BMP-2 and to a lesser degree BMP-6 was demonstrated in both the J744A.1 and RAW 264.1 murine macrophage cell lines and in the

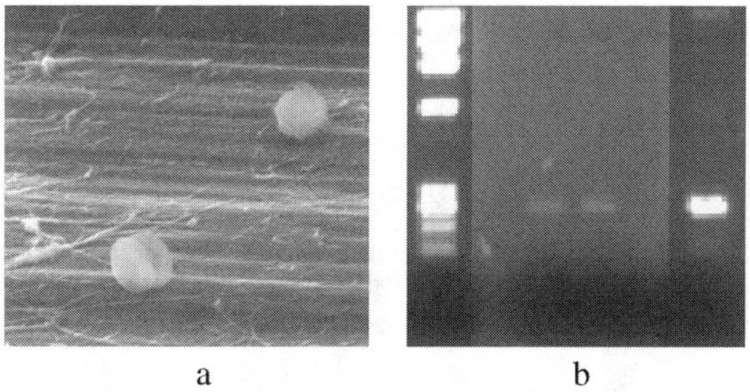

FIGURE 9.3
Reverse transcription polymerase chain reaction identification of macrophage-specific receptor CD14-encoding mRNA expressed by implant adherent cells. (a) Scanning electron micrograph (1000×) reveals that cells of different morphologies are adherent to implants shortly after placement (2 days). (b) Implants were placed in rat tibiae and removed at 1, 2, 5, and 7 days (lanes 1, 2, 3, and 4, respectively). Total RNA from cells lysed from the removed implants was used as the target for CD14-specific reverse transcription and amplification (lane 5). One tenth of each reaction was separated in a 1.2% agarose gel and stained with ethidium bromide. Reaction products from each day are presented. The product from the J744A.1 macrophage total RNA is the same molecular size (MØ).

human TPH-1 monocyte cell line[20] (Figure 9.4). Conditioned media from J744A.1 cell lines further increased the osteoblastic differentiation of human mesenchymal stem cells along the osteoblastic lineage. Significantly, when measured at early timepoints at the level of alkaline phosphatase activity, this positive effect of macrophage-conditioned media on human mesenchymal stem cell alkaline phosphatase expression was partially blocked by the inclusion of anti-BMP-2 antibodies in the culture media (Figure 9.5). The partial response to blocking may be due to the additional stimulation of

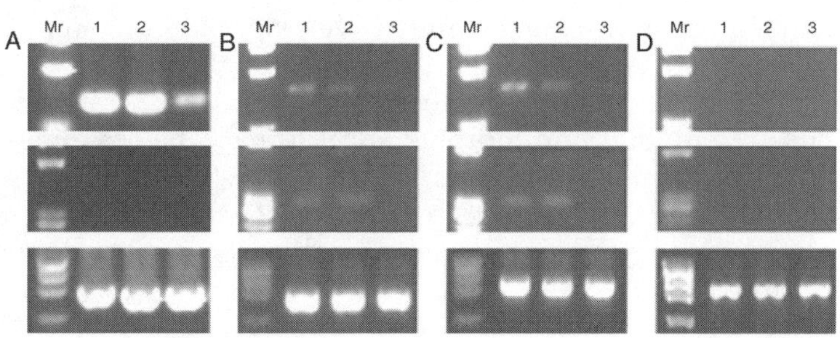

FIGURE 9.4
BMP expression in cultured macrophages. Reverse transcription polymerase chain reaction was used to amplify BMP-2, BMP-6, and actin mRNA present in total RNA isolated from different macrophage cell lines: mouse J774A.1 (A), mouse RAW264 (B), human THP-1 (C); and mouse NIH3T3 fibroblastic cell line (D). The relative abundance of BMP-2 (top panel), BMP-6 (middle panel), and actin (bottom panel) is shown. Expression of BMP by each cell line can be compared among cells treated with MCP-1 (lane 2), LPS (lane 3), or not treated (lane 1).

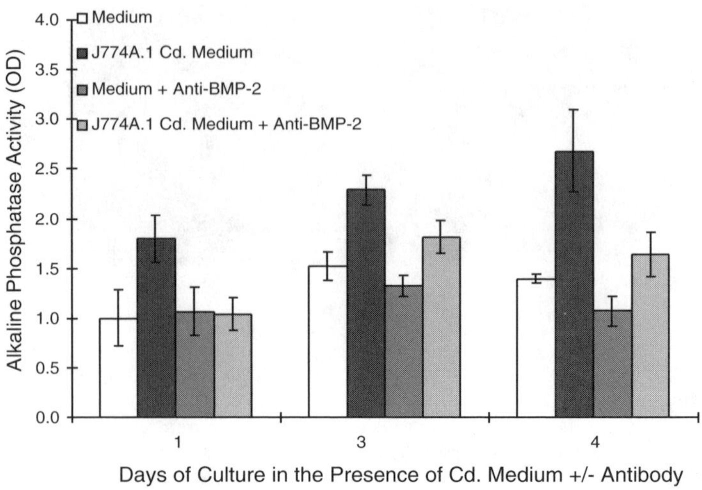

FIGURE 9.5
Effect of macrophage-conditioned media on hMSC alkaline phosphatase expression. Effects of J744A.1 conditioned medium on hMSC alkaline phosphatase expression is compared to effect of media only, and media or conditioned media containing anti-BMP-2 antibody (as shown). Note effect of J744.1 macrophage conditioned media is limited by addition of anti-BMP-2 antibody. Adapted from Takebe, J. et al., *J. Biomed. Mater. Res.*, 64A, 207–216, 2003.

human mesenchymal stems cell by transforming growth factor (TGF)-β1 also secreted by macrophages into conditioned media.

To further implicate monocytes/macrophages in the modulation of tissue responses to endosseous implant surfaces, the effect of surface topography on monocyte/macrophage BMP expression was also investigated.[21] If monocytes/macrophages contribute to the osteoinductive responses at various endosseous implant surfaces, then monocyte/macrophage BMP expression should be modulated by c.p. titanium surface topography.

Preliminary proof of a relationship between c.p. titanium surface topography and macrophage BMP expression was sought using a cell culture model. First, J744A.1 macrophage adhesion to various c.p. titanium surfaces was defined in temporal and morphological terms. The scanning electron microscopy (SEM) evaluation of macrophage adhesion to specular polished, machined, and grit-blasted surfaces confirmed the surface-specific nature of the monocytes. Monocyte adhesion and spreading on c.p. titanium surfaces of different topographies were dramatically different (Figure 9.6). Smooth surfaces did not support rapid adhesion and spreading. Only after 24 hours was spreading observed. In contrast, machined surfaces and, to a much greater degree, the grit-blasted surfaces, promoted more rapid adhesion and extensive spreading by 24 hours.

The topography-dependent interactions of cultured macrophages with the c.p. titanium surfaces were also associated with the topography-dependent ability of macrophages to produce BMP-2 mRNA. When total RNA from macrophages cultured on polished, machined, and grit-blasted c.p. titanium

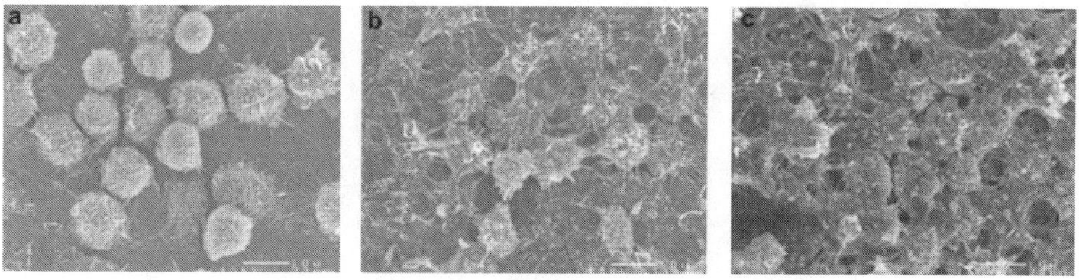

FIGURE 9.6
Morphological assessment of murine macrophage adhesion to c.p. titanium surfaces. Cells were plated onto specular-polished (a), machined (b), and grit-blasted (c) c.p. titanium disks in media containing 10% fetal calf serum. After 24 hours, the cultures were fixed and prepared for scanning electron microscopy. Note the absence of spreading by cells adherent to the specular-polished surface (a). Adapted from Takebe, J. et al., *J. Biomed. Mater. Res.*, 64A, 207–216, 2003.

surfaces was used as the target for BMP-2-specific reverse transcription PCR, BMP-2 expression was absent in macrophages cultured for 24 hours on polished surfaces and was greatest for macrophages cultured in parallel on grit-blasted c.p. titanium surfaces (Figure 9.7).

This surface-related modulation of BMP-2 expression was not observed when MC3T3-E1 or 2T3 osteoblastic cells were cultured for 24 hours on identically prepared substrates (not shown). Moreover, the striking cell adhesion differences observed for macrophages adherent to these surfaces was not observed for the osteoblastic cells. After 8 hours in serum-containing media, both cell lines demonstrated similar adhesion and spreading. Low levels of BMP-2 mRNA were expressed by the murine osteoblastic cell lines at this time point in culture. The absence of significant BMP-2 or BMP-6 expression by the osteoblastic cells shortly following their adhesion to c.p. titanium surfaces as well as the surface-specific and relatively high levels of BMP-2 expression by the cultured macrophages led to speculation of an adjunct or

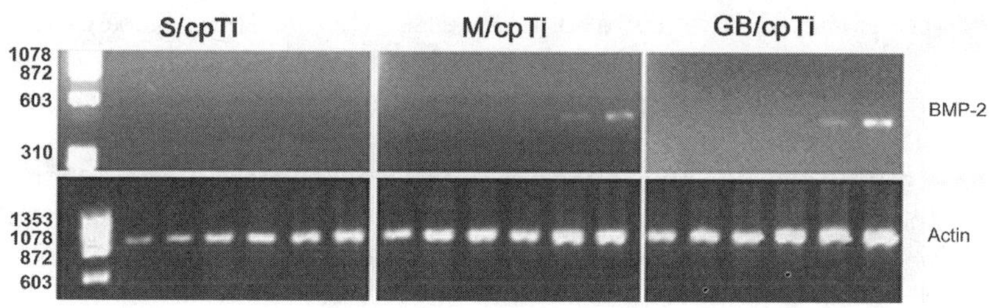

FIGURE 9.7
Reverse transcription polymerase chain reaction quantification of BMP-2 expression by murine macrophages adherent to c.p. titanium surfaces prepared as specular-polished (S/cpTi), machined (M/cpTi), and grit-blasted (GB/cpTi) surfaces. The composite represents reaction products for cells grown on each surface visualized by transilluminated ethidium bromide-stained agarose gel electrophoresis. Each panel contains six lanes loaded with one tenth of the PCR product from cycles 20, 22, 24, 26, 28, and 30 (left to right). Molecular markers are present in the far left lane. The absence of BMP-2 expression on S/cpTi surfaces was confirmed at a higher PCR cycle number. Adapted from Takebe, J. et al., *J. Biomed. Mater. Res.*, 64A, 207–216, 2003.

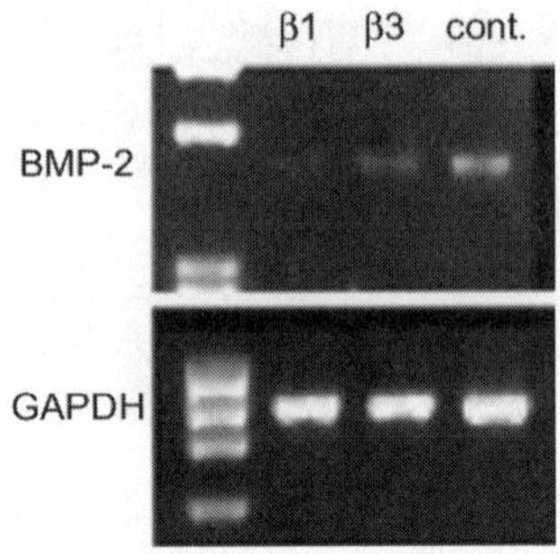

FIGURE 9.8
Possible role for integrin-mediated signaling of surface-dependent BMP-2 expression by J744A.1 macrophages. J774A.1 cells were cultured on TCP surfaces for 24 hours in the presence of anti-β1 (CD29), anti-β3 (CD61), or normal rabbit serum (control). Total RNA was extracted, cDNA synthesized, and PCR reactions were performed using BMP-2 or GAPDH primers. Aliquots (10 × 1) were removed after 30 amplification cycles and analyzed by transillumination of agarose gel electrophoresis.

principal role for macrophages in contributing osteoinductive signals to the biological conditioning of the freshly implanted c.p. titanium endosseous implant surface. This is one possible mechanism by which surface topography effects dramatic increases in the bone formed at endosseous implant surfaces.

To begin to appreciate the molecular processes that may control the macrophage's expression of BMP-2, the adhesion-dependent nature of the macrophage was explored further. The differentiating macrophage is known to utilize both the β1 and β3 integrin receptors (as well as other classes of receptors) in its interactions with specific tissues. Inclusion of antibodies specific to the β1 integrin in the culture media inhibited spreading and BMP-2 expression (Figure 9.8).

The level of BMP-2 mRNA expressed by J774A.1 macrophages adherent to c.p. titanium surfaces is dependent upon macrophage interaction with the surface using the β1 integrin and to a lesser degree the β3 integrin. Two extracellular matrix proteins that serve as insoluble ligands for these receptors are serum fibronectin and serum vitronectin.[22] Thus, extravasated monocytes resident in the fibrin clot may subsequently adhere to the implant surface conditioned for this event through early interaction with blood. These adherent macrophages may serve as osteoinductive agents to guide wound healing at the endosseous implant.

Beyond osteoinduction, the macrophage may serve an additional role in preparation of the dental implant surface for population by bone-forming cells. Investigations of bone interfaces by McKee and Nanci[23] have established that a prominent feature of bone interfaces and the implant–bone interface is the immunohistochemically-defined presence of BSP and osteopontin. The macrophage is able to produce and secrete osteopontin. In preliminary investigations, it was also confirmed that cultured macrophages produce and secrete osteopontin on c.p. titanium substrates (data not shown). Thus, the macrophage may contribute to the biological conditioning

TABLE 9.2

Factors Implicating Macrophages in Commercially Pure (c.p.) Titanium Surface-Related Osteogenesis

1. Macrophages have a defined central role in wound healing.[19]
2. Monocyte and macrophage populations of the c.p. titanium surface precede osteoprotegenitor cell adhesion.[18]
3. Macrophages are able to produce BMPs.[20]
4. Macrophages produce bone-related adhesive extracellular matrix proteins.[23]
5. Macrophage BMP expression increases with increasing surface roughness.[43]

of the implant–bone interface by contributing to the induction of osteoprogenitor cells, their chemotaxis, and the adhesion of bone-forming osteoprogenitors to an interface largely devoid of type I collagen (Table 9.2).

If monocyte/macrophages are to be implicated in a central role for successful bone formation at an implant surface, is there evidence that they can also play a pivotal role in failure of osseointegration? The etiology of fibrous scar formation is partially a function of macrophages[24] and its contribution to high TGF-β levels in the healing tissue. Blocking this pathway improves wound healing.[25] In fact, macrophages have a central role in mediating fibrosis[26] induced by particulate debris. Macrophage opsonization and engulfment of particulate materials are associated with induction of fibroblasts and fibrosis. In this regard, it is important to note that particulate-induced fibrosis is one aspect of hip implant failure. Similar fibrosis is noted around titanium or hydroxyapatite particles shed from coated implants upon placement.[27]

While recent reports demonstrate a possible role for osteoblastic cells in response to this particulate material, the macrophage likely plays a central role in the pathophysiology of all fibrotic disease. It remains to be determined whether the macrophage occupies a pivotal contributory position in the formation of an osseous versus a fibrotic interface at an endosseous implant.

It is not clear whether or how nonosteogenic cells also contribute to the process of osseointegration. A clear role for T cells is defined in cutaneous wound healing.[28] However, it is conceivable that local cellular responses contribute to the relative absence of bone resorption in the medullary region of bone following implant placement. Future investigation of local regulatory events may be expanded to include other cells and mechanisms, for example, T-cell expression of osteoprotegerin ligand as a local mechanism of promoting bone resorption in rheumatoid arthritis and periodontitis.[29,30]

9.5 Early Responses to Osteoinductive Signals

Evidence of bone formation at an implant suggests that woven bone formation commences within 7 to 14 days after placement.[13] Before this, recruitment and induction of a progenitor population of cells are required. While some cells are derived from endosteum, the resident bone marrow mesenchymal stem cells contribute to this new population of osteoblastic cells.[31,32] Thus, a relevant model of the early bone formation phase of osseointegration may include assessment of the interaction of human mesenchymal stem cells (hMSCs) with the c.p. titanium surface and how surface topography per se affects MSC differentiation along the osteoblastic lineage.

The *in vitro* differentiation of the hMSC is a well defined model of osteoblastic differentiation.[33] When cultured in the presence of dexamethasone and in media supplemented with ascorbic acid and β-glycerophosphate, the hMSC is able to produce a mineralizing matrix replete with bone matrix proteins expressed in a temporal pattern consistent with bone formation *in vivo*.

Figure 9.9 offers a simple representation of some aspects of osteoblastic differentiation. A single cell (leftmost) represents an undifferentiated MSC. Both positive (e.g., BMPs) and negative factors (e.g., noggin) are active in controlling osteoinduction. The induction of two key transcription factors (osterix and Cbfa-1(RunX2)) is associated with the commitment of this cell along the osteoblastic lineage.

Proliferation of these committed precursors is in part influenced by numerous growth factors and cytokines (e.g., fibroblast growth factor-2). At the time of implant placement, many different local factors contribute to the positive and negative influences on MSC osteoinduction and proliferation. It is not clear how the presence of an implant surface of one or another topographic character and chemistry influences these essential first steps. A present partially defined genetic program is subsequently followed by the committed osteoprogenitor such that a sequential pattern of extracellular matrix proteins is produced and secreted by the osteoblastic cell. Cell interaction with these proteins is considered important to the process of differentiation[34] and by inference, similar cellular interactions with implant surfaces have been suggested to alter or enhance osteoblast bone matrix

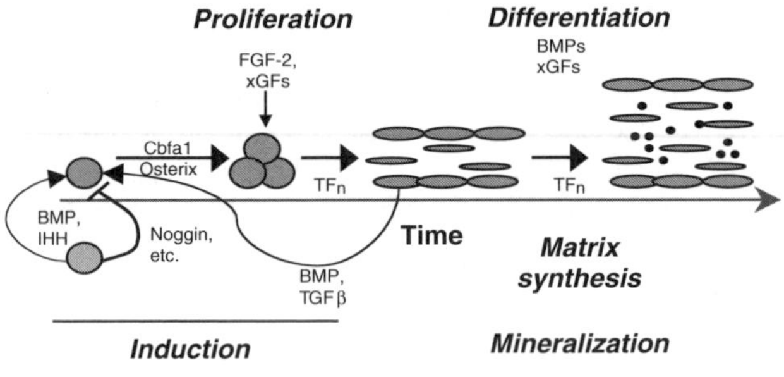

FIGURE 9.9
A simple model of induction and differentiation of osteoblasts from a precursor cell. It shows the function of time (2 to 4 weeks, from left to right) and the roles of many different factors on the induction, proliferation, and differentiation of osteoblasts. Assumed is an underlying genetic program that is initiated or suppressed and one that may be influenced by these and other factors. How this general program is influenced by the local environment established by a c.p. titanium implant after surgical placement into bone is presently not well defined. xGF = various growth factors, TF_n = numerous transcription factors.

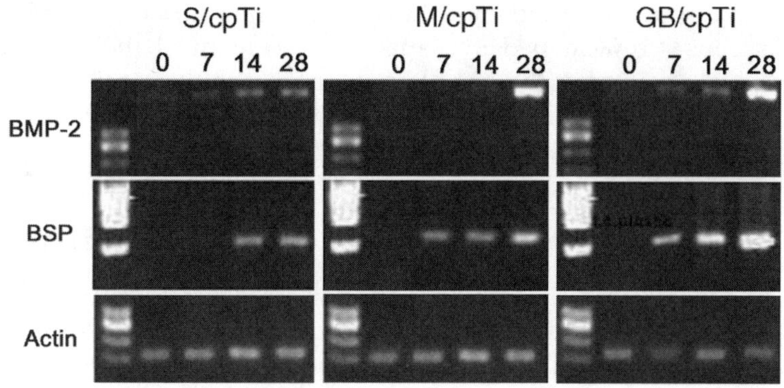

FIGURE 9.10
Reverse transcription polymerase chain reation amplification of BMP-2, BSP and actin mRNAs expressed by hMSCs cultured on polished (S/cpTi), machined (M/cpTi) or grit-blasted (GB/cpTi) disks. Relative abundance of specific products are shown for mRNAs isolated 0, 7, 14 or 28 days after plating on the different cpTi disks. Adapted from Takebe, J. et al., *J. Biomed. Mater. Res.*, 64A, 207–216, 2003.

formation at the implant–bone interface. Eventually, osteoblastic differentiation is terminated and most osteoblastic cells are removed by the process of apoptosis, but only after the collagenous matrix has mineralized.

If hMSCs are recruited to a c.p. titanium surface, do they then produce BMPs and serve as osteoinductive agents? Does surface topography influence subsequent bone matrix expression? To begin to investigate these possibilities, hMSCs were cultured on c.p. titanium surfaces of varying topographies for which a relationship between altered surface topography and increased bone formation as an *in vivo* outcome had been measured in a rat tibia model.[35]

Using total RNA isolated by direct lysis of cells cultured on the c.p. titanium surfaces for 0 to 28 days, cDNA was synthesized using Superscript reverse transcriptase and 1-μg portions of resulting cDNA were then used as targets for PCR reactions programmed using human BMP-2 or BSP-specific primers. Reaction products were separated in 1.2% agarose gels and were viewed by transillumination of ethidium bromide-stained products (Figure 9.10). The results indicate that incipient (0- to 7-day) BMP-2 and BMP-6 expression is not dramatically changed by the interaction of cultured hMSCs with c.p. titanium surfaces of differing topography.

The osteoblastic differentiation of hMSCs was confirmed by evaluation of BSP gene expression. BSP is an adhesive bone matrix protein expressed just prior to mineralization of osteoid.[36] When BSP–osteoblast interactions were blocked using anti-BSP antibodies, further osteoblastic differentiation did not occur.[37] BSP expression is a marker of irreversible commitment to osteogenesis. As shown in Figure 9.10, BSP expression was elevated and accelerated when hMSCs were grown on the grit-blasted surfaces. Implied is the more rapid and robust differentiation by the hMSCs cultured on the grit-blasted versus machined or specular-polished surfaces. Interpretation of these results to the *in vivo* situation is difficult. When these same surfaces were imparted to endosseous screw-shaped implants, enhancement of the implant bone interface was revealed at the grit-blasted surfaces in the rat tibia model.[35]

9.6 Potential Specialization of Bone Formation at Implants

There are several potential explanations for the different rates and extents of osteoblastic differentiation observed for hMSCs grown on different surfaces. One explanation is autocrine regulation occurring after initial induction (days 14 through 28 in culture) and evidence of greater BMP-2 expression on "rougher" surfaces at these times is available.[38]

The basis for this autocrine regulation may involve the central transcriptional regulators that control BMP expression. Currently, the RunX2 family of transcription factors[39] and a novel mediator of osteoinduction, osterix,[40] are implicated. (Refer to Chapter 8 in this book.) Of further obvious importance is the role of signal transduction mediated by the adhesion phenomenon. Integrins[41] and syndecans that mediate adhesive extracellular matrix protein–cell interactions are known to be altered by surface topography and the mechanisms of signal transduction from these receptors to the BMPs and bone-specific promoters are now coming to light.[42]

Yet there remains a set of undefined data and unknown genes that may also be important in this process of hMSC induction and osteoblastic differentiation at c.p. titanium interfaces. Key osteoblastic transcriptional regulators and signal transduction proteins have been discovered by conventional approaches. The hMSC cell culture model offers a large number of cells that yield sufficient materials for genomic approaches to discovery. Surface-selective gene expression events await further discovery.

While gene and protein arrays offer high throughput methods for examining broad-based cell responses to surface modification, they offer answers only in terms of what is known. Both functional and informatic approaches to cloning can be applied readily to cell culture models and verified *in vivo*. Proteomic approaches served by the growing availability of protein arrays and mass spectrometry may supplement new information by standard informatic and knowledge environment approaches. Because of the complex nature (multiple cell types, etc.) of the forming implant tissue interface, a bioinformatics approach may offer distinct advantages over single gene assays of the process.

9.7 Summary

The morphologic temporal assessment of cellular and molecular events that occur at endosseous c.p. titanium implants indicates that a heterogeneous population of cells is formed and markedly changed in the first days following implant placement. Molecular evidence demonstrates that macrophages are among the populations of cells adherent early to the *in vivo* implant tissue interface.

The macrophage contributes to the orchestration of subsequent wound healing events and may contribute BMPs as local osteoinductive signals to the implant–tissue interface. Cell culture studies indicate that macrophage BMP expression is dependent upon c.p. titanium surface topography such that topographically enhanced surfaces support higher macrophage BMP expression. Subsequent to population of the surface by platelets, red blood cells, and macrophages, the fibrin clot is replaced by a noncollagenous matrix supporting undifferentiated hMSC adhesion. When hMSC osteoblastic differentiation was examined *in vitro*, more rapid differentiation occurred on topographically enhanced surfaces when compared to machined or specular-polished surfaces. Osteoblast differentiation initiated by inductive signals is subject to continued modulation attributable to surface topography.

The models used to investigate bone formed at an endosseous implant must accurately represent the processes that occur *in vivo*. At least two different populations of cells (inducer and responder) might be considered as targets for future improvements in endosseous implant technology. Further engineering of implant surfaces for clinical improvement may be well served by utilizing novel engineering approaches (e.g., nanotechnology) for surface modification and by directing these efforts at accurate targets that represent and may ultimately effect substantial and accurate biological endpoints.

References

1. Lindh, T. et al., A meta-analysis of implants in partial edentulism, *Clin. Oral Implants Res.*, 9, 80, 1998.
2. Fiorellini, J.P., Martuscelli, G., and Weber, H.P., Longitudinal studies of implant systems, *Periodontol. 2000*, 17, 125, 1998.
3. Lekholm, U., Surgical considerations and possible shortcomings of host sites, *J. Prosthet. Dent.*, 79, 43, 1998.
4. Cooper, L.F., Biologic determinants of bone formation for osseointegration: clues for future clinical improvements, *J. Prosthet. Dent.*, 80, 439, 1998.
5. Stanford, C.M. and Brand, R.A., Toward an understanding of implant occlusion and strain adaptive bone modeling and remodeling, *J. Prosthet. Dent.*, 81, 553, 1999.
6. Ivanoff, C.J. et al., Histologic evaluation of the bone integration of $TiO_{(2)}$ blasted and turned titanium microimplants in humans, *Clin. Oral Implants Res.*, 12, 128, 2001.
7. Trisi, P., Rao, W., and Rebaudi, A., A histometric comparison of smooth and rough titanium implants in human low-density jawbone, *Int. J. Oral Maxillofac. Implants*, 14, 689, 1999.
8. Lazzara, R.J. et al., A human histologic analysis of osseotite and machined surfaces using implants with two opposing surfaces, *Int. J. Periodont. Restor. Dent.*, 19, 117, 1999.

9. Jensen, O.T. and Sennerby, L., Histologic analysis of clinically retrieved titanium microimplants placed in conjunction with maxillary sinus floor augmentation, *Int. J. Oral Maxillofac. Implants*, 13, 513, 1998.
10. Einhorn, T.A., Clinically applied models of bone regeneration in tissue engineering research. *Clin. Orthop.*, 367, S59, 1999.
11. Cooper, L.F. et al., Generalizations regarding the process and phenomenon of osseointegration. II. *In vitro* studies, *Int. J. Oral Maxillofac. Implants*, 13, 163, 1998.
12. Kieswetter, K. et al., The role of implant surface characteristics in the healing of bone, *Crit. Rev. Oral Biol. Med.*, 7, 329, 1996.
13. Masuda, T. et al., Cell and matrix reactions at titanium implants in surgically prepared rat tibiae, *Int. J. Oral Maxillofac. Implants*, 12, 472, 1997.
14. Park, J.Y. and Davies, J.E., Red blood cell and platelet interactions with titanium implant surfaces, *Clin. Oral Implants Res.*, 11, 530, 2000.
15. Davies, J.E., Mechanisms of endosseous integration, *Int. J. Prosthodont.*, 11, 391, 1998.
16. Slater, M. et al., Involvement of platelets in stimulating osteogenic activity, *J. Orthop. Res.*, 13, 655, 1995.
17. Low, Q.E. et al., Wound healing in MIP-1α(-/-) and MCP-1(-/-) mice, *Am. J. Pathol.*, 159, 457, 2001.
18. Sennerby, L., Thomsen, P., and Ericson, L.E., Early tissue response to titanium implants inserted in rabbit cortical bone. II. Ultrastructural observations, *J. Mater. Sci. Mater. Med.*, 4, 494, 1993.
19. DiPietro, L.A., Wound healing: the role of the macrophage and other immune cells, *Shock.*, 4, 233, 1995.
20. Masuda, T. et al., Generalizations regarding the process and phenomenon of osseointegration. I. *In vivo* studies, *Int. J. Oral Maxillofac. Implants*, 13, 17, 1998.
21. Champagne, C.M. et al., Macrophage cell lines produce osteoinductive signals that include bone morphogenetic protein-2, *Bone*, 30, 26, 2002.
22. Berton, G. and Lowell, C.A., Integrin signalling in neutrophils and macrophages, *Cell Signal*, 11, 621, 1999.
23. McKee, M.D. and Nanci, A., Secretion of osteopontin by macrophages and its accumulation at tissue surfaces during wound healing in mineralized tissues: a potential requirement for macrophage adhesion and phagocytosis, *Anat. Rec.*, 245, 394, 1996.
24. Danon, D., Kowatch, M.A., and Roth, G.S., Promotion of wound repair in old mice by local injection of macrophages, *Proc. Natl. Acad. Sci. U.S.A.*, 86, 2018, 1989.
25. Shah, M., Foreman, D.M., and Ferguson, M.W., Neutralisation of TGF-beta 1 and TGF-beta 2 or exogenous addition of TGF-beta 3 to cutaneous rat wounds reduces scarring, *J. Cell Sci.*, 108, 985, 1995.
26. Kovacs, E.J. and DiPietro, L.A., Fibrogenic cytokines and connective tissue production, *FASEB J.*, 11, 854, 1994.
27. Watzek, G., *Endosseous Implants: Scientific and Clinical Aspects*, Quintessence Publishing, Chicago, 1995.
28. Martin, C.W. and Muir, I.F., The role of lymphocytes in wound healing, *Br. J. Plast. Surg.*, 43, 655, 1990.
29. Teng, Y.T. et al., Functional human T-cell immunity and osteoprotegerin ligand control alveolar bone destruction in periodontal infection, *J. Clin. Invest.*, 106, R59, 2000.

30. Kong, Y.Y. et al., Activated T cells regulate bone loss and joint destruction in adjuvant arthritis through osteoprotegerin ligand, *Nature*, 402, 304, 1999.
31. Aubin, J.E., Advances in the osteoblast lineage, *Biochem. Cell Biol.*, 76, 899, 1998.
32. Bruder, S.P. et al., Mesenchymal stem cells in osteobiology and applied bone regeneration, *Clin. Orthop.*, 355, S247, 1998.
33. Kadiyala, S. et al., Culture expanded canine mesenchymal stem cells possess osteochondrogenic potential *in vivo* and *in vitro*, *Cell Transplant*, 6, 125, 1997.
34. Damsky, C.H., Extracellular matrix–integrin interactions in osteoblast function and tissue remodeling, *Bone*, 25, 95, 1999.
35. Abron, A. et al., Evaluation of a predictive model for implant surface topography effects on early osseointegration in the rat tibia model, *J. Prosthet. Dent.*, 85, 40, 2001.
36. Ganss, B., Kim, R.H., and Sodek, J., Bone sialoprotein, *Crit. Rev. Oral Biol. Med.*, 10, 79, 1999.
37. Cooper, L.F. et al., Spatiotemporal assessment of fetal bovine osteoblast culture differentiation indicates a role for BSP in promoting differentiation, *J. Bone Miner. Res.*, 13, 620, 1998.
38. Takebe, J., Champagne, C.M., and Cooper, L.F., *J. Biomater. Rel. Res.*, in press, 2002.
39. Yamaguchi, A., Komori, T., and Suda, T., Regulation of osteoblast differentiation mediated by bone morphogenetic proteins, hedgehogs, and Cbfa1, *Endocr. Rev.*, 21, 393, 2000.
40. Nakashima, K. et al., The novel zinc finger-containing transcription factor osterix is required for osteoblast differentiation and bone formation, *Cell*, 108, 17, 2002.
41. Damsky, C.H., Extracellular matrix–integrin interactions in osteoblast function and tissue remodeling, *Bone*, 25, 95, 1999.
42. Franceschi, R.T., The developmental control of osteoblast-specific gene expression: role of specific transcription factors and the extracellular matrix environment, *Crit. Rev. Oral Biol. Med.*, 10, 40, 1999.
43. Takebe, J. et al., Titanium surface topography alters cell shape and modulates bone morphogenetic protein 2 expression in the J774A.1 macrophage cell line, *J. Biomed. Mater. Res.*, 64A, 207–216, 2003.

10

A Selection of Oral Implant Materials Based on Experimental Studies

Peter Thomsen and Carina B. Johansson

CONTENTS

10.1 Introduction 183
10.2 Commercially Pure Titanium 184
10.3 Titanium Alloys 187
 10.3.1 Ti-6Al-4V 187
 10.3.2 Titanium Alloys Other Than Ti-6Al-4V 187
10.4 Surface-Modified c.p. Titanium and Ti-6Al-4V 188
10.5 Tantalum 189
10.6 Niobium 192
10.7 Zirconium 194
10.8 Hafnium 195
10.9 Vitallium (Cobalt/Chromium Alloy) 196
10.10 Summary 198
Acknowledgments 199
References 199

10.1 Introduction

A large number of factors must be taken into account before the selection of a material for implantation in the human body. In the development work of oral titanium implants *ad modum* Brånemark, the following six factors were considered to be of importance for a reliable outcome of an osseointegrated implant[1]:

0-8493-1474-7/03/$0.00+$1.50

1. Material
2. Design
3. Surface structure
4. Host tissue
5. Surgical technique
6. Loading

Three of these factors are related to the biomaterial, whereas the remaining three are related to conditions of the host and surgical skill.

The interplay between the material and the surrounding tissue and the outcome of this response are of prime concern. Surgical trauma, inflammation, tissue repair, and regeneration constitute the hallmarks of the biological processes that develop around an implanted material. The mechanisms that regulate these processes at the interface of a synthetic material are not fully understood.

Accumulating evidence suggests that both chemical and topographical properties of the material are of importance. Nevertheless, a greater insight into the meaning of the term *biocompatibility* is required. Today, the most widely used definition of biocompatibility is the consensus definition: "The ability to perform with an appropriate host response in a specific application."[2]

In relation to other metals, titanium is considered an inert, corrosion-resistant metal with adequate mechanical properties. Its suitability as an element for bone anchorage and the transfer of loads is well recognized in odontology. In fact, this material revolutionized the treatment of edentia. Although the concept of inertness has been discussed (see Williams, Chapter 23 of this volume, Ratner,[3] and Williams[4]), it is evident that in search for materials for parts of medical devices to be in contact with or implanted in human tissues, titanium is often the material of choice.

In this respect, the field of oral implantology does not differ from other clinical areas. In fact, current development as exemplified in the release of new materials into the oral implant market, is almost exclusively devoted to surface modifications of titanium. It is therefore appropriate to discuss titanium and some modifications of titanium surfaces briefly, and also to discuss in a more comprehensive manner whether evidence indicates that other metals may perform with appropriate host tissue responses and thus may be equally good candidates for bone-anchored oral implants.

10.2 Commercially Pure Titanium

Commercially pure (c.p.) or unalloyed titanium exists in grades 1, 2, 3, and 4. While the contents of C, N, and H are similar, the amounts of Fe and O

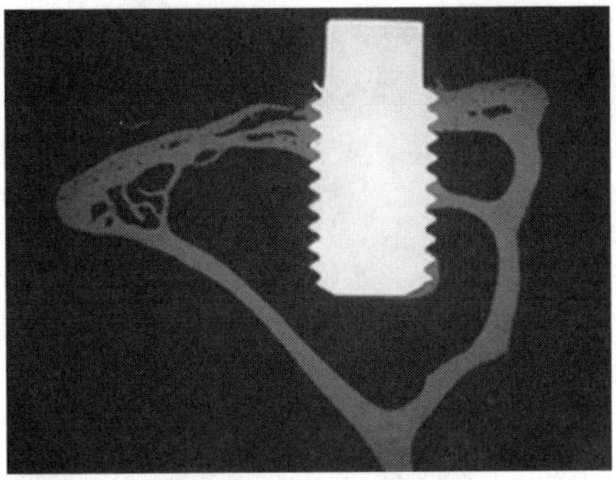

FIGURE 10.1
Microradiographed 100-μm thick undecalcified cut-and-ground section with a c.p. titanium implant inserted in the cortical bone of a rabbit for 3 months. The outer implant diameter is 3.7 mm.

present increase somewhat with the grades. Grade 5 titanium is combined with aluminum and vanadium to produce an alloy known as Ti-6Al-4V.

In 1940, Bothe and coworkers[5] presented an animal study in which bone tissue grew in close contact to a pure titanium implant. Extensive global research since then has explored the TiO_2 passivation film and its corrosion resistance and demonstrated its biocompatibility, clinical success, and utility. TiO_2 is now a material of choice for the fabrication of several oral implant systems due in part at least to its ability to become osseointegrated. As examples, the bone tissue reactions to c.p. titanium implants can be observed in Figures 10.1 through 10.4.

It is beyond the scope of this chapter to discuss the biological response to titanium. Readers interested in the properties of titanium material and subsequent biological responses are referred to selected reviews and articles[6-19] and Ph.D. theses[20-36] based on our research.

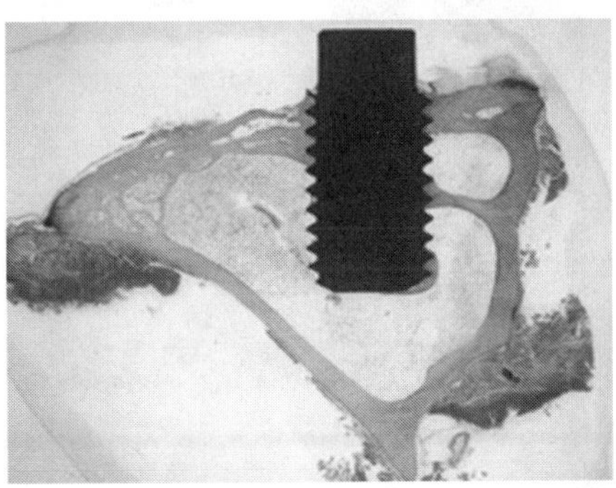

FIGURE 10.2
Same sample shown in Figure 10.1. This section is 10 μm thick and histologically stained with toluidine blue mixed with pyronin G.

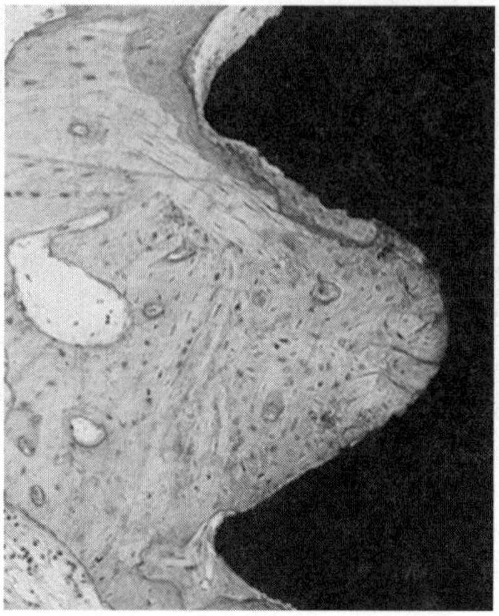

FIGURE 10.3
A c.p. titanium implant retrieved after 6 weeks of insertion in rabbit bone. A close contact of the bone tissue to implant can be observed inside the thread while the thread tips are surrounded with soft tissue. The distance between the thread peaks is 600 μm.

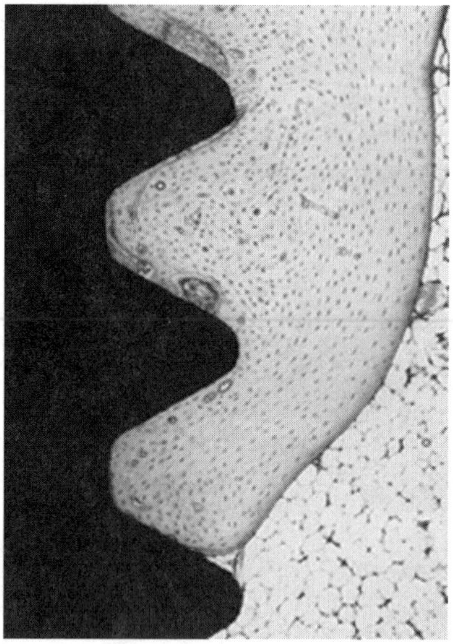

FIGURE 10.4
A c.p. titanium implant after 6 months of insertion in rabbit tibia. Note that the bone in this sample is more mature than the bone tissue inside the threads in the 6-week sample pictured above (Figure 10.3).

10.3 Titanium Alloys

10.3.1 Ti-6Al-4V

It is beyond the scope of this chapter to cover the literature about Ti-6Al-4V. In brief, this alloy has been used since the mid 1970s, particularly to fabricate orthopedic implants. The literature review in the thesis by Johansson[20] concluded that a lack of data supported "better" hard tissue reactions to the alloy compared to the pure titanium. Most recent scientific papers include more specific documentation about materials and methods used. One oral implant system that seems to work well is the the Endopore system discussed by Pilliar (Chapter 3, this volume).

Several investigations have compared c.p. titanium to Ti-6Al-4V implants after various times of insertion in rabbit bone. It has been shown that turned implants of c.p. titanium had significantly higher removal torque values than Ti-6Al-4V screws (23 versus 16 Ncm, respectively) and significantly higher bony contacts (59 versus 50%) after 3 months of insertion.[37] The implant surface roughnesses were essentially similar, as demonstrated by Taylor Hobson Form Talysurf (Rank Taylor Hobson Ltd., UK) measurements (Rz 5.2 for the alloy compared to 4.1 for the c.p. Ti). Titanium ions could be detected by secondary ion mass spectroscopy (SIMS) in the tissues surrounding both types of implants while aluminum ions (and vanadium in very small amounts) could be observed outside the alloy implants. No obvious qualitative differences could be observed on the cut and ground sections. Regardless of material, multinucleated giant cells and macrophages were revealed in close vicinity to the implant materials.

In yet another study comparing similar types of implants with similar surface roughnesses as measured by TopScan three-dimensional equipment (Heidelburg Instruments GmbH, Germany) (mean Sa values 0.7 and 0.6 μm for c.p. Ti and the alloy samples, respectively) and using similar techniques as in the study by Johansson et al.,[37] the 6- and 12-month biomechanical results for c.p. titanium were significantly higher compared to the alloy screws.[38] Comparisons of the 1-month data did not reveal any significant differences between the materials. The bony contact measurements revealed a tendency for higher percentages around the c.p. titanium implants, but no significant differences. Qualitatively, the implants became more integrated in bone tissue over time, but no qualitative differences could be observed between the implant materials.

10.3.2 Titanium Alloys Other Than Ti-6Al-4V

In addition to alloys containing vanadium, other titanium alloys have been evaluated under experimental conditions. Examples include Ti-5Al-2.5Fe, Ti-6Al-7Nb, and Ti-6Al-6Nb-1Ta. Experimental studies performed by Perren et al.[39] showed no major differences in biocompatibility between Ti-5Al-2.5Fe, Ti-

6Al-7Nb, or Ti-6Al-6Nb-1Ta in comparison with c.p. titanium and Ti-6Al-4V after 1, 3, and 9 weeks' subcutaneous implantation in mice. The Ti-5Al-2.5Fe alloy was introduced in 1980 and marketed as Tikrutan LT35 for hip prostheses. Similarly, the Ti-6Al-7Nb T67 alloy (Protasul-100, Sulzer Orthopedics, Austin, TX) has been used for hip arthroplasty components since 1986. The use of vanadium-free titanium alloys in oral implantology has been limited.

10.4 Surface-Modified c.p. Titanium and Ti-6Al-4V

Han and coworkers[40] performed qualitative and quantitative comparisons of bone tissue reactions to c.p. titanium and Ti-6Al-4V implants, blasted with TiO_2 particles of mean sizes of 25 and 75 μm after 3 months of insertion in rabbit bone. The smoother implants had a mean Sa value of 1.1 μm and the rough ones around 1.5 μm. In general, the rough implants were better integrated than the smooth ones. Biomechanically the c.p. titanium implants revealed significantly higher removal torques than the corresponding alloy implants. Both groups (smooth and rough surfaces) demonstrated higher bony contact percentages around the c.p. titanium implants, whereas the bone areas were slightly higher around the alloy implants. Histomorphometrically, no statistically significant difference between the materials was found.

Nitrogen ion-treated and nonion-implanted commercially pure titanium and Ti-6Al-4V implants were inserted for 3 months in rabbit cortical bone. The histomorphometrical results did not reveal any significant differences between the materials. However, the untreated c.p. titanium had a tendency to be better integrated than untreated alloy implants although no significant differences were found (bone contacts of 26 versus 21%, respectively). Ion implantation on the other hand resulted in poorer integration (24 versus 18%, respectively).[41]

An implant surface is spontaneously covered with an oxide layer. The surface oxide properties of titanium implants have been investigated in several *in vivo* experiments.[27,35] Morphometric evaluation of different machined, electropolished, and electropolished anodized titanium implants in rabbit tibiae revealed the highest bone contact for anodized titanium with a 180 nm crystalline oxide.[42] Ultrastructural observations 7 and 12 weeks after insertion in rabbit tibiae[43] have shown that the previously observed amorphous layer and a lamina limitans forming the border of mineralized bone toward the machined titanium implant[44] were present also around electropolished and anodically oxidized (180-nm oxide thickness) titanium.

The electropolished implants that were additionally oxidized (180-nm oxide thickness) showed a higher degree of mineralization compared with the smooth, electropolished implants (2- to 4-nm oxide thickness). Thus, the combination of increased surface topography and oxide thickness presented favorable conditions for bone growth. A long-term (1-year) study,[45] using surface modifications (machined, machined plus anodized, electropolished, electropolished plus anodized) that were relatively smooth compared to blasted and plasma-sprayed surfaces, revealed a high degree of bone–implant contact and a large amount of bone within threads. Taken together, the studies by Larsson and coworkers showed that titanium implants, irrespective of surface topography, oxide thickness, and chemical composition, all became osseointegrated. However, the rate of bone formation was influenced.

Sul and coworkers[46,47] performed quantitative biomechanical and histomorphometrical tests on anodized and nonanodized screw-shaped c.p. titanium implants after 6 weeks of insertion in rabbit cortical bone. Significant differences were noted with both observation methods, when implants with oxides of 600 to 1000 nm compared to thinner oxides (17 and 200 nm) were used.

Titanium surface oxide, through its ability to bind (e.g., with calcium or fluoride), may favor mineralization, which in turn may be beneficial for bone formation.[48] Ellingsen (Chapter 18, this volume) discusses chemical modification in greater detail. Recent studies on bone tissue reactions to screw-shaped implants containing oxides with altered chemistry (addition of S, P, and Ca) compared to the turned control TiO_2 implants revealed that the three former implants performed significantly better compared to controls. Calcium-deposited oxidized titanium implants demonstrated the strongest bone response of all tested implants.[49,50] Figures 10.5 and 10.6 represent an undecalcified cut-and-ground section from an oxidized implant after 6 weeks of insertion in rabbit bone. The section is treated for the visualization and observation of alkaline and acid phosphatase activity. Readers interested in more details about this method are referred to papers by Johansson et al.[51] and Röser et al.[52] Those with further interest in the *in vivo* effects of surface modifications of titanium are referred to the review by Larsson et al,[6] and the thesis by Sul.[35]

10.5 Tantalum

Scientific interest in the *in vivo* effects of tantalum started more than 60 years ago when Burke[53] introduced the metal to surgery. Subsequent *in vitro* studies on the effects of tantalum on cells showed that it and titanium had less effect on the proliferation rates of fibroblasts than aluminium oxide debris and its combination with stainless steel and gold which caused inhibition of cell growth.[54] Similar conclusions were reached by Zetner and coworkers[55] who showed insignificant effects of titanium and tantalum, whereas Vitallium™ and gold (Au) caused significant decreases of fibroblast growth.

Experimental studies *in vivo* on the tissue response to tantalum included performance both in bone and soft tissue. Initial studies in canine bone and soft tissues indicated that tantalum was encapsulated by fibrous tissue (also

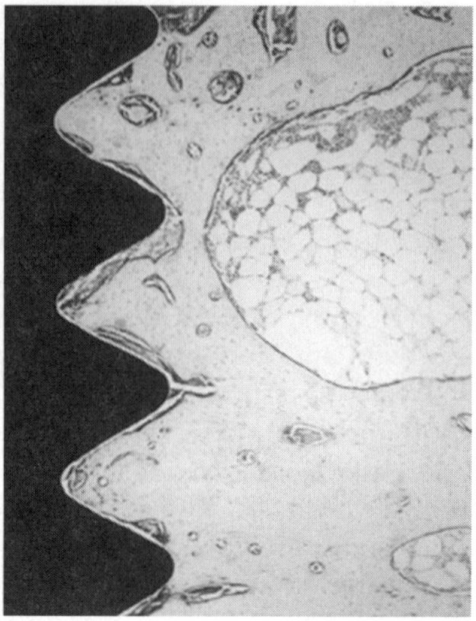

FIGURE 10.5
A cut-and-ground section of an oxidized titanium implant after 6 weeks of insertion in rabbit cortical bone. This section is stained for visualization of alkaline and acidic phosphatase activity. Remodeling areas are observed around the thread tips. The distance between the thread peaks is 500 μm.

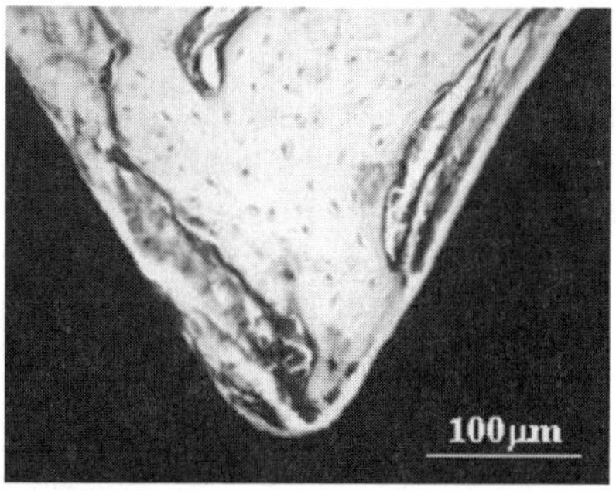

FIGURE 10.6
Higher magnification of a thread area from Figure 10.5. Remodeling areas can be observed inside the threads. The stained cells in the soft tissue areas in close vicinity to the implant surfaces are most likely macrophages. Scale bar = 100 μm.

in bone)[56] but without evidence of bone or soft tissue irritation in follow-up periods up to 3 1/2 months.[53] Subsequent studies in soft tissues indicated that placement of tantalum in rabbit muscle resulted in a fibrous encapsulation that was thicker than around c.p. titanium and titanium alloys.[57]

A series of comparative studies performed in different laboratories show that tantalum has interesting properties in a bone environment. Rabbit bone reactions to porous and surface-structured tantalum, niobium, and stainless steel were examined after 3 weeks, 6 weeks, and 6 months.[58] A growth of osseous tissue right up to the implants and into the pores was demonstrated.

Tantalum and niobium were regarded as favorable compared to stainless steel since they had superior biocompatibility and corrosion resistance in comparison to stainless steel.

Zetner and coworkers[55] found support for their conclusion that "tantalum as well as titanium can be regarded as inert and highly biocompatible materials." Bone responses to tantalum, gold, Vitallium, and plasma-sprayed titanium as coatings on Vitallium foils were examined after 4, 8, and 16 weeks of insertion in a canine jaw. At 4 weeks, new bone formation was observed but formation was reduced where detached metal particles of tantalum and titanium were observed. Tantalum implants were in close connection with bone after 8 weeks in contrast to the other metal implants and remained in tight bone contact after 16 weeks.

Bone tissue reactions to tantalum, niobium, and aluminium oxide in canine jaw were reported to be in favor of tantalum, without, however, presenting supportive numerical data.[59] Studies on tantalum, niobium, and stainless steel wires used for the fixation of experimentally induced fractures in rabbit tibiae did not reveal any differences with respect to bone formation under aseptic conditions after 4 weeks.[60] In contrast, more abundant bone formation was evident under septic conditions around tantalum as compared to niobium and, in particular, stainless steel. The use of tantalum balls as markers in bone was examined by Alberius.[61] Scanning electron microscopical observations after 2, 4, and 16 weeks showed increasing bone support without fibrous tissue encapsulation.

Tantalum was regarded as inert and osseointegration was suggested. Studies on uncemented tantalum and niobium femoral stems in canine hip joint replacement inserted up to 18 months were reported by Plenk and coworkers.[62] The majority of tantalum stems had tight bone contacts without fibrous tissue. Despite some complications associated with the ball head and the proximal portion of the stem, it was concluded that tantalum and niobium were suitable metals for the manufacture of human joint replacements.

More recent light microscopic and ultrastructural interfacial observations of tantalum, niobium, and c.p. titanium in rabbit bone after 3 months demonstrated similar bone reactions at cylindrical polycarbonate plastic implants with 100-nm metal-sputtered films.[63]

Transcortical porous implants of tantalum with pore sizes of 430 and 650 μm were inserted in canine models for 4, 16, and 52 weeks in the former group and 2, 3, 4, 16, and 52 weeks in the latter group.[64] In general, the tissue responses (i.e., the extent of bone in-growth in percent as a function of pore size and time) were similar (13% at 2 weeks) regardless of pore size. However, the smaller-pore implants showed a more complete in-growth after 52 weeks (80%). This was significant compared to the larger-pore samples (71%).

A series of *in vitro* and *in vivo* animal experiments were conducted within a European Community Biomed-2 project entitled "Novel Surface Structures on Improved Metals." The materials involved were commercially pure titanium (c.p. Ti), niobium (c.p. Nb), and tantalum (c.p. Ta) and Ti-6Al-7Nb. Three different surfaces were prepared: (1) ground (Ra +/ –0.35 μm), (2) microblasted (Ra+/–0.7 μm), and (3) reactive ion-etched (RIE) (Ra +/– 1.1 μm). The results on osteoblasts cultured *in vitro* indicated an advantage of the ground samples of c.p. Ti. Blasted samples drastically decreased cell activity (alkaline phosphatase/DNA) in all groups while reactive ion etching was in favor for all but the c.p. Nb group.[65]

In a subsequent *in vivo* study, cylinder-shaped implants of similar materials and surface treatments were inserted in rabbit bone for 6 weeks.[66] The ground samples had an average Sa value of 0.22 μm and when etched, the surface roughness increased to 0.43 μm. The blasted implants revealed a mean value of 0.40 μm compared to 0.43 μm after etching. There was a greater difference in surface roughness between ground and RIE surfaces (the latter having much rougher surfaces) than between blasted and RIE surfaces (quite similar in terms of microsurface roughness).

The undecalcified cut-and-ground sections demonstrated that the implants were integrated in a similar manner in rabbit bone. The RIE implants demonstrated a tendency of higher bony contacts compared to the nonetched ones. In yet another *in vivo* study, with a follow up of 12 weeks in rabbit bone, a comparison of novel macrosurface-structured wafer-shaped implant surfaces of c.p. Ti (Sa = 1.12 μm), c.p. Ta (Sa = 0.81 μm), and c.p. Nb (Sa = 1.52 μm) revealed a similar integration, i.e., about 30% of the implant surfaces were in contact with bone tissue.[67]

In summary, *in vitro* observations indicate that the proliferation of cells is not negatively affected by tantalum, which appears to exert effects similar to those of titanium. However, the number, different cell types, and different cellular properties studied are still very few. Taken together, the recent experimental animal studies on tantalum show that favorable tissue reactions, comparable to those of c.p. titanium, are demonstrated when tantalum is inserted in bone.

Interestingly, very early observations cited above demonstrated that when tantalum and titanium were presented in a particulate form, new bone formation was hampered. These observations show that the design of the material and its surface has a proven importance: bone resorption prevails once particles are generated. In dentistry, in contrast to orthopedics, particulate-induced loosening has not been a major finding.

10.6 Niobium

The chemical and mechanical properties of niobium are similar to those of tantalum.[68,69] The modulus of elasticity of niobium (1.1×10^{11} Pa) is closer to that of bone (0.1×10^{11} Pa) in comparison with most other metals. Further, niobium (and tantalum) are highly corrosion-resistant.[62,69-70]

As discussed above (see Section 10.5), niobium, stainless steel, and tantalum were implanted (porous and grooved cylinder) in rabbit tibiae and evaluated after 3 to 6 weeks and 3 to 6 months.[58] A growth of osseous tissue into the pores was found after 3 weeks, whereas after 6 weeks, a reduction of bone formation was observed. All three types of implant materials were enveloped by newly formed bone. Examination of only the niobium and tantalum cylinders after 3 and 6 months revealed a reduction of the surrounding bone tissue. The authors concluded that niobium and tantalum were just as biocompatible as stainless steel.

Niobium and tantalum were examined for their possible usefulness as materials in femoral stems. Canine experiments showed that tight bone contact without intervening layers of connective tissue was evident along the entire lengths in all the niobium stems. The authors therefore concluded that niobium was an "extremely promising material for this implant application."[70] Radiographic and morphometrical examination of bone reactions to cementless niobium femoral stems in dogs after periods ranging from 2 to 33 months revealed that a spongy bone anchorage developed and was able to withstand functional loading despite some decrease of bone mass.[71]

No major differences in the bone reaction to niobium, tantalum, and c.p. titanium-coated polycarbonate plastic plugs were detected 3 months after insertion in rabbit tibial bone.[72] However, macrophages and multinuclear giant cells were observed in association with detached fragments of niobium. Most likely these fragments were due to accidental detachment from the underlying substrate. Similar observations were not noted for Ta and c.p. Ti.

Screw-shaped c.p. Nb and Ti implants were investigated in an *in vivo* rabbit bone model.[73] Biomechanical tests revealed that the niobium implants were significantly more stable than c.p. Ti (33 versus 25 Ncm, respectively) in bone. The histomorphometrical results, on the other hand, did not demonstrate any significant differences in the bone contact between the materials (mean 41 and 37% bone-to-metal contacts, respectively). No obvious qualitative morphological differences in bone interface response were observed.

Surface roughness investigations obtained from Form Talysurf measurements demonstrated similar values (Ra values of 4.1 for both implants); however, scanning electron microscopy demonstrated a relatively rough c.p. niobium surface — probably due to the softness of the material. Investigations of the latter showed an approximate hardness in Vickers of 92 (10 kg) for c.p. Nb and 145 (10 kg) for c.p. Ti. Figures 10.7 and 10.8 are histological depictions of undecalcified bone with Nb implants after 3 months of insertion.

Although soft tissue response to material is not the subject of the present chapter, it is worth mentioning that niobium implants 6 months after insertion in rabbit muscle exhibited fibrous capsule formations thicker than those formed by titanium and its alloys.[57] Further, significantly higher numbers of macrophages were found around niobium and tantalum in comparison with c.p. titanium and aluminum after 1 to 52 weeks in rat muscle.[74]

In summary, available light microscopic evidence suggests that c.p. niobium in bone is equally well tolerated as stainless steel, tantalum, and tita-

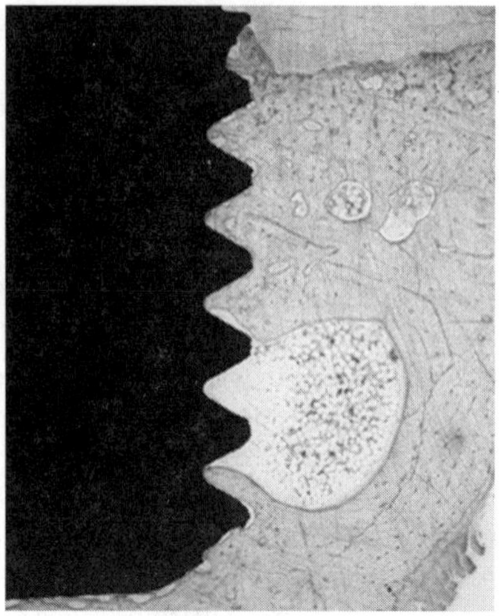

FIGURE 10.7
This c.p. niobium implant was inserted in rabbit cortical bone for 3 months. Compared to the c.p. titanium implants, the tissue reactions were similar. The distance between the thread peaks is 600 μm.

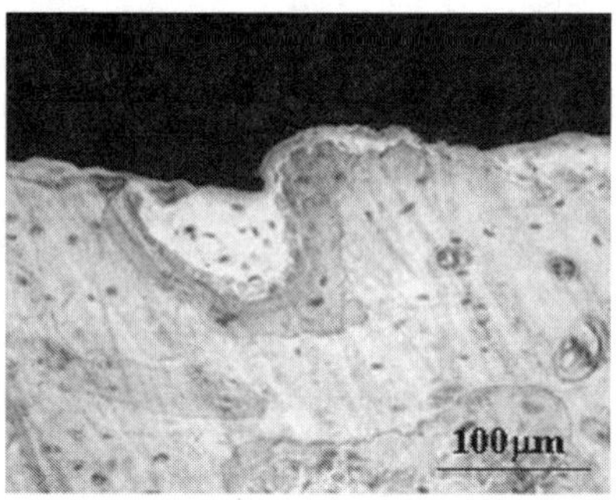

FIGURE 10.8
Higher magnification of an area from the apical region shown in Figure 10.7. Note the rough surface irregularities of the soft niobium implant and the multinucleated giant cells in close relation to the implant. Bone formation with osteoblasts and bone resorptive surface can be observed. Scale bar = 100 μm.

nium. Similarly, ultrastructural observations have suggested that niobium, tantalum, and c.p. titanium are similarly accepted by bone tissue.

10.7 Zirconium

Experiments on Zircalloy (Zr 98%, Sn 1.5%, Fe 0.15%, Cr 0.1%), Vitallium, stainless steel, Ti-6Al-4V, and c.p. titanium revealed little or no corrosion in any specimen.[75] Until recent years, few studies focused on tissue response to zirconium and Zircalloy materials. A qualitative ultrastructural interfacial analysis of c.p. zirconium and c.p. titanium coatings on plastic plugs inserted for 6 months in rabbit bone showed that both materials were well accepted and no adverse reactions or fibrous encapsulations were demonstrated.[76] A slightly thicker amorphous layer of noncollagenous material was detected between the calcified bone and Zr than around Ti.[76,77] A histomorphometric evaluation showed that Ti and Zr had similar bone area and bone–implant contacts after 1 and 6 months, in contrast to Au.[77]

Rod-shaped implants of Ti, Zr, and Vi, with similar rugosity (Ra = 0.6, 0.8, and 0.9, respectively) were inserted in rabbit bone and tested in terms of push-out at 4 and 24 weeks.[78] The push-out data were rather similar between the groups and increased over time; values were 1.9, 1.1, and 1.3 MPa, respectively, after 24 weeks.

In a study by Johansson and coworkers[79] screw-shaped implants of Zr and c.p. Ti were inserted for 3 months in rabbit bone. Several quantitative comparisons of data were performed. The microsurface roughness values were rather similar (Ra = 0.8 and 0.6 for c.p. Ti and Zr, respectively). No significant differences were observed in biomechanical tests; mean removal torque was 26 Ncm for both materials. The bony contact and bone area quantifications went in the same direction and did not result in any significant differences. The authors concluded that the materials were equally well accepted in bone after 12 weeks.

10.8 Hafnium

In relation to the other metals discussed above, very little information is available on the use of hafnium (Hf) in a biologic environment.

Wire-shaped implants (mean Ra = 155 nm) of titanium, hafnium, niobium, tantalum, and rhenium were investigated after 2 and 4 weeks of subcutaneous insertion and in femur bone marrow in rats.[80] The authors reported all implants were encapsulated in fibrous connective tissue after 2 weeks and became thinner after 4 weeks, with the absence of inflammatory response. The bony contacts were rather similar after 2 weeks (about 10% around all implants) compared to the 4-week follow-up when Ti and Ta demonstrated the largest integration (about 40%). No metal dissolution could be observed in soft or hard tissue. The authors concluded that all the tested materials had "good biocompatibility and osteoconductivity."

Cylinder-shaped implants of Hf with 1.24% Zr content and c.p. Ti were inserted in a rat soft tissue model for 8 days, 6 weeks, and 12 weeks.[81] No qualitative or quantitative differences were observed. The latter involved measurements of fibrous capsule width and the numbers and distributions of macrophages. In the second part of the paper, the authors reported bone

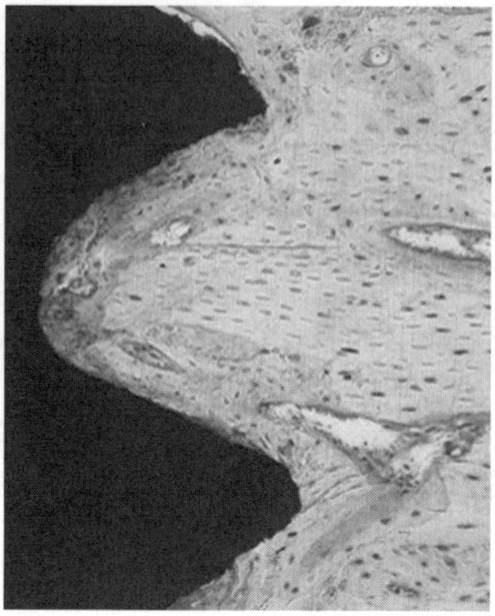

FIGURE 10.9
Hafnium implant inserted in the contralateral leg of the rabbit shown in Figure 10.3 also for 6 weeks. Qualitatively, similar tissue reactions were observed around c.p. titanium and hafnium implants. The distance between the thread peaks is 600 μm.

tissue reactions to screw-shaped implants for 6, 12, and 24 weeks. No significant differences in bone-to-metal contact or bone area measurements of the materials were observed at any time. The conclusion was that "Hf is a highly interesting metal for biomedical applications." Figures 10.9 through 10.11 demonstrate bone morphology around Hf implants inserted in rabbit bone at 6 weeks and 6 months.

10.9 Vitallium (Cobalt/Chromium Alloy)

Vitallium has been used as an orthopedic and dental implant material for about 80 years. Bone studies dating back to the early 1940s include reports on good bone apposition to Vitallium screws but lack quantitative data.[82] It was reported that Vitallium implants were associated with greater extraction forces than unthreaded Ti implants (7.2 kp versus 5.8 kp, respectively).[83] The same authors reported similar qualitative tissue reactions to both materials on thick-ground (300 to 500 μm) sections. In other qualitative histological comparisons of bone to implants made of Vitallium, stainless steel, Ti-6Al-4V, and c.p. titanium, the authors reported that the tissue reactions were similar to all materials.[84-86]

Screw-shaped implants of Vitallium and c.p. titanium were inserted in rabbit bone for 3 months prior to biomechanical and histomorphometrical tests.[87] Both *in vivo* tests revealed the c.p. titanium implant to be significantly

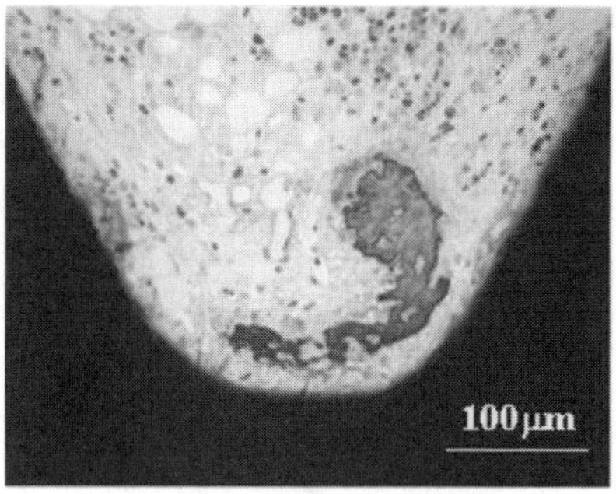

FIGURE 10.10
De novo bone formation can be observed inside this hafnium implant thread (6 weeks after implantation). Irrespective of material, this phenomenon can clearly be observed, especially in implant areas inside the marrow cavity. Scale bar = 100 μm.

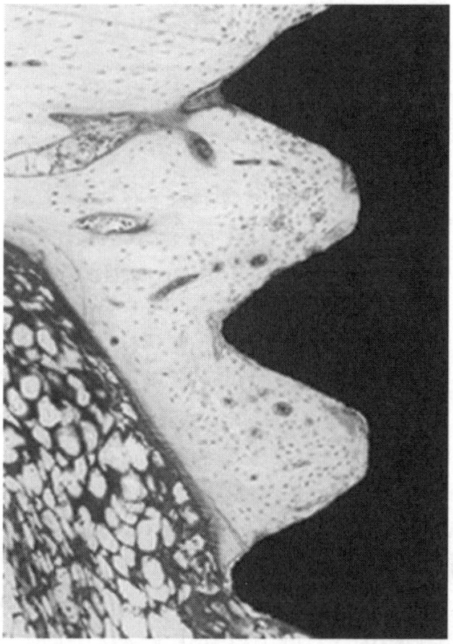

FIGURE 10.11
Cut-and-ground section of a hafnium implant 6 months after insertion. The tissue reaction is similar to that of c.p. titanium (Figure 10.4).

better integrated in bone than the Vitallium implants. One reason for the biomechanical results may be that the c.p. titanium screws were rougher (mean Ra = 4.1) than the Vitallium (mean Ra = 1.7, as deduced from Form Talysurf measurements). Qualitative observations on the cut-and-ground sections revealed multinucleated giant cells in close vicinity to the implants, irrespective of materials. Figure 10.12 shows this observation for a cut-and-ground Vitallium implant.

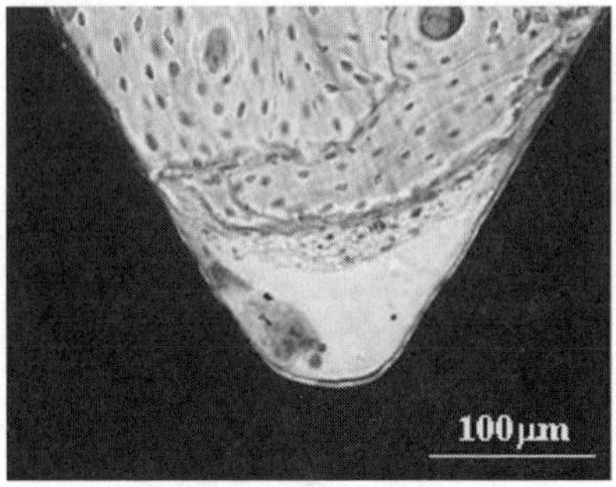

FIGURE 10.12
Implant made of cobalt–cromium (Vitallium). As compared to the niobium implant in Figure 10.8, the Vitallium implant is smooth although one can observe a multinucleated giant cell with black particles internalized. Irrespective of materials, these cells are observed, sometimes darker or lighter stained and, as in this case, as an elongated droplet formation. Scale bar = 100 μm.

10.10 Summary

This review discussing the performances of selected metals under animal experimental conditions suggests that titanium, its alloys, and several other metals have excellent hard tissue biocompatibilities. As judged from the scientific literature covering comparisons of these materials, no biological observations suggest that these materials would differ for instance in their general biologic properties. Thus, bearing in mind that we do not really understand the meaning of the term *inertness*, it is assumed that Ta, Nb, Zr, and Hf all may possess the beneficial *bio-inertness* generally ascribed to Ti. Further research on these materials and host responses is therefore of interest.

A major difference between Ti on one hand, and Ta, Nb, Zr, and Hf on the other is that the clinical community has much more experience and long-term appraisal data showing titanium as a safe and functional implant material. Not as much information is available about the others. Further, it is assumed that research and development costs and the expenses of regulatory approval for titanium and its modifications are more favorable than for the group including Ta, Nb, Zr, and Hf. This has implications also for the industrial development and clinical introduction of new oral implant materials.

Much emphasis today is put on the importance of titanium surface modifications and alleged improvement of clinical results. An analysis of the published literature on the biologic performance of surface-modified titanium does not reveal a uniform picture. Instead, a variety of conclusions and even contradictory results can be found.[6] In fact, rapidly introduced modifications of titanium are intimately coupled to market strategies and an anticipation that they cannot perform worse than currently available so-called golden standards. It is therefore evident that the potential benefits or drawbacks of such modifications will await further results of controlled clinical studies. In a recent editorial, similar concerns were expressed. Albrektsson stated that "It is definitely time to focus more on surgical and prosthodontic skills than continuing the present overemphasis on different hardware parameters."[88]

Although future improvements of implant surfaces will include alterations of material surface properties, it is equally important to understand the local host's response and optimize surgical techniques. It is likely Ti and several other oxide-bearing metals may serve as surfaces for such an approach.

Acknowledgments

The authors are grateful for the financial support of The Swedish Research Council (Grants 9495 and 6533), the EU HIPEDHIPS II project, the Swedish National Board for Technical Development (Vinnova), the Swedish National Board for Laboratory Animals (CFN), the Handlanden Hjalmar Svensson Foundation, the Wilhelm and Martina Lundgren Foundation, and the Eivind and Elsa K-son Sylvan Foundation. We also wish to thank our colleagues and coworkers in previous and ongoing projects who made this presentation possible.

References

1. Albrektsson, T. et al., Osseointegrated titanium implants: requirements for ensuring long-lasting, direct bone-to-implant anchorage in man, *Acta Orthop. Scand.*, 52, 155, 1981.
2. Williams, D.F., Ed., Definitions in biomaterials, in *Progress in Biomedical Engineering*, Elsevier, Amsterdam, 1987.
3. Ratner, B.D., A perspective on titanium biocompatibility, in *Titanium in Medicine*, Brunette, D.M. et al., Eds., Springer Verlag, Heidelberg, 2001, chap. 1.
4. Williams, D.F., Titanium for medical applications, in *Titanium in Medicine*, Brunette, D.M. et al., Eds., Springer Verlag, Heidelberg, 2001, chap. 2.
5. Bothe, R.T., Beaton, L.E., and Davenport, H.A., Reactions of bone to multiple metallic implants, *Surg. Gynecol. Obstet.*, 71, 589, 1940.
6. Larsson, C. et al., The titanium–bone interface *in vivo*, in *Titanium in Medicine*, Brunette, D.M. et al., Eds., Springer Verlag, Heidelberg, 2001, chap. 18.
7. Brunski, J., Puleo, D., and Nanci, A., Biomaterials and biomechanics of oral and maxillofacial implants: current status and future developments, *Int. J. Oral Maxillofac. Implants*, 15, 15, 2000.
8. Brunette, D. and Chehroudi, B., The effects of the surface topography of micromachined titanium substrata on cell behavior *in vitro* and *in vivo*, *J. Biomech. Eng.*, 121, 49, 1999.

9. Kienapfel, H. et al., Implant fixation by bone in-growth, *J. Arthroplast.*, 14, 55, 1999.
10. Cooper, L., Biologic determinants of bone formation for osseointegration: clues for future clinical improvements, *J. Prosthet. Dent.*, 80, 439, 1998.
11. Klinger, M. et al., Proteoglycans at the bone–implant interface, *Crit. Rev. Oral Biol. Med.*, 9, 449, 1998.
12. Pilliar, R., Overview of surface variability of metallic endosseous dental implants: textures and porous surface-structured designs, *Implant Dent.*, 7, 305, 1998.
13. Steinemann, S., Titanium: the material of choice? *Periodontology 2000*, 17, 7, 1998.
14. Wen, X., Wang, X., and Zhang, N. Microrough surface of metallic biomaterials: a literature review, *Bio-Med. Mater. Eng.*, 6, 173, 1996.
15. Schwartz, Z. and Boyan, B. Underlying mechanisms at the bone–biomaterial interface, *J. Cell. Biochem.*, 56, 340, 1994.
16. Linder, L., Ultrastructure of the bone–cement and the bone–metal interface, *Clin. Orthop.*, 276, 147, 1992.
17. Roberts, W. and Garetto, L., Physiology of osseous and fibrous integration, *Alpha Omegan*, 85, 57, 1992.
18. Keller, J., Oral biology and dental implants, *Adv. Dent. Res.*, 13, 1, 1999.
19. Davies, J., Mechanisms of endosseous integration, *Int. J. Prosthodont.*, 11, 391, 1998.
20. Johansson, C.B., On Tissue Reactions to Metal Implants, Ph.D. thesis, Göteborg University, Göteborg, Sweden, 1991.
21. Sennerby, L., On the Bone Tissue Response to Titanium Implants, Ph.D. thesis, Göteborg University, Göteborg, Sweden, 1991.
22. Eriksson, A., Inflammatory Reactions at Biomaterial Surfaces, Ph.D. thesis, Göteborg University, Göteborg, Sweden, 1993.
23. Gottlander, M., On Hard Tissue Reactions to Hydroxyapatite-Coated Titanium Implants, Ph.D. thesis, Göteborg University, Göteborg, Sweden, 1994.
24. Holgers, K.-M., Soft Tissue Reactions around Clinical Skin-Penetrating Titanium Implants, Ph.D. thesis, Göteborg University, Göteborg, Sweden, 1994.
25. Brånemark, R., A Biomechanical Study of Osseointegration: *in Vivo* Measurements in Rat, Rabbit, Dog, and Man, Ph.D. thesis, Göteborg University, Göteborg, Sweden, 1996.
26. Wennerberg, A., On Surface Roughness and Implant Incorporation, Ph.D. thesis, Göteborg University, Göteborg, Sweden, 1996.
27. Larsson, C., The Interface between Bone and Metals with Different Surface Properties: Light Microscopic and Ultrastructural Studies, Ph.D. thesis, Göteborg University, Göteborg, Sweden, 1997.
28. Meredith, N., On the Clinical Measurements of Implant Stability and Osseointegration, Ph.D. thesis, Göteborg University, Göteborg, Sweden, 1997.
29. Ivanoff, C-J., On Surgical and Implant-Related Factors Influencing Integration and Function of Titanium Implants: Experimental and Clinical Aspects, Ph.D. thesis, Göteborg University, Göteborg, Sweden, 1999.
30. Friberg, B., On Bone Quality and Implant Stability Measurements, Ph.D. thesis, Göteborg University, Göteborg, Sweden, 1999.
31. Esposito, M., On Biological Failures of Osseointegrated Oral Implants, Ph.D. thesis, Göteborg University, Göteborg, Sweden, 1999.
32. Liljensten, E., On Bone Grafts and Bond Substitutes Adjacent to Titanium Implants, Ph.D. thesis, Göteborg University, Göteborg, Sweden, 1999.

33. Gretzer, C., Macrophage–Material Surface Interactions, Ph.D. thesis, Göteborg University, Göteborg, Sweden, 2000.
34. Höstner, C., On the Bone Response to Different Implant Textures: A Three-Dimensional Analysis of Roughness, Wavelength and Surface Pattern of Experimental Implants, Ph.D. thesis, Göteborg University, Göteborg, Sweden, 2001.
35. Sul, Y.-T., On the Bone Response to Oxidized Titanium Implants: The Role of Microporous Structure and Chemical Composition of the Surface Oxide in Enhanced Osseointegration, Ph.D. thesis, Göteborg University, Göteborg, Sweden, 2002.
36. Franke-Stenport, V., On Growth Factors and Titanium Implant Integration in Bone, Ph.D. thesis, Göteborg University, Göteborg, Sweden, 2002.
37. Johansson, C.B. et al., Tissue reactions to titanium–6 aluminum–4 vanadium alloy, *Eur. J. Exp. Musculoskel. Res.*, 1, 161, 1992.
38. Johansson, C.B. et al., Quantitative comparison of machined commercially pure (c.p.) titanium and titanium–6 aluminium– 4 vanadium (Ti6Al4V) implants in rabbit bone, *J. Oral Maxillofac. Implants*, 13, 315, 1998.
39. Perren, S.M. et al., Quantitative evaluation of biocompatibility of vanadium-free titanium alloy, in *Biological and Biomechanical Performance of Biomaterials*, Christel, P. et al., Eds., Elsevier, Amsterdam, 1986, p. 397.
40. Han, C.-H. et al., Quantitative and qualitative investigations of surface enlarged titanium and titanium alloy implants, *Clin. Oral Implants Res.*, 9, 1, 1998.
41. Johansson, C.B. et al., Commercially pure titanium and Ti-6Al-4V implants with and without nitrogen ion implantation: surface characterization and quantitative studies in rabbit cortical bone, *J. Mater. Sci. Mater. Med.*, 4, 132, 1993.
42. Larsson, C. et al., Bone response to surface-modified titanium implants: studies on electropolished implants with different oxide thicknesses and morphology, *Biomaterials*, 15, 1062, 1994.
43. Larsson, C., Thomsen, P., and Ericson, L.E., The ultrastructure of the interface zone between bone and surface modified titanium, in manuscript, 2002.
44. Sennerby, L., Thomsen, P., and Ericson, L.E., Ultrastructure of the bone–titanium interface in rabbits, *J. Mater. Sci. Mater. Med.*, 3, 262, 1992.
45. Larsson, C. et al., Bone response to surface modified titanium implants: studies on the response after one year to machined and electropolished implants with different oxide thicknesses, *J. Mater. Sci. Mater. Med.*, 8, 721, 1997.
46. Sul, Y.-T. et al., Resonance frequency and removal torque analysis of implants with turned and anodised surface oxides, *Clin. Oral Implants Res.*, 13, 252, 2002.
47. Sul, Y.-T. et al., Qualitative and quantitative observations of bone tissue reactions to anodised implants, *Biomaterials*, 23, 1809, 2002.
48. Hanawa, T., Titanium and its oxide film: a substrate for formation of apatite, in *The Bone-Biomaterial Interface*, Davies, J.E., Ed., University of Toronto Press, Toronto, 1991, chap. 4.
49. Sul, Y.-T. et al., Bone reactions to oxidized titanium implants with electrochemical anion sulphuric acid and phosphoric acid incorporation, *Clin. Implant. Dent. Rel. Res.*, 4, 478, 2002.
50. Sul, Y.-T., Johansson, C.B., and Albrektsson, T., Oxidized titanium screws coated with calcium ions and their performance in rabbit bone, *JOMI*, 17, 625, 2002.
51. Johansson, C.B. et al., Bone tissue formation and integration of titanium implants: an evaluation with newly developed enzyme and immunohistochemical techniques, *Clin. Implant. Dent. Rel. Res.*, 1, 33, 1999.

52. Röser, K. et al., A new approach to demonstrate cellular activity in bone formation adjacent to implants, *J. Biomed. Mater. Res.*, 51, 280, 2000.
53. Burke, G.L., The corrosion of metals in tissues and an introduction to tantalum, *Can. Med. Assn. J.*, August 1940, p. 125.
54. Plenk, H., Jr., Evaluation of the effects of ceramic and different metallic implant materials on the growth rate of human fibroblast cultures, in *Evaluation of Biomaterials,* Winter, G.D. et al., Eds., *Advances in Biomaterials,* John Wiley & Sons, Chichester, 1980, vol. 1, chap. 42.
55. Zetner, K., Plenk, J., Jr., and Strassl, H., Tissue and cell reactions *in vivo* and *in vitro* to different metals for dental implants, in *Dental Implants, Materials and Systems*, Heimke, G., Ed., Hanser Verlag, Munich, 1980, p. 15.
56. Carney, H.M., An experimental study with tantalum, *Proc. Exper. Biol. Med.*, 51, 147, 1942.
57. Laing, P.G., Ferguson, A.B, and Hodge, E.S., Tissue reactions in rabbit muscle exposed to metallic implants, *J. Biomed. Mater. Res.*, 1, 135, 1967.
58. Pflüger, G. et al., Bone reaction to porous and grooved stainless steel, tantalum and niobium implants, in *Biomaterials*, Winter, G.D. et al, Eds., *Advances in Biomaterials,* John Wiley & Sons, Chichester, 1980, vol. 3, chap. 8, p. 45.
59. Strassl, H., Porteder, H., and Zetner, K., Vergleich zweier Iimplantatwerkstoffgruppen (Metall-Keramik) am selben Objekt: Eine vergleichende tierexperimentelle Studie, *Orale Implantol. Organ. DGZI*, 10, 73, 1982.
60. Rabenseifner, L. et al., Ist die Knochenbruchheilung bei den gewebeverträglichen Implantatwerkstoffen Tantal und Niob gegenüber Stahlimplantaten verändert? *Z. Orthop.*, 122, 349, 1984.
61. Alberius, P., Bone reaction to tantalum markers: a scanning electron microscopic study, *Acta Anat.*, 115, 310, 1983.
62. Plenk, H., Jr. et al., Mechanical and biological suitability of niobium for skeletal implants, 9th Annual Meeting, Society for Biomaterials, Birmingham, Alabama, April–May 1983, p. 74.
63. Johansson, C.B. et al., Ultrastructural differences of the interface zone between bone and Ti-6Al-4V or commercially pure titanium, *J. Biomed. Eng.*, 11, 3, 1989.
64. Bobyn, J.D. et al., Characteristics of bone ingrowth and interface mechanics of a new porous tantalum biomaterial, *J. Bone Joint Surg. (Br.),* 81B, 907, 1999.
65. Pypen, C.M. et al., Influence of microblasting and reactive ion etching of niobium, tantalum, titanium and Ti-6Al-7Nb on osteoblast activity, abstr., *European Society for Biomaterials*, Abstract, The Hague, 1998.
66. Johansson, C.B. et al., Surface characterization of blasted and reactive ion etched Ti, Nb, Ta and Ti-6Al-7Nb implants and their endosteal tissue response in rabbit tibia, abstr., 15th European Conference on Biomaterials, European Society for Biomaterials, Bordeaux, France, Abstract, 1999.
67. Johansson, C.B. et al., *In vivo* evaluation of the tissue response to wafer-structured, microblasted and reactive ion-etched titanium, niobium and tantalum implants in rabbit bone, abstr., 27th Annual Meeting, Society for Biomaterials, St. Paul, MN, Abstract, 2001.
68. Schider, S. and Bildstein, H., Tantalum and niobium as potential prosthetic materials, in *Biomaterials,* Winter, G.D. et al., Eds., *Advances in Biomaterials,* John Wiley & Sons, Chichester, 1980, vol. 3, chap. 3, p. 13.
69. Pflüger, G. et al., Niobium as candidate material for surgical implants, World Congress on Medical Physics and Biomedical Engineering, Hamburg, Abstract, 1982.

70. Plenk, H., Jr. et al., Long-term anchorage of cementless tantalum and niobium femoral stems in canine hip joint replacement, in *Biomaterials and Biomechanics*, Ducheyne, P. et al., Eds., Elsevier, Amsterdam, 1984, p. 61.
71. Gottsauner-Wolf, G. et al., Histomorphometrical and roentgenological evaluations of bone reactions to cementless niobium femoral stems in dogs, in *Biomaterials and Clinical Applications*, Pizzoferrato, A. et al., Eds., Elsevier, Amsterdam, 1987, p. 753.
72. Johansson, C.B., Albrektsson, T., and Thomsen, P., Removal torques of screw-shaped c.p. titanium and Ti-6Al-4V implants in rabbit bone, in *Clinical Implant Materials*, Heimke, G. et al., Eds., *Advances in Biomaterials*, Elsevier, Amsterdam, 1990, 9, 87.
73. Johansson, C.B. and Albrektsson, T., A removal torque and a histomorphometric study of commercially pure niobium and titanium implants in rabbit bone, *Clin. Oral Implant Res.*, 2, 24, 1991.
74. Therin, M., Meunier, A., and Christel, P., A histomorphometric comparison of the muscular tissue reaction to stainless steel, pure titanium and titanium alloy implant materials, *J. Mater. Sci Mater. Med.*, 2, 1, 1991.
75. Galante, J. and Rostoker, W., Corrosion-related failures in metallic implants, *Clin. Orthop. Relat. Res.*, 86, 237, 1972.
76. Albrektsson, T., Hansson, H.-A., and Ivarsson, B., Interface analysis of titanium and zirconium bone implants, *Biomaterials*, 6, 97, 1985.
77. Thomsen, P. et al., Structure of the interface between rabbit cortical bone and implants of gold, zirconium and titanium, *J. Mater. Sci. Mater. Med.*, 8, 653, 1997.
78. Niki, M. et al., Comparative push-out data of bioactive and non-bioactive materials of similar rugosity, in *The Bone–Biomaterial Interface*, Davies, J.E., Ed., University of Toronto Press, Toronto, 1991, p. 350.
79. Johansson, C.B., Wennerberg, A., and Albrektsson, T., A quantitative comparison of screw shaped commercially pure titanium and zirconium implants in rabbit tibia, *J. Mater. Sci. Mater. Med.*, 5, 340, 1994.
80. Matsuno, H. et al., Biocompatibility and osteogenesis of refractory metals, titanium, hafnium, niobium, tantalum and rhenium, *Biomaterials*, 22, 1253, 2001.
81. Mohammadi, S. et al., Tissue response to hafnium, *J. Mater. Sci. Mater. Med.*, 12, 603, 2001.
82. Bernier, L. and Canby, C.P., Histologic studies on the reactions of alveolar bone to Vitallium implants, *J. Am. Dent. Assn.*, 30, 188, 1943.
83. Linder, L. and Lundskog, J., Incorporation of stainless steel, titanium and Vitallium in bone, *Injury*, 6, 4, 1976.
84. Agadir, M. and Lindgren, U., Mechanical fixation of cobalt–chromium and stainless steel implants in rats, *Acta Orthop. Scand.*, 235 (suppl. 1), 51, 1990.
85. Linder, L., Osseointegration of metallic implants. I. Light microscopy in the rabbit, *Acta Orthop. Scand.*, 60, 129, 1989.
86. Linder, L., Carlsson, Å., and Brånemark, P.-I., Osseointegrated ankle joint replacement: a 2-year follow-up of the first case, abstr., *Svensk Ortopedisk Förenings årsmöte*, Kalmar, 5–7/9, 1990.
87. Johansson, C.B., Sennerby, L., and Albrektsson, T., A removal torque and a histomorphometric study of bone tissue reactions to commercially pure titanium and Vitallium® implants, *Int. J. Oral Maxillofac. Implant.*, 6, 437, 1992.
88. Albrektsson, T., Is surgical skill more important for clinical success than changes in implant hardware? *Clin. Implant Dent. Rel. Res.*, 3, 174, 2001.

11

Possibilities of Improving Implants and Regenerating Dentoalveolar Tissues by Tissue Engineering Using Stem Cells and Growth Factors

Irma Thesleff and Mark Tummers

CONTENTS

11.1 Introduction 205
11.2 Stem Cells and Their Potential in Tissue Regeneration 206
  11.2.1 Adult Stem Cells 206
  11.2.2 Embryonic Stem Cells 207
  11.2.3 Future Visions of Stem Cell Therapy 209
11.3 Use of Bioactive Signal Molecules in Induction of Stem Cell Differentiation 210
11.4 Possibilities for Improving or Replacing Implants through Tissue Engineering 212
  11.4.1 Improvement of Implant Performance: Stimulation of Bone and Periodontal Tissue Regeneration around Implants 212
  11.4.2 Replacement of Implants: Growing Roots or Teeth from Stem Cells 213
    11.4.2.1 Regeneration of Roots 213
    11.4.2.2 Regeneration of Whole Teeth 214
References 216

11.1 Introduction

Recent scientific breakthroughs have raised expectations that adult tissues can be replaced biologically by means of regenerative medicine rather than

0-8493-1474-7/03/$0.00+$1.50

by artificial parts, implants, and prostheses. It is hoped that it will be possible to regenerate tissues destroyed by diseases such as cancer, diabetes, and periodontal disease, and that congenitally missing tissues and perhaps even whole organs can be generated. In dentistry the hopes are to regenerate dentoalveolar tissues including alveolar bone, periodontal ligament, dentin, and enamel, and perhaps even to grow whole new teeth.

Like all new therapies, the practice of tissue engineering is based on previous fundamental research dating back decades. The understanding of the molecular mechanisms of normal embryonic development is elementary when tissues and organs are to be regenerated in patients. This knowledge derives from a long research tradition in the field of developmental biology, in particular, from experimental analyses of the mechanisms that regulate organ development and cell differentiation in vertebrate embryos. The present immense interest in the prospects of tissue engineering is due to recent advances in stem cell biology and in the field of signaling molecules — the so-called growth and differentiation factors. We shall first focus on the important recent discoveries in these fields of research, then discuss the possibilities of regenerating dental tissues and improving implants via stem cell therapies and bioactive signal molecules that stimulate tooth morphogenesis, cell differentiation, and production of dentoalveolar hard tissues.

11.2 Stem Cells and Their Potential in Tissue Regeneration

Stem cells have the capacity to self-renew and give rise to differentiated progeny. In early embryos, all cells are totipotent stem cells because they have the ability to form all tissues of the organism. As cells differentiate during advancing embryonic development, they progressively lose their plasticity, and their capacity to differentiate into other directions becomes restricted. However, adult tissues still contain stem cells that contribute to renewal and regeneration.

11.2.1 Adult Stem Cells

Stem cells are present in all continuously renewing structures such as hematopoietic tissue, skin, bone, and intestinal epithelium. In addition, stem cells must be present in tissues such as liver and muscle that regenerate after injury. Interestingly, recent evidence indicates that stem cells are much more widely distributed than previously believed. In particular, the identification of stem cells in the adult brain has led to dramatically increased research activity in the field of neuroscience and to hopes that stem cell therapies may be used to cure brain damage in Alzheimer´s and Parkinson´s diseases, for example.

Odontoblast and ameloblast stem cells have been identified recently in teeth. Mesenchymal stem cells were found in adult dental pulp.[1] When clones of cultured dental pulp cells were transplanted to muscle, they differentiated into odontoblasts and formed dentine matrix. In similar experiments, stromal stem cells present in bone marrow differentiated into osteoblasts and gave rise to bone after transplantation.[2] Dental epithelial stem cells were identified by our laboratory in the cervical loop epithelium in the germinative ends of rodent incisors.[3] These teeth erupt continuously and enamel production continues throughout the lives of the animals. Thus, by definition stem cells are required for ameloblasts to be present.

Most stem cells have no known markers that can be used for localization in tissues. However, evidence from a variety of studies indicates that the cells reside in specific locations called stem cell niches.[4,5] The microenvironment in these niches supports the maintenance of stem cell characteristics as well as their self-renewal. The differentiation of the cells first to transit amplifying cells and then to terminally differentiated cell types is stimulated by specific signal molecules called growth and differentiation factors. For example, in the case of dental epithelial stem cells, their niche is in the center of cervical loop epithelium, and their maintenance and differentiation into ameloblasts are regulated by signals from the dental mesenchyme.[3] Fibroblast growth factor-10 (FGF-10) was identified as a necessary signal.[6]

Usually the stem cells in different tissues give rise to one or a few cell types. For example, stem cells in hair follicles give rise to hair matrix cells, sebaceous gland cells, and epidermal cells of the skin.[7] However, evidence from many studies indicates that stem cells in adult tissues may have the potential to give rise to a variety of different cell types. This has been shown by transplanting labelled stem cells to chick or mouse embryos. It appears that when stem cells are removed from their original niche and encounter a new environment, they can be reprogrammed and cross lineage boundaries. For instance, brain stem cells may give rise to hematopoietic cells, and bone marrow cells may give rise to epithelium.[8,9]

Epidermal stem cells, on the other hand, can contribute to ectodermal, mesenchymal, and neural crest-derived tissues.[10] Hence, it seems stem cells have much more plasticity in their reprogrammable capacity than previously thought. However, at present, no practical methods are available for the isolation of stem cells from their niches in adult tissues, and hence it is not possible to collect them for tissue engineering purposes.

11.2.2 Embryonic Stem Cells

Stem cells from human embryos have recently become alternative sources for the regeneration of human tissues. It has been known for more than a century that the cells in the early vertebrate embryo are totipotent, i.e., they have the capacity to form all tissues. For example, one isolated cell of an eight-cell embryo can give rise to a whole organism. In the blastocyst stage embryo, the cells of the inner cell mass contribute to all tissues of the embryo.[11] It has been already possible for 20 years to culture inner mass cells from mouse embryos as continuous growing stem cell lines.

These stem cell lines have formed and still form the basis for the production of transgenic mice in which specific genes are targeted and modified. For instance, so-called knockout mice, in which the function of a specific gene is deleted, are produced by using the technique of gene targeting in embryonic stem cells. When the modified cells are mixed with cells from the inner cell mass of a wild-type mouse embryo, they contribute to the newly formed embryo and can differentiate to all embryonic tissues. Some of these cells will end up in the germ line and then the genetic modification can be passed on to the offspring.

Successful culture of stem cells from human embryos was reported for the first time in 1998.[12] Since then, the technical and ethical aspects of their use in tissue engineering have been actively discussed in professional journals and in the media. For the first time it is possible to analyze the differentiation of human embryonic cells experimentally. Although the mechanisms of embryonic development are astonishingly similar for all mammals including mice and humans, differences exist and it is very important for the development of stem cell technologies to learn these differences because small regulatory differences during development can ultimately lead to hugely different end results.

The first application for human embryonic stem cell lines and the first order of business will therefore be the fundamental study of human development and cellular differentiation.[13] This will be essential for the generation of knowledge on how to differentiate tissues and maybe even organs from human cells in the future. It is apparent that this will be a long endeavor requiring much effort before we have sufficient knowledge about the molecular mechanisms of human cell differentiation.

The vision for the future is that the human embryonic stem cells will serve as sources of cells for tissue regeneration. Stem cells could be exposed to specific combinations of growth and differentiation factors *in vitro*, which would induce their differentiation to desired directions (Figure 11.1). Different types of tissues could then be grown in culture and later transplanted to patients. Another possibility is that the totipotent embryonic stem cells could be implanted directly to patient tissues, where they would differentiate into specific cell types after encountering the appropriate niche.

One problem of using embryonic stem cell lines for tissue engineering is the potential rejection of these cells by the patient. It is, at least theoretically, possible to overcome this problem by producing embryonic stem cells from the patient's own cells by so-called therapeutic cloning. The basis for this is a nuclear transfer technique based on the one developed to clone Dolly, the first sheep to be cloned. The nucleus of a somatic cell of the patient is transferred to an enucleated oocyte cultured until the blastocyst stage *in vitro*, and a stem cell line is derived from the blastocyst. Since the nucleus contains the genetic information of the patient, any tissue produced by this method

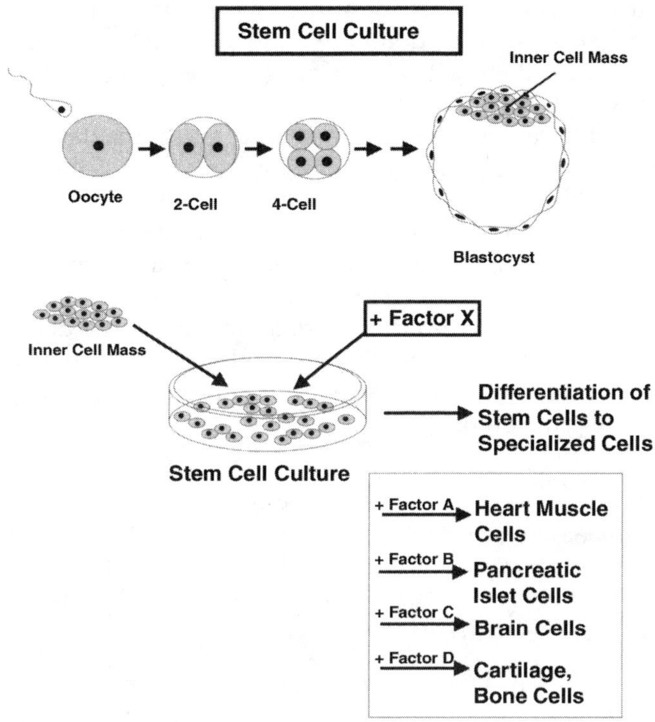

FIGURE 11.1
Stem cell culture. Fertilized oocytes are cultured until the blastocyst stage. Cells of the inner cell mass that will give rise to the embryo are cultured. By adding specific growth and differentiation factors to the culture medium, stem cells are induced to differentiate into certain specialized cell types.

will be immunologically identical and not rejected by the patient. The technology behind the method is obviously demanding, and at present the technology only partially exists. Thus, therapeutic cloning is not yet feasible in practice. In addition, it requires donated oocytes, and raises a number of ethical issues currently under discussion.

11.2.3 Future Visions of Stem Cell Therapy

The optimal way to produce stem cells would be to generate undifferentiated cells from a patient's own differentiated tissue and hence avoid the use of donated human oocytes and human embryonic stem cells. In fact, recent findings suggesting a previously unanticipated level of plasticity in some adult cells and their capacity to differentiate into multiple directions (see above) give some indication that this could be possible in the future.

The cloning of Dolly also showed that the cytoplasm of the oocyte provides an environment that can turn back the developmental clock of a transplanted adult nucleus so that it "forgets" its previous state and history and becomes totipotent. If we learn enough about the factors that turn back the cellular clock, it may be possible to dedifferentiate adult cells experimentally, for example, by treating them with a set of specific chemicals. A possible scenario for future stem cell therapy could be as simple as taking a skin biopsy of the patient, dedifferentiating his cells *in vitro*, and transplanting them back to the right niche in the patient where they would differentiate and replace lost tissue.

Evidence also indicates that damaged tissues may exert chemotactic influences on stem cells and that stem cells might be guided specifically to sites where they are needed for tissue regeneration. Alternatively, dedifferentiated skin cells could be induced to differentiate in culture to a desired direction using specific "cocktails" of bioactive molecules. For example, heart muscle, bone, or brain cells could be induced and subsequently transplanted to a site of tissue destruction or loss.

11.3 Use of Bioactive Signal Molecules in Induction of Stem Cell Differentiation

The ability to induce differentiation of stem cells to desired directions is still a major challenge in stem cell research. Whether the stem cells are derived from embryos or from adult tissues, the molecular mechanisms that guide the differentiation of various types of cells must be understood in order to be able to regenerate specific tissues. The mechanisms that regulate morphogenesis and cell differentiation in the developing embryos have been subjects of intensive research for many decades.

One of the pioneers in this field was Hans Spemann, who won a Nobel Prize in 1935 for studies he performed in the early 1900s on amphibian embryos. He showed that inductive signals generated in one embryonic tissue can regulate differentiation of neighboring tissues.[11] These findings initiated a long search for the identities of the actual inductive signals and it was only after the technological advances in molecular biology that the molecular nature of the signals was discovered. The last 15 years have been an era of extreme activity in the field of developmental biology, and a number of scientific breakthroughs have contributed to the current understanding of the molecular signals regulating cell differentiation.

It is now evident that most signals are small secreted molecules called growth factors or differentiation factors. They are hormone-like molecules that act from outside of the cell, and through binding to specific receptors, they regulate gene expression which subsequently affects cellular differentiation (Figure 11.2). The currently most actively studied growth and differentiation factor families are listed in Table 11.1. Growth and differentiation factors exert a variety of effects on cells and, typically, the same molecules affect the differentiation of many cell types and organs.

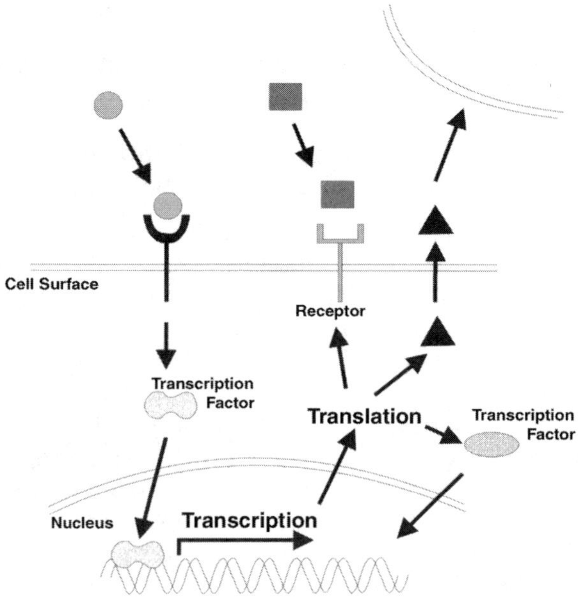

FIGURE 11.2
Growth and differentiation factors from outside the cell transduce their signals through specific transmembrane receptors into the cell. The signals are then forwarded to the nuclei where they activate transcription of specific genes. The mRNAs of these genes are translated into functional proteins, for instance, into receptors, signaling molecules, or transcription factors. The transcription factors will modulate the expression of certain genes in the same cell. The receptors will move to the cell membrane and are then capable of receiving signals from outside the cell. New signaling molecules will be transported out of the cell and can communicate hence with other cells.

TABLE 11.1

Families of Growth and Differentiation Factors
Transforming growth factor β (TGF β)
Bone morphogenetic protein (BMP)
Wnt
Fibroblast growth factor (FGF)
Hedgehog
Platelet-derived growth factor (PDGF)
Insulin-like growth factor (IGF)
Epidermal growth factor (EGF)

The understanding of the regulation of cell differentiation by growth and differentiation factors has increased rapidly during recent years. There are even some examples of successful use these bioactive molecules in the stimulation of mouse embryonic stem cell differentiation. However, we are still far from the ability to apply specific cocktails of factors to undifferentiated cells and stimulate their differentiation into specific pathways and thereby produce desired replacement tissues for experimental animals or human patients.

11.4 Possibilities for Improving or Replacing Implants through Tissue Engineering

11.4.1 Improvement of Implant Performance: Stimulation of Bone and Periodontal Tissue Regeneration around Implants

Bone is a unique tissue in that it undergoes constant turnover resulting from apposition by osteoblasts and resorption by osteoclasts. It also has fantastic ability to regenerate after injury. It has been known for a long time that bone matrix is rich in growth and differentiation factors, and today the molecular natures of the most important of these factors are known. They can stimulate the differentiation of stem cells into bone-forming osteoblasts.

The ability of bone matrix to stimulate the formation of new bone was experimentally proven several decades ago by transplanting demineralized bone matrix into muscle.[14] After many decades of intense biochemical research, the active substance known as bone morphogenetic protein (BMP) was finally isolated and cloned.[15] More than 15 BMPs are known at present and many induce bone and cartilage formation *in vivo* when transplanted with carrier substances to muscle. They also induce the differentiation of osteoblasts and chondrocytes in a variety of cultured cells *in vitro*.

Animal experiments over many years have shown that BMPs are involved in the physiological regeneration of bone. They have the capacity to stimulate formation in different bones including jawbones, and thus they also stimulate alveolar bone formation around teeth. BMPs also induce the regeneration of periodontal attachment, and they apparently have stimulatory effects on cementoblast differentiation.[16] In addition, BMPs induce the differentiation of odontoblasts and dentine regeneration.[17] BMPs have also been shown to induce cementogenesis and the formation and insertion of Sharpey's fibers.[18] Clinical trials in humans are presently testing the effects of BMPs on bone formation in various orthopedic applications as well as on regeneration of dentin and periodontal ligament. In conclusion, BMPs are growth and differentiation factors that can stimulate the differentiation of bone marrow stem cells into osteoblasts, pulpal stem cells into odontoblasts, and dental follicle cells into cementoblasts (Figure 11.3).

It is conceivable that BMPs will be the first bioactive molecules to be used for stimulation of bone formation around implants. As described above, evidence shows that stem cells are guided to sites of tissue injury and hence it is conceivable that the trauma caused by implant surgery will attract stem cells that differentiate into osteoblasts and form new bone. Coating the implant surface with BMP and perhaps other bioactive molecules will stimulate the differentiation of the stem cells into osteoblasts.

Although the improved integrity of bone around the implant is a positive effect, the ankylosis of the implant to bone has considerable negative effects. Particularly when implants are used in growing children, it would be a great improvement if an implant could erupt with neighboring teeth and

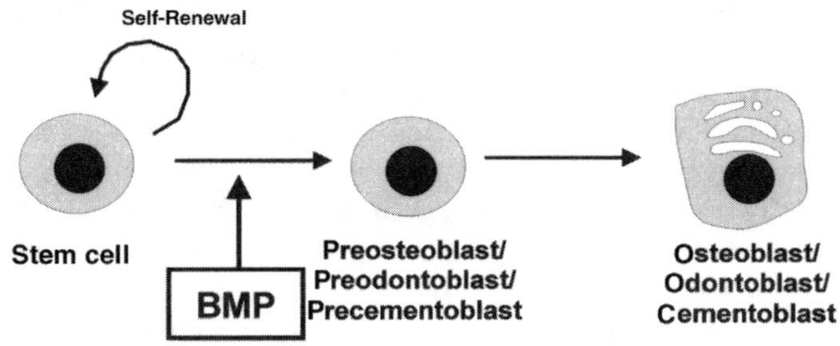

FIGURE 11.3
Maintenance and differentiation of stem cells. During stem cell divisions, new stem cells and cells that will differentiate are created. In this case, BMPs are capable of inducing the differentiation of stem cells into preosteoblasts, preodontoblasts, or precementoblasts that will then continue differentiating into mature osteoblasts, odontoblasts, and cementoblasts, respectively.

stimulate alveolar bone growth. This obviously requires a functioning periodontal ligament.

The regeneration of a periodontal ligament between the implant and alveolar bone is a challenge for future research. The periodontal ligament is a complex structure in which the necessary elements for function include at least the cementum on the root surface and the periodontal fibers connecting the cementum to alveolar bone. These tissues differentiate from the dental follicle surrounding the developing tooth germ, and the specific characteristics of these cells are poorly understood. Although cementoblasts greatly resemble osteoblasts and there is evidence that BMPs stimulate their differentiation and periodontal regeneration, it is unlikely that BMP alone can stimulate the regeneration of cementum and periodontal ligament formation on the surface of an implant.

More research is needed on characterization of cementoblasts in order to understand how the stem cells of osteoblasts and cementoblasts differ and what the specific requirements for cementum formation are. Similarly, it is completely unclear how periodontal fibers and periodontal cells can be regenerated and what the characteristics of their stem cells are. Finally, we do not know the function of the epithelial cell rests of Malassez that form a network at the root surface. It is possible that they are required for some periodontal ligament function, and that they too need to be regenerated on the implant surface.

11.4.2 Replacement of Implants: Growing Roots or Teeth from Stem Cells

11.4.2.1 Regeneration of Roots

The regeneration of three-dimensional anatomical structures of certain size and shape is much more demanding than the regeneration of a single tissue like bone or dentin. Molds have been used for the production of desired shapes and sizes of bones in experimental animals.[19] Muscle flaps placed inside small silicone molds in the shapes of various bones transformed to bone in the presence of BMPs. Although this method may have potential, for example, in enhancement of alveolar bone growth, it clearly cannot be used for creating new roots.

It is obvious that if such bony structures are implanted to the jaw, they will integrate with bone and undergo remodelling. In general, although it may sound attractive to bioengineer real roots from stem cells for implant replacement, this may not be a feasible goal. This is because roots always develop after the formation of the tooth crown during normal development, and it is difficult to imagine how the process of root formation could be initiated in the absence of a crown. Therefore, the only realistic way to engineer a root that could replace an implant is to grow a whole tooth.

11.4.2.2 Regeneration of Whole Teeth

The regeneration of whole organs that consist of several different cell types is difficult. Organogenesis is a complicated sequential process in which the complexity of form increases with time and the process of cell differentiation is tightly associated with morphogenesis. It is obvious that the regeneration of an organ requires that the process is started from the initiation stage.

While this is a demanding goal, it may not be as distant as it appeared a few years ago due to the rapid increase in our understanding of the molecular mechanisms that regulate the development of embryonic organs in general and of teeth in particular. Teeth develop from oral ectoderm and the underlying mesenchymal cells, and at the time of tooth initiation, the epithelial and mesenchymal cells are undifferentiated. Dental epithelium consists of cuboidal cells forming the thickened dental lamina and the dental mesenchymal cells underneath are morphologically similar to the rest of the jaw mesenchyme. A chain of signaling events mainly taking place between the epithelium and mesenchyme of the tooth germ guides morphogenesis through several stages, each increasing in complexity, and this development is also accompanied by advancing differentiation of cells.[20]

Numerous molecules involved in the complex process of tooth morphogenesis have been identified during the last 20 years. Our laboratory created a database on the expression patterns of genes associated with tooth morphogenesis (http://bite-it.helsinki.fi). Patterns of more than 200 genes are shown in this database.

Many growth and differentiation factors act as signals mediating the morphogenetic cell–cell interactions during tooth development. For instance, our laboratory discovered signaling centers (called enamel knots) in the tooth germ epithelium. The knots are composed of small aggregates of epithelial cells that simultaneously produce more than 10 growth and differentiation factors.[21] The enamel knots regulate the formation of tooth cusps and are therefore important organizing centers of tooth development.

The targets of the signals regulating tooth development have been identified in some cases, and hence the molecular and genetic networks regulating

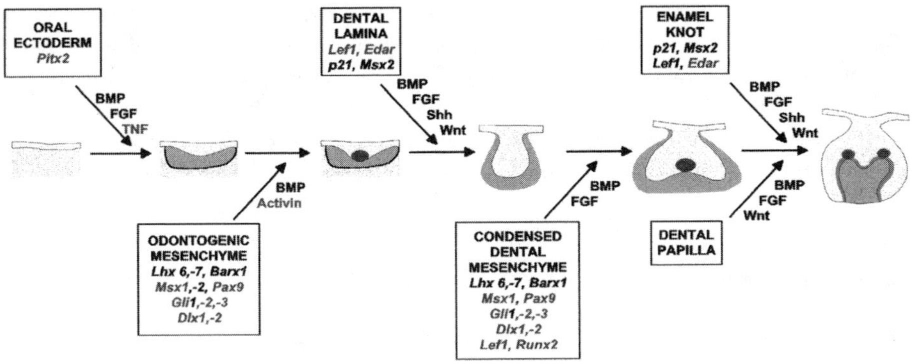

FIGURE 11.4
Signaling between mesenchyme and epithelium plays an important role in the development of the tooth. The same growth and differentiation factors regulate different stages of development. The top panels show epithelial signals and the bottom panels mesenchymal signals. In the boxes are transcription factors regulated by the signals. The grey letters indicate genes shown to be necessary for tooth development in mice.

odontogenesis are starting to be understood. Figure 11.4 shows the molecular cascades regulating early tooth morphogenesis.

Despite the accumulation of molecular information and increased understanding of the regulation of tooth development, it is not clear how teeth can be grown in practice. Perhaps one day we will be able to isolate cells that have the capacity to form teeth and perhaps then tooth development can be inititated *in vitro*. Multipotential stem cells could be obtained from a patient or from embryos by some of the methods described above. Alternatively, it may be possible to use dental stem cells that have the capacity to regulate tooth morphogenesis. Odontoblast stem cells were recently discovered in the dental pulp. These cells may be used in the future for the production of dentin, but it is also possible that they possess the ability of early dental mesenchymal cells that can direct tooth morphogenesis. After its initiation, the tooth germ could be transplanted to the mouth or could be cultured *in vitro*.

In another scenario, tooth development could be initiated *in vivo* by applying specific growth and differentiation factors to the site of the missing tooth or to another site from which the tooth could be transplanted later to the final location. We developed some years ago a technique whereby growth factors are introduced locally to embryonic tissue *in vitro* by small agarose beads that release the factors to surrounding cells.[22] Could it be possible to induce the formation of new teeth *in vivo* by such beads?

It is intriguing that FGF-releasing beads induced extra limbs in chicken embryos when implanted in the flanks between the wings and legs.[23] Additional credibility to the potential feasibility of tooth regeneration comes from the notion that teeth are continuously replaced in certain animals like fish or amphibians. Furthermore, teeth are often found in human teratomas. These tumors consist of a variety of differentiated tissues and it is noteworthy that the teeth found in these tumors often have normal shapes and structures. This indicates that the program for development may be present very early in tooth-forming tissue and is therefore not influenced by surrounding tissues to a significant extent. Hence, the challenge now is to increase the understanding of the process of tooth initiation and the characteristics of dental stem cells in order to succeed in the induction of tooth formation and dental regeneration.

References

1. Gronthos, S. et al., Postnatal human dental pulp stem cells (DPSCs) *in vitro* and *in vivo*, *Proc. Natl. Acad. Sci. U.S.A.*, 97, 13625, 2000.
2. Bianco, P. and Robey, P.G., Stem cells in tissue engineering, *Nature*, 414, 118, 2001.
3. Harada, H. et al., Localization of putative stem cells in dental epithelium and their association with notch and FGF signaling, *J. Cell Biol.*, 147, 105, 1999.
4. Watt, F.M. and Hogan, B.L., Out of Eden: stem cells and their niches, *Science*, 287, 1427, 2000.
5. Spradling, A., Drummond-Barbosa, D., and Kai, T., Stem cells find their niche, *Nature*, 414, 98, 2001.
6. Harada, H. et al., FGF-10 maintains stem cell compartment in developing mouse incisors, *Development*, 129, 1533, 2002.
7. Fuchs, E. and Segre, J.A., Stem cells: a new lease on life, *Cell*, 100, 143, 2000.
8. Bjornson, C.R. et al., Turning brain into blood: a hematopoietic fate adopted by adult neural stem cells *in vivo*, *Science*, 283, 534, 1999.
9. Anderson, D.J., Gage, F.H., and Weissman, I.L., Can stem cells cross lineage boundaries? *Nature Med.*, 7, 393, 2001.
10. Liang, L. and Bickenbach, J.R., Somatic epidermal stem cells can produce multiple cell lineages during development, *Stem Cells*, 20, 21, 2002.
11. Gilbert, S.F., *Developmental Biology*, 6th ed., Sinauer Associates, Sunderland, MA, 2000.
12. Thomson, J.A. et al., Embryonic stem cell lines derived from human blastocysts, *Science*, 282, 1145, 1998.
13. Donovan, P.J. and Gearhart, J., The end of the beginning for pluripotent stem cells, *Nature*, 414, 92, 2001.
14. Urist, M.R., Bone: formation by autoinduction, *Science*, 150, 893, 1965.
15. Wozney, J.M. et al., Novel regulators of bone formation: molecular clones and activities, *Science*, 242, 1528, 1988.
16. Talwar, R. et al., Effects of carrier release kinetics on bone morphogenetic protein-2-induced periodontal regeneration *in vivo*, *J. Clin. Periodont.*, 28, 340, 2001.
17. Rutherford, R.B. et al., Induction of reparative dentine formation in monkeys by recombinant human osteogenic protein-1, *Arch. Oral Biol.*, 38, 571, 1993.
18. Ripamonti, U. et al., Induction of cementogenesis by recombinant human osteogenic protein-1 (hop-1/bmp-7) in the baboon (*Papio ursinus*), *Arch. Oral Biol.*, 41, 121, 1996.
19. Khouri, R.K., Koudsi, B., and Reddi, H., Tissue transformation into bone *in vivo*: a potential practical application, *JAMA*, 266, 1953, 1991.

20. Thesleff, I. and Nieminen, P., Tooth morphogenesis and cell differentiation, *Curr. Opin. Cell Biol.*, 8, 844, 1996.
21. Jernvall, J. and Thesleff, I., Reiterative signaling and patterning during mammalian tooth morphogenesis, *Mech. Dev.*, 92, 19, 2000.
22. Vainio, S. et al., Identification of BMP-4 as a signal mediating secondary induction between epithelial and mesenchymal tissues during early tooth development, *Cell*, 75, 45, 1993.
23. Cohn, M.J. et al., Fibroblast growth factors induce additional limb development from the flank of chick embryos, *Cell*, 80, 739, 1995.

12

Critical Issues in Endosseous Peri-Implant Wound Healing

John E. Davies and Jun Y. Park

CONTENTS

12.1 Introduction 219
12.2 Osteoconduction 221
12.3 *De Novo* Bone Formation 222
12.4 Bone Bonding 226
12.5 Concluding Remarks 226
References 227

12.1 Introduction

The mechanisms by which endosseous implants become integrated in bone can be subdivided into three separate phenomena: *osteoconduction, bone formation,* and *bone remodeling,* as reviewed in detail elsewhere.[1,2] Of these, osteoconduction and bone formation may have profound effects on treatment outcomes in endosseous implantology through the design of optimized implant surfaces. For this reason, it is reasonable to limit our discussion to the mechanisms by which bone is formed on an implant surface, rather than the growth of bone toward an implant surface. This distinction was explored by Osborn and Newesley,[3] who described two phenomena, distance and contact osteogenesis, by which bone can become juxtaposed to an implant surface.

In distance osteogenesis, new bone is formed on the surfaces of old bone in the peri-implant site. The bone surfaces provide a population of osteogenic cells that lay down new matrix that encroaches on the implant. An essential observation here is that new bone does not form on the implant; the implant becomes surrounded by bone. Thus, in these circumstances, the implant

0-8493-1474-7/03/$0.00+$1.50

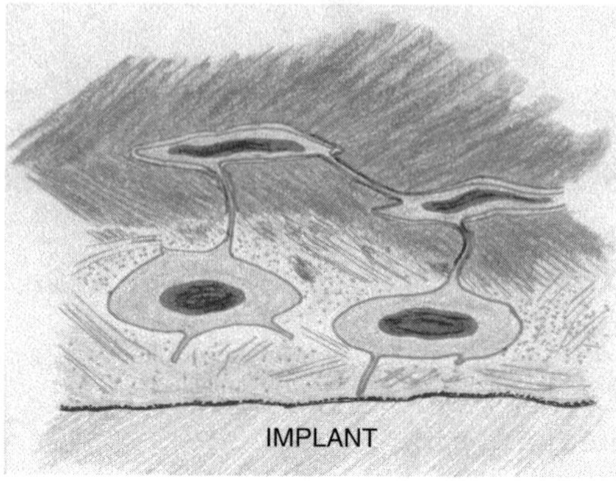

FIGURE 12.1
The consequence of distance osteogenesis. Bone approaches the implant but ultimately is separated from it by a layer of entrapped dead osteoblasts and extracellular ground substance.

surface will always be partially obscured from bone by intervening cells, as illustrated in Figure 12.1.

In contact osteogenesis, new bone forms first on the implant surface. Since no bone is present on the surface of the implant upon implantation, the surface must be colonized by bone cells before bone matrix formation can begin. This is also what happens at bone remodeling sites where a resorption surface of old bone is populated with osteogenic cells before new bone can be laid down. The common factor in these cases is that bone is formed for the first time at these sites by differentiating osteogenic cells. We have called this *de novo* bone formation. Clearly an essential prerequisite of *de novo* bone formation is the recruitment of bone cells to the implant surface. However, the result of *de novo* bone formation is that the implant–bone interface, in an identical fashion to remodeling bone surfaces, will be occupied by a cement line matrix (Figure 12.2) as first described by von Ebner in 1875.[4]

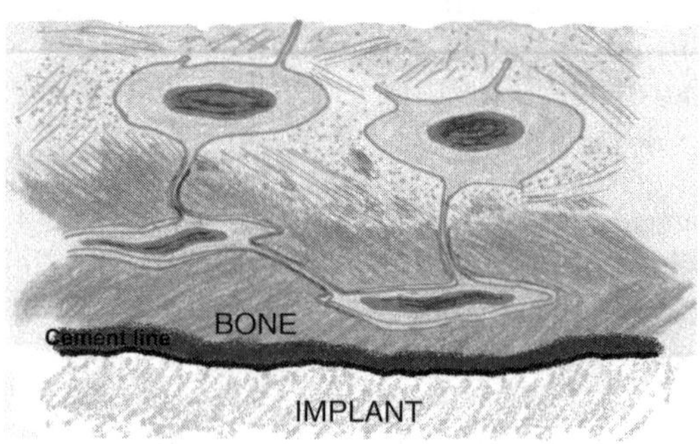

FIGURE 12.2
The consequence of contact osteogenesis. *De novo* bone matrix secreted by differentiating osteogenic cells is laid down directly on the implant surface. In this case, the first matrix formed will be the collagen-free, mineralized, cement line.

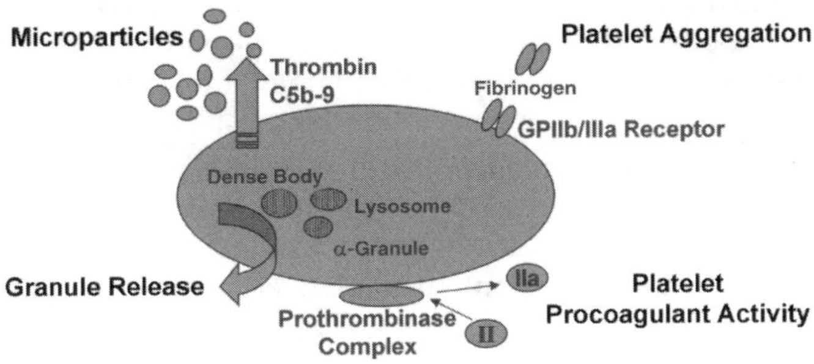

FIGURE 12.3
Platelets become activated by contact with implant surfaces. The degree of activation is a function of the implant surface. Upon activation, the platelets release microparticles and granules containing a wide range of growth factors and cytokines that stimulate cell migration into the healing compartment and the differentiation of these healing-capable cells. (*Source:* Gemmell, C.H. and Park, J.Y., in *Bone Engineering*, em squared, Toronto, Canada, 2000, p. 108. With permission.)

While both distance and contact osteogenesis will result in the juxtaposition of bone to the implant surface, the biological significance of these different healing reactions is of critical importance in attempting to unravel the role of implant design in endosseous integration and elucidating the differences in structure and composition of the bone–implant interface. For rapid peri-implant healing in class III and class IV bone, optimizing contact osteogenesis by implant surface design to ensure early stability is of considerable importance.[2,5]

12.2 Osteoconduction

As mentioned above, contact osteogenesis relies upon the migration of differentiating osteogenic cells to the implant surface. Typically, differentiating osteogenic cells are derived at bone remodeling sites from undifferentiated perivascular connective tissue cells. However, a more complex environment characterizes the peri-implant healing site since it will be occupied transiently by blood.

We have to consider, then, the interactions of blood cells, particularly platelets, with the implant surface. The activation of platelets is particularly important in early healing since it results in the release of cytokines, growth factors, and microparticles (Figure 12.3) that are known to accelerate wound healing, although the exact mechanisms have yet to be elucidated. Our recent work has shown that:

1. Microtextured implant surfaces promote more platelet adhesion than smoother implant surfaces.[6]

2. Microtextured implant surfaces activate platelets to a greater extent than smoother implant surfaces.[7] This is seen in the expression of P-selectin (a membrane-bound platelet molecule) and platelet microparticle formation, as seen in Figure 12.4.
3. Platelets activated on microtextured candidate implant surfaces will up-regulate neutrophils — the first leukocyte population to enter the wound site during the acute inflammatory phase of healing — to a greater extent than platelets activated on smoother surfaces (Figure 12.5).[8]

As seen in fracture healing, the migration of bone cells in peri-implant healing will occur through the fibrin of a blood clot. Since fibrin, the reaction product of thrombin and fibrinogen released into the healing site, can be expected to adhere to almost all surfaces, osteogenic cell migration may be expected toward any implanted material. However, as is well known from dermal wound healing models, connective tissue cell migration is concomitant with wound contraction.[9] Indeed, the migration of cells through fibrin will cause retraction of the fibrin scaffold. Thus, the ability of an implant surface to retain fibrin during this wound contraction phase of healing is critical in determining whether the migrating cells will reach the former. Implant surface design plays an important role in fibrin retention as illustrated in Figure 12.6.

Thus, bone cells will reach the implant surface by migration through fibrin, and these cells will then be available to synthesize *de novo* bone on the implant surface. In so doing, they also stop migrating, and other cells still in migratory mode will gain the contiguous implant surface and secrete bone. The histological result will present itself as the apparent "flowing" of bone over the implant surface as seen in Figure 12.7. However, it should be emphasized that the bone matrix itself has no inherent capacity to "flow" and the histological appearance is created by the matrix secretory activities of previously migratory osteogenic cells.

Thus, the phenomenon of osteoconduction critically relies upon the migration and recruitment of differentiating osteogenic cells to and over the implant surface. The implant surface design can have a profound influence on osteoconduction not only by modulating the levels of platelet activation, but also by maintaining the anchorage of the temporary scaffold through which these cells reach the implant surface. It can be predicted that roughened surfaces will promote osteoconduction by both increasing available surface area for fibrin attachment, and by providing surface features with which fibrin can become entangled.

12.3 *De Novo* Bone Formation

The initial stage of bone formation at remodeling sites is the secretion by osteogenic cells of the cement line matrix.[4,10] This is a collagen-free, miner-

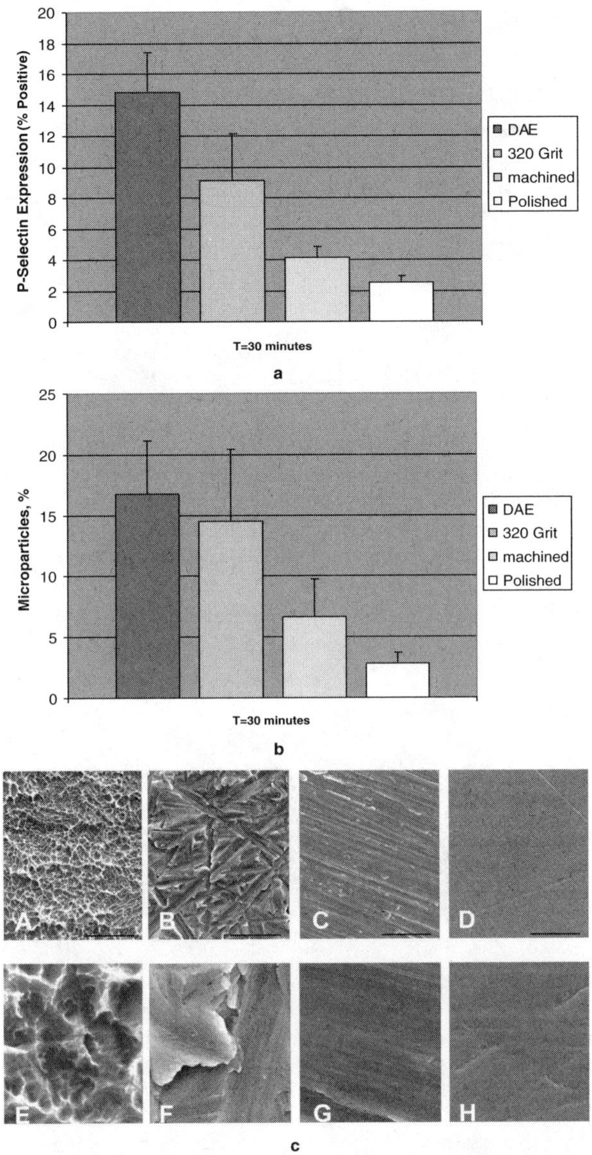

FIGURE 12.4
Activation of platelets through contact (30 minutes at 37°C) with various surfaces shown in panels A through H. Errors bars in graphs = standard error. Top: percentage P-selectin (CD62p) expression derived from flow cytometric analysis using a fluorescently tagged CD62p-specific antibody. Middle: percentage microparticle (MP) release. Bottom: scanning electron micrographs of titanium surfaces employed. A through D: low magnification: 2,000×; bar = 15 μm. E through H: high magnification: 15,000×; bar = 2 μm. A and E: dual acid-etched (DAE) c.p. Ti. B and F: 320-grit abraded c.p. Ti. C and G: machined c.p. Ti. D and H: polished c.p. Ti. Both DAE and 320-grit surfaces show enhanced levels of surface microtexture in comparison to machined and polished samples. (*Source:* Park, J.Y., Ph.D. thesis, University of Toronto, Canada, 2003. With permission.)

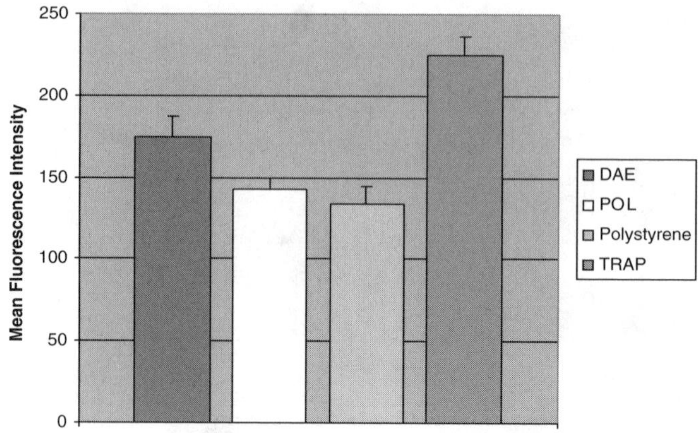

FIGURE 12.5
Platelets activated by contact with dual acid-etched titanium (DAE), polished titanium (POL), and polystyrene up-regulated neutrophils (as measured by CD11b expression) to different extents. Platelets from microtextured DAE surface induced significant enhancement of CD11b over platelets from polished or polystyrene surfaces. Thrombin receptor agonist peptide (TRAP)-activated platelets provided maximum positive controls. Bars = standard error. (*Source:* Park, J.Y., Ph.D. thesis, University of Toronto, Canada, 2003. With permission.)

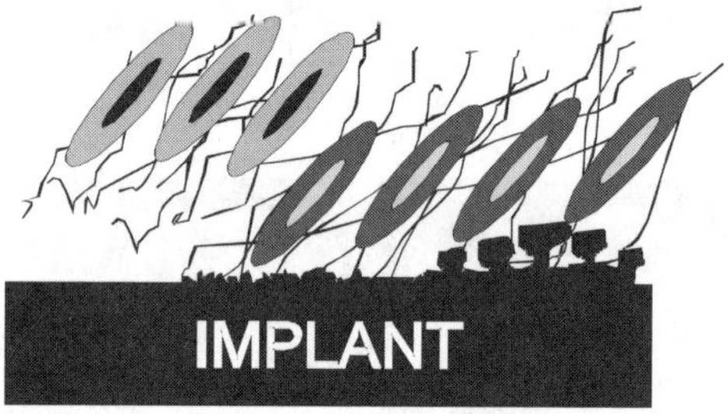

FIGURE 12.6
Fibrin retention by the implant is critical in allowing osteogenic cells to migrate to the implant surface where they can elaborate bone matrix. Failure of fibrin retention, as seen on the left, will result in cessation of osteogenic cell migration distant from the implant surface. On the contrary, retention results in osteogenic cells reaching the implant surface as seen on the right. Many different implant surface topographies will be fibrin-retentive.

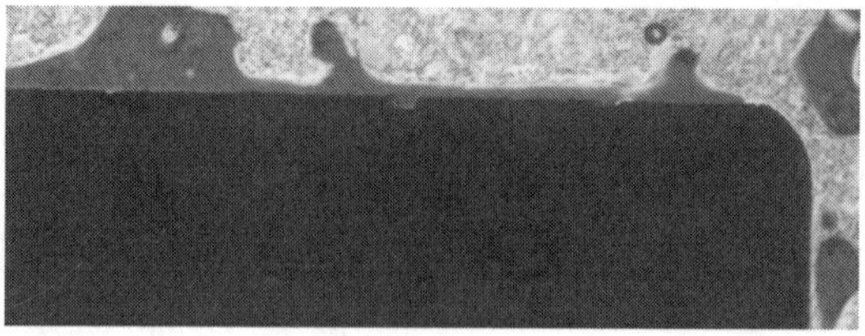

FIGURE 12.7
Bone matrix has no ability to "flow" or "spread" over an implant surface, so the apparently contradictory histological appearance is actually caused by the matrix secretion activities of osteogenic cells that previously migrated over or were recruited to the implant surface.

alized interfacial matrix laid down between old bone and new bone. Despite the early description of this prominent histological feature in bone, the cement line interface eluded both structural and compositional characterization for over a century, but is now widely accepted as the tissue that occupies the bone–implant interface formed through contact osteogenesis.

This *de novo* bone formation cascade is a four-stage process confirmed by both *in vitro* and *in vivo* experiments.[10] Briefly, differentiating osteogenic cells initially secrete a collagen-free organic matrix that provides nucleation sites for calcium phosphate mineralization. We identified two noncollagenous bone proteins, osteopontin and bone sialoprotein, in this initial organic phase. Calcium phosphate nucleation is followed by crystal growth and the initiation of collagen fiber assembly, as seen in an *in vivo* example in Figure 12.8. Finally, calcification of the collagen compartment will occur. Thus, in this process of *de novo* bone formation, the collagen compartment of bone will be separated from the underlying substratum by a collagen-free calcified tissue layer containing noncollagenous bone proteins. This layer is approximately 0.5 μm thick, as are cement lines that form the interface between old and new bone at reversal sites.

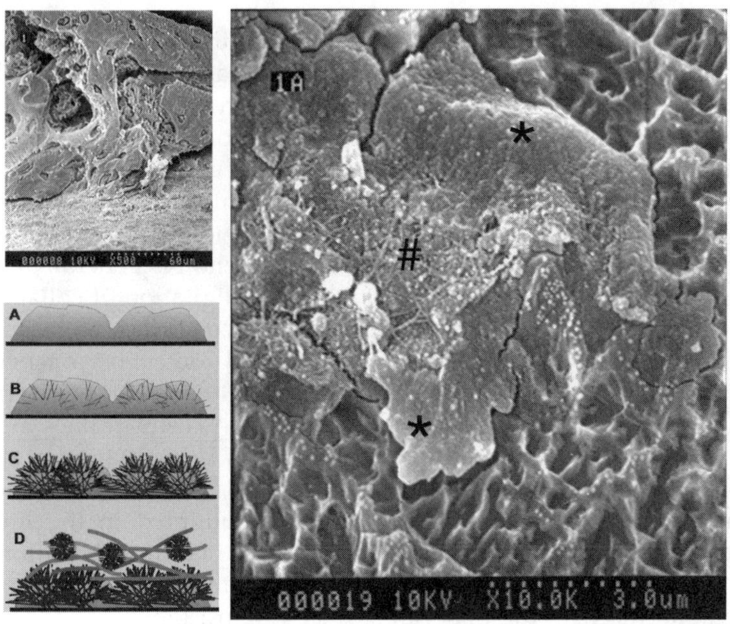

FIGURE 12.8
Top left: low magnification view of bone–implant interface. The bone is clearly distinguishable by the presence of osteocyte lacunae and vascular canals. Field width = 188 μ. Bottom left: sequence of interfacial matrix elaboration events is summarized. This illustration shows how the collagen in bone is separated from the underlying substrate by the cement line matrix. Right: at the bone–implant interface, the bone cement line matrices (*) are directly apposed to a dual acid-etched titanium implant surface *in vivo*. Collagen can be seen to be assembling on the cement line matrix (#). Field width = 9.5 μ.

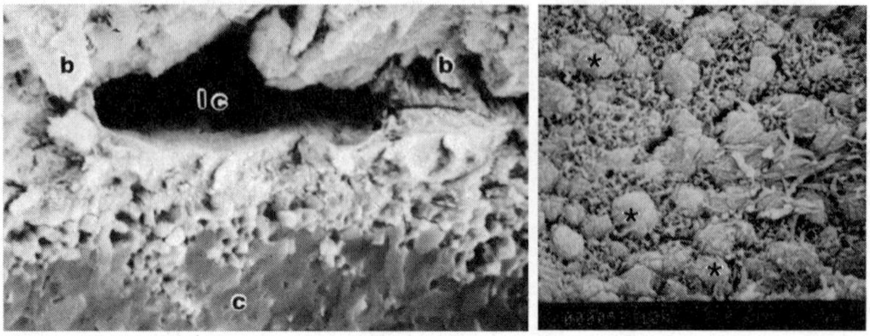

FIGURE 12.9
Left: scanning electron micrograph of the bone–hydroxyapatite (HA) implant interface showing interdigitation of the bone matrix with the surface microporosity of the implant. b = bone; lc = osteocyte lacuna; c = ceramic HA implant. Field width = 20 μ. Right: *In vitro* modeling reveals that individual globules of the interfacial cement line matrix interdigitate with the surface. Field width = 9 μ.

12.4 Bone Bonding

When *de novo* bone forms on an implant surface in the manner described (this biological cascade has been shown to occur on many candidate implants *in vivo* including metals and ceramics), then such an interfacial matrix can be expected with endosseous implants of all material compositions. Nevertheless, since the pioneering work of Hench,[11] two classes of endosseous implants have been identified: bonding, and nonbonding. While metals such as titanium are nonbonding, calcium phosphate materials are considered bone-bonding.

The mechanism for the bone-bonding phenomenon is generally accepted as a chemical interaction that results in the interdigitation of collagen from the bony compartment with the chemically active surface of the implant. Clearly, in the cases of *de novo* bone formation and contact osteogenesis, this mechanism is inconceivable since the first extracellular matrix elaborated by bone cells at the implant surface is collagen-free. As cement lines are found on both nonbonding and bonding biomaterials, a re-evaluation of the phenomenon of bone bonding is essential. In brief, while chemical hypotheses to explain bone bonding have been generally adopted in the literature, experimental evidence demonstrates that in cases of *de novo* bone formation at implant surfaces, bonding is achieved by micromechanical interdigitation of the cement line with the material surface (Figure 12.9).[12]

12.5 Concluding Remarks

While many aspects of peri-implant healing still need to be elucidated, it is now possible to deconvolute this biological reaction cascade phenomenologically and experimentally into three distinct phases. The first, osteoconduction, relies on the migration of differentiating osteogenic cells to the implant surface. The second, *de novo* bone formation, results in a mineralized interfacial matrix equivalent to that seen in cement lines in natural bone tissue. The third healing phase, bone remodeling, will also, at discrete sites, create a bone–implant interface comprising *de novo* bone formation.

Implant surface design will have a profound effect on osteoconduction, while the surface topography of the implant will play a critical role in bone bonding concomitant with the *de* novo bone formation seen in contact osteogenesis. Among the most important areas still to explore are the knock-on effects generated by the implant surface and initiated by platelet activation that result in accelerated osteogenic cell migration. We have provided preliminary evidence that the degree of activation of platelets as a function of implant surface topography can differentially affect neutrophil up-regulation, but neutrophils are short-lived in the healing compartment, and new evidence is needed to link these early events to the increased contact osteogenesis reported with textured implant surfaces. Similarly, bone healing will not occur without the generation of new vasculature in the peri-implant healing site. We know almost nothing today about peri-implant angiogenesis and how it may be affected by implant surface design.

Treatment outcomes employing endosseous implants will be critically dependent upon implant surface designs that optimize biological responses during each of these three distinct integration mechanisms.

References

1. Davies, J.E., Mechanisms of endosseous integration, *Int. J. Prosthondont.*, 11, 391, 1998.
2, Davies, J.E. and Hosseini, M.M., Histodynamics of endosseous wound healing, in *Bone Engineering*, Davies, J.E, Ed., em squared, Toronto, 2000, p. 1.
3. Osborn, J.F. and Newesely, H., Dynamic aspects of the implant–bone interface, in *Dental Implants: Materials and Systems*, Heimke, G., Ed., Carl Hanser Verlag, München, 1980, p. 111.
4. von Ebner, V., Über den feineren Bau der Knochensubstanz, *S.B. Akad. Wiss. Math. Nat. Kl. Abt. III*, 72, 49, 1875.
5. Lazzara, R.J., Bone response to dual acid-etched and machined titanium implant surfaces, in *Bone Engineering*, Davies, J.E., Ed., em squared, Toronto, 2000, p. 381.
6. Park, J.Y. and Davies, J.E., Red blood cell and platelet interactions with titanium implant surfaces, *J. Clin. Oral Implant Res.*, 11, 530, 2000.
7. Park, J., Gemmell, C.H., and Davies, J.E., Platelet interactions with titanium: modulation of platelet activity by surface topography, *Biomaterials*, 19, 2671, 2001.
8. Park, J.Y., Blood Interactions with Titanium Implant Surfaces, Ph.D. Thesis, University of Toronto, Canada, 2003.

9. Schultz, R.J., *The Language of Fractures*, 2nd ed., Williams & Willkins, Baltimore, 1990, p. 1.
10. Davies, J.E., *In vitro* modeling of the bone/implant interface, *Anat. Rec.*, 245, 426, 1996.
11. Hench, L.L. and Wilson, J., Surface-active biomaterials, *Science*, 226, 630, 1984.
12. Dziedzic, D.M. et al., Osteoconduction on, and bonding to, calcium phosphate ceramic implants, *Mat. Res. Soc. Symp. Proc.*, 414, 147, 1996.

Section IV

Extracellular Matrix Biology and Biomineralization in Bone Formation and Implant Integration

13

Initiation and Modulation of Crystal Growth in Skeletal Tissues: Role of Extracellular Matrix

Colin Robinson, Roger C. Shore, Simon R. Wood, Steven J. Brookes, D. Alistair Smith, and Jennifer Kirkham

CONTENTS

13.1 Introduction....232
13.1.1 Biphasic Development: The Organic Matrix....232
13.1.2 Initiation of Crystal Deposition....232
13.1.3 Modulation of Crystal Growth....233
13.1.4 Initiation versus Inhibition....233
13.2 Role of Organic Matrix....234
13.2.1 Bone....234
13.2.1.1 Collagen....234
13.2.1.2 Bone Sialoprotein (BSP-2)....235
13.2.1.3 Osteopontin (BSP-1)....237
13.2.1.4 Bone Acidic Glycoprotein (BAG-75)....237
13.2.2 Dentine....238
13.2.2.1 Collagen....238
13.2.2.2 Dentine Sialoprotein (DSP)....238
13.2.2.3 Phosphophoryn (Dentine Phosphoprotein or DPP)....238
13.2.2.4 Dentine Sialophosphoprotein....239
13.2.3 Enamel....240
13.2.3.1 Amelogenin....240
13.2.3.2 Enamelin....240
13.2.3.3 Possible Combined Role of Enamel Matrix Proteins....241
13.3 Summary....242
References....242

0-8493-1474-7/03/$0.00+$1.50

13.1 Introduction

Skeletal tissues comprise an inorganic mineral phase usually embedded in an extracellular organic, usually proteinaceous, matrix. Cells may be but are not always present within the tissue or at its periphery. The mineral phase is usually crystalline and in mammalian skeletal tissues, comprises a poorly crystallized, highly substituted calcium hydroxyapatite.

The size, morphology, arrangement, and, to a large extent, chemistry of these hydroxyapatite crystals are related to the tissue in which they are formed, their locations within the tissue, and the stage of tissue development from which they derive. Enamel crystals are, for example, very large (~800 nm × 500 nm × 400 nm) compared with bone (~500 nm × 500 nm × 5 nm). Carbonate concentration in enamel ranges from ~2 to ~4%, whereas in bone it may range from 4 to 6%. Fluoride content is invariably higher in the crystals of the outer periphery of the tissues and in enamel; fluoride, carbonate, and magnesium levels are much higher in newly formed crystals than in those from later developmental stages.

It is clear therefore that the deposition of mineral crystals in the skeletal tissues, bone, dentine, cementum, and enamel involves processes that specifically locate the crystals, determine their size and morphology, and in some way prescribe their chemistry.

13.1.1 Biphasic Development: The Organic Matrix

Almost all mineralized tissues deposit mineral via a biphasic process. The first phase is the deposition by specific tissue cells of a broadly tissue-specific organic matrix with a molecular architecture characteristic of the tissue. This also delimits the external tissue morphology.

The second phase involves the initiation and growth of hydroxyapatite crystals within the matrix. The molecular architecture of the matrix exerts considerable influence over the disposition and nature of the mineral phase. In some cases, the distinction between these two phases is very clear, for example, in dentine and bone where predentine and osteoid, respectively, represent precursor stages of unmineralized matrix. In enamel, this temporal interval is much less obvious, with crystals appearing almost immediately near cells that are elaborating matrix. The extracellular organic matrix is thus considered the key determinant that modulates mineral deposition.

Development of the mineral phase can also be considered a two-step process: initiation followed by crystal growth.

13.1.2 Initiation of Crystal Deposition

This event involves the clustering and dehydration of inorganic ions to form the first mineral nucleus. Mineral initiation requires supersaturation of the local environment with regard to a calcium phosphate phase that is presumably under control of local cells. However, supersaturation alone cannot dictate the ultrastructural locations of individual crystals within the tissue nor their size and morphology, both of which are ubiquitous features of biological mineralization and thought to be achieved by specifically located initiation sites resident within the organic matrix.

Unless ions are deposited on a template comprising a stereospecific array of charges resembling a hydroxyapatite surface, such initial ion clusters are unlikely to be apatitic. They are more likely to be amorphous, i.e., showing no long-range order,[1,2] although on the basis of juxtaposition of opposite charges, it is likely that some short-range order will exist.

Normally, unless such clusters are stabilized, for example, by carbonate, magnesium, or an interacting organic molecule, hydroxyapatite will ultimately develop because it is the most thermodynamically stable calcium phosphate under biological conditions. Such transformation to apatite from precursors may well be an important controlled step in crystal development. Indeed, modification or removal of specific extracellular matrix molecules is emerging as a component of the crystal development process.

13.1.3 Modulation of Crystal Growth

Once critical radius has been achieved by clustering calcium, phosphate, and other ions at the initiation site, crystal growth/development ensues. This is most likely accompanied by ionic rearrangement either from short-range order (amorphous) material and/or through intermediate species such as octacalcium phosphate or brushite-like phases.[3,4] The existence of such specific phases for any length of time is still a matter of debate. However, it seems likely that the phases are transient assemblies of calcium and phosphate ions.

Control of growth would be effected by a physical constraint on the size of the compartment available to the growing crystal or binding of specific protein entities to particular crystal surfaces. Either constraint would limit growth by preventing access of further ions to the surface growth sites or by stabilizing the lattice structure to the point where growth is severely inhibited. Growth control could be effected by hydrolysis of an inorganic crystal growth inhibitor such as pyrophosphate[5] or by protein degradation and removal as is very clearly the case with enamel, where the matrix is almost entirely removed at the final stages of tissue development concomitant with massive crystal growth.[6]

Such features would be able to control final crystal size and binding of modulating molecules to specific crystal faces and could also play a role in determining crystal morphology.

13.1.4 Initiation versus Inhibition

It is worth making the point at this stage that interaction with mineral per se may either initiate mineral deposition and facilitate growth or inhibit it.

Inhibition becomes important when it affects specific crystal faces and thus modulates morphology and size.

Initial nuclei may serve as chemical foci for crystal initiation, but if binding is too restrictive, they may allow insufficient ion mobility and result in inhibition of crystal development. Mineral binding is not therefore a natural indicator of mineral initiation.

The specific activity of matrix molecules in terms of initiation or inhibition may be determined also by local environment. For example, dentine phosphoprotein (DPP) in solution was a potent inhibitor of nucleation, whereas when covalently bound to a solid support, it functioned as an initiator.[7,8] This may be due to the fact that when affixed to a support, only one face of the nucleus is protein bound, leaving other faces exposed to solution and the possibility of growth. On the other hand, the conformation of the protein and its state of charge when bound may differ from its state in solution, changing its intrinsic behavior from initiation to inhibition. This could be viewed as a change from initiation to growth modulation.

13.2 Role of Organic Matrix

This section discusses, in the light of the above definitions, the possible roles of specific extracellular matrix components in each of the mineralized tissues (bone, dentine, cementum, and enamel). Since this review is relatively short, it focuses only on selected proteins for which we have reasonable evidence of roles in crystal initiation and/or growth.

13.2.1 Bone

13.2.1.1 Collagen

In mesenchymal tissues (bone, dentine, and cementum), the bulk of the extracellular organic matrix is type 1 collagen. While soft unmineralized tissue type 1 collagens contain rather different cross-links and often retain glycosylaminoglycans (GAGs) and other associated molecules, the mineralized tissue collagens differ among themselves only in, for example, distribution and perhaps degree of cross-linking.

Dentine collagen is rather more stable than that of bone.[9] Such highly stable cross-linking tends to reside at the telopeptide region of the collagen molecule[10] in the area of the overlap and hole zones. This would prevent rupture of the fibrils/fibers by growth of excessively large crystals and as indicated below, constrain the sizes of mineral crystals.

Earliest visible mineral loci are classically seen in the hole zone regions of collagen, i.e., in the gaps between nonabutting ends of tropocollagen molecules.[11,12] The mechanism for this is not unequivocally clear. Purified collagen does not appear to mineralize well *in vitro*.[7,8,13] Therefore it is presumed that additional entities, possibly noncollagenous proteins or GAGs serve this function. Unequivocal localization of noncollagenous proteins within collagen fibrils has not been demonstrated. Indeed, it is difficult to see how the proposed initiating entities could be accommodated. Given the small spaces between tropocollagen molecules, such molecules would need to be incorporated during fibrillogenesis.

It is therefore likely that initiation sites within collagen rely on groupings resident on the collagen itself. Although there are no large numbers of charged amino acid side chains on the collagen molecule, charged groups in the hole zones could provide nonspecific nucleation sites that promote formation of initial calcium and phosphate clusters.

The side chains on collagen molecules are known to project from the helix surface; perhaps within the confines of the hole zone, only one or two charged groups are necessary.[13] The amino and carboxy terminals of the collagen molecules may provide sufficient charge density. Little is, in fact, known about the internal environment of the hole zone. Its size, however, of the order of 1 to 2 nm diameter × ~40 nm,[14,15] would not accommodate many hydrated calcium or phosphate ions across its width.

Together with the ordered hydration layer of the collagen, the effective solution volume in hole zones may be very small, leading to high supersaturation values. Such small poorly formed crystals could easily constitute nuclei for the precipitation of minerals within the fibrils, perhaps in contiguous hole zone domains.[16]

In addition to the proposed intrafibrillar mineral, much of the hydroxyapatite formed exists between the collagen fibrils.[12,16] Thus, surface charge on the collagen per se or more likely at exposed hole zone/overlap sites on the fibril surface may well function as initiation sites.[12,13,16,17] The overlap zones are known to be relatively highly charged and may also bind other organic components. It is here that non-collagenous molecules may be more clearly implicated as initiators and modulators of crystal growth with collagen as a scaffold in and around which the mineralization process can occur.

Figure 13.1 shows the structure of mineralized vertebrate tissue collagen and the dimensions of collagen molecules, intermolecular areas, hole zone spacing, and locations of minerals.

13.2.1.2 Bone Sialoprotein (BSP-2)

13.2.1.2.1 Location

BSP-2, based on its temporospatial expression coinciding with the appearance of mineral crystals, is considered a prime candidate for initiation of mineralization in bone.[18] It is highly specific to mineralized tissues, and in hypertrophic cartilage[19] it appears simultaneously with mineral deposition. *In situ* hybridization has also demonstrated its expression by osteoblasts actively engaged in mineral deposition.[20] BSP-2 did not appear to be expressed in other areas of these tissues. It has been located in several forms of calcifying carcinomas including breast, lung, and prostate neoplasms.[21,22]

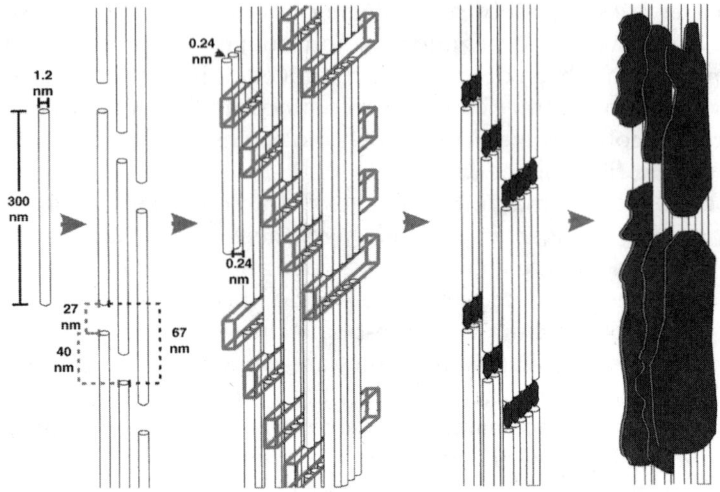

FIGURE 13.1
Structure of mineralized tissue collagen. Dimensions of collagen molecules (300 nm × 1.2 nm diameter) and hole zones (27 nm × ~3 nm diameter) are indicated. Only one or two hydrated calcium (~0.8 nm) and hydrated phosphate (~1.5 nm) ions could be accommodated across the hole zones. Space created by alignment of hole zone region and mineral nuclei present in hole zones and as extended intrafibrillar mineral plates are also shown. (*Source:* Based on Landis, W., *Conn. Tiss. Res.*, 34, 239, 1996. With permission.)

13.2.1.2.2 Mechanism

BSP-2 is a 300-amino acid residue sialoprotein that carries ten serine and two tyrosine phosphorylation sites. Seven sulfated tyrosine residues are also present. Near the amino terminus are two highly conserved contiguous sequences of glutamic acid residues. The entire molecule is therefore rather acidic and has a large number of anionic side chains. Figure 13.2 illustrates the structure of bone sialoprotein including the functional side chains.

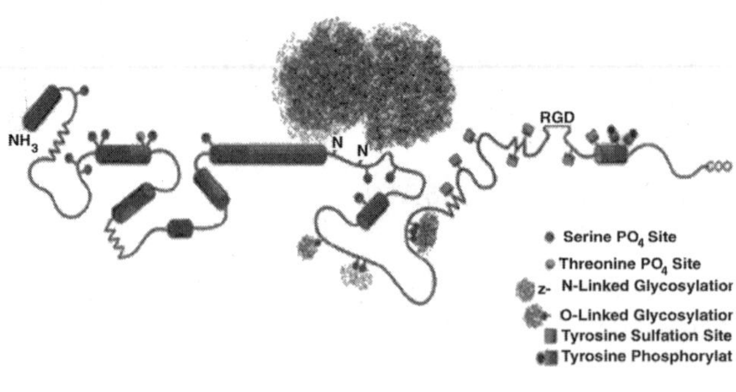

FIGURE 13.2
Proposed structure of bone sialoprotein showing functional side-chains. Cylinders indicate contiguous anionic sequences. (From Gauss, B., Kim, R.H., and Sodek, J., *Crit. Rev. Oral Biol. Med.*, 10, 79–98, 1999.)

In vitro studies have shown that only BSP-2 was able to nucleate hydroxyapatite.[23] No other noncollagenous protein from bone was able to do this. In view of suggestions that serine phosphate residues may play a role in apatite nucleation, dephosphorylated BSP was examined for mineral initiation. It had little effect, suggesting that phosphate residues are not critical for mineral initiation by this molecule.[23,24]

Recent work with site-directed mutagenesis targeted the glutamic acid residues. One of the two polyglutamate domains was replaced with polyalanine, which retains a helical structure and has no charge density, or by polyaspartate, which maintains charge density but not helical structure. Both decreased but did not abolish mineral initiation activity. However, replacement of both contiguous glutamic acid domains with polyalanine removed all activity.[25]

The implications are that anionic charge density is important in mineral crystal initiation and may be rather more important than protein conformation. From this, it is possible to suggest that initiation in this case may be nonepitactic. As far as BSP is concerned, this appears to be related to clusters of anionic groups, viz., contiguous glutamic acid residues in the amino acid sequence. While an association of BSP with type I collagen seems to be the case, specific stereochemical relationships with collagen have not yet been demonstrated.

13.2.1.3 Osteopontin (BSP-1)

13.2.1.3.1 Location

BSP-1 appears in the bone matrix just prior to mineralization. It is a 44- to 75-kDa phosphorylated glycoprotein that possesses contiguous aspartic acid side chains and a cell-binding region GRDGS.

13.2.1.3.2 Mechanism

While BSP-1 binds to mineral, it has been shown to inhibit hydroxyapatite formation rather than initiate it, probably via interaction with phosphorylated residues.[26,27] Later work has suggested that the carboxylate groups may be important,[28] and some evidence is available for preferential interaction with the 100-crystal face plane.[29] Since removal would be necessary for growth to occur, it may be more important to modulate morphology by facilitating growth, preferentially in the c-axis direction.[29] However, since this tends to be the preferred mode of growth of calcium hydroxyapatite crystals, it might be argued that BSP-1 simply facilitates a preferred growth habit.

13.2.1.4 Bone Acidic Glycoprotein (BAG-75)

13.2.1.4.1 Location

BAG-75 is certainly present in mineralizing bone matrix and more especially in growth plate cartilage.[30] More precise location in terms of mineral deposition is still unclear.

13.2.1.4.2 Mechanism

BAG-75 is a 75-kDa molecule containing 7% sialic acid and 8% phosphate. It is an acidic/anionic molecule and 30% of its residues are anionic. Sequence homology is shared with phosphophorin, osteopontin, and BSP and it may share structural similarities. It binds calcium ions, hydroxyapatite, and collagen.[31] It may function as an initiator and/or inhibitor of hydroxyapatite deposition. There is as yet no definitive indication of a precise function.

13.2.2 Dentine

13.2.2.1 Collagen

Type 1 collagen is the main matrix component for dentine. The same arguments apply to both mineralization of dentine collagen and of bone as described above. However, it is perhaps worth remarking that the more stable and highly cross-linked dentine collagen[9,10] may be associated with the greater degree of mineral content in dentine. Such additional stability may be required to prevent fibril disruption.

13.2.2.2 Dentine Sialoprotein (DSP)

13.2.2.2.1 Location

DSP, like its bone counterpart, accumulates at the histological sites of mineral deposition, in this case, at the mineralizing front.

13.2.2.2.2 Mechanism

DSP is a 53-kDa glycoprotein, similar in many ways to osteopontin (see above) and dentine phosphoprotein-1 (DMP-1, Bag-75). All are rich in aspartic and glutamic acid residues and have considerable numbers of sialic acid residues. There is, however, no RGD, i.e., cell attachment sequence and levels of phosphorylation are relatively low compared for example with DPP.

Unlike BSP, DSP has a much less demonstrable effect on mineral modulation — either initiation or inhibition. When DSP-treated hydroxyapatite crystals were investigated, some inhibition of growth was observed,[32] arguing perhaps for a small modulating effect on crystal growth.

13.2.2.3 Phosphophoryn (Dentine Phosphoprotein or DPP)

13.2.2.3.1 Location

DPP is specific to dentine. It appears to be secreted at the mineralizing front, i.e., at the junction between predentine and dentine proper where, after attachment to collagen, it may initiate extrafibrillar mineral deposition.[7,8]

13.2.2.3.2 Mechanism

DPP has a molecular size 90 to 95 kDa, contains mainly phosphoserine and aspartic acid residues in a repeating series of Pse, Pse, Asp, Pse, and Asp

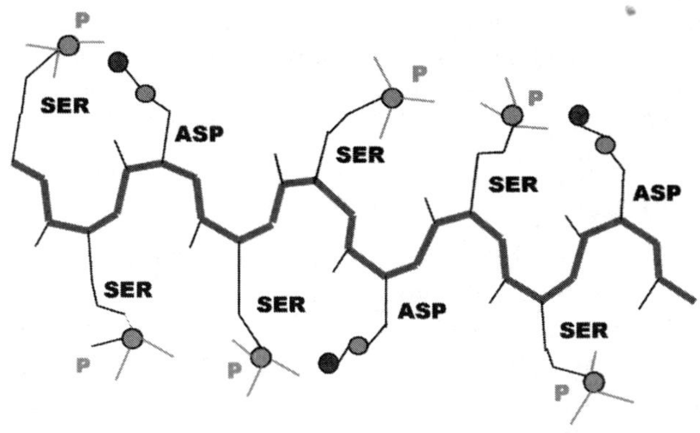

FIGURE 13.3
Portion of amino-acid sequence of dentine phosophoprotein (DPP) showing proposed array of aspartic acid carboxyl and some serine phosphate groups. (From: George, A., *J. Biol. Chem.*, 271, 32069, 1996. With permission.)

sequences, and has 220 phosphorylation sites. Modeling of this structure suggests that it exhibits Pse on opposite sides of the peptide backbone with the following aspartic residue on the same side as the first Pse. This regular array of anionic charges could well function as a heterogeneous nucleus if not a quasitemplate for calcium phosphate deposition.[33,34] Figure 13.3 illustrates the proposed structure of DPP and the disposition of aspartic acid and phosphoserine side chains.

Measurement of chemical shifts on DPP bound to apatite suggests that this extended structure approximated to a β-pleated sheet. Such an extended structure would allow maximum coverage of the crystal surface.[33,34]

It must be borne in mind, however, that a conformation seen on the surface of mineral crystal may be a result of crystal surface facilitation of a particular protein conformation rather than the other way around. Long et al.[35] demonstrated that a hydroxyapatite-binding peptide incorporating serine phosphate (DpSpEEK) tended to form an extended structure on crystal surfaces rather than an alpha helix.

DPP is unusual in that it behaves differently in solution compared with its behavior when immobilized. When free in solution, DPP is an effective inhibitor of apatite crystal development. When attached to a solid support, it acts effectively as an initiation site.[7,8] This suggests that the conformation or immediate environment of the protein may be an important factor in mineral crystal initiation. It is also possible that immobilized proteins attach only to one face or side of a growing mineral entity, permitting unencumbered faces to grow. In solution, however, free DPP would have access to all crystal growth sites and when bound could inhibit growth.

13.2.2.4 Dentine Sialophosphoprotein

DPP and DSP have been ascribed to one gene product although an entire dentine sialophosphoprotein entity has not yet been isolated from tissue such that cleavage must occur early if it occurs at all. One possibility is that the cleavage is in fact an activation step for mineral initiation. See Long et al.[35,36]

13.2.3 Enamel

The proteins of dental enamel are worth discussing at this point. While not a mesenchymal tissue, dental enamel is nevertheless the most highly mineralized of the skeletal tissues. Specific nucleators have not been identified within this matrix but it is known that many of these molecules will inhibit growth, if not initiation. As a result, it has been speculated that initiation occurs at the dentine or that stable mineral/protein nanoparticles are systematically destabilized and degraded to allow crystal to initiate and then grow.[37]

13.2.3.1 Amelogenin

The primary protein of enamel is amelogenin, a ~19-kDa self-aggregating hydrophobic protein with little ability to nucleate hydroxyapatite. It is processed rapidly as it leaves the cell by endogenous metalloproteases and is ultimately almost completely degraded and removed from tissue.[6,36] Since amelogenin-processing products larger than ~20 kDa associate with minerals, they may serve as supports for growing crystals.[38,39] However, since their removal is a prerequisite for final crystal growth,[38,40,41] it appears that they might exert an inhibitory effect on crystal thickness and width.[41-43]

The nature of binding is not clear. Electrostatic binding is suggested by the selective binding to regular charge domains on apatite crystal surfaces.[44] In view of the hydrophobic nature of amelogenins, it has been suggested that this may drive them from the solution onto the apatite surface. Binding to positively charged crystal surfaces could reflect binding to domains less highly charged than interdomain regions. In support of this, it is interesting to note that fluoridated apatite tends to retain protein in developing enamel and has been reported as having a more hydrophobic surface than its non-fluoridated counterpart.[45]

13.2.3.2 Enamelin

Enamelin is an 89-kDa protein at a concentration of about 2% in the enamel matrix; however, it has the distinction among all enamel matrix proteins that at least part of it (a 32-kDa processing product) binds tightly to hydroxyapatite.[46,47] This fragment contains two of the three phosphorylated serines reported for this molecule. Examination of the amino acid sequence has revealed that enamelin is acidic/anionic in character and has a relatively high number of side chains of glutamate and aspartate, often in contiguous groups of two or three. Its precise effect on initiation and crystal growth is unknown.

13.2.3.3 Possible Combined Role of Enamel Matrix Proteins

Investigations using freeze etching technology suggest that the matrix structure takes the form of collinear spheres of similar width to ultimate enamel hydroxyapatite crystals.[48] It was suggested that the spheres comprise mineral ion/matrix colloidal particles/nanospheres with mineral ions associated with anionic charges within the spheres. A good candidate for this role is enamelin since it is very acidic and is known to bind to mineral.[46,47] The association of amelogenin with mineral would facilitate this process.

Processing/degradation of the matrix would fragment stretches of anionic groups on enamelin and render the aggregates of amelogenin more soluble. This would tend to reduce mineral binding, permitting mineral ion clustering and precipitation. Subsequent fusion of contiguous mineral nuclei from each cluster would then give rise to the elongated crystals typical of enamel.[37] The reduction of binding to mineral by amelogenin degradation products and progressive degradation of enamelin during enamel development support this view.[38,39] This is also supported by atomic field and confocal microscopy studies that revealed spherical structures on secretory stage crystals.[49] It was also suggested that repeated charge domains on crystal surfaces seen after matrix removal represented ionic memories of the original subunits.[37,50] Figure 13.4 consists of scanning probe microscopy images of hydroxyapatite crystallites from developing enamel. The images show charge density banding described above and associated adsorbed amelogenin matrix protein.

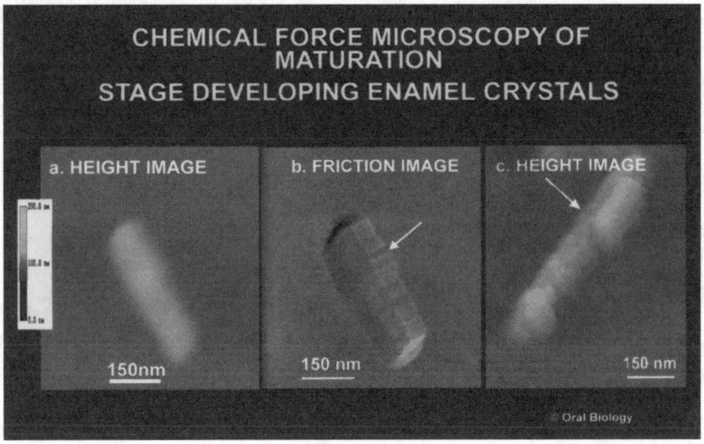

FIGURE 13.4
Atomic force microscope images of hydroxyapatite crystals from maturation stage of dental enamel. (a) Height image. (b) Friction image showing repeating bands of positive and less positive (or negative) charge. (c) Height image of maturation-stage crystal exposed to recombinant amelogenin, the major protein of developing enamel matrix. Pattern of amelogenin bonding corresponds to pattern of charge bonding in (b). (From Kirkham, J. et al., *J. Dent. Res.*, 79, 1945, 2000. With permission.)

13.3 Summary

With regard to mineralization, many extracellular matrix proteins have the potential to serve as centers of mineral initiation, probably by generating mineral ion clusters that are then free to develop into crystals. The size and morphology of such crystals may be defined by the space available, such as the hole zones in collagen or interfibrillar volume. By adherence of proteins to specific faces, it is also possible to influence morphology. Since, however, most rapidly growing faces tend to disappear, this could also have an effect on crystal size.

The nature of nucleating entities is emerging as clusters of acidic side chains forming anionic domains on peptide backbones. However, glutamic acid and serine phosphate seem to be more effective in this respect than aspartic acid, implying that longer side chains are more effective than shorter ones. This may reflect the greater flexibility and freedom of movement of the anionic entities. Bound ions may thus have sufficient freedom of movement to form preferred stable mineral phases. More tightly bound mineral ions may be stabilized at the ion cluster stage, effectively inhibiting further growth.

The anionic domains that seem to characterize putative initiating entities would also imply the presence of a negative ion field. This could confer even greater cation (calcium) mobility on the protein surfaces, allowing them to assemble and reassemble with phosphate to form stable mineral nuclei.

Stereospecific arrays of protein anionic groups might well nucleate crystals directly, but the mobility of such side chains might make this less likely than a short-range order ion cluster. However, the binding of stereospecific arrays of such groups to existing crystal faces could well exert the opposite effect in stabilizing the face and possibly obscuring growth sites. In this context, stereospecific interaction might be more likely to offer a modulating role than initiating crystal deposition (for a review, see Kirkham et al.).[51]

References

1. Posner, A.S. and Betts, F., Synthetic amorphous calcium phosphate and its relation to bone mineral structure, *Accounts Chem. Res.*, 8, 273, 1975.
2. Posner, A.S., The mineral of bone, *Clin. Orthopaed. Rel. Res.*, 200, 87, 1985.
3. Bodier-Houlle, P. et al., First experimental evidence for human dentine crystal formation involving conversion of octacalcium phosphate to hydroxyapatite, *Acta. Crystallogr. D. Biol.*, 54, 1377, 1998.
4. Roufosse, A.H. et al., Identification of brushite, in newly deposited bone mineral from embryonic chicks, *J. Ultrastruct. Res.*, 68, 235, 1979.
5. Caswee, A.M. et al., Hypophosphatasia and the extracellular metabolism of inorganic pyrophosphate: clinical and laboratory aspects, *CRC Crit. Rev. Clin. Lab. Sci.*, 28, 175, 1991.

6. Robinson, C. et al., Changes in the protein components of rat incisor enamel during tooth development, *Arch. Oral Biol.*, 28, 993, 1983.
7. Saito, T. et al., Mineral induction by immobilised phosphoproteins, *Bone*, 4, 30, 1997.
8. Saito, T. et al., *In vitro* apatite induction by phosphophoryn immobilised on modified collagen fibrils, *J. Bone Miner. Res.*, 8, 1615, 2000.
9. Kuboki, Y. and Mechanic, G.L., Comparative molecular distribution of cross-links in bone and dentine collagen: structure–function relationships, *Calcif. Tiss. Int.*, 3, 306, 1982.
10. Robins, S.P. and Brady, J.D., Collagen cross-linking and metabolism, in *Principles of Bone Biology*, vol. 2, Bilezikian, J.P., Raisz, L.G., and Rodan, G.D., Eds., Academic Press, San Diego, 2002.
11. Robinson, R.A. and Watson, M.L., Collagen-crystal relationships in bone as seen in the electron microscope, *Anat. Rec.*, 114, 383, 1952.
12. Landis, W.J. et al., Mineral and organic matrix interaction in normally calcifying tendon visualised in three dimensions by high voltage electron microscopic tomography and graphic image reconstruction, *J. Struct. Biol.*, 110, 39, 1993.
13. Saito, T., Yamauchi, M., and Crenshaw, M.A., Apatite induction by insoluble dentine collagen, *J. Bone Miner. Res.*, 2, 2650, 1998.
14. Rhee, S., Lee, J.D., and Tanaka, J., Nucleation of hydroxyapatite crystals through chemical interaction with collagen, *J. Am. Ceram. Soc.*, 83, 11, 2890, 2000.
15. Miller, A., Collagen: the organic matrix of bone., *Philos. Trans. R. Soc. London Ser. B*, 304, 455, 1984.
16. Lees, S., Considerations regarding the structure of the mammalian mineralised osteoid from the viewpoint of the generalised packing model, *Connect. Tiss. Res.*, 16, 281, 1987.
17. Landis, W.J. et al., Mineralisation of collagen may occur on fibril surfaces: evidence from conventional and high voltage electron microscopy and three-dimensional imaging, *J. Ultrastruct. Biol.*, 116, 24, 1966.
18. Chen, J., Shapiro, H.S., and Sodek, J., Developmental expression of bone sialoprotein mRNA in rat mineralised connective tissues, *J. Bone Miner. Res.*, 7, 987, 1992.
19. Galotto, M. et al., Hypertrophic chondrocytes undergo further differentiation to osteoblast like cells and participate in the initial bone formation in developing chick embryo, *J. Bone Miner. Res.*, 9, 1239, 1994.
20. Zhu, X.L. et al., Synthesis and processing of bone sialoproteins during *de novo* bone formation *in vitro*, *Biochem. Cell Biol.*, 79, 737, 2001.
21. Bellahacene, A. and Castronovo, V., Expression of bone matrix proteins in human breast cancer: potential roles in microcalcification formation and in the genesis of bone metastases, *Bull. Cancer*, 84, 17, 1997.
22. Bellahacene, A. et al., Expression of bone sialoprotein in human lung cancer, *Calcif. Tiss. Int.*, 61, 183, 1990.
23. Hunter, G.K. and Goldberg, H.A., Nucleation of hydroxyapatite by bone sialoprotein, *Proc. Natl. Acad. Sci. U.S.A.*, 90, 8562, 1993.
24. Hunter, G.K. and Goldberg, H.A., Modulation of crystal formation by bone phosphoproteins: role of glutamic acid-rich sequences in the nucleation of hydroxyapatite, *Biochem. J.*, 15, 175, 1994.
25. Harris, N.L. et al., Functional analysis of bone sialoprotein: identification of the hydroxyapatite-nucleating and cell-binding domains by recombinant peptide expression and site directed mutagenesis, *Bone*, 27, 795, 2000.

26. Hunter, G.K., Kyle, L., and Goldberg, H.A., Modulation of crystal formation by bone phosphoprotein: structural specificity of the osteopontin-mediated inhibition of hydroxyapatite formation, *Biochem. J.*, 300, 723, 1994.
27. Boskey, A.L. et al., Osteopontin–hydroxyapatite interactions *in vitro*: inhibition of hydroxyapatite formation and growth in a gelatin gel, *Bone Miner.*, 22, 147, 1993.
28. Goldberg, H.A. et al., Binding of bone sialoprotein, osteopontin and synthetic polypeptides to hydroxyapatite, *Connect. Tiss. Res.*, 42, 25, 2001.
29. Fujisawa, R. and Kuboki, Y., Preferential adsorption of dentine and bone acidic proteins on the (100) face of hydroxyapatite crystals, *Biochim. Biophys. Acta*, 1075, 56060, 1991.
30. Gorski, J.P. et al., Bone acidic glycoprotein-75 is a major synthetic product of osteoblastic cells and localised as 75- and/or 50-kDa forms in mineralised phases of bone and growth plate and in serum, *J. Biol. Chem.*, 265, 14956, 1990.
31. Gorski, J.F. and Shimizu, K., Isolation of a new phosphorylated glycoprotein from mineralised phase of bone that exhibits limited homology to adhesive protein osteopontin, *J. Biol. Chem.*, 263, 15938, 1988.
32. Boskey, A. et al., Dentin sialoprotein (DSP) has limited effects on *in vitro* apatite formation and growth, *Calcif. Tiss. Int.*, 6, 472, 2000.
33. Dahlin, S., Angstrom, J., and Linde, A., Dentine phosphoprotein sequence motifs and molecular modelling: conformational adaptation to mineral crystals, *Eur. J. Oral Sci.*, 106, 239, 1998.
34. Fujisawa, R. and Kuboki, Y., Conformation of dentin phosphophoryn adsorbed on hydroxyapatite crystals, *Eur. J. Oral Sci.*, 106 (Suppl.), 249, 1998.
35. Long, J.R. et al., A peptide that inhibits hydroxyapatite growth is in an extended conformation on the crystal surface, *Proc. Natl. Acad. Sci. U.S.A.*, 21, 12083, 1998.
36. D'Souza, R.N. et al., Gene expression patterns of murine dentin matrix protein-1 (DMP-1) and dentin sialophosphoprotein (DSPP) suggest different developmental functions *in vivo*, *J. Bone Miner. Res.*, 12, 2040, 1990.
37. Robinson, C. et al., Subunit structures in hydroxyapatite crystal development in enamel: implications for amelogenesis imperfecta, *Connect. Tiss. Res.*, in press, 2002.
38. Robinson, C. et al., The developing enamel matrix nature and function, *Eur. J. Oral Sci.*, 106 (Suppl.), 282, 1998.
39. Brookes, S.J. et al., Biochemistry and molecular biology of amelogenin proteins of developing enamel, *Arch. Oral Biol.*, 40, 1, 1995.
40. Fincham, A.G. and Moradian-Oldak, J., Recent advances in amelogenin biochemistry, *Connect. Tiss. Res.*, 32, 119, 1997.
41. Robinson, C. et al., Extracellular matrix processing of enamel matrix proteins and the control of crystal growth, *J. Biol. Buccale*, 18, 355, 1990.
42. Aoba, T. et al., Possible roles of partial sequences at N- and C- termini of amelogenin protein: enamel interaction, *J. Dent. Res.*, 9, 133, 1989.
43. Wallwork, M.L. et al., Binding of matrix proteins to developing enamel crystals: an atomic force microscopy study, *Langmuir*, 17, 2508, 2001.
44. Wu, W. and Nancollas, G.H., Kinetics and surface energy approaches to the crystallisation of synthetic and biological calcium phosphates, *Phosph. Sulf. Silicon*, 144, 125,1999.
45. Ijima, M. et al., Effects of bovine amelogenins on the crystal morphology of octacalcium phosphate in a model system of tooth enamel formation, *J. Cryst. Growth*, 222, 615, 2001.

46. Tanabe, T. et al., Properties of phosphorylated 32-kDa nonamelogenin proteins isolated from porcine secretory enamel, *Calcif. Tiss. Int.*, 46, 20, 1990.
47. Fukae, M. et al., Primary structure of porcine 89-kDa enamelin, *Adv. Dent. Res.*, 10, 11, 1996.
48. Robinson, C., Fuchs, P., and Weatherell, J.A., The appearance of developing rat incisor enamel using a freeze fracturing technique, *J. Cryst. Growth*, 53, 160, 1981.
49. Kirkham, J. et al., Atomic force microscopy studies of crystal surface topology during enamel development, *Connect. Tiss. Res.*, 38, 91, 1998.
50. Kirkham, J. et al., Evidence for charge domains on developing enamel crystal surfaces, *J. Dent. Res.*, 79, 1943, 2000.
51. Kirkham, J. et al., Physico-chemical properties of crystal surfaces in matrix-mineral interactions during mammalian biomineralisation, *Curr. Opin. Colloid. Interface Sci.*, in press, 2002.

14

Use of a Matrix Scaffold for Tissue Engineering and Bone Regeneration

P. Mark Bartold and Yin Xiao

CONTENTS

14.1 Introduction....247
14.2 Materials and Methods....248
  14.2.1 Osteoblast Cultures....248
  14.2.2 Cell Culture in Collagen Sponges....248
  14.2.3 Wound Model....249
  14.2.4 Histological Assessment....249
  14.2.5 Densitometric Assessments....249
  14.2.6 Immunohistochemistry....249
  14.2.7 Real-Time Polymerase Chain Reaction (RT-PCR)....250
  14.2.8 *In Situ* Hybridization....251
14.3 Results....251
  14.3.1 Expression of Bone Marker Proteins....251
  14.3.2 Densitometric Assessments....252
  14.3.3 Histological Evaluation....255
  14.3.4 Identification of Bone-Forming Cells....256
14.4 Discussion....256
Acknowledgments....258
References....258

14.1 Introduction

The regeneration of bone defects resulting from tumors, diseases, infections, trauma, biochemical disorders, and abnormal skeletal development poses a significant clinical challenge. Over the years, many bone graft substitutes including autografts, allografts, and synthetic materials have been devel-

0-8493-1474-7/03/$0.00+$1.50

oped.[1] The relative shortage and traumatic harvesting procedures required for autografts, together with the potential for disease transmission and adverse host immune reactions against allografts, have increased the need to develop synthetic bone substitutes.

Current permanent synthetic grafts are limited by inflammatory reactions to debris of wear and by osteolysis of surrounding bone.[2] Such limitations of current therapies have inspired a search for improved methods for repairing skeletal defects.

Tissue engineering is an emerging interdisciplinary field involving use of principles of the life sciences and engineering toward the formation of three-dimensional tissue substitutes by culturing cells on natural or synthetic polymer scaffolds. After implantation into patients, such engineered devices help to create or restore the lost tissue or organ function.[3]

The three essential ingredients for morphogenesis and tissue engineering are cellular components, growth and differentiation factors, and a scaffold or three-dimensional matrix.[4] The cellular components must not only be present; they must be able also to give rise to new structural tissue. They can be introduced from an exogenous cell source or recruited from the local environment of implantation. Growth and differentiation factors may be essential to guide the appropriate development of the cellular components.[5] These factors may be produced by transferred cells or provided exogenously as purified proteins. A scaffolding matrix must be introduced to provide a substrate for cellular attachment, proliferation, and differentiation.[4]

In this chapter, we demonstrate how cells from alveolar bone retain their osteogenic properties in a three-dimensional collagen scaffold and subsequently synthesize a bone matrix which, after implantation, can induce new bone formation in critical size calvarial bone defects.

14.2 Materials and Methods

14.2.1 Osteoblast Cultures

Human osteoblasts were isolated from alveolar bone by explant culture.[6,7] Normal human alveolar bone specimens were obtained from healthy young patients and were first treated by collagenase digestion and then used as explants for establishment of cell culture. The cells obtained were subcultured and characterized by morphological and functional criteria. Normal human gingival fibroblasts and periodontal ligament fibroblasts were obtained from gingival and periodontal ligament using methods described previously.[8]

14.2.2 Cell Culture in Collagen Sponges

Cells were seeded onto collagen sponges (ICN Biomedical products, Costa Mesa, CA). Such sponges contain specially designed pore sizes that allow cell penetration deep into the sponges. The sponges containing cells were cultured in six-well cell culture plates for 6 days. The cell culture media were changed to mineralization media containing 50 μg/ml ascorbic acid, 10 mM β-glycerophosphate, and 10 μM dexamethasone for a further 6 weeks. Collagen sponges alone in the same culture conditions were used as controls.

14.2.3 Wound Model

Collagen sponges (4 × 4 × 1 mm) were placed into calvarial critical-sized bony defects in SCID mice (Animal Resource Centre, Western Australia) anesthetized with intraperitoneal injection of a 1:1:8 solution of ketamine hydrochloride (Troy Laboratories, New South Wales, Australia), xylazine (Troy Laboratories) and 0.9% physiological saline. The periosteum was dissected from the bone surface and a calvarial bone defect 3.5 mm in diameter was created on the parietal bone using a trephine bur in a slow-speed dental drill. The implant was placed precisely into the defect, and soft tissue above the defect was closed with skin staples.

14.2.4 Histological Assessment

For histological examination, collagen sponges, with or without cells, after 6 weeks' culture were fixed, embedded in paraffin, and serial 5-μm sections were cut. Animals were sacrificed 4 weeks after surgery and the defect areas were dissected. After radiographic and direct light microscope examinations of bone density of the defect sites, tissue biopsies were fixed and the tissues were decalcified in EDTA. Tissues were then embedded in paraffin and serial sections of 5 μm were cut and stained with hematoxylin and eosin. Collagen sponge slices were also stained using von Kossa staining for examination of calcium deposition.

14.2.5 Densitometric Assessments

Radiographs were taken of the defect sites, scanned, and captured using the NIH Image Analysis program (Version 1.76). The optical densities of the defect areas were measured and ratios obtained by comparison to adjacent normal bone density.

14.2.6 Immunohistochemistry

Table 14.1 lists antibodies used for these studies. Sections were incubated with optimal dilution of primary antibodies for alkaline phosphatase (ALP, 1:200), bone morphogenetic proteins (BMP-2 and BMP-4, 1:100), osteocalcin (OCN, 1:2000), osteopontin (OPN, 1:2000), and bone sialoprotein (BSP, 1:100) overnight at 4°C. Sections were then incubated with a biotinylated swine

TABLE 14.1
Sources of Antibodies

Protein	Antibody	Source
Alkaline phosphatase (ALP)	Antihuman ALP	Sigma-Aldrich St Louis, MO
Bone morphogenetic proteins (BMP-2 and BMP-4)	Goat antihuman BMP-2 and BMP-4	Santa Cruz Biotechnology Inc. Santa Cruz, CA
Osteocalcin (OCN)	Goat antihuman OCN	Biomedical Technologies Inc. Stoughton, MA
Osteopontin (OPN	Rabbit antihuman OPN	Dr. L.W. Fisher National Institutes of Health Bethesda, MD
Bone sialoprotein (BSP)	Rabbit antihuman BSP	Dr. L.W. Fisher National Institutes of Health Bethesda, MD

antibody reactive against mouse, rabbit, and goat IgG (Dako Multilink, Carpinteria, CA) for 15 minutes, and then incubated with horseradish periodase-conjugated avidin–biotin complex (ABC) for 15 minutes. Antibody complexes were visualized after the addition of buffered diaminobenzidine (DAB). Sections were then lightly counterstained with Mayer's hematoxylin and Scott's blue. Controls included omission of the primary or secondary (antimouse IgG) antibody and use of an irrelevant antibody (antiCD-15).

14.2.7 Real-Time Polymerase Chain Reaction (RT-PCR)

The primers designed for RT-PCR are listed in Table 14.2. Total RNA was isolated using RNA isolation reagent (Advanced Biotechnology, Foster, RI) and the concentration was determined spectrophotometrically. First-strand cDNA was synthesized using M-MLV reverse transcriptase (Promega, Madison, WI) with oligo dT as a primer. Primers were selected for each target gene, using Primer Express software (Applied Biosystems, Foster City, CA). The PCR reaction mix contained cDNA, primers, and SYBR green master

TABLE 14.2
Primers for Real-Time Polymerase Chain Reaction

Gene	Forward	Reverse	Product Size (bps)
ALP	CGTGGCTAAGAATGTCATCATGTT	TGGTGGAGCTGACCCTTGA	89
β-2M	ACTTTGTCACAGCCCAAGATAGTTAA	AAATGCGGCATCTTCAACCT	76
BMP-2	AAAACGTCAAGCCAAACACAAA	GTCCACGTACAAAGGGTGTCTCT	72
BMP-4	GCCAAGCGTAGCCCTAAGC	GTGGCGCCGGCAGTT	65
BSP	GGCCTGTGCTTTCTCAATGAA	GCCTGTACTTAAAGACCCCATTTTC	96
OCN	GCAAAGGTGCAGCCTTTGTG	GGCTCCCAGCCATTGATACAG	80
OPN	ACATCCAGTACCCTGATGCTACAG	GGCCTTGTATGCACCATTCA	347

mix (Applied Biosystems), which also provides nucleotides, PCR buffer, AmpliTaq Gold DNA polymerase, double-strand DNA fluorescent dye, and ROX internal passive reference dye).

For each cDNA sample, a *no RT* control was run in the PCR reaction. Results were normalized by being expressed relative to the amount of β-2 microglobulin (β-2M) mRNA determined in each sample.

14.2.8 *In Situ* Hybridization

To verify the origins of cells that formed bone tissue in this study, *in situ* hybridization (ISH) was performed by using a human-specific fluorescein-labeled oligonucleotide probe (InnoGenex, San Ramon, CA) that detects *Alu* repeat sequences found in human chromosomes. Tissues were dewaxed with Rnase-free reagents, then treated with proteinase K and heated to a boil in a microwave.

The slices were post-fixed and a ready-to-use probe solution was added onto the sections. After posthybridization washes, the bound probe was detected by serial addition of a biotinylated antifluorescein antibody (InnoGenex), followed by streptavidin–horseradish peroxidase conjugate, and finally DAB for visualization. All slices were lightly counterstained with eosin.

14.3 Results

14.3.1 Expression of Bone Marker Proteins

The collagen sponge provided a three-dimensional culture environment and allowed cells to penetrate deep into the pores. After 5 to 6 weeks of culture in mineralizing media, BMP-2, BMP-4, BSP, OCN, and OPN were monitored with regard to their gene expression and protein levels. Figure 14.1 shows that the mRNA levels for these proteins were significantly up-regulated ($P = <0.05$, ANOVA) in the three-dimensional cultures compared with the two-dimensional cultures. Moreover, in three-dimensional cultures in mineralizing media, the bone marker mRNAs were also significantly increased ($P = <0.05$, ANOVA) in comparison with normal culture media.

The levels of protein expression of ALP, BMP-2, BMP-4, BSP, OCN, and OPN in the collagen sponges were determined using immunohistochemical methods (Figure 14.2). BMP-2 and BMP-4 were mostly localized in the cells and their surrounding matrices. ALP, BSP, OCN, and OPN were also located to the cells and their matrices and around the collagen sponge fibers.

Calcium deposition was monitored in the collagen sponges seeded with osteoblasts cultured in mineralized media. No positive staining was found in the sponges seeded with human gingival fibroblasts (Figure 14.3). The sponges containing osteoblasts demonstrated significant calcium deposits.

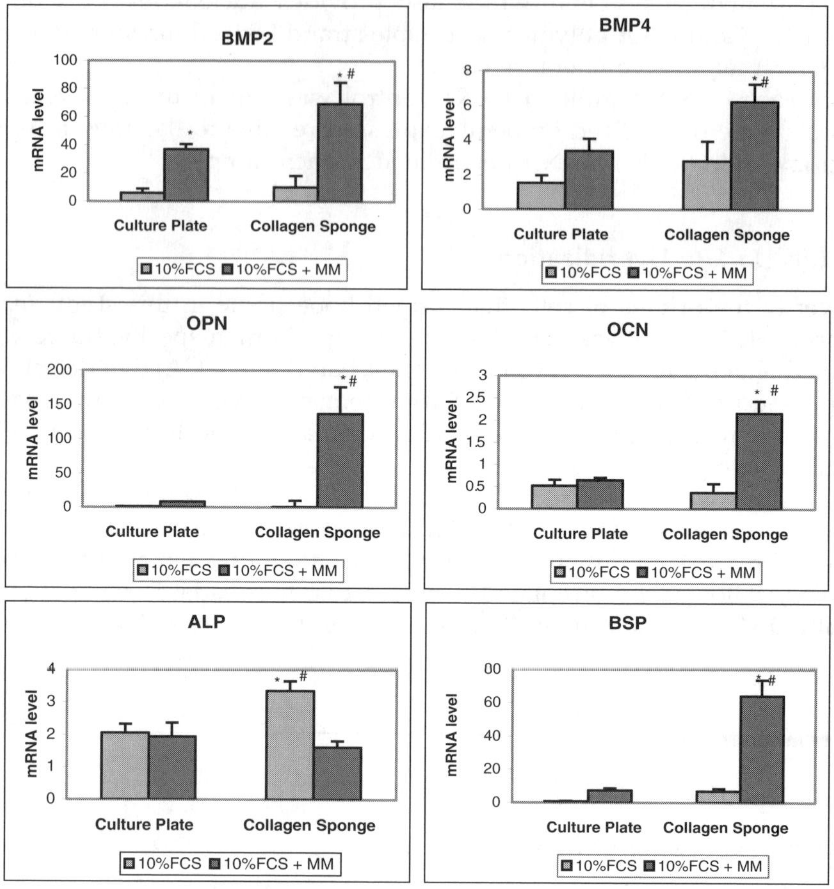

FIGURE 14.1
Regulation of mRNA of bone-related proteins from osteoblasts cultured under different conditions. Osteoblasts cultured in three-dimensional collagen sponges in mineralized culture media (MM) resulted in a significant up-regulation of BMP-2, BMP-4, OPN, OCN, and BSP mRNA. Extracted RNA was analyzed by RT-PCR for BMP-2, BMP-4, OPN, OCN, ALP, BSP, and β2-M. C_T values were converted to nanograms input RNA for each gene and the final results were expressed relative to the β2-M value for each sample. Data points represent mean ± standard deviation of triplicate values. * = $P < 0.05$ relative to normal culture media. # = $P < 0.05$ relative to tissue culture plate.

Calcium was deposited on the collagen fibers and also in the newly formed cell matrices.

14.3.2 Densitometric Assessments

Four weeks after the surgery, the bone defects were examined and photographed using light microscopy at 20× magnification. (Examples of the light microscopy and radiographs are shown in Figure 4a.) Obvious increases in

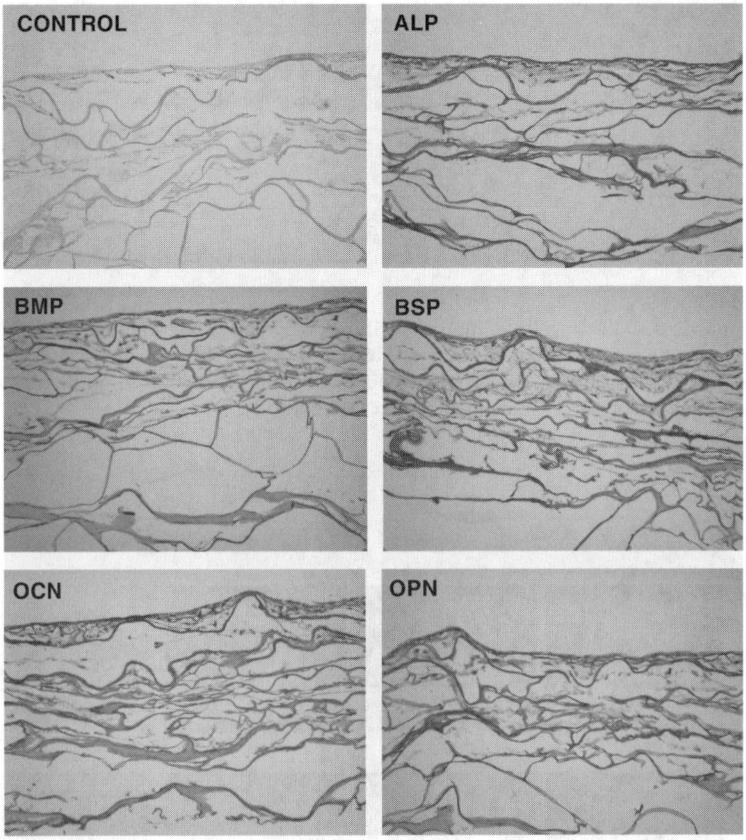

FIGURE 14.2
(See color insert.) Bone matrix proteins expressed in collagen sponges in osteoblast culture. Control: no staining was detected in negative control stained with irrelevant antibody. BMP: sections were stained with goat antihuman BMP-2 and BMP-4 polyclonal antibody. OCN: sections were stained with goat antihuman OCN polyclonal antibody. ALP: sections were stained with monoclonal antihuman ALP antibody. BSP: sections were stained with rabbit antihuman BSP antibody (LF-6). OPN: sections were stained with rabbit antihuman OPN antibody (LF-7).

light opacity and radiopacity were noted in the group of bone defects filled with collagen sponge containing osteoblasts. Light microscopy revealed that the bone defects filled with collagen sponge alone or collagen sponge containing human gingival fibroblasts produced more fibrous tissue deposition, compared with defects that did not receive collagen sponges. Bone densities (Figure 14.4b) in the defect areas filled with collagen sponges containing osteoblast-derived matrices were significantly higher compared to unfilled bone defects, defects filled with collagen sponges alone, and collagen sponges impregnated with human gingival fibroblasts ($P = <0.05$). No significant differences were found in the groups of bone defects without

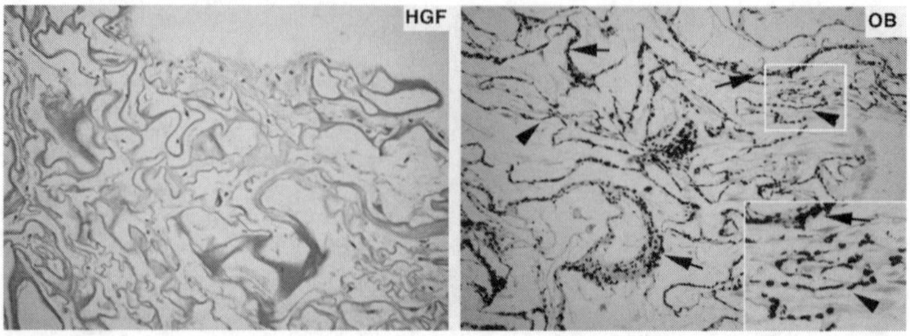

FIGURE 14.3
Collagen matrices and extracellular matrix calcification by von Kossa staining. HGF: no calcium deposition was detected in human gingival fibroblasts cultured in collagen matrices. OB: Osteoblasts cultured in collagen matrices resulted in calcium deposition in both collagen fibrils (arrow) and newly formed extracellular matrix (arrowhead).

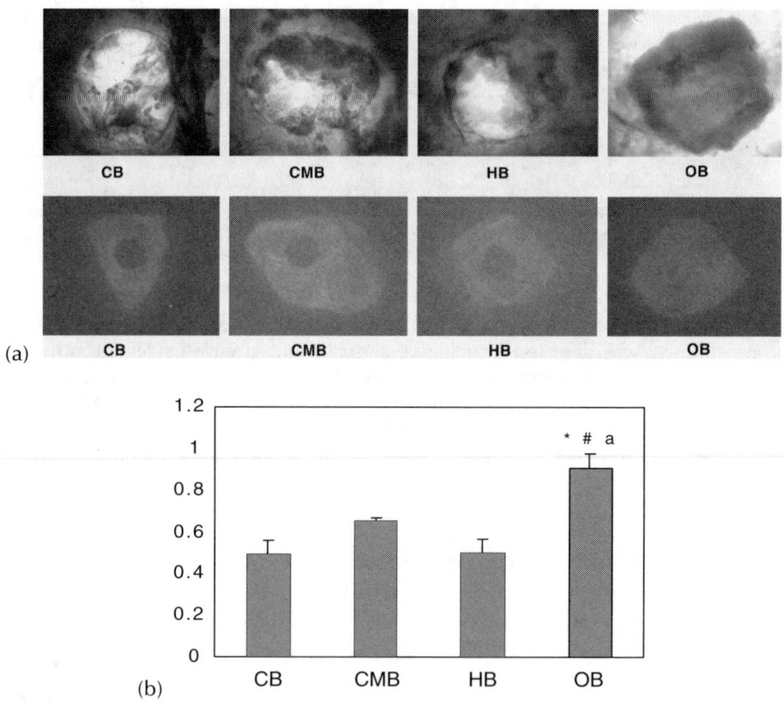

FIGURE 14.4
Light microscopy images and radiographs reveal bone defects filled with or without collagen sponges in conjunction with HGF or osteoblasts. CB: bone defect without filling. CMB: bone defect filled with collagen sponge alone. HB: bone defect filled with collagen sponge plus HGF. OB: bone defect filled with collagen sponge plus osteoblasts.

filling, bone defects filled with collagen sponge alone, and bone defects filled with collagen sponge impregnated with human gingival fibroblasts (P = >0.05).

14.3.3 Histological Evaluation

No histological evidence of inflammatory reaction was found in any of the treatment groups (Figure 14.5). Unfilled calvarial defects were covered with thin fibrous connective tissue sheets without new bone formation. Bone defects filled with collagen sponge alone showed increased amounts of fibrous tissue and cells within the defects. New bone formation was noted in the defects containing implanted human osteoblasts in collagen sponges, whereas human gingival fibroblasts did not appear to induce new bone formation. In the calvarial defects treated with sponges containing osteoblasts, newly formed bone tissue was found in the central areas of the defects. In addition, mineralized bony trabeculae surrounded by osteoblasts were found. No cartilage was observed in bone defects in any of the groups.

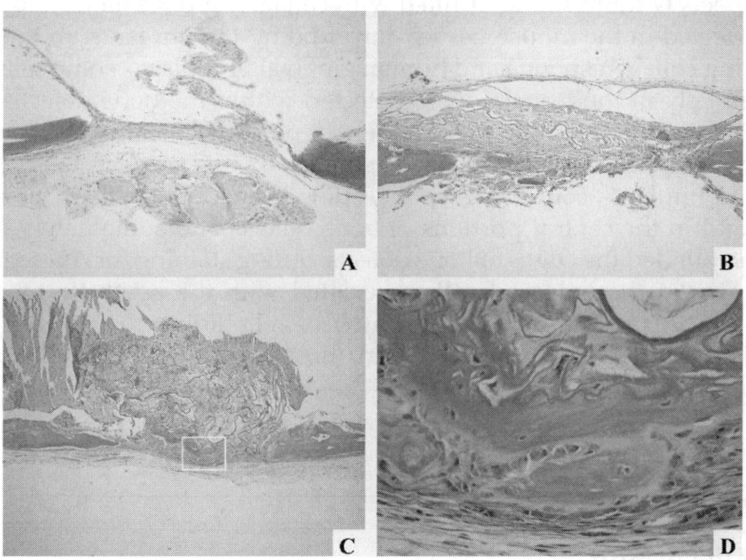

FIGURE 14.5
(See color insert.) Histological evaluation of tissue reaction after 4 weeks implantation of osteoblasts in bone defects. A: bone defect without filling showed no new bone formation and no obvious osteoblast activity in the rims of defects. B: bone defects filled with collagen sponge plus HGF resulted in more fibrous tissue in defect areas; no new bone formation was detected. C and D: bone defects filled with collagen sponge plus osteoblasts resulted in new bone formation in the central parts of the defects; active osteoblasts lining the new bone matrix and the rims of defects were detected. D: high magnification of the central part of bone defect.

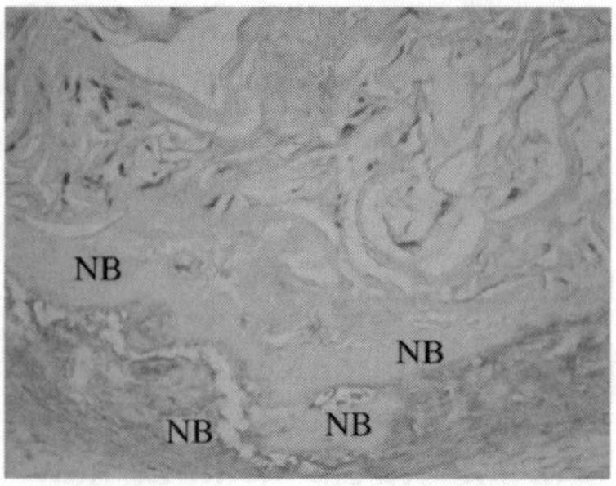

FIGURE 14.6
In situ hybridization of human-specific *Alu* sequence in tissue sections with osteoblast implantation. NB: new bone. Arrow: collagen fibrils of implanted collagen sponges. Arrowhead: positive hybridization signal of *Alu* sequence in the nuclei of the cells associated with newly formed bone tissue.

14.3.4 Identification of Bone-Forming Cells

The origins of the bone-forming cells within the defects were determined by *in situ* hybridization to trace the human-specific *Alu* sequence (Figure 14.6). No hybridization signals were found in the sections from control groups of bone defects without filling or filled with collagen sponge alone. No signals were detected in the mouse tissues surrounding the implants. In the group containing collagen sponge and human gingival fibroblasts, some cells staining positively in their nuclei were detected within the bone defects. These cells were surrounded by large numbers of negatively stained cells embedded among the collagen fibrils of the sponge.

For the implants containing sponge plus human osteoblasts, new bone was found in the central portions of bone defects and some newly formed bone surrounded the edges of bone defects. Strong staining for *Alu* sequences was shown in the nuclei of cells associated with the newly formed bone tissue, and this was particularly located to cells lining the newly formed bone. However, other osteoblasts and most of the osteocytes within the newly formed bone failed to stain for the *Alu* sequence.

14.4 Discussion

To enable successful cell implantation into bone defects, an ideal carrier is necessary to act as a scaffold for cell proliferation and differentiation at the transplantation sites. Since type I collagen is the major component of bone matrix, a number of studies attempted to use type I collagen as a scaffold material to construct bone tissue and demonstrated that this collagen exhibits favorable effects on attachment, proliferation, and differentiation of human osteoblastic cell lines.[9-11]

We found that osteoblasts cultured in collagen sponge expressed highly differentiated osteoblastic phenotypes compared with osteoblasts cultured on the plastic surfaces of tissue culture plates. The remarkable up-regulation of bone-related markers at both the mRNA and protein levels demonstrated that the three-dimensional collagen matrices encouraged the expression of osteogenic phenotype. Moreover, calcium deposition (von Kossa staining) verified the different mineralizing potentials of osteoblasts and gingival fibroblasts when cultured in collagen sponges. These results indicate that collagen matrices appear to enhance the osteoblastic phenotypes of cells derived from alveolar bone and exhibit accelerated mineralization in a manner similar to osteoblasts from other sources.[11,12]

Animal models of calvarial bone critical defects have been used for comparisons of different osteopromotive materials.[13-15] Implantation of sponges containing osteoblasts was used to develop a bone repair device that would promote new bone formation from grafted osteoblasts, support the recruitment of osteoprogenitor cells into a repair site, and initiate osteogenesis. Delivery and migration of osteoprogenitor cells into bone defect areas is a requirement for repair because these cells secrete specific extracellular matrix components.[16] This study revealed that implantation of human osteoblasts seeded in an engineered device into calvarial bone defects induced the proliferation and differentiation of mesenchymal cells into osteoblasts that resulted in formation of new bone.

Osteoconduction is the replacement of a mineralized tissue with host bone and is sometimes described as "creeping substitution" whereby the osteoconductive agent, serving as a passive scaffold, is gradually resorbed and replaced by new bone growing in from the margins.[17,18] The repair noted in our model mainly occurred in the central portion of the defect, with minor amounts of new bone formation at the rim of the host bone. Without osteoblast implantation, no new bone formation was detected in the central part of the bone defect and only a small number cells differentiated into osteoblasts that synthesized a small amount of new bone adjacent to the defect. The origins of the bone-forming cells were determined to be both the grafted cells and the host mesenchymal cells subsequently differentiating into osteoblasts. Implants with differentiated osteoblasts and developed matrix were not only involved in direct bone formation, but also appeared to exert an osteoinductive role, inducing differentiation of host mesenchymal cells into osteoprogenitor cells during the repair of the critical-sized bone defects. This finding further confirms that the healing of critical-sized bone defects is not accomplished by the extension of bone growth from previously differentiated bone cells of the host bone or by the unique properties of the surfaces of certain synthetic or natural materials by stimulating the motility of cells.[19]

The process of osteoinduction implies the recruitment of immature cells and the stimulation of these cells to develop into preosteoblasts.[20] For regeneration of skeletal tissues, an implant must contain a high concentration of progenitor cells or differentiated cells and bioactive factors to attract reparative cells to the sites.[21,22] Several *in vitro* experiments demonstrated that

BMPs can induce or stimulate differentiation of osteoblasts in various cell lines.[5,23] In the present study, most bone-related molecules were found to be highly expressed by the osteoblasts cultured in the collagen matrices. Thus, after implantation, the cell and matrix complex exerted an osteoinductive role on the differentiation of mesenchymal cells into osteoblasts and resulted in new bone tissue formation.

In conclusion, the implantation of a complex of cells derived from alveolar bones and their extracellular matrices can lead to new bone formation and exert an osteoinductive influence on surrounding tissues. Such an approach offers a novel means of triggering endogenous response cascades leading to the recruitment of cells, their subsequent differentiation into osteoblasts, and production of new bone.

Acknowledgments

The work described in this chapter was supported by a grant from the National Health and Medical Research Council of Australia.

References

1. Holy, C.E., Shoichet, M.S., and Davies, J.E., Engineering three-dimensional bone tissue *in vitro* using biodegradable scaffolds: investigating initial cell-seeding density and culture period, *J. Biomed. Mater. Res.*, 51, 376, 2000.
2. Robinson, D. et al., Inflammatory reactions associated with a calcium sulfate bone substitute, *Ann. Transplant.*, 4, 91, 1999.
3. Vancanti, C.A. and Mikos, A.G., Letter from the editors, *Tissue Eng.*, 1, 1, 1995.
4. Bruder, S.P. and Fox, B.S., Tissue engineering of bone: cell-based strategies, *Clin. Orthop.*, 367 (Suppl.), 68, 1999.
5. Tamura, S. et al., The effects of transplantation of osteoblastic cells with bone morphogenetic protein (BMP)/carrier complex on bone repair, *Bone*, 29, 169, 2001.
6. Bouvier, M. et al., Isolation and characterization of rat alveolar bone cells, *Cell. Mol. Biol.*, 37, 509, 1991.
7. Worapamorn, W. et al., Cell surface proteoglycan expression by human periodontal cells, *Connect. Tissue Res.*, 41, 57, 2000.
8. Bartold, P.M. and Page, R.C., Isolation and characterization of proteoglycans synthesized by adult human gingival fibroblasts *in vitro*, *Arch. Biochem. Biophys.*, 253, 399, 1987.
9. Bhatnagar, R.S. et al., Design of biomimetic habitats for tissue engineering with P-15, a synthetic peptide analogue of collagen, *Tissue Eng.*, 5, 53, 1999.
10. Masi, L. et al., Adhesion, growth, and matrix production by osteoblasts on collagen substrata, *Calcif. Tissue Int.*, 51, 202, 1992.

11. Yamanouchi, K. et al., Bone formation by transplanted human osteoblasts cultured within collagen sponge with dexamethasone *in vitro*, *J. Bone Miner. Res.*, 16, 857, 2001.
12. Lynch, M.P. et al., The influence of type I collagen on the development and maintenance of the osteoblast phenotype in primary and passaged rat calvarial osteoblasts: modification of expression of genes supporting cell growth, adhesion, and extracellular matrix mineralization, *Exp. Cell Res.*, 216, 35, 1995.
13. Einhorn, T.A., Clinically applied models of bone regeneration in tissue engineering research, *Clin. Orthop.*, 367 (Suppl.), S59, 1999.
14. Bosch, C., Melsen, B., and Vargervik, K., Importance of the critical-size bone defect in testing bone-regenerating materials, *J. Craniofac. Surg.*, 9, 310, 1998.
15. Tholpady, S.S. et al., Repair of an osseous facial critical-size defect using augmented fibrin sealant, *Laryngoscope*, 109, 1585, 1999.
16. Mizuno, M. et al., Bone sialoprotein (BSP) is a crucial factor for the expression of osteoblastic phenotypes of bone marrow cells cultured on type I collagen matrix, *Calcif. Tissue Int.*, 66, 388, 2000.
17. Urist, M.R., Bone Transplants and Implants: Fundamental and Clinical Bone Physiology, Lippincott, Philadelphia, 1980, p. 331.
18. Whang, K. et al., Engineering bone regeneration with bioabsorbable scaffolds with novel microarchitecture, *Tissue Eng.*, 5, 35, 1999.
19. Wang, J. and Glimcher, J., Characterization of matrix-induced osteogenesis in rat calvarial bone defects: II. Origins of bone-forming cells, *Calcif. Tissue Int.*, 65, 486, 1999.
20. Albrektsson, T. and Johansson, C., Osteoinduction, osteoconduction and osseointegration, *Eur. Spine J.*, 10 (Suppl. 2), S96, 2001.
21. Lucas, P.A. and Caplan, A.I., The extravascular fluid dynamics of the chick wing bud, *Dev. Biol.*, 126, 7, 1988.
22. Caplan, A.I. and Goldberg, V.M., Principles of tissue engineered regeneration of skeletal tissues, *Clin. Orthop.*, 367 (Suppl.), S12, 1999.
23. Katagiri, T. et al., The non-osteogenic mouse pluripotent cell line, C3H10t1/2, is induced to differentiate into osteoblastic cells by recombinant human bone morphogenetic protein-2, *Biochem. Biophys. Res. Commun.*, 172, 295, 1990.

15

Inducing Bone Growth Using Extracellular Matrix Proteins

Staale Petter Lyngstadaas, Jan Eirik Ellingsen, Axel Spahr, and Ivan Slaby

CONTENTS

15.1 Introduction 261
15.2 Surface Molecular Recognition 265
15.3 Growth Factors and Extracellular Matrix Proteins 268
15.4 Enamel Matrix Proteins for Bone Growth 270
15.4.1 Amelogenins 271
15.4.2 Amelin and Ameloblastin 274
15.5 Conclusion 275
References 277

15.1 Introduction

In the rapidly progressing fields of biomedicine and biotechnology, much effort has been focused on tissue engineering for creating biological alternatives to transplanted tissues, implants, and prostheses. In most tissue engineering strategies, a highly porous artificial extracellular matrix or scaffold is required to accommodate mammalian cells and direct their growth and hence tissue regeneration in three dimensions.[1] When seeded with specific cells like stem cells or genetically enhanced cells, such tissue engineering bioscaffolds are regarded as promising and powerful strategies for tissue and organ regeneration.[2,3]

The use of three-dimensional scaffolds for skeletal tissue engineering has been limited because of their lack of mechanical strength and firm structures and their inherent instability when loaded.[4] These limitations and the time required by current tissue engineering strategies for cellular growth, matrix deposition, and biomineralization before functional loading begins make

0-8493-1474-7/03/$0.00+$1.50

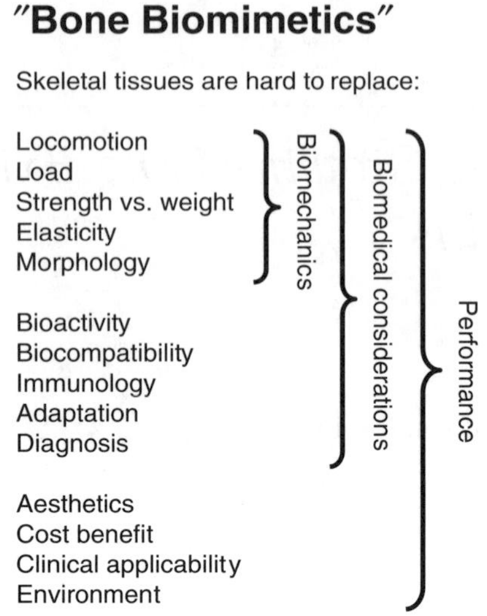

FIGURE 15.1
Replacing lost or damaged skeletal structures in the adult body is mechanically and biologically challenging. The biomaterial used should be able to resist loading immediately after implantation. Moreover, to function satisfactorily in the body, the implant should comprise biomechanical and biomedical properties that ensure a satisfactory long-term clinical outcome. The implant in question must comply also with additional requirements related to diagnosis (biological and mechanical failures should be detected at an earliest possible time point) and aesthetics, and should be easy to place to minimize surgical trauma. Finally, an implant should fulfill public needs with regard to applicability, health, economy, and environmentally friendly manufacture.

these strategies suboptimal for treatment of large defects in loaded bones in the adult body (Figure 15.1).[5]

Metal implants and prostheses on the other hand, having both the structures and mechanical strength necessary for direct function in heavily loaded organs as in joints and jaws, lack important features such as osteogenic or osteoconductive capacity and active surfaces for specific cell binding and growth. Moreover, a medical implant often induces formation of a poorly vascularized collagenous capsule that eventually can lead to implant failure. This process, often referred to as foreign body reaction, develops in response to almost all implanted biomaterials and consists of overlapping phases similar to those in wound healing and tissue repair processes.[6]

Lately, the use of microrough surface topography has reduced the extent of fibrous encapsulation of implants and increased the biomechanical properties of the implant–bone interface.[7,8] However, even though reduced in degree, the problem of foreign body reaction still exerts a major clinical impact and is considered an important issue in all implant treatment strategies including applications in orthopedics and dentistry.

Other strategies for improving biocompatibility and osteoconductive capacity of metal implants in bone include surface modification by inorganic

Strategies for Hard Tissue Maintenance

Historical and clinical order ↓

- Mechanical
  - Debridement
  - Cements
  - Fixation and immobilization
  - Macro and micro structured surface
- Systemic treatments
  - Infection control
  - Treatment for osteoporosis, etc.
  - Prophylaxis (vitamins, minerals, etc.)
- Bone fillers
  - "Bioglass", Inorganic minerals (HAp)
  - Synthetic matrices and membranes (GTR)
- Bio-strategies

FIGURE 15.2
Biological strategy for improving implant performance is both historically and clinically the "last choice." Biological strategies are employed usually when the risk of failure is high or when all other treatments have failed. This significantly reduces the benefit of biostrategy for the average patient, and also reduces efficacy and the possibility for a good clinical outcome in cases where biomedical approaches are used. However, as biostrategies are proven safe, reliable, and applicable in clinically demanding cases, the use of biological approaches will become more common. Only then, when biostrategy has become the "first choice" treatment, will its full potential be evident.

mineral coatings, plasma spraying, and particulates or cements containing a diversity of calcium salts, mainly calcium phosphates, sulfates, or carbonates (Figure 15.2). The idea behind these strategies is to make the metal surface look more like bone and, by doing so, trick the body into integrating the implanted structure in surrounding bone rather than isolating the structure by encapsulation. The success criterion for this strategy is two-sided. To be osteoconductive, a mineral deposition must have chemical and structural characteristics suitable for eliciting the wanted cell activity (i.e., osteogenesis) resulting in full osseointegration. Secondly, the mineral deposition must have internal strength and bind to the underlying metal surface strongly enough to endure the shear forces produced by implant loading. Many calcium phosphate-based biomaterials have been shown to have outstanding biological properties. They have compositions similar to bone minerals and have the ability to induce hydroxyapatite-like depositions on their surfaces.

Many materials also promote cellular functions and expression, leading to formation of strong bone–biomaterial interfaces. In addition, several of these calcium-based biomaterials are osteoconductive, that is, they provide appropriate templates for bone formation.[9,10] These materials are not, however, able to induce new bone formation when applied ectopically, and are thus not regarded as osteoinductive biomaterials on their own. Moreover, the biggest obstacle in using calcium minerals for improving metal implant

Bio-Strategies for Bone

- Living tissue and cells:
  - Auto-,allo- and Xenografts
  - Blood plates
  - Cultured cells in matrices
- "Passive"
  - Collagen membranes
  - Demineralized bone
  - Inorganic bone
- "Bioactive"
  - Hard tissue matrix proteins
  - RGD containing peptides
  - Plasma extracts
  - Growth factors

FIGURE 15.3
Several biologic approaches have been explored for templating or induction of bone growth. These range from "classical" tissue engineering techniques using living tissue or cells to inert barriers of biodegradable materials for guided tissue growth. Among the more potent strategies for use with metal implants are the growth factors and extracellular matrix molecules that provide signals to cells in the wound area to differentiate and proliferate into bone-forming tissues.

performance has not been biological performance, but rather it is the strength of the metal–mineral interface. Much effort has been put into designing calcium–mineral coatings that can resist the destructive forces resulting from implant loading and usage. However, in clinical situations, these coatings have proved to be too brittle and weak. Crackling and peeling occur frequently, often resulting in a strong secondary foreign body reaction and subsequent implant failure. Today, calcium-based biomaterials are mostly used as bioactive space fillers for regeneration of bone in critical-sized defects and for bone augmentation procedures (Figure 15.3).[11]

The lesson learned from earlier experiments and clinical studies with modified implant surfaces is that the interaction of the implant with its biological environment, the formation of the implant material–tissue interface, and the long-term outcome of implant integration in the human body are strongly connected with the surface properties of the implanted device and the ability of the organism to respond positively to such surfaces.[12]

True integration of metal implants in bone requires that osteoinductive signals are produced in the peri-implant tissue immediately after implantation. Such osteoinductive signals are mostly attributed to bone morphogenetic proteins (BMPs), a subfamily within the transforming growth factor-beta (TGF-β) superfamily of growth factors. These signals, believed initially to be expressed from macrophages during the initial bone healing, initiate a cascade reaction that ideally should lead to osseointegration of the implanted structure.[13] The outcome of the implant procedure (i.e., failure or osseointegration) is thus dictated by the initial tissue response to the surface of the implant.

All other modes for success in osseointegration are secondary to this single stage. With this in mind, it is clear that the optimal implant surface should provide instant epigenetic signals for cells exposed to the surface to express combinations of growth factors and signal molecules optimized for rapid osseous wound healing and subsequent integration of the osseous implant. The major challenge in implantology today is therefore to combine current knowledge in materials science, tissue engineering, and biology to design metal implant surfaces capable of providing epigenetic signals to cells to elicit proper biological responses that favor bone healing and osseointegration over adverse effects and suboptimal treatment outcomes.

15.2 Surface Molecular Recognition

When an implant is brought in contact with the body, its surface is instantly (within seconds) covered by a proteinaceous biofilm precipitating from tissue fluids, ruptured cells, and blood (Figure 15.4). The nature of this biofilm depends strongly on the surface characteristics of the implanted device, in particular the surface hydrophobicity, the zeta potential, and the surface charge density.[14] The composition and thickness of this biofilm will strongly influence or even occult the effect of any surface modification made to the implant to improve biological performance.

Thus, to be successful in designing surfaces that signal to cells, care must be taken also to provide a surface that ideally restricts assembly of detrimental biofilms without hindering accretion of positive biofilm components like fibrin, soluble collagens, growth factors, coagulation factors, cell homing factors, and some enzymes.

Investigations of the roles of zeta potentials and surface charge density have shown that extracellular organic matrix proteins are the main surface charge regulators in hard tissues. In contrast to mineral depositions, these organic matrix molecules stabilize and pattern the mineral–tissue interface in bone and control the formation of the interfacial structure and thus the stability of the tissue–mineral complex.[14] In sum, the implant surface exposed to cells is a composite bioactive surface resulting partly from the chemical and structural characteristics of the underlying implant and partly from the composition and thickness of the acquired biofilm.

Tissue damage, for example, resulting from implant surgery, rapidly (within minutes to hours) attracts cells to limit the damage and start the wound healing and repair processes. The cells attracted to the implant surface are not blind. They "see" the surface and each other by probing the surroundings with a complex mixture of cell surface structures commonly known as receptors and ligands that mediate cell adhesion, cell signaling,

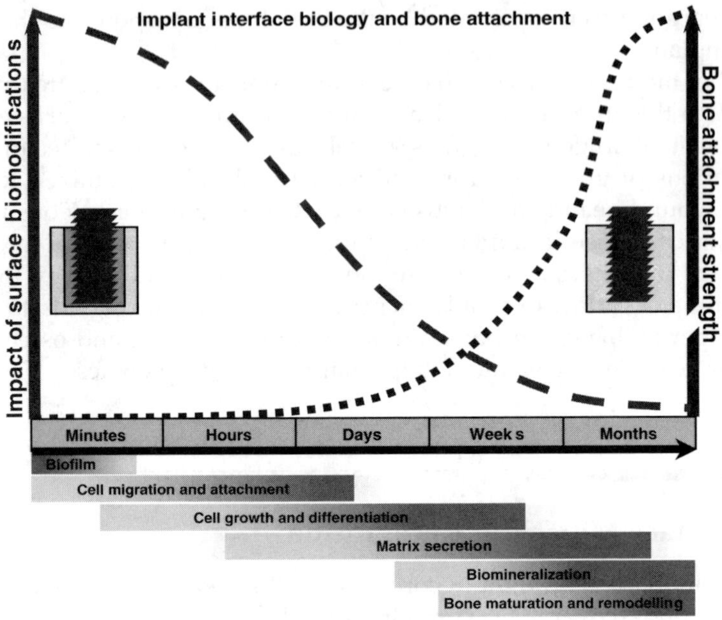

FIGURE 15.4
When an implant is placed into living bone, ensuing events have profound effects on how the implanted structure is integrated in the recipient tissue. Biological strategies are used for influencing these events to improve wound healing and bone formation and subsequently improve the integration of the implant in bone. The impact of the biostrategy is greatest in the very beginning of the healing process when biomolecules can be used to engineer biofilm formation or signal specific cells to colonize the implant surface and differentiate into bone-forming cells. Biostrategies become less effective when introduced later in the healing process. After ECM biomineralization commences, little can be added to the process. To improve the clinical outcome of implant treatment using biomolecules, they must be present at the surface from the start, and aim at patterning and/or promoting important cellular processes at the implant–tissue interface during early healing phases.

and communication.[15] Receptors and ligands are protein molecules that fit one another much like a lock and a key. Receptors are typically transmembrane proteins. The central part of the molecule is confined to the lipid bilayer of the cell membrane; the remainder extends beyond the membrane outside and inside of the cell.

Ligands may be integral to the membranes of other cells, parts of the extracellular matrix or an implant surface structure, or they can simply diffuse freely in the medium outside the cell. The milieu outside the cell varies with location and condition, and is usually quite complex. It consists of insoluble proteins and glycosaminoglycans that together form a matrix, a variety of different cell types, and several water-soluble molecules like ions, organic compounds, and peptides.

The cell surface–extracellular milieu interactions are analogous to a compound cellular Velcro™. Cells attach to the matrix, to structures on the implant surface, and to each other to form the structure of a tissue. The ligands presented by the milieu provide an address code for a cell to adhere to or migrate from or an epigenetic signal for a certain cell to proliferate, grow, differentiate, undergo structural alterations, or die. The signals from a ligated receptor may be transmitted directly to the nucleus to activate or inactivate gene transcription or mRNA translation, or the signal may activate cellular kinases that can affect a wide range of cellular processes including more secretion of growth factors and matrix molecules that can replenish the extracellular ligand stocks and reinforce the ongoing signal cascade.

Alternatively, a receptor ligated to the extracellular matrix may provide a direct link to the internal cytoskeleton that, much like the skeleton of an organism, provides structural integrity and dictates migratory behavior and shape of the cell. This is the case for some integrin receptors that connect the extracellular matrix protein fibronectin to the intracellular molecules talin and vinculin that, in turn, latch onto actin, a major cytoskeleton component.[15] In this way, an integrin receptor binding to the extracellular matrix or to a fibronectin-coated implant can directly affect the shape and internal structure of the attached cell. Integrins have also been suggested to play important roles when cells adhere directly onto metals like titanium, and it has been shown that the nature of a metal alloy can influence the expression pattern of the involved integrins.[16]

In a third scenario, ligands presented on the surface of one cell recruit a second cell type into the tissue. This type of recruitment is the basis for the immune system to function, and is the way lymphocytes are recruited from the circulatory system to initiate wound healing and repair processes, including osseous healing around implants.

Each type of cell has its own unique pattern and combinations of surface recognition molecules, and is genetically preprogrammed to launch responses when certain surface structures are encountered. In addition, many different families of receptors are present on the surface of a single cell, and a large variety of ligands are displayed in the extracellular milieu. In fact, several extracellular matrix proteins contain multiple domains that make up a set of different ligands for different cells or even different receptors on the same cell surface. Such ligand clustering serves to control overall receptor occupancy because the binding energy of a ligated matrix receptor increases in the presence of neighboring ligated receptors. This gives rise to a strong ligand distribution effect by which juxtaposition of substrate-immobilized matrix ligands leads to a nonlinear positive receptor response to increasing ligand density.[17]

This complexity in ligand presentation and the diversity of receptors on the cell surfaces make it difficult to pinpoint the individual roles of each ligand–receptor pair during intricate processes like wound healing and histogenesis. The complexity also makes it difficult to improve biological performance of implants by using free-floating ligands like hormones or growth factors, that specifically target single receptors whose binding equilibria are little influenced by neighboring ligand–receptor complexes. On the other hand, the redundancy and synergy in the ligand–receptor system for substrate immobilized ligands and surface recognition ensures robustness and stability to the process of osseous healing and repair. Thus, if properly utilized, a substrate-immobilized multidomain extracellular matrix protein, a synthetic biomimetic material, or a combination of such molecules could form the basis for new biomodified implant surfaces that take advantage of how the spatial distribution of ligands controls cell responses and initiates focal contact formation.

15.3 Growth Factors and Extracellular Matrix Proteins

Bone is formed by a series of complex events involving secretion and biomineralization of extracellular matrix proteins. The events are rigidly controlled and orchestrated by cells with specific functions to maintain the integrity of the bone.[9] The bone-forming cells grow, differentiate, and maintain their levels of differentiation through a network of epigenetic signals from other cells and from the surrounding extracellular matrix. Growth factors (GFs) make up the predominant class of intercellular signal molecules. GFs are generally classified according to their ability to influence proliferation or differentiation or both.

However, it is now well established that these effects are not constant for each GF, but vary with concentration, cell type, and developmental stage of the cells or tissues in question.[18] Moreover, most, if not all GFs act in concert to vary differentiation and proliferation of cells as part of interdependent morphogenetic networks. This allows each GF to exhibit multiple functions simply by up- or down-regulating the expression of additional GFs.

A number of growth factors were tested for their effects on bone formation and implant osseointegration.[13,19-25] Of significant interest is the TGF-β superfamily of polypeptide factors that can control both cell growth and differentiation, according to cell type and state of differentiation,[18] and directly affect expression of receptors involved in surface recognition and cellular attachment to titanium implants.[25] The TGF-β superfamily includes bone morphogenetic proteins (BMPs), a subfamily of molecules directly involved in bone growth, morphogenesis, and maintenance.[26]

BMPs are multifunctional molecules that can promote ectopic bone formation and modulate the expression and organization of osteoblastic cell proteins. BMP-2 treatment of osteoblastic cells has been shown to significantly affect the cytoskeletal and extracellular matrix organization, and promote cellular adhesion to titanium surfaces by increasing the expression of fibronectin and integrin receptor subunits with a subsequent rise in focal adhesion kinase (p125FAK) activity.[19] There is little doubt that BMP signaling is required for proper bone wound healing and integration of implants in bone. The cellular origin of these osteoinductive signals after wounding of adult bone has only partly been elucidated. It has been shown that macrophages arriving at the wound are capable of regulating and controlling osteoinduction and osseous wound healing through expression of BMPs.[13]

The importance of growth factors in general and BMPs in particular for bone formation and repair can hardly be overestimated. Nevertheless, numerous attempts to use GFs for improving the osteogenic capacities of implanted biomaterials have failed to reach the clinic to date. The reason for this somewhat disappointing situation is most probably found in the intrinsic nature of these molecules. GFs are by nature free-floating, short-lived signals that initiate or modulate small incremental changes in cells as part of cascade reactions. The effects of the signals vary dramatically by cell type, stage, location, condition of surrounding tissues, and the presence of other GFs.

Moreover, GFs are "temporal" signals that are not immobilized substrates for focal adhesion, nor are their cellular receptors designed for cell attachment. It should therefore not come as a surprise that application of a single GF does not provide a signal potent enough to significantly improve implant integration in bone. Consequently, to take full advantage of GFs, the problem must be attacked at a more fundamental level where one can trigger an orchestrated cascade of GF expression that provides a full-scale, local signal for cells to kick-start and maintain osteogenesis at a high level over a clinically significant time period.

One possible route for triggering developmental-like cascades of GF expression for bone growth is to take advantage of the surface molecular recognition apparatus for extracellular matrix ligands discussed earlier. Because receptor binding of immobilized conglomerations of juxtaposed matrix ligands provides both a strong synergistic signal for GF expression and a focal adhesion site for cell attachment, the surface molecular recognition apparatus is possibly one master switch by which GF expression cascades can be initiated and spatially regulated. Thus, incorporating into the implant surface the epigenetic signals that mimic the naturally occurring clustered ligands present in mineralizing extracellular matrices for cells to "see" would be a big leap toward the ideal osteoinductive implant.

The extracellular matrix (ECM) molecules in mineralizing hard tissues are prominent components of the cell-signaling system. There is a definitive continuum between cells and the matrix, beginning with the membrane-bound receptors participating in surface recognition and attachment, other transmembrane molecules for cellular attachment (anchorage proteins and attachment factors), and molecules such as fibronectin and laminin that have attachment domains with affinities to both cells and structural elements such as collagens or even metal or mineral surfaces.[27-30]

Thus, the ECM molecules are directly connected to cell machinery, and subtle changes in surfaces or in the ECM can be sensed and acted upon by the attaching cells. Several classes of ECM molecules are known, including structural molecules, enzymes, proteoglycans, glycosaminoglycans, protease inhibitors, and blood clotting factors. Together these components make up a dynamic ECM that is constantly degraded and rebuilt in a balanced process that maintains tissue homeostasis and facilitates tissue repair and remodeling.

In mineralizing bone, most matrix molecules are produced by osteoblastic cells. Many of the structural ECM molecules in bone have arginine–glycine–aspartic acid (RGD) sequences where cells can attach via integrin receptors.[31] Several of these molecules including fibronectin, osteonectin, vitronectin, laminin, collagens, osteopontin, bone sialoprotein, dentin sialoprotein, and thrombospondin have been tested for initiation of bone growth and maintenance of bone integrity.[24,32-36] Integrin receptor binding is believed to represent the primary mechanism of the osteoblastic cell–ECM interactions that control cell morphology, proliferation, and differentiation.[37] However, recent studies suggest that RGD-containing molecules must work in concert with BMPs to be able to induce bone growth. Thus, bone induction by implantation of RGD-containing matrices is observed mainly when BMPs are supplied concomitantly. It is defined spatially by the volume of the matrix and limited temporally to only the time when BMPs are present.[38]

Other matrix components that do not express an RGD motif are also directly involved in the formation of mineralized tissues. Heparan sulfate, a glycosaminoglycan, and lumican, a proteoglycan, are both closely associated to the differentiation of osteoblastic cells.[39,40] Other ECM molecules like members of the von Willebrand factor A-domain superfamily play important roles in cartilage and bone structure and function.[41] Matrix metalloproteinases (MMPs) and their corresponding inhibitors, the tissue inhibitors of metalloproteinases (TIMPs), are important components of bone ECM. These proteins are directly responsible for the plasticity and integrity of the bone by providing a system for controlled breakdown and remodeling of insoluble organic matrix components like collagens. Moreover, the MMPs provide secondary signals for bone cell differentiation and function and for angiogenesis during bone healing, simply by the release of soluble signaling peptides from the degrading matrix biomolecules. This release of breakdown products and matrix-bound GFs provides a strong feedback signal from the ECM to the bone cells, which in turn can react by adjusting the rate of bone formation or remodeling through altered expression and secretion of ECM components.[42,43]

It is evident that bone ECM is a biologically active entity containing molecules that may represent breakthroughs in guided interfacial osteogenesis if added to an implant surface.[44] Such molecules, when used for recruiting the surface recognition apparatus and focal adhesion mechanisms for cell–surface interactions, could provide a viable route for biomimetic induction of GF cascades at the bone–implant interface that promote attachment, growth, and repair of hard tissues over a time period consonant with a favorable clinical outcome.[45]

15.4 Enamel Matrix Proteins for Bone Growth

Teeth differ from most other skeletal tissues in that they form directly without a preceding, time-consuming cartilage intermediate. Teeth are also more highly mineralized and more resistant to mechanical, chemical, and biological breakdown. Dental matrix proteins are potent inducers for biomineralization of extracellular matrices and bony tissues.

Mammalian tooth enamel ECM proteins responsible for generating the hardest and most highly mineralized tissue known in nature best exemplify this property. Moreover, since teeth are direct descendants of the prevertebrate exoskeleton that preceded internal bones in evolution, the principal mechanism of action of dental matrix components probably underlies formation of most mineralized structures in the body. This assumption is further strengthened by recent observations that the major ECM proteins in developing enamel can induce and maintain formation and mineralization of other skeletal hard tissues such as bone (Figures 14.5 and 14.6),[46-52] dentin,[46,53,54] root cementum,[55-57] and cartilage.[58]

The potential for dental matrix proteins to trigger innate, dormant developmental processes in adjacent hard tissues makes them ideal therapeutic agents for use with metal implants where direct formation of functional bone or bone-related tissues is required for a successful clinical outcome. In fact, several studies in animals have demonstrated that enamel ECM proteins are capable of enhancing bone formation around titanium implants.[59,60]

15.4.1 Amelogenins

Amelogenin proteins from immature enamel matrix have been successfully employed to restore functional periodontal ligament (PDL), cementum, and alveolar bone in patients with severe tooth attachment loss due to periodontitis.[61,62] The role of amelogenins in PDL formation is further underlined by their presence in initial cementum formation during normal development of tooth attachment.[55,63] However, the details of the mechanisms by which amelogenins promote tissue regeneration are still not known.

The amelogenins constitute a family of hydrophobic proteins derived from a single gene by alternative splicing and controlled post-secretory processing. The amelogenins are known to self-assemble into supramolecular aggregates that form an insoluble extracellular matrix[64] with high affinity for hydroxyapatite and collagens.[65] When applied to surfaces under physiological conditions, the amelogenins precipitate to form a hydrophobic ECM deposit similar in composition and structure to the lining present on the tooth root surface prior to cementum formation.

Once in contact with biological systems, this amelogenin deposit has potential for supporting and patterning surface interactions with cells and adjacent tissues.[63-65] So far amelogenins are the only devices on the market that have potential for actually triggering regenerative responses in PDL cells. If, as several observations suggest,[55,57,63] enamel matrix protein deposition directly precedes hard tissue development in the jaw, enamel matrix-to-cell interaction at pretreated implant surfaces could be used to restart dormant developmental programs in progenitor cells for regeneration of bone.

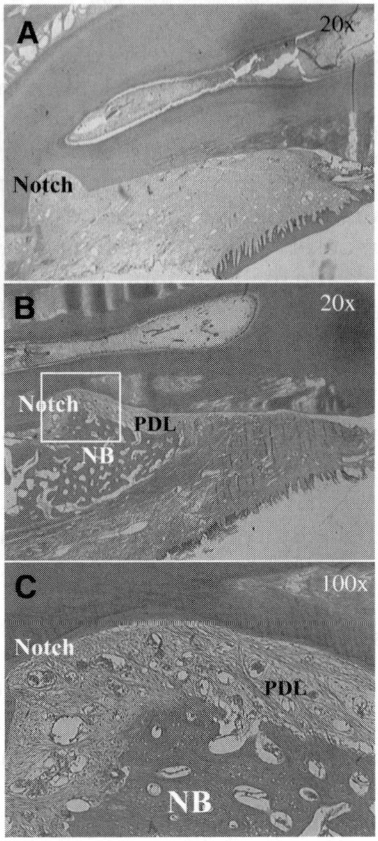

FIGURE 15.5
Histological slide showing regeneration of cementum, periodontal ligament, and alveolar bone using amelogenins extracted from immature pig enamel extracellular matrix in an experimental buccal defect in the permanent third upper premolar of a 3-year-old mini-pig. Amelogenins were obtained by acidic extraction and subsequent purification using a standardized method.[65] Following removal of bone, PDL, and cementum, a notch was made in the root at the bottom of the defect. The denuded root surface was then treated with concentrated EDTA for 2 minutes and rinsed carefully with excess of saline. Amelogenins dissolved in polyglycol alginate (PGA) to a final concentration of 30 mg/ml were then applied on the root in surplus. The flap was repositioned and fixed with sutures. Eight weeks later the pig was sacrificed. The tooth was removed and block-fixed in 4% formaldehyde, decalcinated in 5% trifluoroacetic acid, sectioned, and stained with hematoxylin and eosin. A: in control teeth (contralaterals, split-mouth design) using the same procedure, with application of PGA without amelogenins, the treatment caused formation of a long junctional epithelium all the way down to the notch. No signs of new alveolar bone, cementum, or PDL were observed. B: in amelogenin-treated teeth, new cementum, ligament (PDL), and alveolar bone (NB) are clearly visible. C: enlargement of B. Note new cementum on the root surface and the functional arrangement of the collagen bundles embedded in the new cementum attaching the tooth to the new alveolar bone.

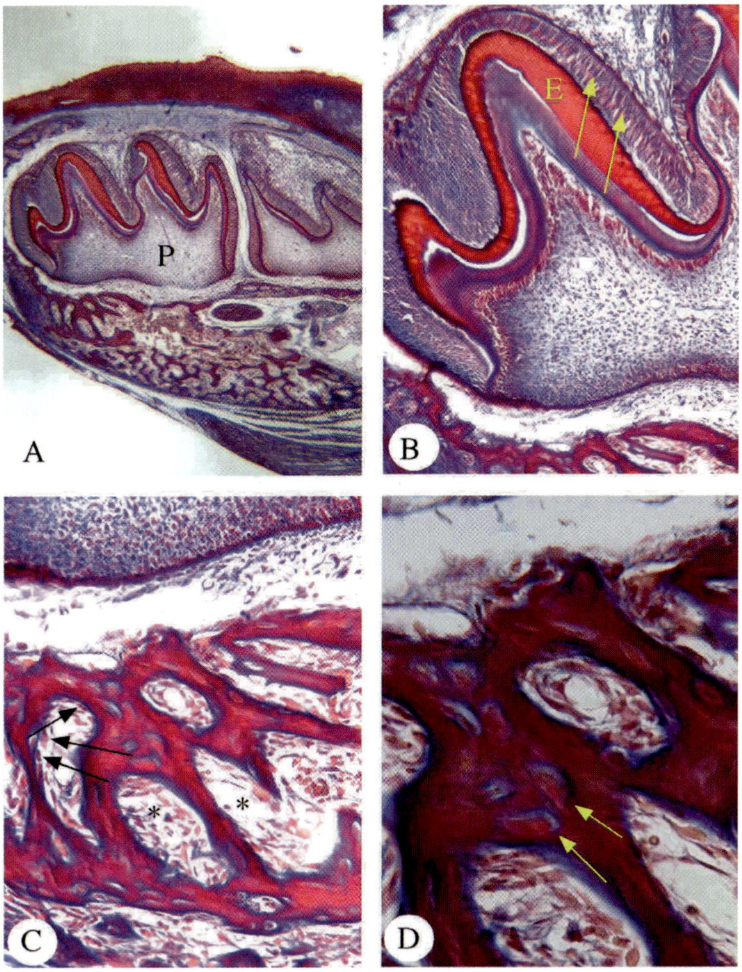

COLOR FIGURE 7.1 The developing cancellous bone from the mandible of a 5-day postnatal mouse. Tissue prepared by Mallory–Heidenhain stain. Panels A and B show dental pulp (P) and enamel (E) of a first molar. Arrows point to osteoblasts in panel C and to osteocytes in panel D. Bone marrow is identified by asterisks. Panels B, C and D are magnified 10, 20, and 40×, respectively.

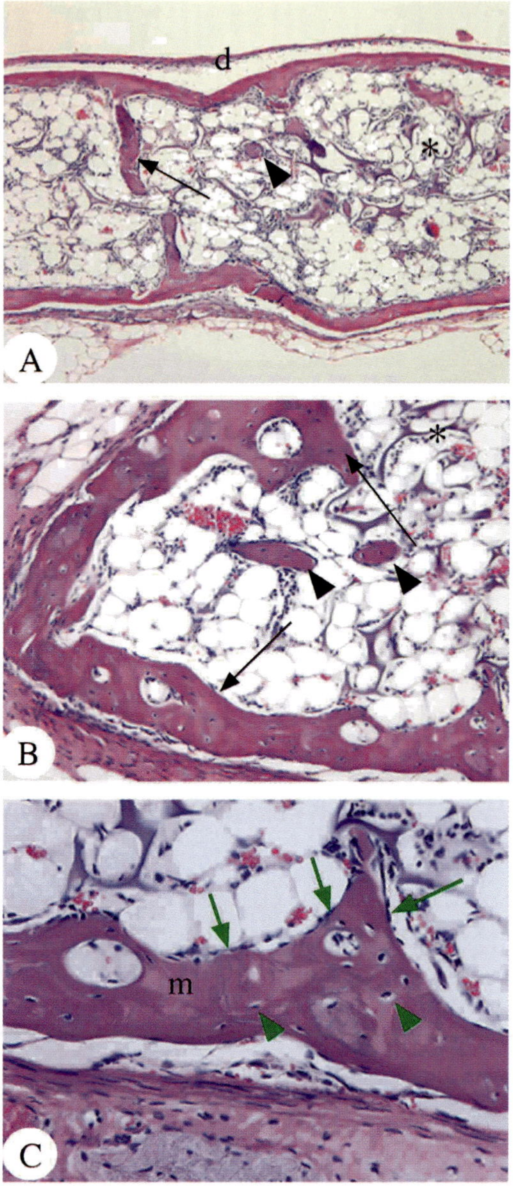

COLOR FIGURE 7.2 Panels A and B: newly formed cancellous bone (black arrows), ossicles (black arrowheads), and marrow cavities (asterisks) are formed after subcutaneous implantation of the adenovirus vector AdCMV-BMP-7 with a bovine bone-derived collagen carrier. Panel A also shows dermis (d). Panel C: bone matrix (m), osteoblasts (green arrows), and osteocytes (green arrowheads) are shown. Panels A, B, and C are magnified 10, 20, and 40×, respectively.

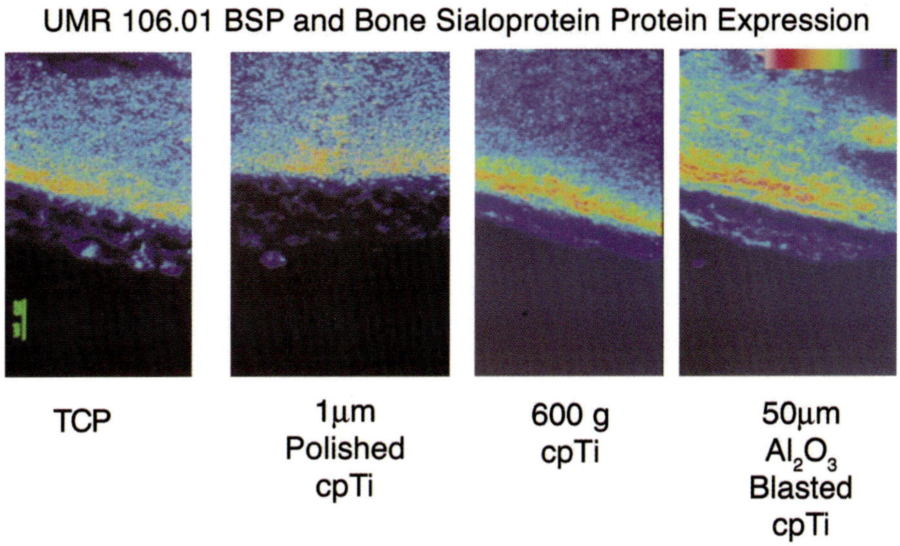

COLOR FIGURE 8.9 Immunofluorescent labeling for bone sialoprotein (BSP). Cultures were grown for 72 hours and frozen-embedded. Embedded cultures were removed and cyto-sectioned. Sections were then labeled with a primary monoclonal antibody to BSP followed by secondary labeling with 1/300 FITC Goat antimouse IgG. Cultures were grown on tissue culture plastic (TCP) or on prepared c.p. Ti surfaces. BSP labeling occurred within a region of the micromass culture above the layer of cells directly in contact with the substratum.

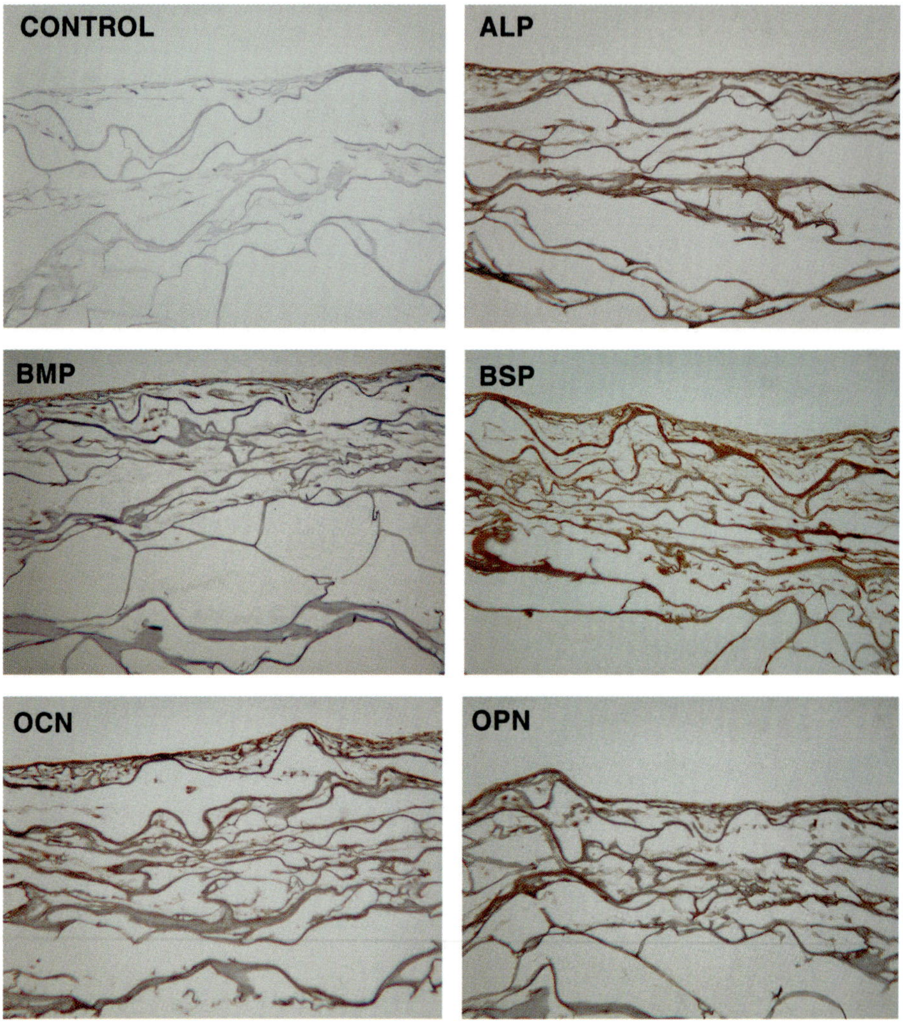

COLOR FIGURE 14.2 Bone matrix proteins expressed in collagen sponges in osteoblast culture. Control: no staining was detected in negative control stained with irrelevant antibody. BMP: sections were stained with goat antihuman BMP-2 and BMP-4 polyclonal antibody. OCN: sections were stained with goat antihuman OCN polyclonal antibody. ALP: sections were stained with monoclonal antihuman ALP antibody. BSP: sections were stained with rabbit antihuman BSP antibody (LF-6). OPN: sections were stained with rabbit antihuman OPN antibody (LF-7).

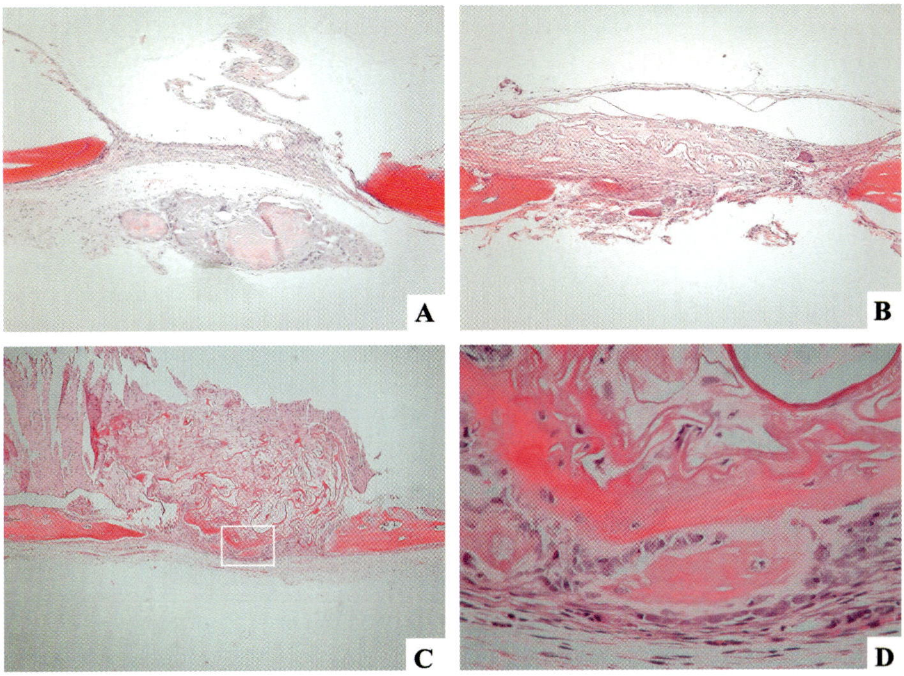

COLOR FIGURE 14.5 Histological evaluation of tissue reaction after 4 weeks' implantation of osteoblasts in bone defects. A: bone defects without filling showed no new bone formation and no obvious osteoblast activity in the rims of defects. B: bone defects filled with collagen sponge plus HGF resulted in more fibrous tissue in defect areas; no new bone formation was detected. C and D: bone defects filled with collagen sponge plus osteoblasts resulted in new bone formation in the central parts of the defects; active osteoblasts lining the new bone matrix and rims of defects were detected. D: high magnification of central part of bone defect.

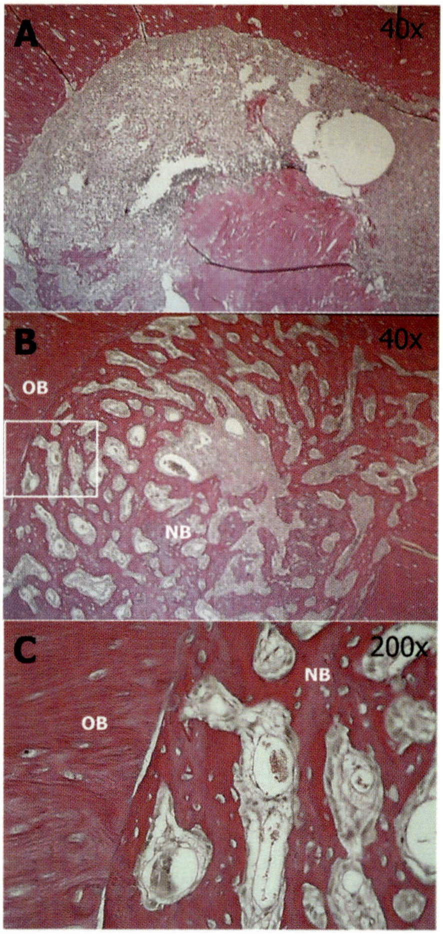

COLOR FIGURE 15.8 Induction of new trabecular bone formation using the enamel extracellular matrix-derived protein amelin (ambn). Critical size bone defects in the form of round holes 2.5 mm in diameter through the ramus of the lower jaws of adult rats (200 gr) were made using a low-speed drill and saline irrigation. Care was taken to remove the periosteum over the hole on both sides to ensure that defects healed by fibrous tissue filling and not by bone formation. After the procedure, a collagen sponge fitted to the size of the defect was used to fill the hole. The overlaying soft tissues were repositioned and the wounds were closed by sutures. After observation for 2 weeks, the rats were sacrificed and the jaw segments containing the defects were removed én bloc, fixed in 4% formaldehyde, decalcinated in 5% trifluoroacetic acid, and sectioned and stained with hematoxylin and eosin. A: in control defects, the collagen sponges were wetted in sterile PBS prior to implantation. This treatment did not induce significant amounts of new bone, and only small amounts of bone growing from the margins out (lower left corner in micrograph) could be observed. These collagen sponges were mostly surrounded by dense, cell-poor, fibrous tissue, sometimes with signs of inflammatory cell infiltrate. The collagen sponges were easily observed in the centers of the defects. B: in experimental defects, the collagen sponges were wetted in a recombinant rat ambn–PBS solution (1 mg rAmbn/ml PBS) immediately before implantation. Recombinant rat amelin was obtained by over-production in *E. coli*73 and purification by affinity chromatography. A rapid formation of new trabecular bone was invariably observed, filling most of the volume of defects (OB = old bone, NB = new bone). C: enlargement of B. Note that new bone formed from the defect out, and not as appositional growth from the old bone margins. The new bone has the appearance of mature trabecular bone with marrow and normal anatomy. However, at this stage the new bone is not fusing with the old bone, suggesting that ambn has the potential to induce trabecular bone formation, at least in the jaw, and could be useful for induction of hard tissue formation around implants.

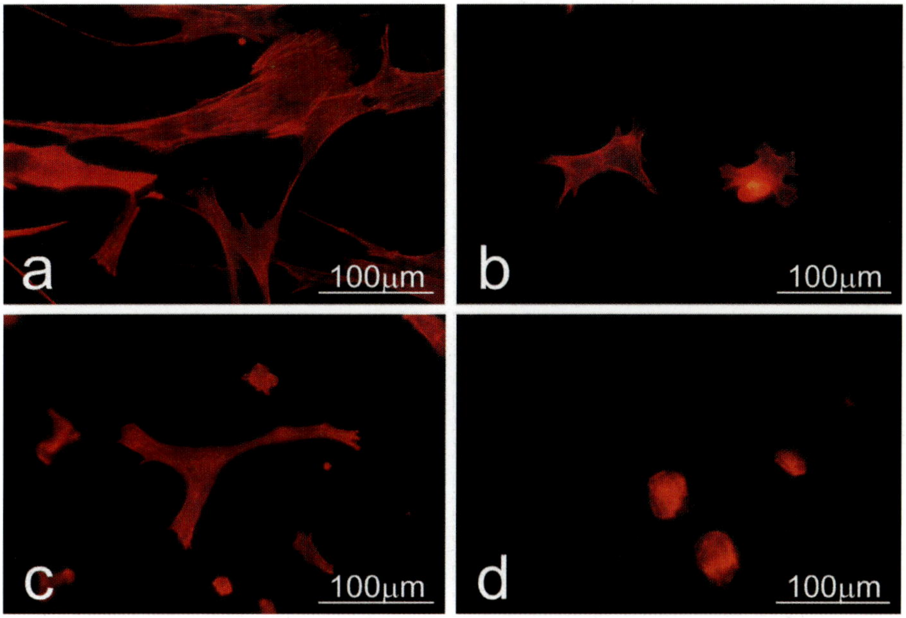

COLOR FIGURE 19.13 Fluorescence microscopy of human foreskin fibroblast cells stained for actin stress fibers on smooth and rough (SLA) titanium surfaces without and with assembled monolayers of poly-L-lysine-g-poly(ethylene glycol) (PLL-g-PEG). (a) smooth/natural oxide film surface; (b) smooth/PLL-g-PEG surface; (c) rough/natural oxide film surface; (d) rough/PLL-g-PEG surface. Cells were seeded at a concentration of 10^4 cells per mL in culture medium with 10% fetal calf serum, incubated for 24 hours, fixed in 10% formalin solution, and fluorescently stained for actin stress fibers with dissolved phalloidin. (*Source:* Tosatti, S. et al., in preparation, 2002. With permission.)

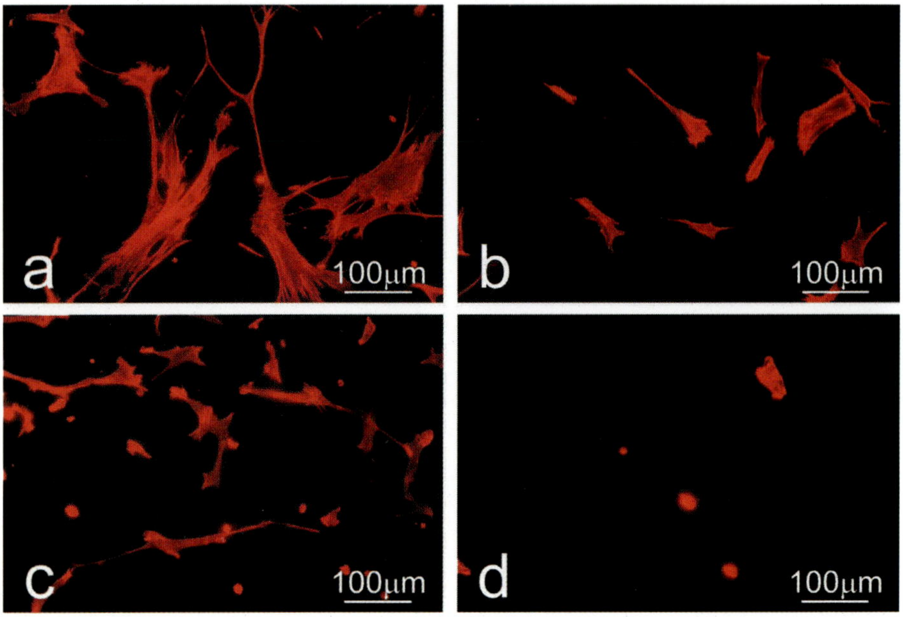

COLOR FIGURE 19.14 Fluorescence microscopy of human foreskin fibroblast cells stained for actin stress fibers on smooth and rough (SLA) titanium surfaces without and with assembled monolayers of poly-L-lysine-g-poly(ethylene glycol) (PLL-g-PEG): (a) smooth/PLL-g-PEG/PEG-RGD 5% (active peptide); (b) smooth/PLL-g-PEG/PEG-RDG 5% (inactive peptide control); (c) rough/PLL-g-PEG/PEG-RGD5% (active peptide); (d) rough/PLL-g-PEG/PEG-RGD 5% (inactive peptide control). Cells were seeded at a concentration of 10^4 cells per mL in culture medium with 10% fetal calf serum, incubated for 24 hours, fixed in 10% formalin solution, and fluorescently stained for actin stress fibers with dissolved phalloidin. (*Source:* Tosatti, S. et al., in preparation, 2002. With permission.)

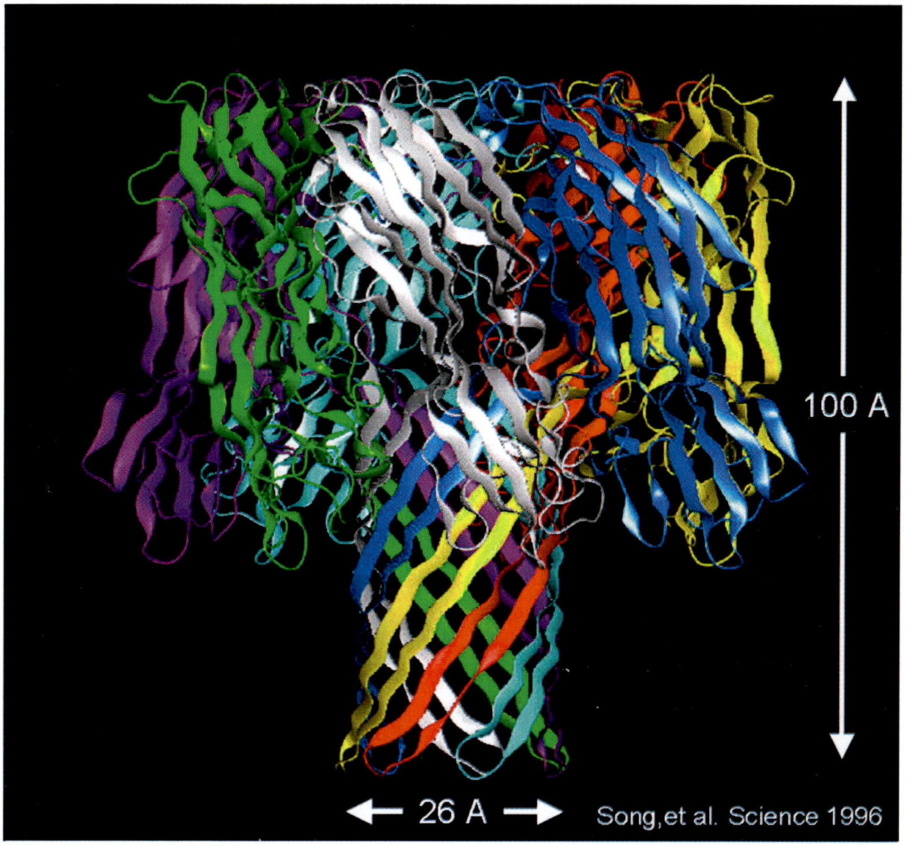

COLOR FIGURE 22.1 Complex of seven polypeptide chains known as a-hemolysin, synthesized by the human *Staphylococcus aureus* pathogen. This mushroom-shaped nanostructure has a pore parallel to the long axis and inserts itself into bilayer membranes of cells. (*Source:* Song, L. et al., *Science*, 274, 1859, 1996. With permission.)

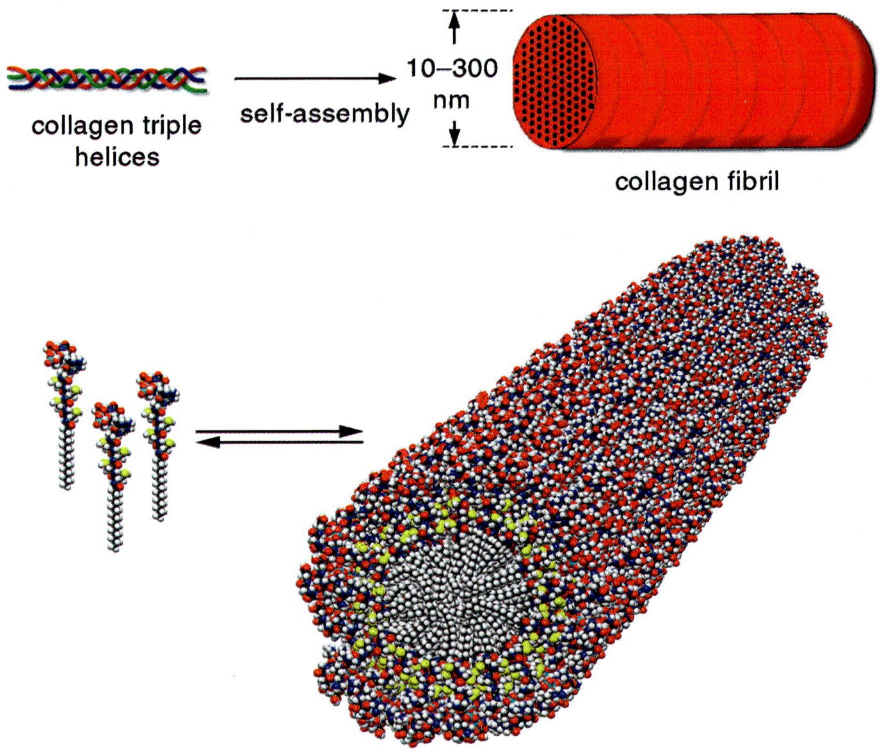

COLOR FIGURE 22.5 Schematic showing how small molecules (bottom left) self-assemble into solid fibers with nanoscale diameters (bottom right). Self-assembly produces nanostructures that mimic the morphology of collagen fibrils — common constituents of extracellular matrices formed through the aggregation of polypeptide triple helices (top).

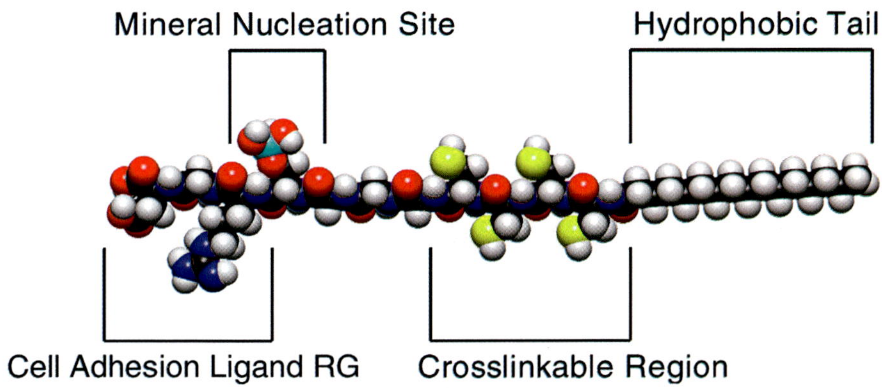

COLOR FIGURE 22.6 Molecular graphics of a molecule designed to generate a synthetic extracellular matrix by self-assembly. The molecule has four important regions: a bioactive tripeptide at one terminus for cell adhesion, a phosphorylated serine residue to generate an array of mineral nucleation sites in the supramolecular structure, a tetrapeptide of cysteine residues to capture covalently the supramolecular nanofiber through disulfide bonds, and a hydrophobic alkyl segment to impart a large amphiphilic moment to the molecule backbone.

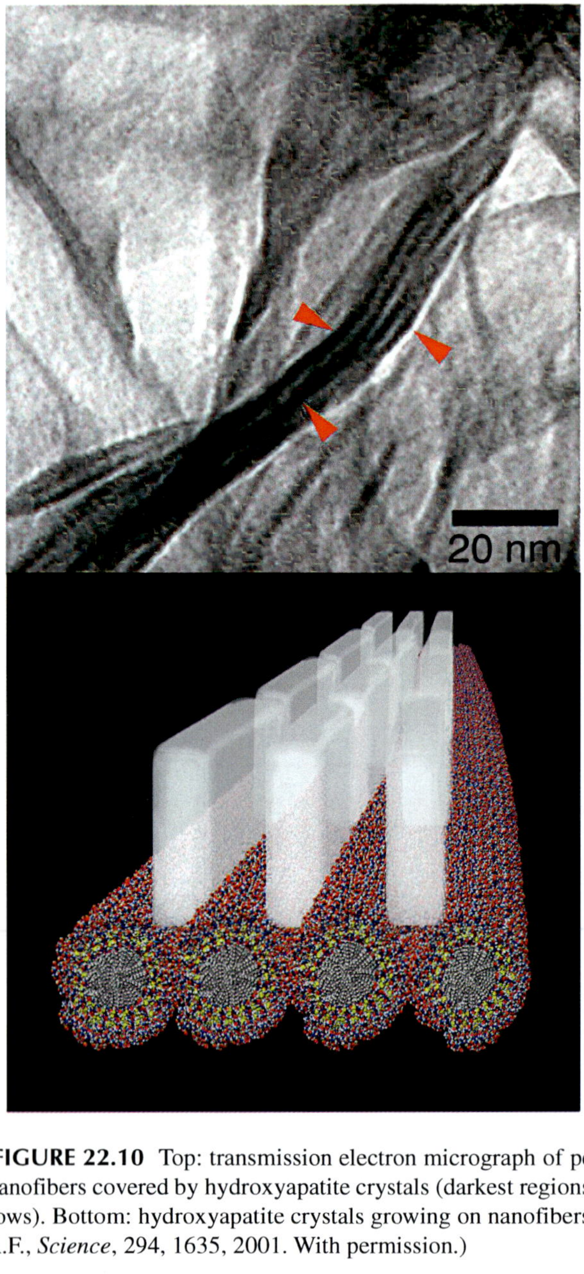

COLOR FIGURE 22.10 Top: transmission electron micrograph of peptide amphiphile nanofibers covered by hydroxyapatite crystals (darkest regions indicated by the arrows). Bottom: hydroxyapatite crystals growing on nanofibers. *(Source:* Service, R.F., *Science*, 294, 1635, 2001. With permission.)

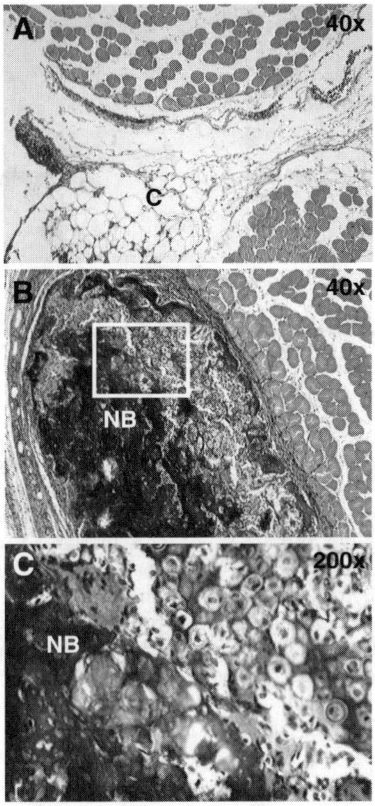

FIGURE 15.6
Collagen sponges implanted in skeletal muscles in the backs of rats. A: control collagen sponges $5 \times 5 \times 5$ mm wetted in PBS were implanted through small incisions into the muscles on the left sides of the spines. After 2 weeks, the implants were removed, fixed in 4% formaldehyde, and sectioned and stained with hematoxylin and eosin. No sign of hard tissue formation was observed in control implants. B: collagen sponges similar to those described in A were wetted in cold PBS containing 10 mg/ml amelogenins[65] and implanted in contralateral positions to the sponges implanted in the control group. After excision and fixing, the implants were decalcinated in 5% trifluoroacetic acid before sectioning and staining with hematoxylin and eosin and alcian blue. Note the new hard tissue forming in and around the collagen sponge. C: enlargement of B showing tissue consisting of newly formed, immature bone and bone-forming cells.

Such responses typically would involve sequential cascades of growth factors that act on the multitude of cells needed to completely reconstitute lost tissues or build new ones. This is in fact observed when amelogenins are added to cultures with human primary PDL cells.[66,67] These experiments have demonstrated that PDL cells increase their proliferation and metabolism in response to amelogenins, and start to express BSP, integrin receptors, and several GFs, including TGF-β1, interleukin 6 (IL-6), and PDGF-AB — all regarded as important mediators of bone healing and neogenesis. Preliminary studies on amelogenin coatings on titanium implants suggest that

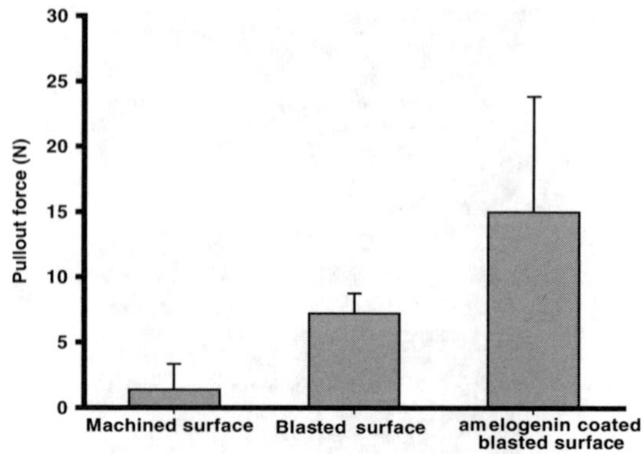

FIGURE 15.7
Pull-out experiment with coin-shaped titanium implants coated with amelogenins[65] and implanted into the cortical bones of rabbit tibiae using a standardized, validated model for measuring bone attachment forces.[8] Negative controls (machined surface), positive controls (blasted surface, 180- to 220-μm particles), and test implants (coated with amelogenins in cold, sterile PBS, 10 mg/ml overnight and air-dried) were implanted using the method of Rønold et al.[8] After 7 weeks of observation, the rabbits were euthanized and the implants exposed. A specially designed jig was then applied to pull each implant loose, while measuring the force needed to detach the titanium coins from the bone. Each group contained 12 animals. Error bars are ±2 standard deviation. The force needed to detach the amelogenin-coated implants was significantly higher than required for both control groups ($p = <0.005$), demonstrating the potential benefit of applying extracellular matrix-derived biomolecules to implant surfaces for improving tissue–implant interface reactions.

these proteins can improve biomineralization, and hence bone attachment, at the bone–implant interface (Figure 15.7). Amelogenins are thus not only promising candidates for ECM-induced bone regeneration, but also in biomimetic strategies for patterning of cell–implant interfaces to improve implant integration and attachment in bone.

15.4.2 Amelin and Ameloblastin

The amelin/ameloblastin protein family is also believed to play a central role in tooth formation and extracellular matrix (ECM) mineralization. The shorter amelin (40 kDa) and longer ameloblastin (55 kDa) are both expressed from one alternatively spliced gene (ambn). They were discovered in the inner enamel and epithelial root sheaths where they are involved in the control of amelogenesis and cementogenesis.[6,68,70-72]

Later studies of amelin and ameloblastin function also demonstrated expression of ambn mRNA in mesenchymal cells of the dental papilla, preodontoblasts, and young odontoblasts at stages prior to onset of mantle dentine mineralization.[73] When the mantle dentin starts to mineralize, the expression of amelin in odontoblasts gradually fades away and translocates to the newly differentiated secretory ameloblasts. The cells of the epithelial root sheath and cells embedded in newly formed cellular cementum have been shown to express amelin mRNA.[69,72] This ambn expression in the epithelial root sheath during apical growth of the tooth root also corresponds with the induction of adjacent odontoblasts and cementoblast differentiation with consequent formation of dentin and cementum.[73,74]

The precise functions of the ambn gene products remain largely unknown. The abundant expression and wide distribution of ambn expression from cells in mineralizing dental tissues suggest that this gene is crucial to the formation of these structures. In the enamel, ambn expression is believed to participate in ameloblast–matrix interactions and the control of enamel architecture by determination of the prism–interprism boundary.[75] In the mesenchymal part of the developing tooth, ambn seems to be involved in cell signaling and differentiation during mantle dentine, root, and cementum formation. Consequently, based on the timing and location of expression, ambn expression may function in extracellular signaling during sequential and reciprocal developmental processes or act in the process of crystal nucleation in the dentine and enamel extra cellular matrices or both.[76]

In a recent study on the formation of a cementum-like tissue onto denuded enamel surfaces by dental follicular cells, it was noted that an excess of osteodentine-like tissue was formed in the dental papillae of experimental teeth. The reparative hard tissue formations were directly preceded by strong ambn expression and secretion of large amounts of amelin in the traumatized area.[53,55] This observation suggests that ambn expression is not only a developmental signal, but is also part of the trauma-induced reparative process in mature hard tissue. This notion is further strengthened by other observations indicating that ambn gene expression is intimately associated with the expression of the osteoblast differentiation factor cbfa-1,[76,78] that amelin and ameloblastin are present in mandibular bone,[77] and that amelin in fact can induce new bone formation in experimental defects (Figure 15.8).

The observation that ambn expression is involved in cell signaling, cell differentiation, and cell–matrix interactions in several types of mineralized tissues is a strong indication that proteins and/or peptides based on the ambn sequence can be utilized for optimizing the implant–bone interface. Further studies on the possible involvement of ambn in bone healing and implant integration are thus justified and could provide yet another route to improve implant performance.

15.5 Conclusion

Even though titanium implants and joint prostheses have shown considerable progress over the last three decades, they are not ideal. The "time to healing" and "time to loading" parameters are still considered unsatisfactory. Moreover, metal implants are still regarded as suboptimal devices with respect to their ability to interact with biological environments without caus-

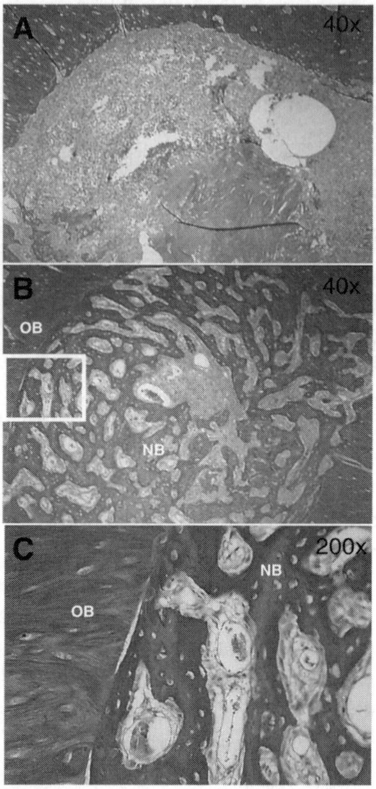

FIGURE 15.8
(See color insert.) Induction of new trabecular bone formation using the enamel extracellular matrix-derived protein amelin (ambn). Critical size bone defects in the form of round holes 2.5 mm in diameter through the ramus of the lower jaws of adult rats (200 gr) were made using a low-speed drill and saline irrigation. Care was taken to remove the periosteum over the hole on both sides to ensure that defects healed by fibrous tissue filling and not by bone formation. After the procedure, a collagen sponge fitted to the size of the defect was used to fill the hole. The overlaying soft tissues were repositioned and the wounds were closed by sutures. After observation for 2 weeks, the rats were sacrificed and the jaw segments containing the defects were removed én bloc, fixed in 4% formaldehyde, decalcinated in 5% trifluoroacetic acid, and sectioned and stained with hematoxylin and eosin. A: in control defects, the collagen sponges were wetted in sterile PBS prior to implantation. This treatment did not induce significant amounts of new bone, and only small amounts of bone growing from the margins out (lower left corner in micrograph) could be observed. These collagen sponges were mostly surrounded by dense, cell-poor, fibrous tissue, sometimes with signs of inflammatory cell infiltrate. The collagen sponges were easily observed in the centers of the defects. B: in experimental defects, the collagen sponges were wetted in a recombinant rat ambn–PBS solution (1 mg rAmbn/ml PBS) immediately before implantation. Recombinant rat amelin was obtained by over-production in *E. coli*[73] and purification by affinity chromatography. A rapid formation of new trabecular bone was invariably observed, filling most of the volume of defects (OB = old bone, NB = new bone). C: enlargement of B. Note that new bone formed from the defect out, and not as appositional growth from the old bone margins. The new bone has the appearance of mature trabecular bone with marrow and normal anatomy. However, at this stage the new bone is not fusing with the old bone, suggesting that ambn has the potential to induce trabecular bone formation, at least in the jaw, and could be useful for induction of hard tissue formation around implants.

ing adverse reactions and failure. Current implants also lack biological properties that stimulate integration and attachment in bone. If bone "regenerative" strategies are to be adopted in orthopedics and implant dentistry, new methods for surface-mediated, direct bone induction will have to be developed.

The rapidly progressing fields of biomedicine and tissue engineering have not yet devised alternatives to metal implants to restore functions in adult skeletal tissues. Thus, to further improve metal implant performance, strategies for making metal surfaces more osteoinductive must be designed. Adding bioactive surface layers to implants and prostheses could improve biocompatibility, osseointegration, and durability required for long-term function in the adult body. Of particular interest are biochemical methods for surface modification that aim at immobilizing biomolecules on the implant surface to induce specific cell and tissue responses. Recruiting GF-producing cells to the bone–implant interface using immobilized ECM proteins to provide Velcro-like surfaces for focal attachment and surface molecular recognition is one potential route to improve the osteogenic capacities of implants.

Among bioactive ECM molecules, the enamel proteins are particularly attractive. These ancient molecules have been shown to induce and control formation of several hard tissues including bone. Moreover, amelogenin, the major enamel ECM protein, is already in clinical use for periodontal ligament and alveolar bone regeneration. If enamel ECM molecules or synthetic analogs can be immobilized on metal surfaces with their bioactivity intact, they should provide a viable biomimetic approach to improved fixation of metal implants in bone.

References

1. Yang, S. et al., The design of scaffolds for use in tissue engineering. II. Rapid prototyping techniques, *Tissue Eng.*, 8, 1, 2002.
2. de Bruijn, J.D. et al., Bone induction by implants with cultured bone marrow cells, *Adv. Dent. Res.*, 13, 74, 1999.
3. Cooper, L.F. et al., Incipient analysis of mesenchymal stem cell-derived osteogenesis, *J. Dent. Res.*, 80, 314, 2001.
4. Butler, D.L., Goldstein, S.A., and Guilak, F., Functional tissue engineering: the role of biomechanics, *J. Biomech. Eng.*, 122, 570, 2000.
5. Badylak, S.F. et al., Marrow-derived cells populate scaffolds composed of xenogeneic extracellular matrix, *Exp. Hematol.*, 29, 1310, 2001.
6. Kyriakides, T.R. et al., Regulation of angiogenesis and matrix remodeling by localized, matrix-mediated antisense gene delivery, *Mol. Ther.*, 3, 842, 2001.
7. Abron, A. et al., Evaluation of a predictive model for implant surface topography effects on early osseointegration in the rat tibia model, *J. Prosthet. Dent.*, 85, 40, 2001.
8. Rønold, H.J. and Ellingsen, J.E., Effect of micro-roughness produced by TiO_2 blasting: tensile testing of bone attachment by using coin-shaped implants, *Biomaterials*, 23, 4211, 2002.

9. LeGeros, R.Z., Properties of osteoconductive biomaterials: calcium phosphates, *Clin. Orthop.*, 395, 81, 2002.
10. Hulshoff, J.E. et al., Interfacial phenomena: an *in vitro* study of the effect of calcium phosphate (CA-P) ceramic on bone formation, *J. Biomed. Mater. Res.*, 40, 464, 1998.
11. Bucholz, R.W., Nonallograft osteoconductive bone graft substitutes, *Clin. Orthop.*, 395, 44, 2002.
12. Lavos-Valereto, I.C. et al., *In vitro* and *in vivo* biocompatibility testing of Ti-6Al-7Nb alloy with and without plasma-sprayed hydroxyapatite coating, *J. Biomed. Mater. Res.*, 58, 727, 2001.
13. Champagne, C.M. et al., Macrophage cell lines produce osteoinductive signals that include bone morphogenetic protein-2, *Bone*, 30, 26, 2002.
14. Kim, Y.W. et al., Effects of organic matrix proteins on the interfacial structure at the bone-biocompatible nacre interface *in vitro*, *Biomaterials*, 23, 2089, 2002.
15. Sampson, N.S., Mrksich, M., and Bertozzi, C.R., Surface molecular recognition, *Proc. Natl. Acad. Sci. U.S.A.*, 98, 12870, 2001.
16. Sinha, R.K. and Tuan, R.S., Regulation of human osteoblast integrin expression by orthopedic implant materials, *Bone*, 18, 451, 1996.
17. Irvine, D.J. et al., Simulations of cell-surface integrin binding to nanoscale-clustered adhesion ligands, *Biophys. J.*, 82, 120, 2002.
18. Langille, R.M. Differentiation of craniofacial mesenchyme, in *Bone: Differentiation and Morphogenesis*, vol. 9, Hall, B.K., Ed., CRC Press, Boca Raton, FL, 1994.
19. Shah, A.K. et al., Mechanism of BMP-2-stimulated adhesion of osteoblastic cells to titanium alloy, *Biol. Cell*, 91, 131, 1999.
20. Stenport, V.F. et al., Systemically administered human growth hormone improves initial implant stability: an experimental study in the rabbit, *Clin. Implant Dent. Relat. Res.*, 3, 135, 2001.
21. Ferretti, C. and Ripamonti, U., Human segmental mandibular defects treated with naturally derived bone morphogenetic proteins, *J. Craniofac. Surg.*, 13, 434, 2002.
22. Laato, M. et al., Interferon-gamma-induced inhibition of wound healing *in vivo* and *in vitro*, *Ann. Chir. Gynaecol.*, 90, 215, 19, 2001.
23. Doukas, J. et al., Matrix immobilization enhances the tissue repair activity of growth factor gene therapy vectors, *Hum. Gene Ther.*, 12, 783, 2001.
24. Salih, E. et al., Natural variation in the extent of phosphorylation of bone phosphoproteins as a function of *in vivo* new bone formation induced by demineralized bone matrix in soft tissue and bony environments, *Biochem. J.*, 364, 465, 2002.
25. Schierano, G. et al., *In vitro* effect of transforming growth factor-beta on adhesion molecule expression by human gingival fibroblasts cultured in the presence of a titanium abutment, *J. Periodontol.*, 72, 1658, 2001.
26. Zhao, M. et al., Bone morphogenetic protein receptor signalling is necessary for normal murine postnatal bone formation, *J. Cell Biol.*, 157, 1049, 2002.
27. Groessner-Schreiber, B. and Tuan, R.S., Enhanced extracellular matrix production and mineralization by osteoblasts cultured on titanium surfaces *in vitro*, *J. Cell Sci.*, 101, 209, 1992.
28. Derhami, K. et al., Quantifying the adherence of fibroblasts to titanium and its enhancement by substrate-attached material, *J. Biomed. Mater. Res.*, 52, 315, 2000.
29. Cook, S.D. et al., The effect of demineralized bone matrix gel on bone ingrowth and fixation of porous implants, *J. Arthroplasty*, 17, 402, 2002.

30. Linez-Bataillon, P. et al., *In vitro* MC3T3 osteoblast adhesion with respect to surface roughness of Ti6Al4V substrates, *Biomol. Eng.*, 19, 133, 2002.
31. Itoh, D. et al., Enhancement of osteogenesis on hydroxyapatite surface coated with synthetic peptide (EEEEEEEPRGDT) *in vitro*, *J. Biomed. Mater. Res.*, 62, 292, 2002.
32. Grzesik, W.J. et al., Age-related changes in human proteoglycans structure: impact of osteogenesis imperfecta, *J. Biol. Chem.*, 277, 43638, 2002.
33. McKee, M.D. and Nanci, A., Osteopontin at mineralised tissue interfaces in bone, teeth and osseointegrated implants: ultrastructural distribution and implications for mineralised tissue formation, turnover and repair, *Microsc. Res. Tech.*, 33, 141, 1996.
34. Ferrara, D. et al., Three-dimensional cultures of normal human osteoblasts: proliferation and differentiation potential *in vitro* and upon ectopic implantation in nude mice, *Bone*, 30, 718, 2002.
35. Karsdal, M.A. et al., MMP-dependent activation of latent TGF-β controls the conversion of osteoblasts into osteocytes by blocking osteoblast apoptosis, *J. Biol. Chem.*, 277, 44061, 2002.
36. Gurevich, O. et al., Fibrin microbeads for isolating and growing bone marrow-derived progenitor cells capable of forming bone tissue, *Tissue Eng.*, 8, 661, 2002.
37. Stephansson, S.N., Byers, B.A., and Garcia, A.J., Enhanced expression of the osteoblastic phenotype on substrates that modulate fibronectin conformation and integrin receptor binding, *Biomaterials*, 23, 2527, 2002.
38. Ebara, S. and Nakayama, K., Mechanism for the action of bone morphogenetic proteins and regulation of their activity, *Spine*, 27, 10, 2002.
39. Chipperfield, H. et al., Heparan sulfates isolated from adult neural progenitor cells can direct phenotypic maturation, *Int. J. Dev. Biol.*, 46, 661, 2002.
40. Raouf, A. et al., Lumican is a major component of the bone matrix, *Matrix Biol.*, 21, 361, 2002.
41. Fitzgerald, J., Tay-Ting, S., and Bateman, J.F., WARP is a new member of the von Willebrand factor A-domain superfamily of extracellular matrix proteins, *FEBS Lett.*, 517, 61, 2002.
42. Weiss, S. et al., Systemic regulation of distraction osteogenesis: a cascade of biochemical factors, *J. Bone Miner. Res.*, 17, 1280, 2002.
43. Wittrant, Y. et al., Osteoprotegrin differentially regulates protease expression in osteoclast cultures, *Biochem. Biophys. Res. Commun.*, 293, 38, 2002.
44. Letic-Gavrilovic, A., Scandurra, R., and Abe, K., Genetic potential of interfacial guided osteogenesis in implant devices, *Dent. Mater. J.*, 19, 99, 2000.
45. Puleo, D.A. and Nanci, A., Understanding and controlling the bone-implant interface, *Biomaterials*, 20, 2311, 1999.
46. Veis, A. et al., Specific amelogenin gene splice products have signalling effects on cells in culture and in implants *in vivo*, *J. Biol. Chem.*, 275, 41263, 2000.
47. Boyan, B.D. et al., Porcine fetal enamel matrix derivative enhances bone formation induced by demineralised freeze dried bone allograft *in vivo*, *J. Periodontol.*, 71, 1278, 2000.
48. Sculean, A. et al., Healing of fenestration-type defects following treatment with guided tissue regeneration or enamel matrix proteins: an experimental study in monkeys, *Clin. Oral Investig.*, 4, 50, 2000.
49. Kawana, F. et al., Porcine enamel matrix derivative enhances trabecular bone regeneration during wound healing of injured rat femur, *Anat. Rec.*, 264, 438, 2001.

50. Tonetti, M.S. et al., Enamel matrix proteins in the regenerative therapy of deep intrabony defects, *J. Clin. Periodontol.*, 29, 317, 2002.
51. Ohyama, M. et al., Effect of enamel matrix derivative on the differentiation of C2C12 cells, *J. Periodontol.*, 73, 543, 2002.
52. Rosen, P.S. and Reynolds, M.A., A retrospective case series comparing the use of demineralised freeze-dried bone allograft and freeze-dried bone allograft combined with enamel matrix derivative for the treatment of advanced osseous lesions, *J. Periodontol.*, 73, 942, 2002.
53. Spahr, A. et al., Expression of amelin and trauma-induced dentin formation, *Clin. Oral Investig.*, 6, 51, 2002.
54. Nakamura, Y. et al., The induction of reparative dentine by enamel proteins, *Int. Endodont. J.*, 35, 407, 2002.
55. Spahr, A. and Hammarstrom, L., Response of dental follicular cells to the exposure of denuded enamel matrix in rat molars, *Eur. J. Oral Sci.*, 107, 360, 1999.
56. Tokiyasu, Y. et al., Enamel factors regulate expression of genes associated with cementoblasts, *J. Periodontol.*, 71, 1829, 2000.
57. Hamamoto, Y. et al., Effects of distribution of the enamel matrix derivative Emdogain in the periodontal tissues of rat molars transplanted to the abdominal wall, *Dent. Traumatol.*, 18, 12, 2002.
58. Dean, D.D. et al., Effect of porcine fetal enamel matrix derivative on chondrocyte proliferation, differentiation, and focal factor production is dependent on cell maturation state, *Cells Tiss. Organs*, 171, 117, 2002.
59. Shimizu-Ishiura, M. et al., Effects of enamel matrix derivative to titanium implantation in rat femurs, *J. Biomed. Mater. Res.*, 60, 269, 2002.
60. Casati, M.Z. et al., Enamel matrix derivative and bone healing after guided bone regeneration in dehiscence-type defects around implants: a histomorphometric study in dogs, *J. Periodontol.*, 73, 789, 2002.
61. Hammarström, L., Heijl, L., and Gestrelius, S., Periodontal regeneration in a buccal dehiscence model in monkeys after application of enamel matrix proteins, *J. Clin. Periodontol.*, 24, 669, 1997.
62. Heijl, L. et al., Enamel matrix derivative (Emdogain®) in the treatment of intrabony periodontal defects, *J. Clin. Periodontol.*, 24, 705, 1997.
63. Hammarström, L., Enamel matrix, cementum development and regeneration, *J. Clin. Periodontol.*, 24, 658, 1997.
64. Fincham, A.G. et al., Self-assembly of a recombinant amelogenin protein generates supramolecular structures, *J. Struct. Biol.*, 112, 103, 1994.
65. Gestrelius, S. et al., Formulation of enamel matrix derivative for surface coating: kinetics and cell colonization, *J. Clin. Periodontol.*, 24, 678, 1997.
66. Lyngstadaas, S.P. et al., Autocrine growth factors in human periodontal ligament cells cultured on enamel matrix derivative, *J. Clin. Periodontol.*, 28, 181, 2001.
67. Suzuki, N. et al., Attachment of human periodontal ligament cells to enamel matrix-derived protein is mediated via interaction between BSP-like molecules and integrin alpha (v) beta-3, *J. Periodontol.*, 72, 1520, 2001.
68. Cerny, R. et al., A novel gene expressed in rat molars: codes for proteins with cell binding domains, *J. Bone Miner. Res.*, 11, 883, 1996.
69. Fong, C.D., Slaby, I., and Hammarström, L., Amelin: an enamel-related protein, transcribed in the cells of the epithelial root sheath, *J. Bone Miner. Res.*, 11, 892, 1996.

70. Fong, C.D. et al., Expression patterns of RNAs for amelin and amelogenin in developing rat molars and incisors, *Adv. Dent. Res.*, 10, 195, 1996.
71. Krebsbach, P.H. et al., Full-length sequence, localization, and chromosomal mapping of ameloblastin: a novel tooth-specific gene, *J. Biol. Chem.*, 271, 4431, 1996.
72. Lee, S.K. et al., Ameloblastin expression in rat incisors and human tooth germs, *Int. J. Dev. Biol.*, 40, 1141, 1996.
73. Fong, C.D. et al., Sequential expression of an amelin gene in mesenchymal and epithelial cells during odontogenesis in rats, *Eur. J. Oral Sci.*, 106, 324, 1998.
74. Bleicher, F. et al., Sequential expression of matrix protein genes in developing rat teeth, *Matrix Biol.*, 18, 133, 1999.
75. Brookes, S.J. et al., Amelin extracellular processing and aggregation during rat incisor amelogenesis, *Arch. Oral Biol.*, 46, 201 2001.
76. Dhamija, S. and Krebsbach, P.H., Role of Cbfa1 in ameloblast gene transcription, *J. Biol. Chem.*, 276, 35159, 2001.
77. Arana-Chavez, V.E. and Nanci, A., High-resolution immunocytochemistry of noncollagenous matrix proteins in rat mandibles processed with microwave irradiation, *J. Histochem. Cytochem.*, 49, 1099, 2001.
78. Zambotti, A. et al., Characterization of an osteoblast-specific enhancer element in the CBFA1 gene, *J. Biol. Chem.*, 277, 41497, 2002.

Section V

Surface Chemistry, Biochemistry, and Molecules: How Do They Interact with Biological Environment?

16

How Surfaces Interact with the Biological Environment

Pentti Tengvall

CONTENTS

16.1 Introduction 285
16.2 The Biomaterial Interface 288
16.3 Protein Adsorption 288
16.4 Blood Plasma–Surface Interactions 289
16.5 Immune System Recognition of Biomaterials 294
16.5.1 Complement 295
16.6 Cells at Interfaces 299
16.7 Final Remarks 301
References 302

16.1 Introduction

Virtually all implant surfaces that contact soft or hard tissues become rapidly coated with a 1- to 10-nm thick protein layer, most often from blood plasma. Such layers have different compositions, depending on the underlying chemistry and topography, and they activate different homeostatic systems. Proteins or their surface-bound proteolytic degradation fragments also offer binding sites to cells, leading to the surface–cell communication necessary for the expression of cell morphology, proliferation, differentiation, and function (see Table 16.1).

Implants inserted into tissues for extended periods of time may be isolated from surrounding tissues by a 50- to 250-μm thick fibrous encapsulation. Poor revascularization is then observed 50 to 100 μm away from the surface.[1-3] Few exceptions have been found to this phenomenon. In one study, 0.02- to 8-μm pore size polytetrafluoroethylene (PTFE) filters were tested subcutane-

0-8493-1474-7/03/$0.00+$1.50

TABLE 16.1

Major Functions and Known Cell Interactions of Selected Proteins Studied on Biomaterials

Protein	Major Function	Cell Receptors	Cell Types
Serum albumin	Body transport and clearance protein; binds to certain cell surfaces (passivates); maintains osmotic balance	gp30 and gp18	Endothelial; hepatocytes?
Fibrinogen (Fib)	Forms fibrin during blood coagulation	CD11b and c; CD41a; CD51; CD61	Platelet; endothelial; myeloid, natural killer; osteoclast; tumor
Fibronectin (FNT)	Extracellular matrix protein that binds cells via RGD sequence	CD49c, d, and e; CD41a; CD61	Platelet; B lymphocyte; monocyte; fibroblast; epithelial; keratinocyte; tumor
Immunoglobulin G (Ig G)	Opsonizes nonself cell surface; activates complement	Fc	PMN; macrophage
P-selectin	Located on activated platelet surfaces and platelet-derived microparticles	PSGL-1	Neutrophils
High molecular weight kininogen (HMWK)	Component of intrinsic pathway of coagulation; binds to negatively charged surfaces		
Lysozyme	Bactericidal activity in body secretions		
α-Lactalbumin	Part of lactose synthetase enzyme		
Ovalbumin	Major protein in egg white		
α-Amylase	Found in saliva; cleaves starch, glycogen, and other polysaccharides		
Complement factor 1q (C1q)	Binds to IgG and IgM; initiates classical complement activation	cC1q-RI; C1q-Rq; gC1q-R	B lymphocyte; T lymphocyte; monocyte/macrophage; PMN; eosinophil; platelet; fibroblast; endothelial; epithelial; smooth muscle; mesengial
Complement factor 3b (C3b)	Key adsorbed complement protein, formed by cleavage of C3 to C3a and C3b	CR1(CD35)	Erythrocyte; phagocyte; B lymphocyte; T lymphocyte; eosonophil
Complement factor 3dg/three-dimensional (C3dg C3d)	Surface-bound complement peptide after proteolytic cleavage of C3b, opsonin	CR2(CD21)	B lymphocyte; T lymphocyte
Complement factor 3bi (iC3b)	Activates phagocytes	CR3(CD11b, CD18)	Phagocyte

ously (s.c.) in a rat model. After a year, increased vascularization was observed outside filters with 5-μm pores compared to outside 0.02-μm filters.[3] In another study, polydimethylsiloxane was implanted s.c. for 4 weeks in thrombospondin 2 (TSP2)-null mice. Increased vascularization but no thinning of the fibrous zone was observed in the implant near the fibrous tissue.[4]

The thickness of the fibrous capsule is believed to be closely connected to both surface topography and mechanical stress, although few conclusive studies have been conducted to correlate topograhical features to total capsule thicknesses. Recently, anodically oxidized titanium with oxide thickness of 600 to 1000 nm, pore size of 1.3 to 2.1 μm^2, and 12.7 to 24.4% porosity and reference chemically pure (c.p.) titanium implants with pore sizes of 17 to 200 nm were implanted for 6 weeks in rabbits. Histomorphometrical analysis displayed more pronounced osteoconductivity at the anodically oxidized surface.[5] When polyurethanes based on 50/50 ε-caprolactone/L-lactide with different porosities were implanted s.c. in rats up to 40 weeks, interconnected micropores of at least 30 μm enabled in-growth of well vascularized cellular connective tissue while smaller micropores became filled with predominantly histiocytic tissue.[6]

In yet another study, the light microscopic thicknesses of the fibrous encapsulations outside 0.2- to 30-μm polypropylene filter sheets were determined after 1 week of s.c. implantation in rats. The thickest encapsulations (up to 280 μm) were observed outside the filters with the smallest pores.[7] Improved but imperfect functional and biological integration between biomaterials and tissues has also been observed with bioactive materials such as Ca–mineral- and bioglass-coated surfaces. It is thus expected that a nonoptimal tissue response is a close-to-universal phenomenon unless a perfect match exists between the material and the surrounding pool of cells. The current hypothesis is that this can be achieved in principle only when an individual's own (stem) cells replace foreign materials and participate in the healing process, i.e., self replaces self in some way.

In order to backtrace possible roots of the material–tissue mismatch, we must consider the organization of tissues, cell–foreign material differences, cell–cell interactions, cell–extracellular matrix interactions and composition, tissue healing and regeneration, inflammation, and hemostasis. The aim of this chapter is not to explain all these issues, but to highlight briefly the within-seconds-to-an-hour interactions between blood plasma and serum and biomaterials. We must admit, however, that after many years of research, no ascertained logical connection of materials, contact activation of humoral systems such as coagulation and complement, and tissue development has been made, simply because the required studies are complex, extend over long periods of time, and overlap pure cell biology — a research field presently in the midst of rapid progress. Despite the lack of fundamental scientific basis, the underlying hypothesis is that early molecular events at surfaces during the wound healing process manifest in different functional integrations in terms of blood compatibility, fibrous encapsulation, neovascularization, and tissue quality. Aspects of prosthesis, interface

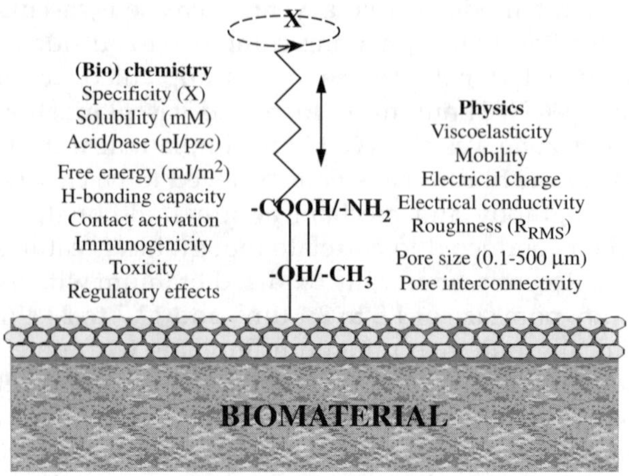

FIGURE 16.1
Surface properties governing behavior of implanted material.

topography, and mechanics are not further considered in this chapter. Instead, we highlight the impacts of chemistry on surface–protein and surface–soft tissue interactions.

16.2 The Biomaterial Interface

The outermost atomic layer of a general biomaterial interface at the moment of insertion is a combination of inorganic or organic oxides and hydroxides with low chemical reactivity and low solubility at physiological conditions. Different surfaces possess different basic water chemistries as represented by their elemental compositions and functionalities, such as –OH, $–CH_3$, $–PO_4$, $–NH_2$, –COOH, and –SiOH groups. This chemistry also gives rise to different free surface energies, water-retaining capacities, surface mobilities, etc. — properties that may or may not be important for blood and tissue responses. Figure 16.1 summarizes a few important surface chemical and physical properties believed to be relevant to *in vivo* behavior of biomaterials.

16.3 Protein Adsorption

Proteins in body fluids accumulate spontaneously at all surfaces sooner or later. A simplified adsorption model reveals that the main adsorption-promoting factor at constant pressure and temperature is the decrease in Gibbs free energy (G) via increased system entropy (S) after, rather than before, adsorption.[8] The two main contributions to increased entropy are suggested to originate from partial dehydration of sorbent and adsorbent surfaces (more free water) and increased internal protein entropy (flexibility) after adsorption. Changes in system enthalpy (H = U + pV), including reaction enthalpy (U), pressure/volume work (pV), and changes in system heat capacity (ΔC_p), are considered less important in this case. Thus, to summarize, adsorption is favored when $\Delta G = \Delta H - T\Delta S < 0$ (exothermic process).

It is indicated in some cases *in vitro* that an adsorption-resisting energy barrier exists at surfaces with high water retention capacity and high mobility (i.e., a large radius of gyration, R), as demonstrated by low protein deposition onto charge-neutral polyethylene glycols (PEGs) or certain sugars such as dextran systems. In the human body, cell membranes, albumin-associating cell surfaces, and mucosas with high oligosaccharide contents behave in a similar manner. However, rigid artificial surfaces, such as oxide-covered metals, ceramics, and polymers with low water-binding capacity, become protein-coated within a fraction of a second of exposure to blood plasma, for example.

Experiments show that low energy (hydrophobic) surfaces deposit more proteins than high energy (hydrophilic) surfaces.[9] The reasons are not well investigated but believed to be coupled to lower water heat of adsorption on hydrophobic surfaces and increased unfolding of adsorbed proteins due to interactions between internal hydrophobic protein domains and the hydrophobic surface, leading to greater denaturation and increased internal protein entropy. Thus, the starting point for further analysis is a protein-coated biomaterial surface that interacts with surrounding cells, which in turn may react differently because of different receptor–protein interactions at different surfaces. This in turn is supposed to affect the early inflammatory process, and so forth; the scenario is shown in Figure 16.2.

16.4 Blood Plasma–Surface Interactions

Experience reveals that blood coagulation can be prevented at biologically active surfaces that mainly inhibit thrombin and factor Xa, such as certain heparin-coated vascular grafts,[10] but not at inert materials or those with low biological activity. The reason for this is simple in principle: the activation and limitation of the coagulation process are actively regulated and tightly controlled processes in concert with plasma proteins and platelets, including several procoagulant and anticoagulant activities regulated by the endothelial linings inside the vessels.

Anticoagulant activities include the release of prostacyclin, thrombomodulin, heparin-like molecules, ecto-ADPase, t-PA, urokinase,[11] and nitric oxide.[12] Procoagulant activity is mediated by platelet-activating factor (PAF),

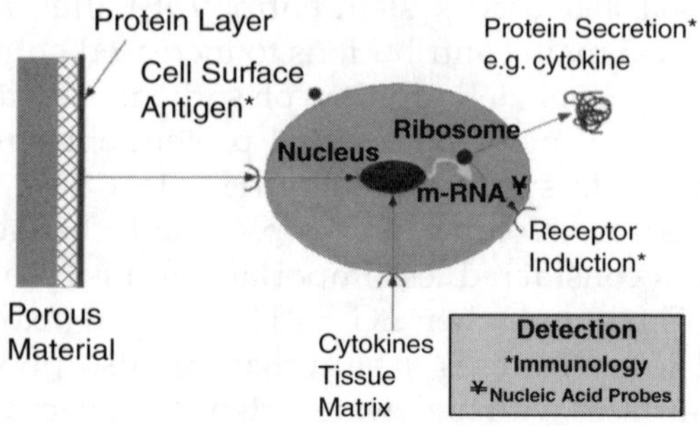

FIGURE 16.2
Biomaterial–tissue interface. Different surfaces induce the production of different signal molecules e.g., via proteolytic activity; cells subsequently expose different membrane receptors and hence interact differently at surfaces with varying protein adsorption patterns and topography. (*Source:* Bjursten, L.M., Lund University, Sweden.)

tissue factor, von Willebrand factor, t-PA inhibitor, and plasma coagulation factors.[11] In clinical practice, heparin, warfarin, hirudin, and their analogs are used to inhibit directly or indirectly the action of thrombin. Platelets and primary hemostasis are controlled through the administration of ASA, ticlopidine, $73Ef_{ab}$, integrelin, and MK-383. This listing is by no means complete and new interactions between components of the humoral and cellular systems are continously discovered. However, attention in this chapter will focus on the interactions between solid nonactive materials and blood proteins, not on hemostasis.

As indicated in the previous section, blood proteins deposit onto virtually all types of artificial surfaces including inorganics, and synthetic and natural polymers. Proteins from three humoral systems (the intrinsic pathway of coagulation, the common pathway of coagulation, and the complement system) are found frequently in adsorbed protein films. The complement system is discussed in Section 16.5.1.

Titanium is an interesting material that activates the intrinsic pathway and is representative of negatively charged surfaces at physiological conditions.[13] As shown in Figure 16.3, titanium deposits approximately 300 ng/cm^2 of plasma proteins. The identity of the absorbed plasma protein achieved by incubation of the plasma-coated surface in polyclonal antibody solution revealed that mainly fibrinogen, high molecular weight kininogen (HMWK), prekallikrein (PKK), coagulation factor-XII (F-XII), immunoglobulin (IgG), and complement factor-1q (C-1q) were adsorbed and antibody was accessible at the surface. Adsorbed fibrinogen took part in primary hemostasis via platelet glycoprotein GP-IIIa and -IIb receptors inducing platelet spreading and activation[14] via primary hemostasis. HMWK, F-XII, and PKK marked the intrinsic pathway of coagulation (contact activation) — an activation that takes place at titanium surfaces and can also be visualized through studies of the generation of activated F-XII and formation of kallikrein from PKK (Figure 16.4).

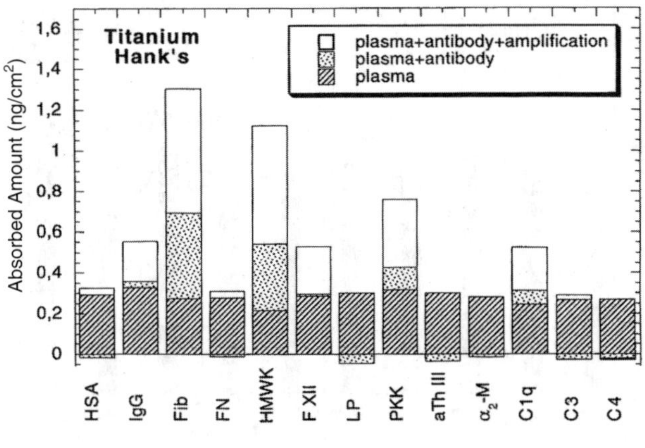

FIGURE 16.3
Ellipsometric *in vitro* measurements showing protein deposition to hydrophilic negatively charged titanium (pI ~4 to 6) after 10 minutes incubation in 67% heparin plasma at room conditions. The dilutions, antibody incubations, and rinsings were made in Hank's buffer. (*Source:* Kanagarazja, S. et al., *Biomaterials*, 17, 2225, 1996. With permission.)

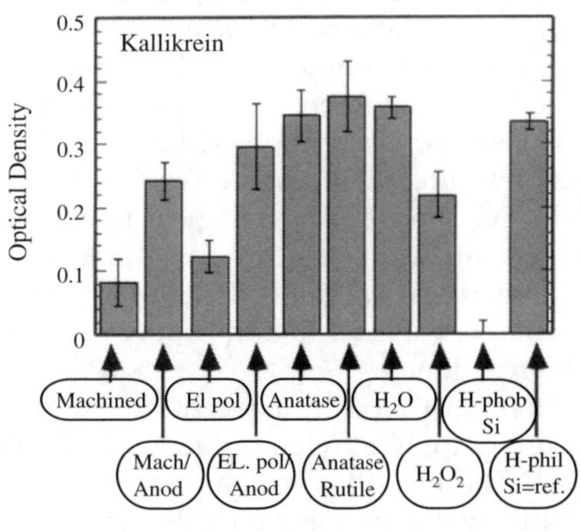

FIGURE 16.4
Kallikrein formation by differently treated titanium surfaces. The samples were incubated for 30 minutes in 10% citrated plasma at room conditions. Kallikrein formation in plasma was detected with a chromogenic substrate (S-2302, Chromogenix AB, Mölndal, Sweden) at 405 nm. Hydrophilic silicon was the positive reference and hydrophobic silicon the negative reference. (*Source:* Wälivaara, B. et al., *Biomaterials*, 15, 827 1994. With permission.)

Aluminum, another well known biomaterial with point-of-zero charge (pzc or surface pI ~8.5) is weakly positively charged under physiological conditions and displays a different ellipsometric plasma protein adsorption pattern when compared to titanium[15] (Figure 16.5). No anti-fibrinogen, anti-HMWK, antiF-XII, or anti-PKK bound onto its plasma protein layer; instead anti-

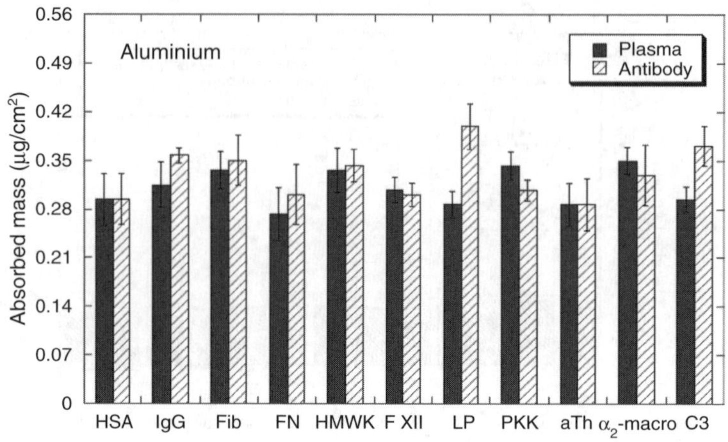

FIGURE 16.5
Heparin plasma deposition to a hydrated aluminum surface at 37°C. Mainly anti-lipoprotein (a-LP) and anti-C3c bound onto the approximately 4- to 5-nm thick (300 ng/cm^2) plasma protein film. (*Source:* Tengvall, P. et al., *Biomaterials*, 19, 935, 1998. With permission.)

lipoprotein (LP) and anti-C3 deposited to some degree. The significance of this difference for blood and tissue compatibility is presently not understood.

When near-charge neutral alkane thiols with 2, 4, or 6 ethylene glycols organized in self-assembled monolayers (oligoethylene glycol-terminated SAMs) on gold were incubated in heparin plasma (Figure 16.6), large differences in protein deposition were observed between the different surfaces and at room versus physiological temperatures.[16] At room temperature, least plasma adsorbed to EG_6, and at physiological temperature onto EG_6 and methoxy surfaces. The interpretation of the adsorption data is that low charge and chemical inertness are not sufficient for the preparation of blood plasma-resistant surfaces; we need to add proper surface mobility and side chain density to the reaction.

This aspect was demonstrated in a recent study in which a positively charged poly(L-lysine)-g-poly(ethylene glycol) (PLL-PEG) backbone was grafted with PEGs.[17] The PLL-PEG was adsorbed and held by coulombic interactions to negatively charged metal oxides and used in serum adsorption experiments.[18] The empirical radius of gyration of the PEG chain was defined as $R_g = 0.181N^{0.58}$ nm, where N = number of repeat units. For PEGs with molecular weights between 2 and 5 kDa, a calculation revealed 1.65 nm $< R_g < 2.82$ nm. If the lateral distance between each PEG side chain is L, $L/2R_g$ represents the extent of surface packing. When $L/2R_g < 1$, the side chain radii of gyration overlap. The best protein suppression data were observed when $L/2R_g \sim 0.5$ in a study using PLL(20)-g(3.5)-PEG(2) and PLL(20)-g(5)-PEG(2) where the PLL backbone was 20 kDa, the PEG side chain 2 kDa, and g (3.5 or 5) indicated the lysine-mer/PEG side chain ratio (Figure 16.7). These polymers displayed a serum adsorption of less than 3 ng/cm^2 on $Si_{0,4}Ti_{0,6}O_2$.

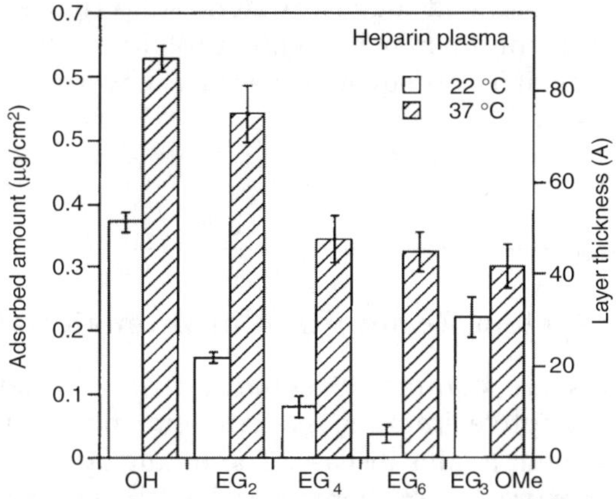

FIGURE 16.6
In vitro deposition of 66% heparin plasma in veronal buffer to near charge-neutral SAMs on Au at 22°C or 37°C after 10 minutes of incubation. Reference surfaces: TOH = 16-mercapto-hexadecanol (HS-$(CH_2)_{16}$-OH); EG_3OMe = methoxy terminated tri(ethylene glycol), (HS-$(CH_2)_{11}$-O-$(CH_2$-CH_2-$O)_3$-CH_3); EG_2, EG_4, and EG_6 = HS-$(CH_2)_{15}$-CONH-$(CH_2$-CH_2-$O)_n$-H; n = 2, 4, or 6. (*Source:* Benesch, J. et al., *J. Biomat. Sci. Polymer Ed.*, 12, 581, 2001. With permission.)

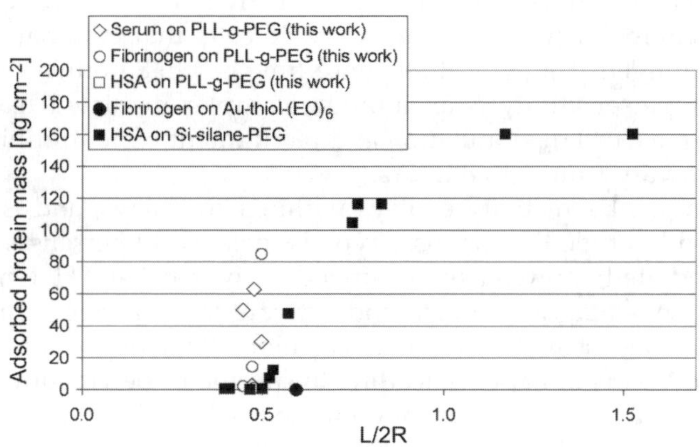

FIGURE 16.7
Serum adsorption onto PEGs with varying surface packing densities ($L/2R_g$). The least adsorption was found during a partial radius of gyration overlap between the grafted PEG side chains, in this case, $L/2R_g$ ~0.5. (*Source:* Kenausis, G.L. et al., *J. Phys. Chem. B*, 104, 3298, 2000. With permission.)

This result is important and suggests that no solid rigid surface, regardless of charge or water retention, may be totally protein-resistant in human body fluids. In retrospect, it is no surprise because few rigid surfaces exist in mammalian tissues.

16.5 Immune System Recognition of Biomaterials

Immune reactions are commonly separated into innate and adapted responses.[18] The adaptive immune system remembers specific infectious agents and can prevent a later disease. The innate system does not change after repeated exposure to an allergen and is therefore less specific. The cellular part of response is mediated mainly by leukocytes (phagocytes and lymphocytes, auxiliary cells), and soluble response mediators are often represented by immunoglobulins (IgGs) and the complement system. Other soluble components are cytokines and interferons.[18] An adapted immune response in an exaggerated or inappropriate form is termed *hypersensitivity.* In reality, the systems work in concert and in parallel to eradicate nonself organic materials such as bacteria and viruses that invade the body.

In type I (IgE-mediated) humoral hypersensitivity response, soluble allergens bind to B lymphocytes that transform into IgE-secreting plasma cells and memory cells. IgE binds to Fc receptors on basophils and mast cells, thereby sensitizing them. Re-exposure to antigens causes them to degranulate and start numerous actions.[18] The typical initiation time for response is 2 to 30 minutes.

Type II is an antibody-mediated hypersensitivity characterized by activation of the complement system or cytotoxic cells that eliminate cells that display the antigen. The typical response time is 5 to 8 hours.

Type III hypersensitivity is an immune complex-mediated reaction that causes local mast cell degranulation and recruitment of neutrophils. Typical rection times vary from 2 to 8 hours.

Metallic implant sensitivity evolves within 1 to 3 days, and is generally associated with a type IV response. Type IV delayed hypersensitivity is cell (T-DTH)-mediated; previously sensitized activated T-DTH lymphocytes release cytokines that accumulate and activate macrophages. This type of hypersensitivity is most likely mediated by biomaterial degradation products that may form parts of haptens, leading to specific responses downstream.[19]

Without a doubt, the most severe immune response in which the complement system of lymphokines and T (T_{helper} and T_{killer}) cells work in a concerted action is elicited by natural materials such as transplanted organs (grafts) expressing histocompatibility antigens different from those of the recipient. It is surprising and interesting to observe that the more distant the foreign body chemistry is, the fewer apparent signs we find of cell-mediated immune rejection.

On the contrary, in the case of end-stage renal disease (ESRD), patients subjected to chronic hemodialysis may show signs of immune suppression.[20] Few reports to date indicate immune reactions against polymeric biomaterials.[21] The exceptions are PMMA (bone cement) and silicone elastomers. However, type IV hypersensitivity has been reported for metallic biomaterials such as Co, Cr, and Ni,[21] and questions have also been raised regarding the use of dental amalgams and gold.

Reactions elicited by silicone mammary replacement materials have remained the focus of controversy and are by far the most studied immune responses elicited by biomaterials. Early reports dealing with silicone implant materials, especially polydimethylsiloxane, cited immune phenomena and immunogenicity.[22,23] The immune functions of 40 individuals who underwent silicone breast augmentation for periods longer than 10 years were compared to those of 40 sex- and age-matched controls.[24] The study indicated abnormalities in the $T_{helper/suppressor}$ ratio, increased autoimmunity, and increased production of immune complexes. Test results from a blind study including serum from 111 patients with and without breast implants demonstrated statistically significant elevations of antisilicone antibodies compared with the unimplanted control group.[25] Silicone gels were, by virtue of adjuvant-like behavior, claimed to give rise to formation of autoantibodies to rat thyroglobulin and bovine collagen II.[26] However, other studies failed to find connections between immunological reactions and biomaterials.

The diverging reactions reported for silicone breast implant materials may be explained partially by differencies in a genetic predisposition to react with the material. When 199 subjects were evaluated by HLA (human leucocyte antigen) typing, 68% of the symptomatic patients (n = 77), 35% of asymptomatic women with implants (n = 37), 52% of healthy female volunteers without implants (n = 54), and 65% of fibromyalgia patients without implants (n = 31) were HLA-DR53-positive, suggesting that symptomatic patients with implants share some genetic characteristics.[27]

In summary, the above results indicate that most implants are recognized as antigens due to the presence of surface-denatured proteins, but do not produce immune responses in the classical sense. Such surfaces interact normally with the complement system designed by nature to clear worn-out or denatured organic materials (e.g., bacteria, fungi, viruses, and proteins) from the system. To a nonimmunologist, the biomaterials inside the body resemble frustrated complement-mediated clearance processes.

16.5.1 Complement

The deposition of complement has been analyzed on few biomedical materials. Interestingly, despite the lack of ascertained classical signs of immune response coupled to a massive leukocyte infiltration to or formation of antibodies against biomaterials, the complement system interacts with all types of surfaces that deposit appreciable amounts of partially denatured proteins. Surfaces that bind low amounts of proteins may be, for example, PEG- or

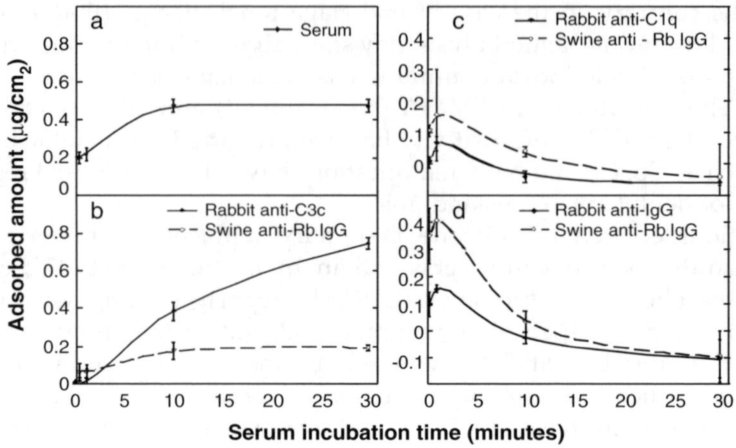

FIGURE 16.8

(a) Serum deposition to titanium; (b) binding of anti-C3c to the serum layer; (c) binding of anti-C1q to the serum layer; and (d) binding of anti-IgG to the serum layer. The Ti surfaces were incubated in 100% native human serum at 37°C. Rinsing, polyclonal antibody dilutions (1/50v/v), and 30-minute incubations were done in Hank's buffer. Quantitations were made by *in situ* null ellipsometry. (*Source:* Wälivaara, B. et al., *J. Biomater. Sci. Polymer Ed.*, 8, 41, 1996. With permission.)

polyethyleneoxid (PEO)-grafted materials, dextrans, and other charge-neutral water-retaining molecules with high surface mobilities.

Titanium represents a rigid negatively charged surface, and showed temporally increased binding of serum proteins *in vitro*[28] (Figure 16.8a). The protein layer bound with time-increasing amounts of polyclonal anti-C3c, indicating clearly that titanium is complement-opsonized after contact with blood serum (Figure 16.8b). Interestingly, after short serum incubations, anti-C1q and anti-IgG (Figures 16.8c and 16.8d) also bound to the protein film, suggesting that the activation took place via the classical pathway of complement.[29] However, if we compare the absolute deposited amounts of serum and antibodies with those of model activator surfaces such as IgG coatings, titanium appears to be a relatively weak complement activator.

In similar experiments in which titanium was replaced by chromium, hydrated Cr bound even less serum and lower amounts of anti-C3c. When the surface cleaning was performed in ethanol, more serum and anti-C3c bound in. The result underlines again the importance of proper surface cleaning procedure prior to the insertion of implants, in this case related to blood.

In a similar fashion, hydrated aluminum exhibited increasing deposits of serum protein over time[15] (Figure 16.9a). The amounts were intermediate — between those of a low activator, immobilized HSA, and the positive reference, immobilized IgG.

In subsequent complement antibody incubations, increasing serum deposition was observed parallel with increased anti-C3c binding into the serum layer, indicating that complement also opsonized this surface (Figure 16.9b).

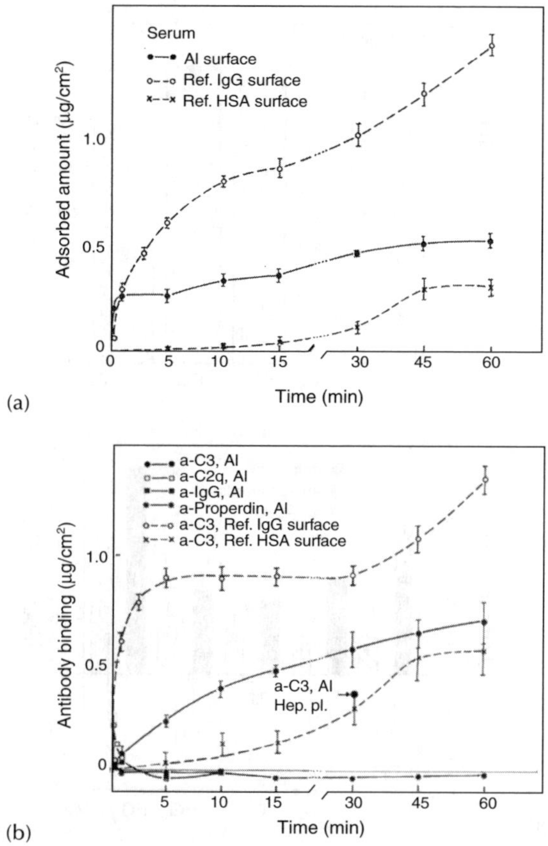

FIGURE 16.9
(a) Serum protein deposition onto hydrated aluminum. The *in situ* ellipsometric amounts of serum increased slowly during 60 minutes of incubation in whole human serum. Rinsing was done in Hank's buffer. (b) Deposition of selected complement antibodies onto the surfaces shown in (a). Observe that the serum layer on aluminum bound anti-C3c but not antiproperdin. Anti-IgG and anti-C1q bound after very short serum incubations. (*Source:* Tengvall, P. et al., *Biomaterials*, 19, 935, 1998. With permission.)

Experiments with C1q-depleted serum revealed that anti-C3c was deposited only after C1q reconstitution, suggesting a mild or rapid transient classical activation type of behavior. Further experiments with a dilution series of serum in Hank's buffer at a constant 1-minute incubation displayed increased deposition of anti-C1q at 1:2 to 1:4 dilutions. This further underlined the transient classical activation pattern.

When the oligo(ethylene glycol) (OEG) surfaces shown in Figure 16.6 were incubated in serum (Figure 16.10a) and subsequently in polyclonal anti-C3c, antiproperdin, and anti-C3d (32 kDa, the final surface-bound degradation product of proteolytically cleaved surface-bound C3b), surprising observations were made (Figure 16.10b): unexpectedly thick serum layers equalling

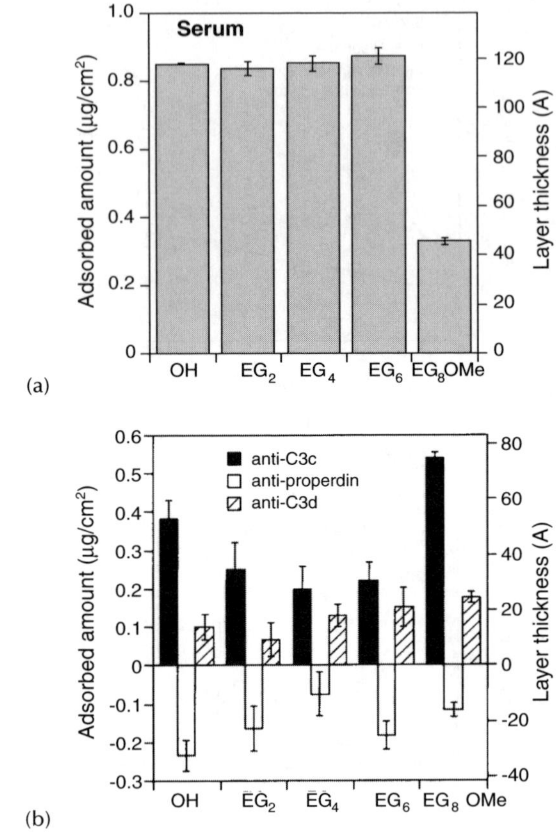

FIGURE 16.10
(a) Serum deposition to closely packed oligo(ethylene glycol) self-assembled monolayers on gold after 30 minutes' incubation at 37°C in 67% serum in veronal buffer with 0.15 mM Ca added (VB^{++}). (b) Net binding of selected polyclonal complement antibodies onto the OEG surfaces shown in Figures 16.6 and 16.10a. Ellipsometric quantitations after incubations at 37°C in 1/50 (v/v) diluted antibody solutions in VB^{++}-buffer for 30 minutes. Negative sign indicates loss of adsorbed mass upon antibody incubation. (*Source:* Benesch, J. et al., *J. Biomat. Sci. Polymer Ed.*, 12, 581, 2001. With permission.)

two to three monolayers bound to OEG surfaces, and more than twice the amount found on the reference EG_3_methoxy surface. It appeared upon closer analysis that charge-neutral OEG surfaces bound large amounts of anti-C3c and anti-C3d, but surprisingly no antiproperdin. The current interpretation of the data is that complement becomes transiently activated (and down-regulated) also on self-assembled OEG surfaces, but the exposure of relatively closely packed charge-neutral layers is not sufficient to resist adsorption and denaturation with a concomitant complement deposition.

This also closes the loop for the search of blood plasma-resistant surfaces in some respects. It appears that *in vitro* protein and complement-resistant surfaces can be prepared through a proper combination of immobilized charge-neutral moieties that possess certain radii of gyration (see Figure 16.7). Thus, the key features seem to be PEG grafting density and its mobility at physiological conditions.

In complement experiments, only the most typical activator surfaces, such as immobilized mercaptoglycerol, mercaptoethanol, IgG, and IgM, indicate the surface presence of stabilized C3 convertases as indicated through the surface binding of antiproperdin after serum or plasma incubation. Two explanations are most likely. In many cases, the probable explanation is the lack of true complement activation at the foreign surface via the early-appearing components of the cascade routes, and C3b likely binds to partially denatured adsorbed proteins via the constantly ongoing spontanous tick-over process to form reactive C3b*. During a short period of time ($T_{1/2}$ ~60 ms), C3b* exposes a reactive thiol ester that reacts with water or adsorbed protein nucleophilic groups. The formation of alternative C3 convertases (C3bBb and C3bBbP) progresses slowly and is constantly down-regulated by interactions of surface-bound C3b (or C3bBb) and the fluid phase C3bBb decay accelerator and cofactor for the cleavage of C3b, factor H, and the C3b-cleaving protease, factor-I. C3b is cleaved to form surface-bound C3dg and C3d.

In the second scenario, surface-bound immune complexes in the shape of adsorbed Igs or complex carbohydrates trigger the classical and lectin pathways of activation. This results in the formation of the classical pathway C3 convertase (C4b2a), cleavage of C3, and again, surface-bound C3b participitates in the formation of alternative pathway C3 convertases. If nothing is present to control classical pathway activation, a heavy surface-induced activation will occur. In this case, the C4-binding protein (C4bp) may interact with factor I to cleave C4b, thereby degrading the convertases. However, this action is yet not proven to take place at artificial surfaces although the transient antibody detection of factor H has been observed on titanium and zirconium (Figure 16.11) and indicates a possible common regulation route, at least for negatively charged surfaces.

16.6 Cells at Interfaces

The first cells to appear on a biomaterial surface during blood contact (adsorption), coagulation, and fibrinolytic phases are blood cells, i.e., platelets, monocytes, and polymorphonuclear granulocytes followed by erythrocytes. Platelets participitate very actively in the coagulation process via the primary hemostasis. Blood cells are trapped into the blood clot and fibroblasts, macrophages, and other more specialized cells soon (hours to days) appear at the wound site. Within hours after the initial clotting and fibrinolytic phases are triggered, wound healing proceeds gradually into the inflammatory process.

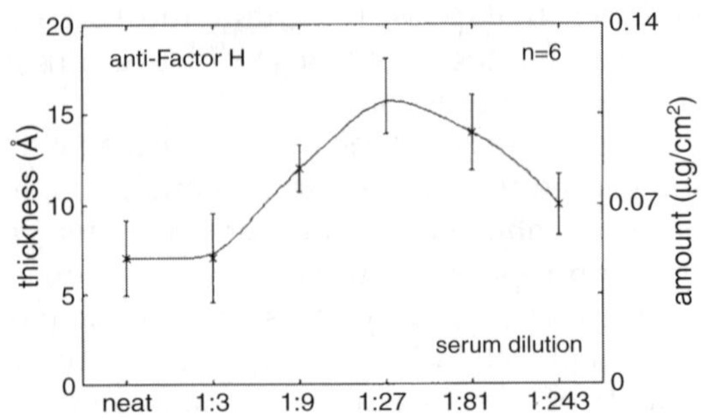

FIGURE 16.11
Binding of antifactor-H to zirconium and titanium after 1-minute incubation in a normal serum dilution series in veronal buffer with Ca^{++} added (VB^{++}). (*Source:* Tengvall, P. et al., *J. Biomed. Mater. Res.*, 57, 285, 2001. With permission.)

A close relationship exists between surface-bound partially denatured proteins or their remains at surfaces after proteolytic cleavage and a variety of membrane-bound cell receptors. See cell types, selected receptors, and their target proteins shown in Table 16.1. During the blood protein adsorption phase and before blood clotting, within minutes, platelets and leukocytes bind onto a surface and participate in the regulation of inflammation and the subsequent wound healing and prosthesis integration processes via signal molecules such as eicosanoids, plasma and lysosomal proteases, platelet-activating factors, growth factors, vasoactive amines, NO, and oxygen metabolites.

The current hypothesis is that the regulation of surface-close cells and tissues is disturbed by the presence of the biomaterial — a large mechanically rigid nonphagocytable immune complex that may lead to consequences such as chronic inflammation, nonspecific low degree immune challenge, down-regulation, and avascular fibrous encapsulation.

What proof shows that cells behave differently near foreign body surfaces than they do in normal tissue? Extensive evidence indicates that foreign bodies become encapsulated or shielded within the body. Researchers are trying to determine why and how this proceeds throughout the healing process. One important previous observation is the so-called frustrated phagocytosis in which inflammatory cells recognize a nonself object (implant surface) too large to be engulfed by the cells. As a consequence, the inflammatory cells seem to remain at the surface or in close vicinity, apparently with a shifted balance in comparison to sham site cells in the regulation of signal molecules, for as long as 24 hours[30] (Figure 16.12).

Not only do the exudate cells display shifted metabolism. When surface-bound cells in the same study were exposed to Luminol, cells on hydrophilic surfaces produced significantly stronger chemiluminescence responses than the other surfaces (Figure 16.13). The results indicate clearly that very early disturbances in the wound healing process occur at implant sites and the response can be modulated by surface physicochemical properties.

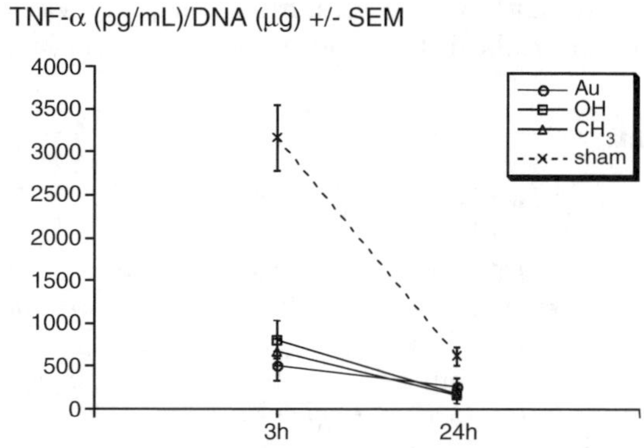

FIGURE 16.12
TNF-α generation by rat exudate cells *ex vivo* after 3 hours and 24 hours of subcutaous implantation of Au surfaces with and without self-assembled monolayers made of $SHC_{16}OH$ (hydrophilic) or $SHC_{15}CH_3$ (hydrophobic). Similar generation trends were observed for IL-α and IL-β. (*Source:* Källtorp, M. et al., *Biomaterials*, 20, 2123, 1999. With permission.)

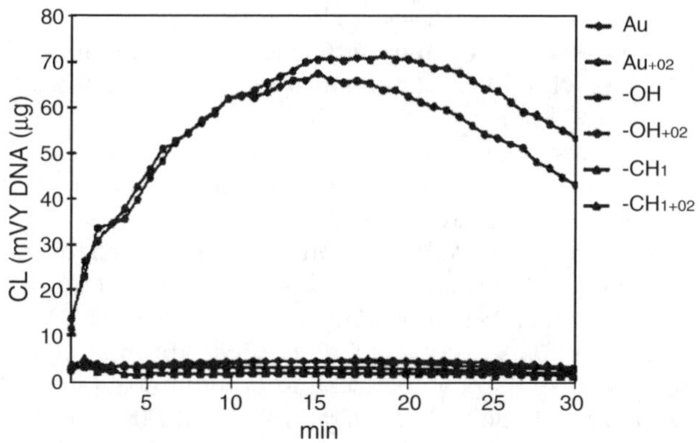

FIGURE 16.13
Luminol-enhanced chemiluminescence *ex vivo* of surface-located cells after 3 hours of subcutanous implantation in rats. (*Source:* Källtorp, M. et al., *Biomaterials*, 20, 2123, 1999. With permission.)

16.7 Final Remarks

Experimental results and literature show clearly that blood plasma and other body fluids deposit proteins onto surfaces. The thickness of the more or less denatured protein film is at nanometer scale. Because of close proximity between proteins and surfaces, cascade reactions such as activation of the intrinsic pathway of coagulation and complement may take place, all depending on the underlying chemical and physical surface properties. The control of the complement system remains a particular challenge for applications of classical materials and for engineered living replacement materials.

References

1. Holgers K.-M. et al,. Titanium in soft tissues, in *Titanium in Medicine: Materials Science, Surface Science, Engineering, Biological Responses, and Medical Applications*, Brunette, D.M. et al., Eds., Springer, Berlin, 2001, chap.16.
2. Larsson, C. et al,. The titanium–bone interface *in vivo*, in *Titanium in Medicine, Materials Science, Surface Science, Engineering, Biological Responses, and Medical Applications*, Brunette, D.M. et al., Eds., Springer, Berlin, 2001, chap.18.
3. Brauker, J.H. et al., Neovascularization of synthetic membranes directed by membrane microarchitecture, *J. Biomed. Mater. Res.*, 29, 1517, 1995.
4. Kyriakides, T.R. et al., Mice that lack the angiogenesis inhibitor, thrombospondin 2, mount an altered foreign body reaction characterized by increased vascularity, *Proc. Natl. Acad. Sci. U.S.A.*, 96, 4449, 1999.
5. Sul, Y.-T. et al., Qualitative and quantitative observations of bone tissue reactions to anodised implants, *Biomaterials*, 23, 1809, 2002.
6. van Tienen, T.G. et al., Tissue ingrowth and degradation of two biodegradable porous polymers with different porosities and pore sizes, *Biomaterials*, 23, 1731, 2002.
7. Olsson, E., Studies on the mechanisms behind the foreign body reaction through detection of TNF-α and newly recruited macrophages, diploma work, Linköping University, Sweden, June 2001.
8. Norde, W. and Haynes, C.A., Reversibility and the mechanism of protein adsorption, in *Proteins at Interfaces II: Fundamentals and Applications*, Horbett, T.A. and Brash, J.L., Eds., ACS Symposium Series. Washington, D.C., 1995, chap. 2.
9. Benesch, J., Askendal, A., and Tengvall, P., Quantification of adsorbed human serum albumin: a comparison between radioimmunoassay (RIA) and simple null ellipsometry, *Coll. Surf. B Biointerfac.*, 18, 71, 2000.
10. Larsson, R., Larm, O., and Olsson, P., The search for thromboresistance using immobilized heparin, *Ann. N.Y. Acad. Sci.*, 516, 102, 1987.
11. Gimbrone, M.A., Vascular endothelium: nature's blood-compatible container, *Ann. N.Y. Acad. Sci.*, 516, 5, 1987.
12. Collier J. and Vallance P., Second messenger role for NO widens to nervous and immune systems, *TIPS*, 10, 427, 1989.
13. Kanagaraja, S. et al., Platelet binding and protein adsorption to titanium and gold after short time exposure to heparinized plasma and whole blood, *Biomaterials*, 17, 2225, 1996.
14. Niewiarowski, S. et al., Fibrinogen interaction with platelet receptors, *Ann. N.Y. Acad. Sci.*, 408, 536, 1983.
15. Tengvall, P., Askendal, A., and Lundström, I., Studies on protein adsorption and activation of complement on hydrated aluminum surfaces *in vitro*, *Biomaterials*, 19, 935, 1998.
16. Benesch, J. et al., Protein adsorption to oligo(ethylene glycol self-assembled monolayers: experiments with fibrinogen, heparinised plasma and serum, *J. Biomater. Sci. Polymer Ed.*, 12, 581, 2001.

17. Kenausis, G.L. et al., Poly(L-lysine)-g-poly(ethylene glycol) layers on metal oxide surfaces: attachment mechanisms and effects of polymer architecture on resistance to protein adsorption, *J. Phys. Chem. B*, 104, 3298, 2000.
18. Roitt, I., Brostoff, J., and Male, D., *Immunology*, 5th ed., Mosby, London, 1998, chap. 23.
19. Hallab, N., Jacobs, J.J., and Black, J., Hypersensitivity to metallic biomaterials: a review of leucocyte migration inhibition assays, *Biomaterials*, 21, 1301, 2000.
20. Lewis, S.L. and Van Epps, D.E., Neutrophil and monocyte alterations in chronic dialysis patients, *Am. J. Kidney Dis.*, 9, 381, 1987.
21. Black, J., Allergic foreign-body response, in *Biological Performance of Materials: Fundamentals of Biocompatibility*, 3rd ed., Marcel Dekker, New York, 1999, chap. 12.
22. Heggers J.P. et al., Biocompatibility of silicone implants, *Ann. Plast. Surg.*, 11, 38, 1983.
23. Kossovsky, N., Heggers, J.P., and Robson, M.C., Experimental demonstration of the immunogenicity of silicone protein complexes, *J. Biomed. Mater. Res.*, 21, 1125, 1987.
24. Vojdani, A., Campbell, A., and Brautbar, N., Immune functional impairment in patients with clinical abnormalities and silicone breast implants, *Toxicol. Ind. Health*, 8, 415, 1992.
25. Wolf, L.E. et al., Human immune responses to polydimethylsiloxane (silicone): screening studies in a breast implant population, *FASEB J.*, 7, 1265, 1993.
26. Naim, J.O., Lanzafame, R.J., and van Oss, C.J., The effect of silicone gel on the immune response, *J. Biomater. Sci. Polym. Ed.*, 7, 123, 1995.
27. Young, V.L. et al., HLA typing in women with breast implants, *Plastic Reconstruct. Surg.*, 96, 1497, 1995.
28. Wälivaara, B. et al., Blood protein interactions with titanium surfaces, *J. Biomater. Sci. Pol. Ed.*, 8, 41, 1996.
29. Tengvall, P., Askendal, A., and Lundström, I., Temporal studies on the deposition of complement on human colostrum IgA and serum IgG immobilized on methylated silicon, *J. Biomed. Mater. Res.*, 35, 81, 1997.
30. Källtorp, M. et al., *In vivo* cell recruitment, cytokine release and chemiluminescence response at gold, and thiol functionalized surfaces, *Biomaterials*, 20, 2123, 1999.

17

Osteocapacities of Calcium Phosphate Ceramics

John A. Jansen, Petra J. ter Brugge, Edwin van der Wal, Arjen M. Vredenberg, and Joop G.C. Wolke

CONTENTS

17.1 Introduction 305
17.2 Osteogenic Lineage 306
17.3 Cell–Substrate Adhesion 307
17.4 Oral Implant Materials 308
17.5 Osteocapacities of CP Ceramics 310
17.6 Sputter Deposition of CaP Coatings 310
17.7 Interface Physics of Sputtered CaP Coatings 311
17.8 *In Vitro* Cell Behavior of Sputtered CaP Coatings 313
17.9 *In Vivo* Bone Behavior of Sputtered CaP Coatings 316
17.10 Conclusion and Final Remarks 317
References 319

17.1 Introduction

Biomaterials can be defined as materials used to replace or reconstruct damaged tissues. With respect to bone-replacing biomaterials, *osseointegration* is the term used to describe an optimal biological interface between the material and the surrounding bone.

Bone formation on an implanted material can be considered as the result of a series of separate stages, involving conditioning of the surface by serum adsorption, followed by cell attachment, proliferation, osteogenic differentiation, and eventually bone remodeling.[1] Among the factors influencing this

0-8493-1474-7/03/$0.00+$1.50

process, biomaterial surface characteristics play important roles. Therefore, knowledge of the precise effects of material surface characteristics is essential when designing bone implant materials.

In this chapter, the bone-forming cells and the effects of calcium phosphate (CaP) ceramics on bone formation will be described.

17.2 Osteogenic Lineage

Bone serves a dual function, i.e., it provides support for the body and acts as a calcium reservoir. Bone is a very dynamic tissue; it is constantly broken down and rebuilt by specialized cells associated with the mineralized bone matrix and called *osteoclasts* and *osteoblasts*, respectively. Although they have different lineages, both cell types originate in the bone marrow.

Two major cell systems are found within bone marrow: (1) the hematopoietic lineage that gives rise to blood cells and osteoclasts and (2) the marrow stroma consisting of a heterogeneous population of cells containing marrow adipocytes, stromal fibroblasts and, near bone surfaces, osteoblasts and bone-lining cells. All these cell types are thought to be the progeny of a common stromal stem cell residing within the stromal compartment that would by definition be characterized as a cell that shows unlimited potential for self-renewal and gives rise to committed progenitors of different cell lines.[2,3]

Little is known about mesenchymal stem cells (MSCs), largely because of the lack of known markers or distinctive morphological characteristics. *MSC* is often used to describe a population of adherent marrow cells with potential to differentiate along different lineages, called colony-forming unit fibroblasts (CFU-Fs),[4] based on the fact that colonies derived from single marrow cells will, with appropriate stimuli, differentiate into several cell types — an indication of the multipotential natures of cells. However, the capacity for self-renewal has not yet been shown in culture, and therefore it is unclear whether CFU-Fs contain stem cells or consist of early uncommitted progenitors.

Attempts to characterize CFU-Fs in ways other than functional assays have been made in the last few years. These studies led to the development of antibodies reacting with markers found on undifferentiated stromal cells. Expression of these markers is lost when the cells differentiate into the different stromal lineages.[5,6] Unfortunately, these markers are not specific for stromal cells and are also found in other tissues.

The precise characteristics of stromal fibroblastic cells *in vivo* are also unclear. Stromal fibroblast cells express high levels of alkaline phosphatase in the primitive bone marrows of prenatal animals, where they provide reservoirs of precursors for prenatal osteogenesis. In the postnatal marrow, the cells generate hematopoietic microenvironment, support hematopoiesis, and also show characteristics of preadipocytes. Thus, the cells are myelo-supportive elements within a multipotential milieu.[2,7]

With progression along the mesenchymal lineage, the precursors are thought to progressively lose the multipotential nature that eventually leads to the formation of committed progenitor cells. *In vitro* studies of bone marrow cells show the existence of a precursor that can differentiate into adipogenic and chondrogenic potential with increased cell doubling.[8]

Differentiation along the osteoblastic lineage has been described to proceed along a number of specific stages. These stages were described based on morphological features, requirements for inducers, and expression of markers *in vitro* and *in vivo*.

Committed osteoprogenitors are identified by functional assays of their capacity to form bone nodules *in vitro*. The cells show limited self-renewal and extensive capacities for proliferation.[9,10] Osteoprogenitor cells are relatively rare, forming less than 0.1% of the total marrow cell population.[11] *In vitro* studies indicate two types of osteoprogenitor cells. The immature type will undergo osteoblastic differentiation only in the presence of specific inducers, whereas the mature type will show spontaneous differentiation in the absence of this inducer.[12]

The osteoprogenitor stage is followed by the preosteoblast stage: cells that stain for alkaline phosphatase, but have not yet acquired many other characteristics of osteoblasts. Preosteoblasts still possess limited capacity for proliferation. The mature osteoblast is a postproliferative, strongly alkaline phosphatase-positive cell found at sites of active matrix production.[13] The osteoblast phenotype is further characterized by the synthesis of bone matrix proteins such as collagen-I, osteocalcin, bone sialoprotein, and osteopontin, and by the ability to mineralize this matrix.

17.3 Cell–Substrate Adhesion

Cells interact with implant materials through a layer of proteins adsorbed onto the material immediately upon implantation. The integrins comprise a large family of cellular adhesion receptors. Integrins are large transmembrane glycoproteins consisting of heterodimers of two subunits, α and β. The combination of the subunits determines ligand specificity.[14]

Integrins are found in specialized cell surface contact sites called focal adhesions or focal contacts. In these structures, integrins span membranes and interact with proteins on both sides of the membranes. The extracellular domain of the integrin heterodimer forms a ligand-binding site that recognizes specific sequences in extracellular matrix (ECM) proteins. Many integrins recognize several proteins, while many ECM proteins act as ligands for more than one integrin. This pattern of overlapping specificity is probably due to the fact that most integrins recognize the arginine–glycine–aspartic acid (RGD) sequence found in many proteins. Several other more restricted recognition sites are also found.[14,15]

The intracellular domain of the β subunit interacts with cytoskeletal proteins and signal transduction proteins. Ligand binding results in generation of intracellular signals that regulate cellular functions such as adhesion, spreading, proliferation, migration, differentiation, and apoptosis.[16,17]

Integrins have been found on all cell types with the exception of erythrocytes. Many studies into the expression of integrins on cells on the osteogenic lineage have been performed. They show that osteogenic cells express a wide variety of integrin subunits.[18-20] Many of these studies show different integrin expression patterns, probably due to the use of cells from different species or anatomical locations, cultured cells, or cells *in vivo*. Furthermore, integrin expression has been shown to change with lineage progression.[20,21]

Interactions of integrins with ECM molecules regulate many cellular functions in osteogenic cells. Interfering with the activity of integrins inhibits attachment of marrow stromal, human, or rat osteoblasts to a variety of ECM proteins.[19,22] Increases in proliferation and expression of osteopontin in osteoblasts are both associated with cell attachment to ECM proteins via integrins.[23] Further, the expression of osteogenic differentiation markers, such as alkaline phosphatase expression, nodule formation, and mineralization, are all inhibited by blocking the activities of specific integrins.[22,24]

Since integrins mediate adhesion of cells and transduce signals from substrates into cells, it is possible that they also mediate the effects of surface characteristics on the cells. Initial interactions of osteogenic cells with different materials may be regulated by different integrins.[25] Integrin expression may be differentially regulated upon adhesion to surfaces with different material characteristics.[26] Finally, formation of focal contacts can be altered, depending on the surface characteristics of the materials to which the cells attach.[27]

17.4 Oral Implant Materials

The success or failure of an oral implant is determined by many variables, including patient bone quality, surgical technique, mechanical loading, and material surface characteristics.

An event that takes place almost immediately upon implantation of a material is the absorption of ions, proteins, lipids, minerals, and sugars from blood and tissue fluids. Cells from the osteogenic lineage attach, spread, proliferate, and differentiate, eventually resulting in bone formation on the implant. In the last step, osteoclasts are recruited and bone is remodeled.[1]

Many different biomaterials can be used for oral implants. These materials differ in characteristics such as surface composition, surface energy, surface

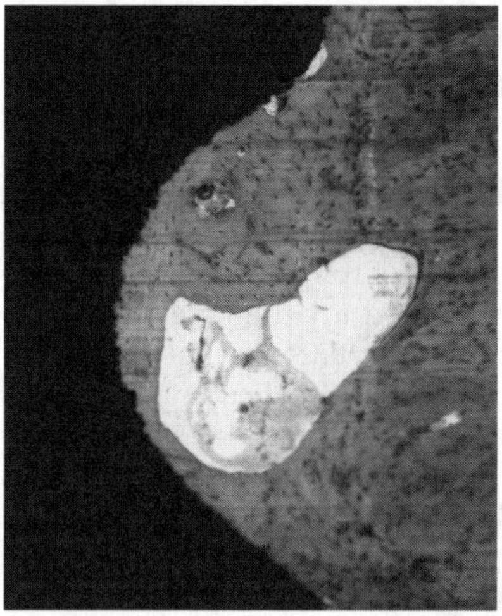

FIGURE 17.1
Histological section showing intimate bone contact with a grit-blasted titanium implant surface. The implant was in place in a human patient about 6 years, and retrieved because of problems with the suprastructure.

charge, surface structure, and surface roughness. Undifferentiated mesenchymal cells are the first cells supposed to encounter the implant material. When an implant is placed into the bone bed, committed osteoprogenitors may also be found around the implant.[1,28] The ability of the cells to attach, migrate, proliferate, differentiate, and eventually form bone depends on the combination of surface characteristics of the implant material.

Titanium is the most widely used material for oral implants due to its excellent biocompatibility. Titanium and its alloys are sometimes classified as bioinert, indicating that they do not induce severe inflammatory responses. Bone formation around titanium implants is called contact osteogenesis. Bone is formed in close contact with the implant but is not attached to the implant. Titanium implants are frequently provided with micrometer scale surface roughness. Various *in vivo* studies show improved bone formation to such surface-roughened implants[29,30] (Figure 17.1). A large number of *in vitro* studies show that increased surface roughness enhances attachment, proliferation, and expression of different markers in osteogenic cells.[31,32] Other reports show no effect of increased surface roughness or indicate that it decreases cell function and bone formation.[33,34]

A titanium implant can also be provided with a coating layer made of calcium phosphate (CaP). This material is considered to be bioactive, meaning that it interacts with surrounding tissue to generate a chemical bond at the bone–implant interface, so-called bonding osteogenesis.[28] Many studies have shown good bone formation around CaP-coated implants, often better formation than around uncoated titanium implants.[29,35,36]

17.5 Osteocapacities of CP Ceramics

Despite the fact that we have known about the beneficial effects of CaP ceramics on bone healing for more than 30 years, the underlying mechanism for this effect is still not clear. One hypothesis is that dissolution of ions from bone-bioactive ceramics followed by a precipitation reaction leads to the formation of a carbonated apatite layer. This new apatite layer resembling bone mineral then stimulates bone formation.[37] High calcium and phosphate concentrations may affect cellular activity directly.[38,39] However, it has been shown that in the presence of serum, dissolution–precipitation reactions around some ceramics are significantly hampered by the presence of the proteins adsorbed to the material.[40] In these materials, formation of carbonated apatite is only found in the presence of cells, suggesting cell-mediated mechanisms.[40]

A second explanation for the bioactivity of CaP is its high affinity for many proteins and growth factors that play roles in bone formation.[41] Initial attachment may be regulated differentially by CaP or titanium surfaces due to differential adsorption of proteins. For example, substrate surface composition can directly influence the types or amounts of proteins adsorbed on the material immediately after implantation.[42-44] Surface composition can also affect protein conformation, which results in changes in the biological activities of the proteins.[45,46]

Direct comparison of CaP and titanium surfaces showed that CaP adsorbs a larger amount of protein from serum than titanium and also adsorbs proteins not found on titanium.[47] Since many of these proteins are involved in cell adhesion to materials, differences in adsorbed protein layers could explain the different biological effects of CaP and titanium surfaces.

Unfortunately, a good comparison of the various bone–implant studies in which CaP ceramic is used is difficult to achieve. The investigated materials vary in composition, crystallinity, and method of manufacturing. Many aspects of a material are determined by production method. For example, variations in CaP composition can lead to different dissolution and precipitation behaviors and can affect bone responses.[40,48] Various techniques can provide a titanium oral implant with a CaP coating.

17.6 Sputter Deposition of CaP Coatings

Sputtering is the process by which atoms or molecules of a material under vacuum are ejected by bombardment of high-energy ions. The dislodged particles deposit on a substrate placed in a vacuum chamber. Techniques include diode, radiofrequent (RF) or direct current (DC), ion beam, and reactive sputtering. However, a drawback inherent to all these techniques is that the deposition rate is low and the process is slow. These problems can be solved by using a magnetically enhanced variant of diode sputtering. Magnetron sputtering is a high rate vacuum coating technique for depositing a wide range of materials (including metals, alloys, and ceramics).

Radiofrequency magnetron sputtering can be used to deposit thin films of hydroxyapatite on titanium substrate at a deposition rate of ~0.5 μm/hr and will produce film thicknesses of 0.5 to 10 μm. A deposited film will have a uniform and dense structure. Further, the coating shows a strong adhesion to the underlying substrate. Another advantage of the technique is that the Ca/P ratio and crystallinity of the deposited coating can be varied easily.[49,50] This means that RF magnetron sputtering is a very suitable technique to deposit standardized CaP coatings on titanium substrates. Since these coatings are very thin, they do not modify the microroughness of the titanium. Therefore, RF magnetron sputter deposition can provide greater understanding of the osteocapacites of CaP ceramics.

17.7 Interface Physics of Sputtered CaP Coatings

The interfacial reaction that occurs during the initial bone-bonding process is a complex phenomenon consisting of multiple sequential processes. One is the formation of a so-called biologically equivalent apatitic surface.[37] We know that remodelling of a CaP coating surface can influence both the final bone formation and bone-bonding behavior. It has been reported that all bioactive ceramics have in common a direct bone bonding that results in a strong bone–material interface,[38] and a relationship exists between resorption behavior and bioactivity of calcium phosphates.

The use of an inorganic equivalent of human blood plasma or simulated body fluid (SBF)[51,52] has been recommended as model system to reveal more about the physical properties of CaP ceramics in physiological environments.

We must emphasize that when the precipitation and dissolution properties of a CaP coating are addressed, different physical processes should be distinguished. First, the concentrations in the bulk of the solution will determine the equilibrium state of the system. Deviations from this state are the driving force for dissolution or precipitation of different CaP phases. Further, the diffusion and convection of species to and from the coating surface, the composition of the adsorption layer and its charge equilibrium, the activation to nucleate the different CaP phases, and the growing and maturing of other CaP phases will have effects. Evidently, the roles of the distinct processes are difficult to unravel, especially when additional parameters such as inhibiting proteins or cells are present in the model system.

In view of the above, we deposited 80-nm thick CaP coatings on silicone substrates using RF magnetron sputtering. Silicon was used to facilitate the

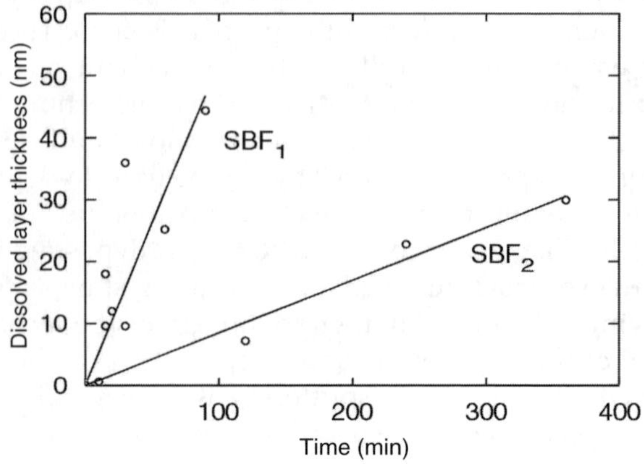

FIGURE 17.2
Equivalent amounts of dissolved coating versus time for sputtered coatings immersed in SBF_1 and SBF_2.

application of ion beam techniques (Rutherford backscattering spectrometry = RBS; elastic recoil detection = ERD) for compositional analysis of the coatings. The produced coatings were found to be extremely smooth and showed very low specific areas. The deposited coatings were completely amorphous. To produce crystalline coatings, a heat treatment of 650°C was applied. It produced highly crystalline (defective) apatite coatings.

A simulated body fluid (SBF_1) was prepared from reagent grade salts according to Kokubo.[51,52] Another SBF with twice the Ca and PO_4 concentrations (SBF_2) was used and gave rise to higher free energy for CaP precipitation. Amorphous CaP coatings were immersed subsequently in SBF_1 and SBF_2 for different periods. Figure 17.2 shows a plot of total dissolved coating contents versus time. The calculated rates of dissolution were $5 \cdot 10^{-1}$ nm min^{-1} and $8 \cdot 10^{-2}$ nm min^{-1} for immersion in SBF_1 and SBF_2, respectively. Ion beam analysis of the coatings revealed that they dissolved in a homogeneous and congruent fashion. Stirring experiments showed that dissolution in SBF_1 was diffusion limited.

Immersion of annealed coatings in SBF_1 at 37°C up to 3 days revealed that the coatings did not degrade and no deposition of CaP occurred. Clearly, the activation barrier for CaP nucleation could not be overcome in SBF_1. Immersion in SBF_2 resulted in the precipitation of CaP; uncoated immersed substrates (including Si, Si_3N_4, and Al_2O_3) were found to be inert. At 20°C, the nucleation was preceded by an induction period of ~1 hour as shown in Figure 17.3.

We calculated a growth rate of ~1.2 nm min^{-1} for immersion at 37°C. No degradation of the coating was found after immersion. Scanning electron microscopy (SEM) showed the formation of plate-like clusters. After providing the surface with nuclei, a continuous growth of CaP in SBF_1 or even in cell culture medium could be obtained.

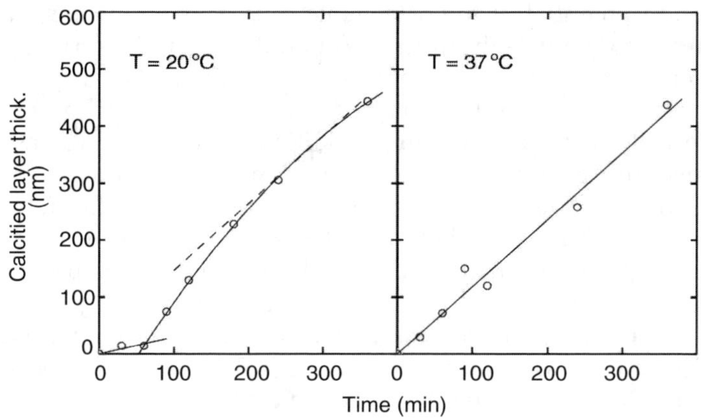

FIGURE 17.3
Equivalent amounts of dissolved coating versus time for sputtered coatings immersed in SBF_2 at 20 and 37°C.

These studies prove that the ability of a CaP coating surface to form a direct calcified layer is determined by the nucleation step. The temperature is critical for the presence and duration of induction time. After nuclei have been formed, growth is possible at much lower supersaturation.

17.8 *In Vitro* Cell Behavior of Sputtered CaP Coatings

Osteogenic cells have to be used to study the osteocapacity of sputtered CaP coatings *in vitro*. Various sources can be used to obtain the required cells and several protocols can be used to perform the studies. However, we noticed that seemingly irrelevant modifications in the cell culture protocol can have significant influence on the final observations. For example, we know that the expression of osteogenic markers is influenced by conditions such as culture medium, addition of growth factors, and serum used.[53-55]

Culture of human osteoblasts in medium containing a defined serum substitute prevents dedifferentiation of cells upon subculture.[56] Also, cells derived from different strains of the same species may show large variations in growth and differentiation. A close relationship exists between hematopoietic and osteogenic cells.

In vitro, hematopoietic bone marrow cells have been shown to alter the expression of cytokines by human osteoblasts in culture.[57] In rat cultures, the number of bone nodules is increased when adherent bone marrow cells are cocultured with the nonadherent fraction[11] of human bone marrow containing cells that stimulate *in vitro* development of osteogenic precursors.[58] Coculture of the adherent fraction with the nonadherent fraction may directly affect the differentiation potential of the osteogenic cells. In view of this, *in vitro* cell culture studies to evaluate the influence of implant material surface properties on the differentiation and growth of osteogenic cells must be designed according to an accurate and well established experimental protocol. In addition, to exclude cell source and culture condition effects as much as possible, experiments must be repeated several times in separate runs.

In 1988, Maniatopoulos et al.[59] cultured bone marrow stromal cells from the femorae of adult rats. They supplemented the culture medium with ascorbic acid, β-glycerophosphate, and dexamethasone. Subsequently, the stromal cells were observed to differentiate along the osteogenic lineage, as revealed by their ability to deposit collagen bundles and form mineralized nodules. Since then, the rat bone marrow (RBM) cells have been used in numerous studies to evaluate the osteogenic potential of CaP ceramics.

For example, in a recent study of ter Brugge et al.,[60] the effect of the crystallinity of sputtered CaP coatings on the proliferation and expression of osteogenic markers by RBM was investigated. It was hypothesized that crystallinity determines the dissolution characteristics of the deposited coating, which in turn can influence its osteocapacity. Surface-roughened titanium was sputter-coated with CaP. The coatings had CaP ratios of 1.77 and were left as prepared or subjected to heat treatment. This generated coatings with different crystallinity levels ranging from amorphous to crystalline. Noncoated surface-roughened and machined titanium substrates were included as reference materials.

RBM cells were cultured up to 16 days on various surfaces. Coated and uncoated substrates without cells were also incubated in culture medium in order to study the effects of material characteristics on dissolution and precipitation phenomena. Low crystallinity CaP-coated substrates showed extensive dissolution and precipitation, whereas only limited dissolution was found for high crystalline coatings. Some CaP precipitation was found on the crystalline coatings and also on the titanium substrates. However, this precipitate was not stable and disappeared after longer culture periods.

Cells on the crystalline coating showed the highest expression of the osteogenic differentiation marker osteocalcin and revealed highest amounts of calcification of cell cultures, followed by the titanium substrates (Figure 17.4). The occurrence of calcification could be associated with the abundant deposition of collagen fibrils. In contrast, no proliferation or differentiation of RBM cells was seen on the amorphous coatings. Evidently, the high level of dissolution of the amorphous coatings inhibits RBM cell proliferation and differentiation.

The biological relevance of the dissolution and precipitation process that occurs on CaP ceramics has been confirmed in other studies. Fourier transform infrared (FTIR) analysis of amorphous-crystalline sputtered CaP coatings showed that during incubation in culture medium, proteins also precipitate on the CaP surface. Proteins are known to fulfill important functions in the mineralization of tissues. They are suggested to be involved as nucleators or inhibitors of hydroxyapatite formation.[61-63]

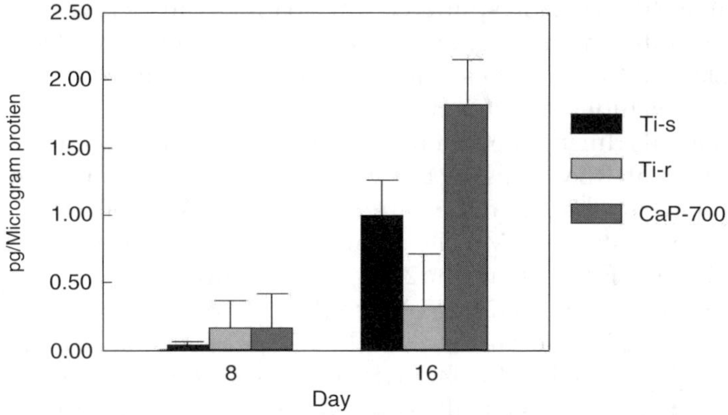

FIGURE 17.4
Osteocalcin expression by rat bone marrow cells after 8 and 16 days of culture on machined (Ti-S), grit-blasted (Ti-R), and CaP sputter-coated (CaP-700) substrates. Expression was normalized for protein content. Values are mean ± standard deviation.

The effects of interfacial dissolution and precipitation are also seen in transmission electron microscopic (TEM) studies of RBM cells cultured on sputtered CaP coatings. TEM examination reveals that at the substrate surface, two distinct layers representing the maintained part original coating and the additional precipitate can be discerned (Figure 17.5). This last layer is less dense. It is covered with an electron-dense (lamina limitans-like) line of approximately 500-nm thickness. Small needle-like foci of mineralization can be observed at this layer.

To further elucidate how a CaP surface can control events such as differentiation, proliferation, and biosynthesis, the initial attachment and spreading behavior and the expression of specific cell-surface adhesion molecules

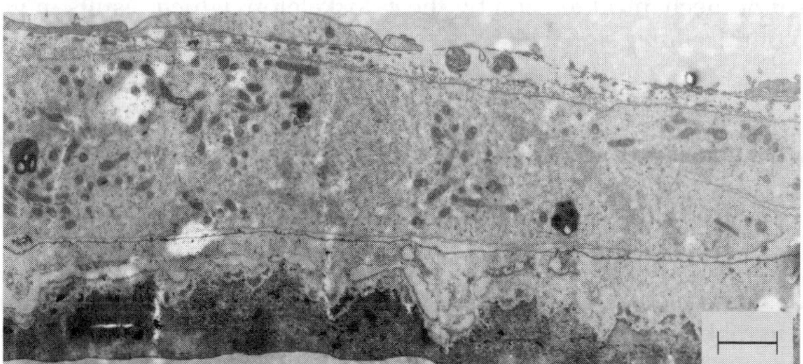

FIGURE 17.5
Transmission electron micrograph of rat bone marrow cells on a CaP sputter-coated substrate. The dense layer represents the original coating. An additional precipitate can be observed on top of the dense layer. An electron-dense line is visible between the cell and the precipitate. Bar = 1.3 μm.

(integrins) of RBM cells on sputtered CaP coatings can be investigated. RBM cells can be cultured on roughened titanium substrates provided with sputtered crystalline CaP coatings. Again, noncoated machined and rough titanium can be included as reference materials.

Measurements during the first 6 hours of incubation showed no difference in attachment of RBM cells to the various materials. Also, no differences were found in expression on the various materials. After 30, 60, 120, and 240 minutes of incubation, RBM cells on all materials expressed α1, α3, α5, α6, and β1 subunits. Expression of α2, α4, and β3 subunits was always absent or very low. Fluorescent staining of the actin cytoskeleton demonstrated that cells spread on all materials and reached larger sizes on smooth titanium than on rough materials. Morphologies of the cells on the materials differed. On smooth titanium, cells usually showed compact bodies with short cellular extensions. On rough materials, cells often showed elongated shapes with many thin cellular extensions.

Although, these results appear not to corroborate other studies,[64,65] we must emphasize that comparison of the various studies is not as straightforward as occasionally suggested. For example, the various studies differ in cell types used, cell seeding densities, and applied surface roughness or CaP ceramic. As mentioned in this section and in Section 17.5, these differences can have a tremendous effect on the final outcome of a study.

Nevertheless, integrin expression seems not to be the major mode by which CaP ceramic affects bone response. Despite the limited relevance of integrin expression, integrin function and subsequent intracellular signalling can still be modulated. This suggestion is made by the observation that cell spreading is different for various substrates. Cell spreading is involved in the regulation of many cellular functions. Inhibition of spreading results in apoptosis and changes in cell spreading are associated with changes in cell proliferation, migration, and differentiation.[66] Spreading may be accompanied by development of mechanical tension by the cytoskeleton, which results in generation of intracellular signals.[67]

17.9 *In Vivo* Bone Behavior of Sputtered CaP Coatings

The effect of crystallinity on the final osteogenic capacity of sputtered CaP coatings has also been confirmed in animal studies. Subcutaneous implantation in rabbits of 0.1, 1.0, and 4.0-μm thick amorphous and crystalline CaP sputter-coated titanium discs revealed that the amorphous coatings were dissolved completely after 4 weeks of implantation. This contrasts with the crystalline coatings that were all still present at 4 weeks.[68] A similar observation was made for CaP sputter-coated titanium discs implanted in more bone-related locations, i.e., subperiosteal in the tibiae of goats.[69] Again, crystalline coatings were still present till 3 weeks after insertion. Further, FTIR analysis showed that the coatings supported the deposition of additional carbonate apatite (CO_3-AP).

Besides these dissolution and degradation studies, various animal studies were performed to evaluate CaP sputter-coated implants.[35,70] In these assays, different animal species and implant locations were used. The thickness of the deposited coatings varied from 0.1 to 4 μm. Also, in most studies the deposited sputter coatings were subjected to additional heat treatment to increase the crystallinity of the CaP films. Roughened noncoated implants usually were included as reference materials. Histological and histomorphometrical analyses of interfacial bone responses revealed that CaP-coated implants inserted in trabecular bones evoked more pronounced bone apposition. However, when the thickness of the deposited coating was less than 0.5 μm, no beneficial influence on bone response was seen. This is probably due to low pH conditions during initial wound healing and can possibly result in early resorption of these thin coatings before any advantageous effect on bone response can be elicited. This theory is supported by a recent study of Koerten and van der Meulen,[71] who demonstrated that even the degradation of 100% crystalline CaP ceramics is pH-dependent with the strongest degradation at pH 4.

The favorable histological response of sputtered CaP coatings has been confirmed by mechanical testing. Torque testing of noncoated and CaP sputter-coated rough titanium implants inserted into the trabecular bones of goats revealed, especially after short (up to 6 weeks) implantation periods, that the coated implants showed higher failure torques than noncoated implants.[72]

Additional information about the *in vivo* interfacial bone response to CaP ceramics can be obtained from ultrastructural studies using transmission electron microscopy (TEM). Unfortunately, technical problems in the preparation of ultrathin sections do not allow the use of sputtered CaP coatings in these studies. Therefore, knowledge must be derived from implant assays with bulk CaP ceramics. Nevertheless, the various reports reveal that bonding occurs between the CaP ceramic and surrounding bone as characterized by the presence of an electron-dense line that covers the CaP ceramic.[73,74] This electron-dense layer shows strong resemblance to the lamina limitans surrounding osteocyte lacunae and canaliculi (approximately 20 nm) in natural bone. The thickness of this layer cited in the various reports ranges from a submicron to a 1-μm thick amorphous zone. This layer is supposed to consist of mineralized proteinaceous bone-like material adsorbed by the hydroxyapatite surface to which the collagen fibers are attached.[75]

17.10 Conclusion and Final Remarks

The successful integration of oral implants into the jawbone can be envisioned as a race against time among the processes of wound healing, fibrosis, and microbial invasion. The stake in this contest is to accomplish a harmonious interface between the implanted material and surrounding bone tissue as characterized by the development of natural tissue structures. Knowledge of the parameters that control the cascade of events involved in tissue response to materials is a prerequisite to becoming a winner. Insight in the ways material properties can stimulate osteoprogenitor cells into differentiation to bone cells and stimulate bone cells to more rapid bone formation is essential.

Currently, we know that CaP ceramic is a material that possesses intrinsic properties to favor realization of a harmonious interface. Although our knowledge of the osteogenic capacity of CaP ceramic has significantly increased during the last 10 years, the complete answers have still not been revealed. Therefore, on basis of available information only, a rudimentary hypothesis (as depicted in Figure 17.6) can be postulated about the bioactive bone behavior of CaP ceramics. The solution for this problem must be the product of even more intense cooperation between engineering and life sciences. An additional argument for the further establishment of such a relationship is that the major question in bone formation and biomaterial bioactivity is the unravelling of the influence of proteins in the nucleation and growth of apatite crystals — a topic positioned at the interface between physics and biology. Eventually, the further improvement of our understanding of bone cell response to specific materials will allow the manufacturing of tailor-made implants that generate predicted tissue responses.

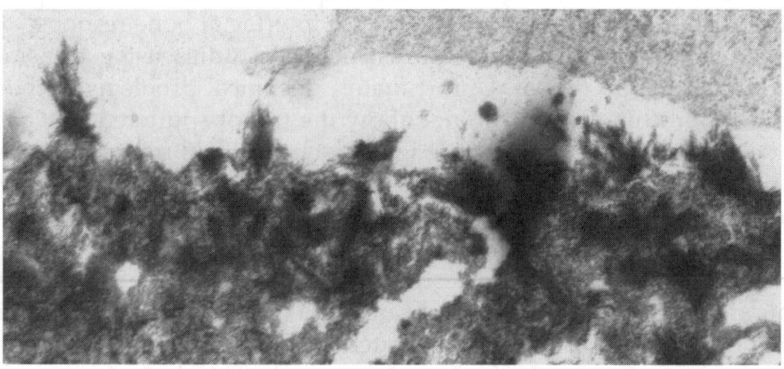

FIGURE 17.6
Step 1: cell adhesion proteins, like fibronectin, that contain the Arg–Gly–Asp (RGD) sequence adhere preferentially to CaP ceramic. Step 2: attached osteogenic cells secrete inorganic cations into the extracellular space between cell membrane and CaP surface. This results in local supersaturation (submicron/nanoscale). Step 3: phosphorylated proteins (i.e., amino acids, like phosphoserine and aspartic acid) initiate HA growth on the ceramic surface. Step 4: osteogenic cells also secrete inorganic cations onto the surface of the cell sheet and a network of collagen fibers is deposited between cell layers. The collagen fibers show repetitive patterns of anionic groups. Apatite growth starts at the collagen bundles. Step 5: three layers can be observed. First is the ceramic surface; second is an apatite layer on top of the ceramic surface (bonding zone); third is bone, characterized by collagen bundles and a mineralized matrix.

References

1. Schwartz, Z. and Boyan, B.D., Underlying mechanisms at the bone–biomaterial interface, *J. Cell. Biochem.*, 56, 340, 1994.
2. Krebsbach, P.H. et al., Bone marrow stromal cells: characterization and clinical application, *Crit. Rev. Oral Biol. Med.*, 10, 165, 1999.
3. Owen, M., Marrow stromal stem cells, *J. Cell Sci.*, 10, 63, 1988.
4. Bruder, S.P., Fink, D.J., and Caplan, A.I., Mesenchymal stem cells in bone development, bone repair and skeletal regeneration therapy, *J. Cell. Biochem.*, 56, 283, 1994.
5. Joyner, C.J., Bennett, A., and Triffit, J.T., Identification and enrichment of human osteoprogenitor cells by using differentiation stage-specific monoclonal antibodies, *Bone*, 21, 1, 1997.
6. Gronthos, S. et al., Differential cell surface expression of the STRO-1 and alkaline phosphatase antigens on discrete developmental stages in primary cultures of human bone, *J. Bone Miner. Res.*, 14, 47, 1999.
7. Bianco, P. and Robey, P.G., Marrow stromal stem cells, *J. Clin. Invest.*, 105, 1663, 2000.
8. Muraglia, A., Cancedda, R., and Quarto, R., Clonal mesenchymal progenitors from human bone marrow differentiate *in vitro* according to a hierarchical model, *J. Cell Sci.*, 113, 1161, 2000.
9. Bellows, C.G., Heersche, J.N.M., and Aubin, J.E., Determination of the capacity for proliferation and differentiation of osteoprogenitor cells in the presence and absence of dexamethasone, *Dev. Biol.*, 140, 132, 1990.
10. McCulloch, C.A.G. et al., Osteogenic progenitor cells in rat bone marrow stromal populations exhibit self-renewal in culture, *Blood*, 9, 1906, 1991.
11. Aubin, J.E., Osteoprogenitor cell frequency in rat bone marrow stromal populations: role for heterotypic cell–cell interactions in osteoblastic differentiation, *J. Cell. Biochem.*, 72, 396, 1999.
12. Long, M.W. et al., Regulation of human bone marrow-derived osteoprogenitor cells by osteogenic growth factors, *J. Clin. Invest.*, 95, 881, 1995.
13. Aubin, J.E., Bone stem cells, *J. Cell. Biochem.*, 30, 73, 1998.
14. Ruoslahti, E. et al., Integrins, *Kidney Int.*, 45, 17, 1994.
15. Hynes, R.O., Integrins: versatility, modulation and signalling in cell adhesion, *Cell*, 69, 11, 1992.
16. Meredith, J.E. et al., The regulation of growth and intracellular signalling by integrins, *Endocrine Rev.*, 17, 207, 1996.
17. Coppolina, M.G. and Dedhar, S., Bi-directional signal transduction by integrin receptors, *Int. J. Biochem. Cell Biol.*, 32, 171, 2000.
18. Gronthos, S. et al., Integrin expression and function on human osteoblast-like cells, *J. Bone Miner. Res.*, 12, 1189, 1997.
19. Castoldi, M. et al., Osteoblastic cells from rat long bone II: adhesion to substrata and integrin expression in primary and propagated cultures, *Biol. Int.*, 21, 7, 1997.
20. Bennett, J.H. et al., Patterns of integrin expression in a human mandibular explant model of osteoblast differentiation, *Arch. Oral Biol.*, 46, 229, 2001.
21. Schneider, G.B., Whitson, S.W., and Cooper, L.F., Restricted and coordinated expression of ß3 integrin and bone sialoprotein during cultured osteoblast differentiation, *Bone*, 24, 321, 1999.

22. Gronthos, S. et al., Integrin-mediated interactions between human bone marrow stromal precursor cells and the extracellular matrix, *Bone*, 28, 174, 2001.
23. Cowles, E.A., Brailey, L.L., and Gronowicz, G.A., Integrin-mediated signalling regulates AP-1 transcription factors and proliferation in osteoblasts, *J. Biomed. Mater. Res.*, 52, 725, 2000.
24. Cheng, S.L. et al., Bone mineralization and osteoblast differentiation are negatively modulated by integrin αvß3, *J. Bone Miner. Res.*, 16, 277, 2001.
25. Okamoto, K. et al., RGD peptides regulate the specific adhesion scheme of osteoblasts to hydroxyapatite but not to titanium, *J. Dent. Res.*, 77, 481, 1998.
26. Gronowitz, G. and McCarthy, M.B., Response of human osteoblasts to implant materials: integrin-mediated adhesion, *J. Orthop. Res.*, 14, 878, 1996.
27. Shah, A.K. et al., High-resolution morphometric analysis of human osteoblastic cell adhesion on clinically relevant orthopedic alloys, *Bone*, 24, 499, 1999.
28. LeGeros, R.Z. and Craig, R.G., Strategies to affect bone remodelling: osseointegration, *J. Bone Miner. Res.*, 8, 583, 1993.
29. Svehla, M. et al., Morphometric and mechanical evaluation of titanium implant integration: comparison of five surface structures, *J. Biomed. Mater. Res.*, 51, 15, 2000.
30. Wennerberg, A. et al., Experimental study of turned and grit-blasted screw-shaped implants with special emphasis on effects of blasting material and surface topography, *Biomaterials*, 17, 15, 1996.
31. Deligianni, D.D. et al., Effect of surface roughness of the titanium alloy Ti-6Al-4V on human bone marrow cell response and on protein adsorption, *Biomaterials*, 22, 1241, 2001.
32. Lincks, J. et al., Response of MG63 osteoblast-like cells to titanium and titanium alloy is dependent on surface roughness and composition, *Biomaterials*, 19, 2219, 1998.
33. Anselme, K. et al., The relative influence of the topography and chemistry of TiAl6V4 surfaces on osteoblastic cell behaviour, *Biomaterials*, 21, 1567, 2000.
34. Vercaigne, S., Wolke, J.G.C. and Jansen, J.A., Histomorphometrical and mechanical evaluation of titanium plasma spray-coated implants placed in the cortical bone of goats, *J. Biomed. Mater. Res.*, 41, 41, 1998.
35. Hayakawa, T. et al., Effect of surface roughness and calcium phosphate coating on the implant/bone response, *Clin. Oral Implant Res.*, 11, 296, 2000.
36. Jansen, J.A. et al., Histological evaluation of the osseous adaptation to titanium and hydroxyapatite-coated titanium implants, *J. Biomed. Mater. Res.*, 25, 973, 1991.
37. Ducheyne, P. and Qui, Q., Bioactive ceramics: the effect of surface reactivity on bone formation and bone cell function, *Biomaterials*, 20, 2287, 1999.
38. Nakade, O. et al., Effect of extracellular calcium on the gene expression of bone morphogenetic protein-2 and -4 of normal human bone cells, *J. Bone Miner. Metabol.*, 19, 13, 2001.
39. Matsuoka, H. et al., *In vitro* analysis of the stimulation of bone formation by highly bioactive apatite- and wollastonite-containing glass-ceramic: released calcium ions promote osteogenic differentiation in osteoblastic ROS17/2.8 cells, *J. Biomed. Mater. Res.*, 47, 176, 1999.
40. Radin, S. et al. Effect of serum proteins and osteoblasts on the surface transformation of a calcium phosphate coating: a physicochemical and ultrastructural study, *J. Biomed. Mater. Res.*, 39, 234, 1998.

41. Ripamonti, U. et al., Osteogenin, a bone morphogenetic protein, adsorbed on porous hydroxyapatite substrata, induces rapid bone differentiation in calvarial defects of adult primates, *Plast. Reconstruct. Surg.*, 90, 382, 1992.
42. Villareal, D.R., Sogal, A., and Ong, J.L., Protein adsorption and osteoblast responses to different calcium phosphate surfaces, *J. Oral Implant.*, 24, 67, 1998.
43. Chang, Y.L. et al., Osteoblastic cell attachment to hydroxyapatite-coated implant surfaces *in vitro, Int. J. Oral Maxiilofac. Implants*, 14, 239, 1999.
44. Webster, T.J. et al., Specific proteins mediate enhanced osteoblast adhesion on nanophase ceramics, *J. Biomed. Mater. Res.*, 51, 475, 2000.
45. Ong, J.L., Chittur, K.K., and Luca, L.C., Dissolution/reprecipitation and protein adsorption studies of calcium phosphate coatings by FTIR/ATR techniques, *J. Biomed. Mater. Res.*, 28, 1337, 1994.
46. Garcia, A.J., Vega, M.D., and Boettiger, D., Modulation of cell proliferation and differentiation through substrate-dependent changes in fibronectin conformation, *Mol. Biol. Cell*, 10, 785, 1999.
47. Zeng, H., Chittur, K.K., and Lacefield, W.R., Analysis of bovine serum albumin adsorption on calcium phosphate and titanium surfaces, *Biomaterials*, 20, 3777, 1999.
48. de Bruijn, J.D., Bovell, Y.P., and van Blitterswijk, C.A., Structural arrangements at the interface between plasma sprayed calcium phosphates and bone, *Biomaterials*, 15, 543, 1994.
49. Jansen, J.A. et al., Application of magnetron sputtering for the production of ceramic coatings on implant materials, *Clin. Oral Imp. Res.*, 4, 28, 1993.
50. Wolke, J.G.C. et al., Study of the surface characteristics of magnetron-sputter calcium phosphate coatings, *J. Biomed. Mater. Res.*, 28, 1477, 1994.
51. Kokubo, T. et al., CaP rich-layer formed on high-strength bioactive glass-ceramic A-W, *J. Biomed. Mater. Res.*, 24, 331, 1990.
52. Kokubo, T. et al., Solution able to reproduce *in vivo* surface-structure changes in bioactive glass ceramic A-W, *J. Biomed. Mater. Res.*, 24, 721, 1990.
53. Jaiswal, N. et al., Osteogenic differentiation of purified, culture expanded human mesenchymal stem cells *in vitro, J. Cell. Biochem.*, 64, 295, 1997.
54. Coelho, M.J., Trigo-Cabral, A., and Fernandes, M.H., Human bone cell cultures in biocompatibility testing. Part I: osteoblastic differentiation of serially passaged human bone marrow cells cultured in αMEM and DMEM, *Biomaterials*, 21, 1087, 2000.
55. Rattner, A. et al., Characterization of human osteoblastic cells: influence of the culture conditions, *In Vitro Cell Dev. Biol. Anim.*, 33, 757, 1997.
56. Schmidt, R. and Kulbe, K.D., Long-term cultivation of human osteoblasts, *Bone Miner.*, 20, 211, 1993.
57. Taichman, R.S. et al., Augmented production of interleukin-6 by normal human osteoblasts in response to CD 34^+ hematopoietic bone marrow cells *in vitro, Blood*, 4, 1165, 1997.
58. Eipers, P.G. et al., Bone marrow accessory cells regulate human bone precursor cell development, *Exp. Hematol.*, 28, 815, 2000.
59. Maniatopoulos, C., Sodek, J., and Melcher, A.H., Bone formation *in vitro* by stromal cells obtained from bone marrow of young adult rats, *Cell Tissue Res.*, 254, 317, 1988.
60. ter Brugge, P.J. and Jansen, J.A., Effect of calcium phosphate coating crystallinity and implant surface roughness on differentiation of rat bone marrow cells, *J. Biomed. Mater. Res.*, 60, 70, 2002.

61. McKee, M.D. and Nanci, A., Ultrastructural, cytochemical and immunocytochemical studies on bone and its interfaces, *Cells Mater.*, 3, 219, 1993.
62. Martin, R.I. and Brown, P.W., Formation of hydroxyapatite in serum, *J. Mater. Sci. Mater. Med.*, 5, 96, 1994.
63. Hunter, G.K. et al., Nucleation and inhibition of hydroxyapatite formation by mineralised tissue proteins, *Biochem. J.*, 317, 59, 1996.
64. Chang, Y.L. et al., Osteoblastic cell attachment to hydroxyapatite-coated implant surfaces *in vitro*, *Int. J. Oral Maxillofac. Implants*, 14, 239, 1999.
65. Okamoto, K. et al., RGD peptides regulate the specific adhesion scheme of osteoblasts to hydroxyapatite but not to titanium, *J. Dent. Res.*, 77, 481, 1998.
66. Webb, K., Hlady, V., and Tresco, P.A., Relationships among cell attachment, spreading, cytoskeletal organization and migration rate for anchorage-dependent cells on model surfaces, *J. Biomed. Mater. Res.*, 49, 362, 2000.
67. Ingber, D.E. et al., Cellular tensegrity: exploring how mechanical changes in the cytoskeleton regulate cell growth, migration and tissue pattern during morphogenesis, *Int. Rev. Cytol.*, 150, 173, 1994.
68. Wolke, J.G.C., de Groot, K., and Jansen, J.A., *In vivo* dissolution behaviour of various RF magnetron-sputtered Ca-P coatings, *J. Biomed. Mater. Res.*, 39, 524, 1998.
69. Wolke, J.G.C., de Groot, K., and Jansen, J.A., Subperiosteal implantation of various RF magnetron-sputtered Ca-P coatings in goats, *J. Biomed. Mater. Res. Appl. Biomater.*, 43, 270, 1998.
70. Vercaigne, S. et al., A histological evaluation of TiO_2-gritblasted and Ca-P magnetron sputter-coated implants placed into the trabecular bone of the goat, part 2, *Clin. Oral Implant Res.*, 11, 314, 2000.
71. Koerten, H.K. and van der Meulen, J., Degradation of calcium phosphate ceramics, *J. Biomed. Mater. Res.*, 44, 78, 1999.
72. Vercaigne, S. et al., A mechanical evaluation of TiO_2-gritblasted and Ca-P magnetron sputter-coated implants placed into the trabecular bone of the goat, part 1, *Clin. Oral Implant Res.*, 11, 305, 2000.
73. de Bruijn, J.D., van Blitterswijk, C.A. and Davies, J.E., Initial bone matrix formation at the hydroxyapatite interface *in vivo*, *J. Biomed. Mater. Res.*, 29, 89, 1995.
74. Kokubo, T. et al., What kinds of materials inhibit bone bonding? in *Bone Engineering*, Davies, J.E., Ed., em squared, Toronto, 2000, chap.16.
75. Hosseini, M.M. et al., The structure and composition of the bone–implant interface, in *Bone Engineering*, Davies, J.E., Ed., em squared incorporated, Toronto, 2000, chap.26.

18

Increasing Biocompatibility by Chemical Modification of Titanium Surfaces

Jan Eirik Ellingsen and Staale Petter Lyngstadaas

CONTENTS

18.1 Introduction 323
18.2 Surface Modifications 324
18.2.1 Electrochemical Oxidation 324
18.2.1.1 Anodized Oxides 324
18.2.1.2 Effects of Surface Roughness 326
18.2.1.3 Nanoscale Morphology 327
18.2.1.4 Ion Implantation of Oxide 327
18.2.2 Fluoride-Modified Oxide 328
18.2.2.1 Experiments with Blasted Implant Surfaces 330
18.2.2.2 Clinical Perspectives 335
18.2.2.3 Discussion 335
References 335

18.1 Introduction

Titanium is the most frequently used material for dental implants and its uses for orthopedic prostheses are continuously increasing. This extensive use is based on the properties of the material, including a combination of corrosion resistance and biocompatibility with satisfactory mechanical performance. Mechanical qualities including fracture resistance or resistance to permanent deformation under long-term dynamic stress are essential. These qualities combined with an elastic modulus that facilitates stress transfer to the bone tissue surrounding the implant material make the biomechanical properties of titanium suitable for use as a load-bearing biomaterial.

Successful long-term stability of the biomaterial in bone tissue relies on several factors; among them is the important surface connection between

0-8493-1474-7/03/$0.00+$1.50

the implant and the bone tissue. This connection can be passive, with no binding between the surface and the tissue; it can be repelling, with establishment of an intermediate interface keeping the bone tissue apart from the implant surface; or a real contact or bond can be established between the surface and the living tissue.

The surface structure, morphology, and chemical and biochemical properties of the biomaterial are important for establishing binding between the bone tissue and the biomaterial. An oxide film 3 to 7 nm thick instantly covers a titanium implant surface when exposed to oxygen in air.[1-4] The naturally formed oxide is often referred to as TiO_2, but characterization of the film reveals different oxide states from the surface and into the metallic titanium.[5-10] The oxide growth is supposed to occur by oxygen diffusion through the existing oxide film toward the metal with a decreasing gradient in the oxygen concentration. Different oxidation states have been identified from the surface to the metallic titanium: TiO_2, Ti_2O_3, and TiO. The environment influences the titanium oxide film and incorporation of both hydroxide and water are reported.[11-17]

The surface oxide layer of titanium is considered essential for the biological performance of this material and the following properties are thought to be important. The oxide should have low solubility, no toxicity, and only a small proportion of charged species in the hydrolysis product. The isoelectric point of the oxide should be 5 to 6, which makes it slightly negative at physiological pH. The dielectric constant should be similar to the dielectric constant of water. The interaction of charged species is therefore similar to that in water.[18-25]

The thickness of this naturally formed oxide film increases slowly over a prolonged period under stable conditions. The rate and thickness of oxide formation are influenced by several factors including temperature and humidity. These properties produce a surface that is passive in biological tissues and performs well clinically, particularly as dental implant material.[26-32]

By observing tissue response to implanted titanium with natural oxides, speculation centers on whether this natural surface has the best qualities that can be gained with titanium or whether it is possible to improve its biological properties. A number of methods have been introduced for modification of the titanium oxide layer. Some of these are well elaborated and show promising results.[33-53]

18.2 Surface Modifications

18.2.1 Electrochemical Oxidation

18.2.1.1 Anodized Oxides

Anodic oxidation makes it possible to control the build-up of the oxide layer by manipulating the different electrochemical parameters. The oxide thickness, crystallinity, crystal structure, and porosity of the oxide film can be modified by changing the electrochemical conditions when performing anodic oxidation.

By using 0.5% KOH solution as an electrolyte and increasing voltage from 10 to 80 V, Ellingsen and Videm reported the formation of increasing thickness of the oxide film from 280 to 2240 Å.[54] These surfaces produced different colors, reflecting the oxide thickness, but electrochemical oxidation on these relative low voltage levels did not change the surface morphology. The authors did not document improvements in the biological response as measured by bone-to-implant attachment and histology.

Larsson et al. used acetic acid as an electrolyte to investigate the effect of galvanostatic anodization of titanium implants and studied further the biological effect of these implants in rabbits.[55-57] They performed the anodization by exposing the test specimens to 1M acetic acid electrolyte at room temperature and at 10 to 80 V. This treatment resulted in the formation of a 20- to 200-nm thick oxide film on the implant surfaces, depending on the voltage and irrespective of whether the implant had a machined or electropolished surface. Anodization resulted in a build-up of the oxide film and as observed by atomic force microscopy, a difference between specimens treated with 10 or 80 V was reported. By using the higher voltage, the group found a rougher appearance of the oxide layer and the surfaces also contained <2-μm diameter pits in the oxide layer. No main differences in the effects on bone healing could, however, be observed between the implants with thin or thicker oxide layers made by anodic oxidation.

By increasing the anodic-forming voltage, major changes in thickness, morphology, and crystallinity of the oxide film can be observed. Anodization with acetic acid as an electrolyte with 100 V resulted in a 202-nm thick amorphous titanium oxide film and negligible changes in porosity. Sul et al. demonstrated that when the anodic-forming voltages were increased to 200, 280, and 380 V, the oxide film thicknesses were increased to 608, 805, and 998 nm, respectively.[58]

The formation of oxide film under these conditions showed additional effects that may have clinical consequences. The films formed at these voltage levels had increasingly more porous structures with crystallinity that changed from amorphous to anatase and further to a combination of anatase and rutile at the highest voltages.

When devices with these characteristics were implanted into rabbit tibiae, a significant increase in bone-to-metal retention as measured by removal torque was recorded when compared to implants with turned surfaces or anodized at low voltage.[59] This significant increase in bone-to-metal retention can, however, be attributed to the increasing porosity of these implants, which was about 20% of the surface area. Porous implant surfaces are shown to have significantly improved retention due to bone growth into the pores and thus a mechanical fixation resistant to loads.

18.2.1.2 Effects of Surface Roughness

Variation of the surface microstructure was reported to influence stress distribution, retention of the implants in bone, and cell responses to the implant surface. The implants with rough surfaces improved bone response, with bone trabeculae growing in a perpendicular direction to the implant surface, an observation reported by several authors. Improved retention in bone was reported also after implantation of rough-surfaced implants.[60-63]

Roughness can be considered on macro-, micro-, or ultra-structural levels, and roughnesses on these different levels will probably exert different effects on the living tissues. Growth of bone into cavities or pores may result in mechanical interlocking of the material with bone, depending on the bone mass and the quality of the bone in the pores.

The optimal pore size to obtain bone in-growth might differ for different materials. An optimal pore size for titanium alloy implants of 100 μm was advocated by Breme et al.[64] When using titanium porous-coated screws of stainless steel with pore sizes of 10 to 40 μm, increased removal torque values were reported.[65] Even if such small pores do not allow a total in-growth of bone, increased retention based on mechanical interlocking can be established.

Surface roughness on a smaller scale was, however, found to be important for integration of bone with the implant surface. These findings indicate that other mechanisms, not purely based on mechanical interlocking, may determine the reactions between bony tissue and biomaterials. *In vitro* cell studies indicate that surface roughness on a micrometer scale influences the functions of the cells, the matrix deposition, and the mineralization — effects that may be more important than retention due to bone in-growth.[66-68] Cells seem to be sensitive to microtopography and appear to be able to use the morphology of the material for orientation and migration,[69-71]

Cell maturation also affects the response to surface roughness. This is in agreement with earlier observations indicating that chondrocytes are affected differently by local factors such as vitamin D and transforming growth factor-β, depending on the stages of cell maturation.[72-75] The differentiation of mesenchymal cells into fibroblasts, chondroblasts, or osteoblasts may therefore be influenced by the microtopography of the material.

The distribution of cortical or cancellous bone and the level of loading to the implant are important parameters that influence identification of ideal surface roughness. An optimal surface roughness has, however, been proposed based on experimental studies. Through a systematic investigation of the effects of surface roughness of implants and responses in rabbit bone, Wennerberg and coworkers concluded that a surface roughness of Sa 1.0 to 1.5 μm seemed to be optimal with regard to retention in bone and bone-to-implant contact as measured by histomorphometry.[76-79]

The roughness created by anodic oxidation with high voltages is in this range. The observation of an improved response of bone to implants with a surface roughness of Sa 1.0 to 1.5 μm is also in accordance with observations by von Recum and van Kooten.[80] These authors reported excellent tissue attachment without signs of inflammation when implanting filter membranes with pore sizes of 1 to 3 μm.

Based on these studies, it seems that a maximum level of biological advantage of increasing roughness on a micrometer scale is between 1.0 and 1.5 μm. This observation corresponds well with observations in *in vitro* cell experiments that bone cells are rugofile and respond positively to such surfaces with increased matrix deposition and mineralization. One reason for this may be that the less rough surfaces to a certain extent stimulate the bony tissue through loading, and the tissue in return responds with increased bone growth. Another interpretation of these observations could be that the rather rough surfaces prepared by coarse particles are recognized as smooth surfaces by the relatively small rugofile bone cells, whereas the 25-μm particles create a true rough surface identified by osteoblasts.

18.2.1.3 Nanoscale Morphology

Although microroughness seems to be an important characteristic for tissue response to biomaterials, observations also indicate a biological response to irregularities on the nanometer level. Via anodic oxidation at high voltages, the surface oxide changes from an amorphous noncrystalline state to a crystalline oxide layer. The oxide crystallinity on the surface of an implant may stimulate the bone-forming cells to increased activity, but little information about this exists in the literature and more studies should be performed. This observation of increased roughness after anodization of titanium was in line with earlier transmission electron microscopy (TEM) studies demonstrating increased pore sizes with increased oxide thickness.[81]

Implants with this thick heterogeneous oxide seemed to produce a slightly improved response in bone, particularly in the first weeks after implantation. This difference could, however, not be observed after longer healing periods. This is in accordance with earlier observations by Ellingsen and Videm that did not show a significant correlation between oxide thickness on titanium implants and bony responses.[54] The latter observation was measured by push-out experiments and histomorphometry after 8-week healing of titanium implants in rabbits. The authors argued that the outermost molecular layers of the biomaterial are the important parameters for bone response, determined by the surface chemistry exposed to the tissue. Morphological changes on a nanometer level may introduce additional effects to the tissue response, which in turn can further improve bone healing.

18.2.1.4 Ion Implantation of Oxide

The build-up of oxide film during anodization can also be influenced by ions in the electrolyte. Ishizawa et al. combined anodic oxidation of titanium at 350 V in an electrolytic solution containing sodium β-glycerophosphate and calcium acetate and hydrothermal treatment in high-pressure steam at

300°C.[82-84] A 1- to 2-mm thick layer of hydroxyapatite (HA) was formed on top of a 5-mm thick layer of Ca and P rich titanium oxide. The group observed significantly increased push-out shear strength compared with spark-anodized implants with Ca- and P-containing oxides. They also reported that the spark-anodized, hydrothermal-treated implants had high osteoconductivity, on the level of plasma-sprayed HA implants.

Introducing Ca or P into the electrolyte solution will incorporate these ions into the oxide layer formed during anodic oxidation and may thus influence biological reactions following implantation. This was presented recently by Sul and coworkers who produced oxide films on titanium implants by anodic oxidation with sulfuric acid or phosphoric acid as an electrolyte.[85] These oxide layers had porous structures with numbers of craters. In one animal study, implants with such surfaces had increased bone-to-metal contact as measured by histomorphometry. The S-containing implant also had increased removal torque. This effect may be due to the changed chemistry of the oxide layer, but may as well be due to the changed surface morphology of these implants as expressed by increased porosity.

Calcium ions can also be incorporated into the oxide layers of titanium implants by ion implantation. With an ion-beam current density of 50 $\mu A/cm^2$ and an acceleration energy of 18 KeV, Hanawa made titanium implants with surfaces characterized as complex oxides of calcium and titanium: $CaTiO_3$ with a surface oxide thickness of 10 nm.[86] After implanting these materials into rat tibiae for 2, 8, and 18 days using tetracycline and calcein markers, the authors reported more new bone formation around these implants compared with untreated implants as early as 2 days post-op. They concluded that the Ca ion-implanted surfaces were superior to pure titanium with respect to bone conduction. They did not discuss the influences of differences in surface morphology on bone responses.

By exposing titanium oxide to calcium phosphate solutions, Ca can be incorporated into the oxide layers of titanium implants. This technique was reported by Takamura in a study comparing this technique with titanium oxide- and Ca-implanted Ti implants in the mandibles of beagles.[87] New bone formation started after 1 week on the surfaces of the old cortex bones of all groups. At 2 weeks, newly formed bone was in contact with all test implants. Ca ion implantation into the oxide layer was suggested as an alternative technique to thicker layers as is common with hydroxyapatite coatings. The problems such as delamination and biodegradation experienced with thicker coatings should not occur with ion implantation.

18.2.2 Fluoride-Modified Oxide

Most effort has focused on modification with or implantation of Ca, P, and even O ions into the titanium oxide layer. These ions were chosen because they are natural parts of the apatite structure in bone. Their incorporation into the titanium oxide film will thus make the film more similar to the bone.

An incorporation of these ions into the titanium oxide film will, however, not necessarily result in osteoconduction and a faster and better integration of the implant and the bone structure.

Modification or treatment with other ions may be more potent either through a stimulation effect by the ion or through structural changes in the surface caused by the ion. One very promising candidate for this purpose is the fluoride ion. The titanium oxide film can be modified with fluoride to produce improved biological response.

Modification of the titanium oxide layer by fluoride at low concentrations causes only small structural changes of the surface. A mean reduction of the Sa value from 1.12 (0.24) to 0.91 (0.14) μm was reported by Johansson et al. after analyzing the surfaces of TiO_2-blasted implants and similar implants with fluoride-modified surfaces.[88] The fluoride-modified blasted implants had slightly smoother surfaces compared with the blasted control implants. Generally, rougher surfaces at micrometer level have improved biological and physiochemical properties, but this slightly smoother surface has other properties important for a bone–implant interaction. One such property is the ability to react with or adsorb calcium and phosphate to the surface. High calcium–phosphate binding capacity may indicate an improved capacity to react with calcified tissues and thus create integration between the implant and bone. The capacity of binding with calcium and phosphate can be tested *in vitro* by exposing the implants to radioactive labeled ^{32}P in a sodium phosphate buffer at pH 7.2.

A significantly higher level of phosphate adsorbed to fluoride-modified titanium implants compared with pure titanium implants after 24 hours in such a test system.[89] These high ^{32}P levels on the surfaces of fluoride-modified implants demonstrated elevated nucleation activity. The ability to induce nucleation of calcium–phosphate on the implant surfaces can also be explored in a saturated calcium–phosphate buffer at 37°C. By monitoring the Ca^{2+} concentration in the solution after introducing the implants into the system, any changes in the stability of the system can be recorded. A drop in Ca^{2+} concentration will indicate that nucleation takes place with formation of calcium–phosphate-containing precipitates on the implant surfaces. Pure titanium implants do not induce precipitation in such a system, even if the surface is blasted by TiO_2 particles to produce a rough surface structure.

After fluoride-modified implants were added to such a system, the concentration of calcium in the solution dropped significantly over time. This indicated that a reaction occurred between the implant surface and the calcium and phosphate in the solution — a desirable reaction in a clinical situation. Scanning electron microscopy following this nucleation test identified several precipitates on the test implant surfaces. Similar precipitates were not visible on the pure titanium implant surfaces. Calcium, phosphorus, and oxygen were identified in these precipitates, indicating that the precipitates formed on the fluoride-modified surfaces contained calcium and phosphate. The exact stoichiometry was not identified.[89]

Much effort has focused on coating titanium implants with calcium and phosphate ions or ceramics with the intent of producing implants with surfaces that mimic nature. These surfaces should bind to calcium phosphates in the body. Studies of fluoride-modified implants have shown that this surface treatment of titanium may be highly beneficial for allowing titanium implants to react with calcified tissues in the body. Whether the effect observed *in vitro* is due to a chemical reaction by incorporated fluoride ions in the titanium oxide layer or a reaction induced by structural changes is not known. Stimulation of physicochemical reactions such as the precipitation of calcium phosphates may occur by still unknown processes. Much focus has been on the surface morphology on the micrometer level, while potent effects may occur due to modifications on the nanometer level.

Similar beneficial effects of fluoride-modified implant surfaces observed *in vitro* have also been observed *in vivo*. Implants with this surface modification were installed in rabbit bone, and the bone reactions were studied with respect to the fixation of the implants to bone and histological analysis. Machined conical-shaped implants were implanted into the ulnae of chinchilla rabbits and allowed to heal for 4 or 8 weeks.[90] Half of the implants had fluoride-modified surfaces and the other half had no modifications and served as controls. The fixation of implants to bones was investigated by a push-out technique and standardized equipment. After 4 and after 8 weeks, the implants with the fluoride-modified surfaces had higher retention to the bone than the control group. Scanning electron microscopy after the pull-out test showed that the test implants had large areas partly covered by bone still attached to the implant surface. This was not observed on the control implants. This finding may be explained by internal fracture of the bone during the extraction procedure due to a higher fixation between the implant and the bone than the internal strength of the bone.

18.2.2.1 Experiments with Blasted Implant Surfaces

The effect of fluoride modification of titanium surface oxide has also been studied with blasted implant surfaces. Due to roughness, higher retention in bone has been documented for blasted surfaces. It was therefore of interest to study whether an additional surface modification of the titanium implant could further increase bone–implant interaction. Bone responses to titanium-threaded implants with three different surface characteristics were investigated and compared: machined surfaces, blasted surfaces (TiO_2 particles), and blasted surfaces (TiO_2 particles) plus fluoride-modified oxide layers. The threaded implants were 4.5 mm in height and 3.5 mm in diameter. The threads had 60-degree angles and gradients of 0.6. The top of each implant had a hexagonal head that fit into a removal torque controller (Figure 18.1).

Twenty-three implants were inserted into the tibial bones of chinchilla rabbits by a standardized technique that included drilling with burs of increasing size and cooling with sterile saline. The soft tissue was sutured in layers and the implants were allowed to heal for 60 days, after which the

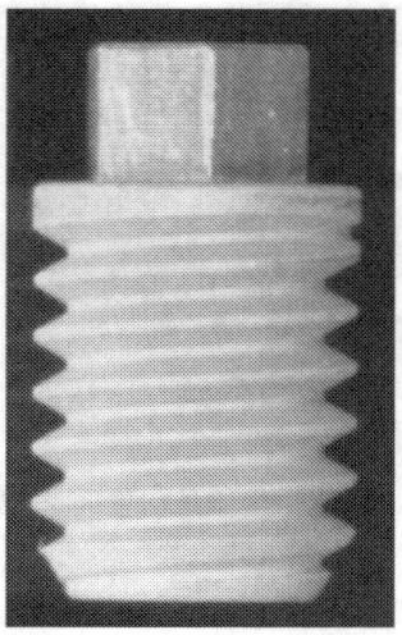

FIGURE 18.1
The titanium implant used in the rabbit study had a height of 4.5 mm and a diameter of 3.5 mm. The threads had 60-degree angles and gradients of 0.6. The hexagonal top fitted into a removal torque controller.

animals were euthanized. The implants were immediately exposed and the fixation in the bone was tested by a removal torque controller using a standardized method. Increasing force was applied until the implants loosened, after which the torque was discontinued and the bone with the implant was processed for histological examination.

The removal torque test revealed significant differences in the attachment among the three test groups (Figure 18.2). The machined implants had a mean removal torque value of 17.2 Ncm (standard deviation = 3.1), whereas

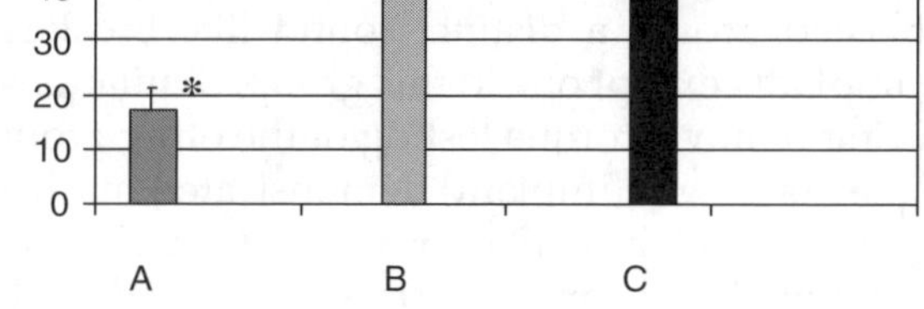

FIGURE 18.2
Mean removal torque values for titanium implants of different surface structure and chemistry recorded after a 60-day healing period in rabbit tibiae. Group A: machined titanium surface. Group B: titanium implant surface blasted with TiO_2 particles. Group C: titanium implant surface blasted with TiO_2 particles and a fluoride-modified surface oxide film. Implants with machined surfaces (A) showed significantly lower retention in bone compared with the two other test groups ($p = <0.005$). The implants with the blasted and fluoride-modified surface film (C) had significantly higher retention in bone compared with the implants with only blasted surfaces and similar microstructures ($p = <0.005$). Clear, fracture-like sounds were heard when 9 of the 10 implants in the group were loosened at maximum torque value.

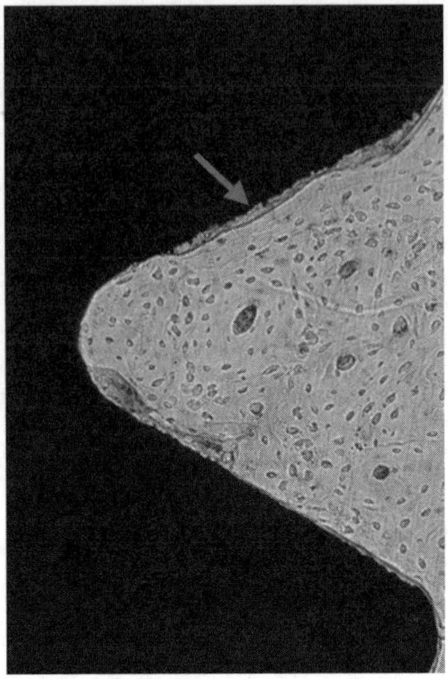

FIGURE 18.3
Histological section showing bone in one thread of a machined surfaced implant (Group A) after the torque test demonstrating bone in close contact with the implant surface; in some areas, the bone separated from the implant surface (arrow).

the blasted implants had an attachment of 56.0 Ncm (standard deviation = 9.0) — significantly higher than the machined implants ($p = <0.005$). Even higher implant retentions were recorded for the blasted implants that had fluoride-modified surface oxide layers. The implants in this group had a mean retention of 69.5 Ncm (standard deviation = 10.5) — significantly higher than the blasted implants ($p = <0.005$).

During measurement of the removal torques of the implants of the fluoride-modified blasted group, a distinct sound like breaking of bone was recorded for all implants except one in this group. Similar observations were not recorded during removal torque testing of the other groups. Histological examination of the bone (with implant) demonstrated marked differences of the groups. The bone had grown into a relative tight connection to the implant in the machined-and-turned surface group and the histological picture was similar to previous reports on this type of surface (Figure 18.3). The blasted implants had tighter bone connections and fewer nonmineralized lacunae than observed in the machined group (Figure 18.4). The implants with blasted and fluoride-modified surface oxides showed a different histological picture. The bone grew in tight contact with the implant surface, but bone growth could also be seen on the implant surface in the central part of the bone, an area that had no bone before the operation. As can be seen in Figure 18.5a, bone lined the surface of the implant in this area as well as the apical part of the implant (Figure 18.5b).

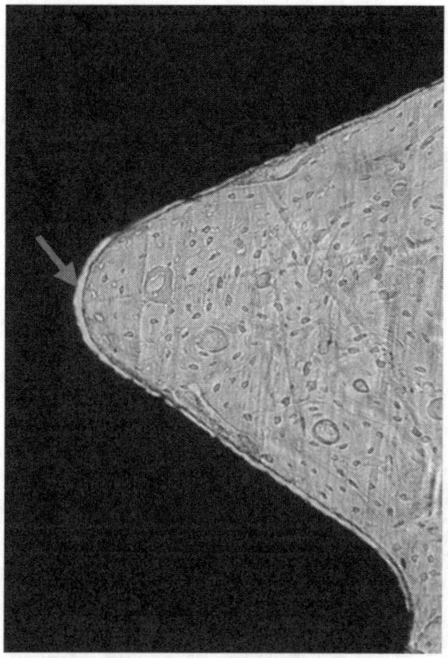

FIGURE 18.4
Histological section showing bone in one thread of an implant with TiO_2-blasted surface (Group B) after the torque test. The bone follows the implant surface geometry, indicating a close bone-to-metal contact. The gap between the bone and the implant surface (arrow) was probably created during the torque test.

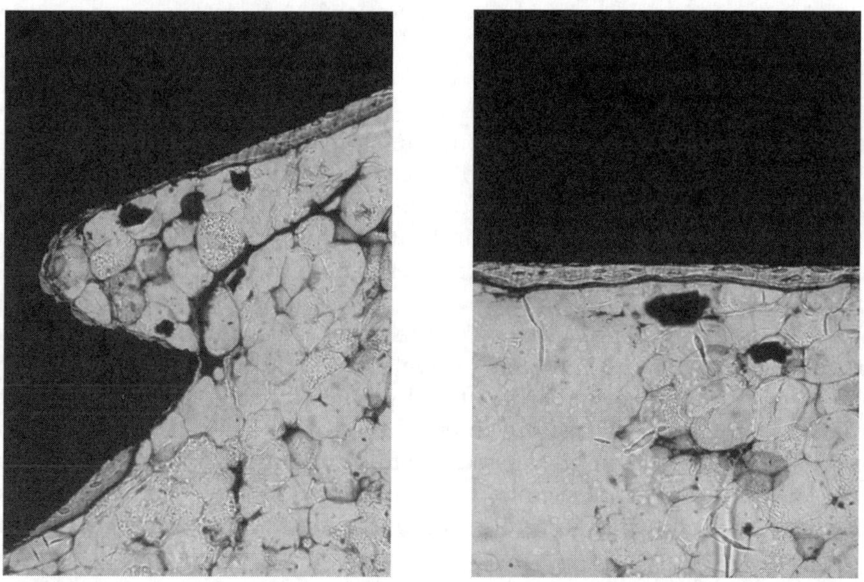

a b

FIGURE 18.5
Histological sections showing bone lining the surface of an implant with TiO_2-blasted and fluoride-modified surface oxide film. The bone also lines the apical part of the implant.

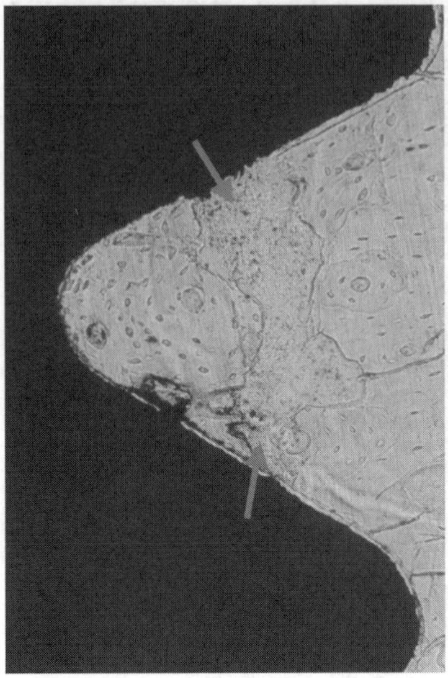

FIGURE 18.6
Histological section of bone in a thread of a titanium implant with TiO_2- blasted and fluoride-modified surface oxide film after the torque test. A tight connection between the bone and implant surface can be observed in the valley of the thread. A fracture line can also be observed demonstrating that a bone had fractured during the removal torque test. This indicates that the binding between bone and the fluoride-modified test implant was higher than the recorded removal torque values.

After a healing period of 60 days, new bone formation was observed extending from the cortical bone along the titanium implant surface. A lining of the implants with new bone in this area as observed on the implants that had blasted and fluoride-modified surfaces is, however, not a common observation. The observation is a strong indication of improved bone response to these surfaces compared to bone responses to both the machined and blasted surfaces.

Another interesting observation of the bone structure was found in the cortical region after the removal torque test of these implants. Normally, bone would have loosened from the implant surface during the removal torque test, but several fracture lines could be observed internally in the bone in the thread area of the blasted and fluoride-modified implants (Figure 18.6). This observation can explain the distinct sound recorded when these implants came loose at high torque values during the test. The mean torque value of these implants was 69.5 Ncm, significantly higher than the torque values of the other groups. A fracture of bone during the removal torque test shows that the bone had a higher retention to the implant surface than the recorded torque value.

18.2.2.2 Clinical Perspectives

From clinical perspectives in dental implantology and in orthopedic surgery, it is of great importance for a patient to have as short a postoperative period as possible and be able to use or load an implant shortly after the operation. It is also desirable to be able to place an implant into bone of nonoptimal quality because nonoptimal bone is often found in the posterior parts of the maxilla.

The development of implants with rough surface structures has improved and widened the indications for implants because such implants have proven to allow better fixation and retention in bone as discussed previously. The observation that bone grows into firm contact with implants with fluoride-modified surfaces and that these implants have increased retention strongly indicates that fluoride-modified implants may further improve clinical results and change clinical protocols. Implants with this surface modification seem to reach a usually accepted level of retention and a higher bone-to-implant contact with shorter healing time than commonly used clinical implants with machined or blasted surfaces.

18.2.2.3 Discussion

The mechanism for this improved bone response may be dual. The fluoride modification may change the titanium oxide by incorporation of fluoride ions and thus lead to improved reaction with the calcified tissue. Fluoride has, at low concentrations, several beneficial effects in bone. Among these are increased incorporation of newly formed collagen into the bone matrix, increased rate of seeding of apatite crystals, increased trabecular bone density, and stimulation of osteoprogenitor cell numbers *in vitro*.[91,92] It is also possible that the observed minor morphological differences between fluoride-modified surfaces and controls may have biological potential that is currently not identified.

Much research has focused on the effect of surface morphology on the micrometer level. Apart from the effect of bone in-growth into the rough structure and subsequent bone interlocking, other mechanisms for this effect have not shown clinical significance. Morphological changes on the nanometer level may exert other effects on the living tissues that are currently not known. More focus will probably be given to this topic in the future and chemical modification and nanostructures may have potential to further improve the integration between biomaterials and biological tissues.

References

1. Lausmaa, J., Surface spectroscopic characterization of titanium implant materials, *J. Electron. Spectrosc. Relat. Phenom.*, 81, 343, 1996.

2. Sittig, C. et al., Surface characterization of implant materials c.p. Ti, Ti-6AL-7Nb and Ti-6Al-4V with different pretreatments, *J. Mater. Sci. Mater. Med.*, 10, 35, 1999.
3. McCafferty, E. and Wightman, J.P., An x-ray photoelectron spectroscopy sputter profile study of the native air-formed oxide film on titanium, *Appl. Surf. Sci.*, 14, 92, 1999.
4. Poilleau, J. et al., Structure and composition of passive titanium oxide films, *Mater. Sci. Eng.*, 47, 235, 1997.
5. Fraker, A.C. et al., Surface preparation and corrosion behavior of titanium alloys for surgical implants, in *Titanium Alloys in Surgical Implants*, Luckey, H.A. and Kubli, F., Eds., Special Technical Publication 796, American Society for Testing & Materials, Philadelphia, 1983, p. 206.
6. Carley, A.F. et al., The identification and characterization of mixed oxide states at oxidized titanium surfaces by analysis of x-ray photoelectron spectra, *J. Chem. Soc. Faraday Trans. I*, 83, 351, 1987.
7. Healy, K.E. and Ducheyne, P., Hydration and preferential molecular adsorption on titanium *in vitro*, *Biomaterials*, 13, 553, 1992.
8. Callen, B.W. et al., Nitric acid passivation of Ti-6AL-4V reduces thickness of surface oxide layer and increases trace element release, *J. Biomed. Mater. Res.*, 29, 279, 1995.
9. Olefjord, I. and Hansson, S., Surface analysis of four dental implant systems, *Int. J. Oral Maxillofac. Implants*, 8, 32, 1993.
10. Machnee, C.H. et al., Identification of oxide layers of commercially pure titanium in response to cleaning procedures, *Int. J. Oral Maxillofac. Implants*, 8, 529, 1993.
11. Bullock, E.L., Patthey, L., and Steinemann, S.G., Clean and hydroxylated rutile TiO_2 (110) surfaces studied by x-ray photoelectron spectroscopy, *Surf. Sci.*, 352, 504, 1996.
12. Boehm, H.P., Acidic and basic properties of hydroxylated metal oxide surfaces, *Discuss. Faraday Soc.*, 52, 264, 1971.
13. Stumm, W. and Sigg, L.M., *Chemistry of the Solid Water Interface Processes at the Mineral Water and Particle Water Interface in Natural Systems*, John Wiley & Sons, New York, 1992.
14. Healy, K.E. and Ducheyne, P., Oxidation kinetics of titanium thin films in model physiological environments, *J. Colloid. Interface Sci.*, 150, 404, 1992.
15. Jobin, M. et al., Hydroxylation and crystallisation of electropolished titanium surface, *Ultramicroscopy*, 42, 637, 1992.
16. Gold, J.M., Schmidt, M., and Steinemann, S.G., XPS study of amino acid adsorption to titanium surfaces, *Helv. Phys. Acta*, 62, 246, 1989.
17. McCafferty, E. and Wightman, J.P., Determination of the concentration of surface hydroxyl groups on metal oxide films by a quantitative XPS method, *Surf. Interface Anal.*, 26, 549, 1998.
18. Tengvall, P. and Lundström, I., Physico-chemical considerations of titanium as a biomaterial, *Clin. Mater.*, 9, 115, 1992.
19. Steinemann, S.G., Corrosion of surgical implants: *in vivo* and *in vitro* tests, in *Evaluations of Biomaterials*, Winter, G.D., Leray, J.L., and de Groot, K., Eds., John Wiley & Sons, New York, 1980, p. 1.
20. Williams, D.F., Electrochemical aspects of corrosion in the physiological environment, in *Fundamental Aspects of Biocompatibility*, Williams, D.F., Ed., CRC Press, Boca Raton, FL, 1981, p. 11.

21. Steinemann, S.G. and Mäusli, P.A., Titanium alloys for surgical implants: biocompatibility from physiochemical principles, in *Proceedings of the Sixth World Conference on Titanium*, Société Francaise de Métallurgie, Les Editions de Physique, Les Ulis, Cannes, 1989, p. 535.
22. Kovacs, P. and Davidson, J.A., Chemical and electrochemical aspects of the biocompatibility of titanium and its alloys, in *Medical Applications of Titanium and its Alloys*, Brown, S.A. and Lemon, J.E., Eds., American Society for Testing & Materials, West Conshohocken, PA, 1996, p. 163.
23. Steinemann, S.G., Tissue compatibility of metals from physicochemical principles, in *Proceedings of a Symposium on the Compatibility of Biomedical Implants*, Kovacs, P. and Istephanous, N.S., Eds., Electrochemical Society, Pennington, NJ, 1994, p. 1.
24. Steinemann, S.G., Titanium: the material of choice? *Periodontology 2000*, 17, 7, 1998.
25. Textor, M. et al., Properties and biological significance of natural oxide films on titanium and its alloys, in *Titanium in Medicine*, Brunette, D.M. et al., Eds., Springer, Heidelberg, 171, 2001.
26. Adell, R. et al., A 15-year study of osseointegrated implants in the treatment of the edentulous jaw, *Int. J. Oral Surg.*, 10, 387, 1981.
27. Adell, R. et al., A long-term follow-up study of osseointegrated implants in the treatment of totally edentulous jaws, *Int. J. Oral Maxillofac. Implants*, 5, 347, 1990.
28. Albrektsson, T. et al., Osseointegrated titanium implants: requirements for ensuring a long-lasting, direct bone-to-implant anchorage in man, *Acta Orthopaed. Scand.*, 52, 155, 1981.
29. Albrektsson, T., On long-term maintenance of the osseointegrated response, *Austral. Prosth. J.*, 7, 15, 1993.
30. Brånemark, P.I. et al., Intraosseous anchorage of dental prostheses. I. Experimental studies, *Scand. J. Plast. Reconstruct. Surg.*, 3, 81, 1969.
31. Brånemark, P.I. et al., Osseointegrated implants in the treatment of the edentulous jaw: experience from a 10-year period, *Scand. J. Plast. Reconstruct. Surg.*, 16, 1, 1977.
32. Buser, D. et al., Tissue integration of one-stage ITI implants: 3-year results of a longitudinal study with hollow-cylinder and hollow-screw implants, *Int. J. Oral Maxillofac. Surg.*, 6, 405, 1991
33. Shirkhanzadeh, M., Nanoporous alkoxy-derived titanium oxide coating: a reactive overlayer for functionalizing titanium surface, *J. Mater. Sci. Mater. Med.*, 9, 355, 1998.
34. Haddow, D.B., James, P.F., and van Noort, R., Sol gel-derived calcium phosphate coatings for biomedical applications, *J. Sol Gel Sci. Tech.*, 13, 261, 1998.
35. Wei, M. et al., Apatite-forming ability of CaO-containing titania, *Biomaterials*, 23, 167, 2002.
36. Kim, H.M. et al., Preparation of bioactive Ti and its alloy via simple chemical surface treatment, *J. Biomed. Mater. Res.*, 32, 409, 1996.
37. Yan, W.Q. et al., Bonding of chemically treated titanium implants to bone, *J. Biomed. Mater. Res.*, 37, 267, 1997.
38. Skripitz, R. and Aspenberg, P., Tensile bond between bone and titanium: a reappraisal of osseointegration, *Acta Orthop. Scand.*, 69, 2, 1998.
39. Nishiguchi, S. et al., Enhancement of bone-bonding strengths of titanium alloy implants by alkali and heat treatments, *J. Biomed. Mater. Res.*, 48, 689, 1999.
40. Nishiguchi, S. et al., The effect of heat treatment on bone-bonding ability of alkali-treated titanium, *Biomaterials*, 20, 491, 1999.

41. Fujibayashi, S. et al., Bioactive titanium: effect of sodium removal on the bone-bonding ability of bioactive titanium prepared by alkali and heat treatment, *J. Biomed. Mater. Res.*, 56, 562, 2001.
42. Hazan, R., Brener, R., and Oron, U., Bone growth to metal implants is regulated by their surface chemical properties, *Biomaterials*, 14, 570, 1993.
43. Hazan, R. and Oron, U., Enhancement of bone-growth into metal screw implanted in the medullary canal of the femur in rats, *J. Orthopaed. Res.*, 11, 655, 1993.
44. Bess, E. et al., Protein adsorption and osteoblast responses to heat-treated titanium surfaces, *Implant. Dent.*, 8, 168, 1999.
45. Bacakova, L. et al., Polishing and coating carbon fiber-reinforced carbon composites with a carbon-titanium layer enhances adhesion and growth of osteoblast-like MG63 cells and vascular smooth muscle cells *in vitro*, *J. Biomed. Mater. Res.*, 54, 567, 2001.
46. Ektessabi, A.M., Surface modification of biomedical implants using ion-beam-assisted sputter deposition, *Nucl. Instr. Meth. Phys. Res. B*, 127–128, 1008, 1997.
47. Hanawa, T. et al., Early bone formation around calcium ion-implanted titanium inserted into rat tibiae, *J. Biomed. Mater. Res.*, 36, 131, 1997.
48. Hanawa, T., *In vivo* metallic biomaterials and surface modification, *Mat. Sci. Eng. A Struct.*, 267, 260, 1999.
49. Keller, J.C., Marshall, G.W., and Brown, I., Effects of Ca ion implantation on bone cell responses, *J. Dent. Res.*, 73, 400, 1994.
50. Krupa, D. et al., Effect of calcium ion implantation on the corrosion resistance and biocompatibility of titanium, *Biomaterials*, 22, 2139, 2001.
51. Pham, M.T. et al., Promoted hydroxyapatite nucleation on titanium ion-implanted with sodium, *Thin Solid Films*, 379, 50, 2000.
52. Pham, M.T. et al., Surface-induced reactivity for titanium by ion implantation, *J. Mater. Sci. Mater. Med.*, 11, 383, 2000.
53. Wang, X.H. et al., *In vivo* and *in vitro* investigation of titanium oxide layers coated on LTI-carbon by IBED, *J. Mater. Sci.*, 36, 2067, 2001.
54. Ellingsen, J.E. and Videm, K., Effect of oxide thickness on the reaction between titanium implants and bone, *Adv. Sci. Tech. Mater. Clin. Appl.*, 12, 543, 1995.
55. Larsson, C. et al., Bone response to surface modified titanium implants: studies on electropolished implants with different oxide thicknesses and morphology, *Biomaterials*, 15, 1062, 1994.
56. Larsson, C. et al., Bone response to surface modified titanium implants: studies on the early tissue response to machined and elctropolished implants with different oxide thicknesses, *Biomaterials*, 17, 605, 1996.
57. Larsson, C. et al., Bone response to surface modifed titanium implants: studies on the tissue response after 1 year to machined and electropolished implants with different oxide thicknesses, *J. Mater. Sci. Mater. Med.*, 8, 1997, 721.
58. Sul, Y.-T. et al., Characteristics of the surface oxides on turned and electrochemically oxidized pure titanium implants up to dielectric breakdown: the oxide thickness, micropore configurations, surface roughness, crystal structure and chemical composition, *Biomaterials*, 23, 491, 2002.
59. Sul, Y.-T. et al., Resonance frequency and removal torque analysis of implants with turned and anodized surface oxides, *Clin. Oral. Implant Res.*, 13, 252, 2002.
60. Bloebaum, R.D. et al., Mineral apposition rates of human cancellous bone at the interface of porous coated implants, *J. Biomed. Mater. Res.*, 28, 537, 1994.

61. Boyan, B.D. et al., The titanium–bone cell interface *in vitro*: the role of the surface in promoting osteointegration, in *Titanium in Medicine*, Brunette, D.M. et al., Eds., Springer, Berlin, 2001, p. 561.
62. Thomas, K.A. and Cook, S.D., An evaluation of variables influencing implant fixation by direct bone apposition, *J. Biomed. Mater. Res.*, 19, 875, 1985.
63. Buser, D. et al., Influence of surface characteristics on bone integration of titanium implants: a histomorphometric study in miniature pigs, *J. Biomed. Mater. Res.*, 25, 889, 1991.
64. Breme, J., Wadewitz, V., and Fürbacher, B., Production and mechanical properties of porous sintered specimens of the implant alloy Ti-Al5-Fe2.5, in *Clinical Implant Materials: Advances in Biomaterials*, Heimke, G., Soltész, U., and Lee, A.J.C., Eds., Elsevier, Amsterdam, 1990, p. 9.
65. Predecki, P. et al., Kinetics of bone growth into cylindrical channels in aluminium oxide and titanium, *J. Biomed. Mat. Res.*, 6, 375, 1972.
66. Boyan, B.D. et al., Effect of titanium surface characteristics on chondrocytes and osteoblasts *in vitro*, *Cells Mater.*, 5, 323, 1995.
67. Martin, J.Y. et al., Effect of titanium surface roughness on proliferation, differentiation and protein synthesis of human osteoblast-like cells (MG63), *J. Biomed. Mater. Res.*, 29, 389, 1995.
68. Schwartz, Z. et al., Effect of titanium surface roughness on chondrocyte proliferation, matrix production, and differentiation depends on the state of cell maturation, *J. Biomed. Mater. Res.*, 30, 145, 1996.
69. Brunette, D.M., The effects of implant surface topography on the behaviour of cells, *Int. J. Oral Maxillofac. Implants*, 3, 231, 1988.
70. Cheroudi, B., Gould, T.R.L., and Brunette, D.M., Effects of a grooved titanium-coated implant surface on epithelial cell behaviour *in vitro* and *in vivo*, *J. Biomed. Mater. Res.*, 23, 1067, 1989.
71. Cheroudi, B., Gould, T.R.L., and Brunette, D.M., Titanium-coated micromachined grooves of different dimensions affect epithelial and connective tissue cells differently *in vivo*, *J. Biomed. Mater. Res.*, 24, 1203, 1990.
72. Schwartz, Z. et al., Production of 1,25-dihydroxyvitamin D_3 and 24,25-dihydroxyvitamin D_3 by growth zone and resting zone chondrocytes is dependent on cell maturation and is regulated by hormones and growth factors, *Endocrinology*, 130, 2495, 1992.
73. Schwartz, Z. et al., Direct effects of transforming growth factor-beta on chondrocytes are modulated by vitamin D metabolites in a cell maturation-specific manner, *Endocrinology*, 132, 1544, 1993.
74. Schwartz, Z. et al., Effect of titanium surface roughness on chondrocyte proliferation, matrix production, and differentiation depends on the state of cell maturation, *J. Biomed. Mater. Res.*, 30, 145, 1996.
75. Sylvia, V.L. et al., Maturation-dependent regulation of protein kinase C activity by vitamin D_3 metabolites in chondrocyte cultures, *J. Cell. Physiol.*, 157, 271, 1993.
76. Wennerberg, A. et al., A histomorphometric and removal torque study of screw-shaped titanium implants with three different surface topographies, *Clin. Oral Implants Res.*, 6, 24, 1995.
77. Wennerberg, A., Albrektsson, T., and Lausmaa, J., Torque and histomorphometric evaluation of c.p. titanium screws blasted with 25- and 75-micron-sized particles of Al_2O_3, *J. Biomed. Mater. Res.*, 30, 251, 1996.

78. Wennerberg, A., Albrektsson, T., and Andersson, B., Bone tissue response to commercially pure titanium implants blasted with fine and coarse particles of aluminum oxide, *Int. J. Oral Maxillofac. Implants,* 11, 38, 1996.
79. Wennerberg, A. et al., Experimental study of turned and grit-blasted screw-shaped implants with special emphasis on effects of blasting materials and surface topography, *Biomaterials,* 17, 15, 1996.
80. Von Recum, A.F. and van Kooten, T.G., The influence of micro-topography on cellular response and the implications for silicone implants, *J. Biomater. Sci. Polymer Ed.*, 7, 181, 1995.
81. Lausmaa, J. et al., Chemical composition and morphology of titanium surface oxides, in *Biomedical Materials,* Williams, J.M., Nichols, M.F., and Zingg, W., Eds., Materials Research Society, Pittsburgh, 1986, p. 351.
82. Ishizawa, H. and Ogino, M., Formation and characterization of anodic titanium oxide films, *J. Biomed. Mater. Res.*, 29, 65, 1995.
83. Ishizawa, H. and Ogino, M., Characterization of thin hydroxyapatite layers formed on anodic titanium oxide films containing Ca and P by hydrothermal treatment, *J. Biomed. Mater. Res.*, 29, 1071, 1995.
84. Ishizawa, H., Fujino, M., and Ogino, M., Mechanical and histological investigation of hydrothermally treated and untreated anodic titanium oxide films containing Ca and P, *J. Biomed. Mater. Res.*, 29, 1459, 1995.
85. Sul, Y.-T. et al., Bone reactions to oxidized titanium implants with electrochemical anion sulphuric acid and phosphoric acid incorporation, *Clin. Implant Dent. Rel. Res.*, 4, 78, 2002.
86. Hanawa, T. et al., Structure of surface-modified layers of calcium-ion-implanted Ti-6Al-4V and Ti-56Ni, *Mater. Trans. JIM.*, 36, 438, 1995.
87. Takamura, R. et al., The bone response of titanium implant with calcium ion implantation, *J. Dent. Res.*, 76, 1177, 1997.
88. Johansson, C.B. et al., Enhanced fixation of bone to fluoride-modified implants, in Trans. Sixth World Biomater. Congr., 2, 601, 2000.
89. Ellingsen, J.E., On the properties of surface-modified titanium, in *Bone Engineering,* Davies, J.E., Ed., em squared, Toronto, 2000, p. 183.
90. Ellingsen, J.E., Pre-treatment of titanium implants with fluoride improves their retention in bone, *J. Mater. Sci. Mater. Med.*, 6, 749, 1995.
91. Anderson, P.A. et al., Response of cortical bone to local controlled release of sodium fluoride: the effect of implant insertion site, *J. Orthopaed. Res.*, 9, 890, 1991.
92. Shteyer, A. et al., Effect of local application of fluoride on healing of experimental bone fractures in rabbits, *Calc. Tissue Res.*, 22, 297, 1977.

19

Use of Molecular Assembly Techniques for Tailoring Chemical Properties of Smooth and Rough Titanium Surfaces

Marcus Textor, Samuele Tosatti, Marco Wieland, and Donald M. Brunette

CONTENTS

19.1 Introduction 342
 19.1.1 Relevance of Surface Properties 342
 19.1.2 Biochemical Surface Modification Techniques 343
 19.1.3 Molecular Assembly Systems: Tools to Control Interfacial Processes and Implant Performance? 345
19.2 Surface Modifications of Titanium by Alkane Phosphate Self-Assembled Monolayers to Control Physicochemical Properties 348
 19.2.1 Background and Surface Technologies 348
 19.2.2 Applications to Smooth and Rough Titanium Surfaces 349
19.3 Molecular Assembly Systems to Control Non-Specific Protein Adsorption and Specific Interactions with Cells 354
 19.3.1 Background and Surface Technologies 354
 19.3.2 Poly(L-Lysine)-*Graft*-Poly(Ethylene Glycol) (PLL-g-PEG) 355
 19.3.3 Applications of PLL-g-PEG Adlayers with and without Grafted Peptides to Smooth and Rough Titanium Surfaces 357
19.4 Conclusions and Outlook 361
Acknowledgments 363
References 363

0-8493-1474-7/03/$0.00+$1.50

19.1 Introduction

19.1.1 Relevance of Surface Properties

Surface properties are important factors in the design of biomedical devices such as implants because early interactions between the synthetic material and the biological environment occur at the surface after implantation. The physical, chemical, and biochemical properties of the implant surface affect processes such as protein adsorption, cell–surface interaction, and cell and tissue development at the interface between the body and the biomaterial, all of which are relevant to the functionality of the device.[1]

Implant surface properties are likely to be of particular relevance the chemical and biological interfacial processes in the early stage after implantation. Nevertheless, it is generally accepted that the early stages are likely to affect host response to the implant and therefore the long-term outcome and success of the surgical intervention.[2,3]

Titanium and titanium alloy devices with surfaces in the "natural" state (i.e., covered by their native oxide films) or as artificially reinforced oxide films (e.g., by anodic oxidation) have a long and successful history because of the general inertness and excellent biocompatibility of titanium oxide.[3,4] In applications where integration of the titanium implant in hard (bone) tissue is of crucial importance, for example, dental implants, artificial hip joints, and osteosynthesis screws, modifications of the topography and roughness have been exploited successfully to influence the differentiation and expression of molecular factors of osteoblast cells *in vitro* and increase the kinetics of formation of close bone apposition and mechanical long-term stability of the implant–body interface *in vivo*. Readers are referred to Esposito, Wennerberg, Brunette, Paine, and Stanford (Chapters 1, 4, 6, 7, and 8, this volume) and to References 5 through 8.

While substantial efforts have been made in the past to optimize the topography of titanium surfaces for bone applications, less clear evidence is available about the importance of the chemical properties of the surface for the healing process and the ability of devices to integrate in host tissue. Even less is known about the combined effect of surface topography and chemistry, implying that an important synergistic potential for optimization is currently unexploited.

What are the arguments to justify investigating the influence of chemical compositions of titanium implant surfaces, either alone or in combination with designed topographies? Four of the possible arguments follow.

First, in an investigation of commercial dental implants, the surface chemical compositions were found to vary widely across the different types and manufacturers. Moreover, unexpected components originated from specific fabrication procedures.[9] Replacing natural (adventitious) or fabrication-related surface contamination with an outer layer of controlled chemical composition could potentially contribute to improved consistency of performance.

Second, in applications where the artificial surface is permanently exposed to blood such as in titanium or nickel–titanium stents, surface treatments would be highly beneficial provided that they were able to reduce the interactions that lead to protein adsorption, complement activation, platelet adhesion and activation, and ultimately to thrombus formation. Readers are referred to Tengvall, Chapter 16, this volume, and to References 3 and 10.

Third, biochemical modification using specific peptides (or more complex biological moieties such as proteins and growth factors) has the potential to affect several aspects of host response including:

1. Selection of specific cells from mixed populations
2. Controlling the strength of cell adhesion, for example, by altering the adhesive–peptide surface density
3. Influencing the rate of cell differentiation or expression of specific phenotypes

Although such concepts for bioactive titanium surfaces are still in research and development stages, several possible approaches may allow implant producers in the future to tailor implant surfaces more specifically to the needs of the particular application rather than simply relying on uncontrolled adsorption of cell-adhesive proteins.[11]

Fourth, calcium phosphate, particularly in the form of hydroxyapatite (HA, the main mineral phase in bone), is an important bio-inorganic material known for its excellent osteoconductive, bone-forming properties. Despite strong interest in combining the bioactive properties of HA with the excellent corrosion and mechanical properties of titanium alloys, we still have no totally satisfactory solution to the use of HA and other phosphates as coatings on metal substrates for clinical applications.

There is a clear interest by surface scientists in developing novel processes that can better fulfill the different requirements for successful use of implants in the biomedical area. Possible modifications range from the incorporation of biofunctional elements to fabrication techniques that allow production of specific precisely controlled three-dimensional shapes to process modifications that increase cost effectiveness under industrial fabrication conditions.

19.1.2 Biochemical Surface Modification Techniques

Biochemical modification can be achieved by a variety of techniques that exploit physical adsorption (through van der Waals, hydrophobic, or electrostatic forces) or chemical binding. Clearly, each approach has advantages and disadvantages. Physical adsorption occurs immediately on contact of a biomolecular solution with a biomaterial surface. Examples such as the adsorption of amino acids, peptides, proteins, and blood components are addressed in other chapters of this book. Some chemical interactions such as ionic and coordination bonds might also be involved in adsorption, but a phase equi-

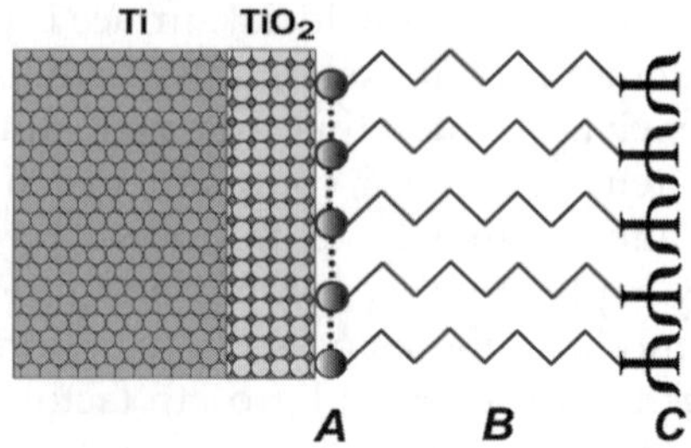

FIGURE 19.1
Biological modification of a titanium surface using thin functional adlayers. A: attachment site by physical or chemical adsorption or covalent linkage with or without cross-polymerization (dashed line). B: spacer to adjust distance of functional group Y from original surface. C: chemical, biochemical, or biological functionality (ψ) such as organofunctional group, peptide, protein. (*Source:* From Xiao, S.J. et al., in *Titanium in Medicine*, Brunette, D.M. et al., Eds., Springer, Berlin, 2001, p. 417. With permission.)

librium exists between the adsorbed species and the solution. Therefore, the adsorption is often reversible and the adsorbed species can easily be washed away with fresh buffers or replaced by other molecules in solution.

Physical and chemical adsorption processes are generally simple to implement experimentally and often allow for retention of biomolecular activity. In contrast, chemical binding involves the covalent attachment of the target molecule to a solid surface. This method is experimentally more delicate, but the resultant irreversible binding with high levels of surface coverage makes this approach more attractive. The bound molecule is much more stable under physiological conditions and is more resistant to disruption under harsh environmental conditions. However, it is important to recognize that in some cases, chemical binding can alter the conformation or orientation of the biomolecule and disturb the bioactive center of the molecule, causing a reduction in activity. Figure 19.1 shows surface modifications based on physical or chemical linkage of ligands to surfaces.

Silanization has often been used on glass or metal oxide surfaces to introduce functional groups that can be further reacted with cross-linkers to incorporate surface-exposed biochemical or biological functions such as peptides or proteins[2,12-15] (Figure 19.2a). While bioligands immobilized to surfaces through silane and cross-linker chemistry may still be biologically active, their potential activity in the presence of serum is likely to be masked by nonspecific protein adsorption. Therefore, strategies have been developed to attach bioligands to surfaces that are inherently resistant toward nonspecific biomolecule adsorption.

Cross-linked polymers have been used on a variety of substrates based on poly(ethylene glycol) (PEG), a compound known to render surfaces resistant to nonspecific adsorption. Thin films based on interpenetrating PEG-containing polymeric networks have been particularly successful in reducing unwanted adsorption and adding specific functions to surfaces.[11,16,17] Their biological functionality has been demonstrated in cell culture investigations using amino acid sequences that specifically interact with integrin- or heparin-active peptides or their synergistic combination. For a review on this topic, see Healy et al.[11]

Due to the covalent nature of surface immobilization, good chemical stability has been achieved under biologically meaningful conditions such as in a full cell culture medium. Figure 19.2b shows a typical surface architecture.

The main drawback of the surface modifications discussed above is complexity — the approach requires several consecutive surface–chemical reactions to be carried out. Apart from substantial costs that may prevent straightforward commercialization and clinical application, it is difficult to achieve sufficient batch-to-batch reproducibility and control bioligand surface density.

19.1.3 Molecular Assembly Systems: Tools to Control Interfacial Processes and Implant Performance?

Molecular self-assembly techniques have attracted substantial attention because of the elegance and simplicity with which well defined surface adlayers or thin films can be produced. One substrate–adlayer system widely studied in the past is gold–alkane thiol, now used routinely to produce model surface systems with controlled wettability (hydrophilicity–hydrophobicity), surface charges, and controlled densities of bioligand functionalities such as peptides, antibodies, and oligonucleotides. Applications are found mainly in the areas of cell–surface interactions,[18] biosensor chip modification, and microchemical and nanochemical surface patterning.[19]

Molecular assembly processes are, however, not limited to gold surfaces. Modifications of metal oxide surfaces using spontaneous adsorption of functional molecules have attracted increased interest in view of their potential usefulness for implants made of titanium, tantalum, or steel and optical sensor chips based on high refractive-indices and transition metal–oxide wave-guiding layers. Two such assembly systems for titanium and other metal oxide surfaces, alkane phosphate self-assembled monolayers (SAMs) (Figure 19.2c) and polycationic PEG-grafted copolymer adlayers (Figure 19.2d), are discussed in more detail below.

The interest in using such systems for biotechnological applications is threefold. First, they are useful for producing model surfaces with truly controlled physicochemical or biochemical properties. One particularly interesting aspect is the possibility of independent study of the effects of surface topography and surface chemical composition on biological response (Figure 19.3). Molecular assembly systems have the advantage of relying on spontaneous adsorption from solution controlled purely by physicochemical principles. Therefore, even complex surface topographies can be combined with tailored surface chemistry as long as the structures are wet by the assembly solution. Since the thickness of a typical assembled monolayer is a few nanometers, while the biologically most relevant topog-

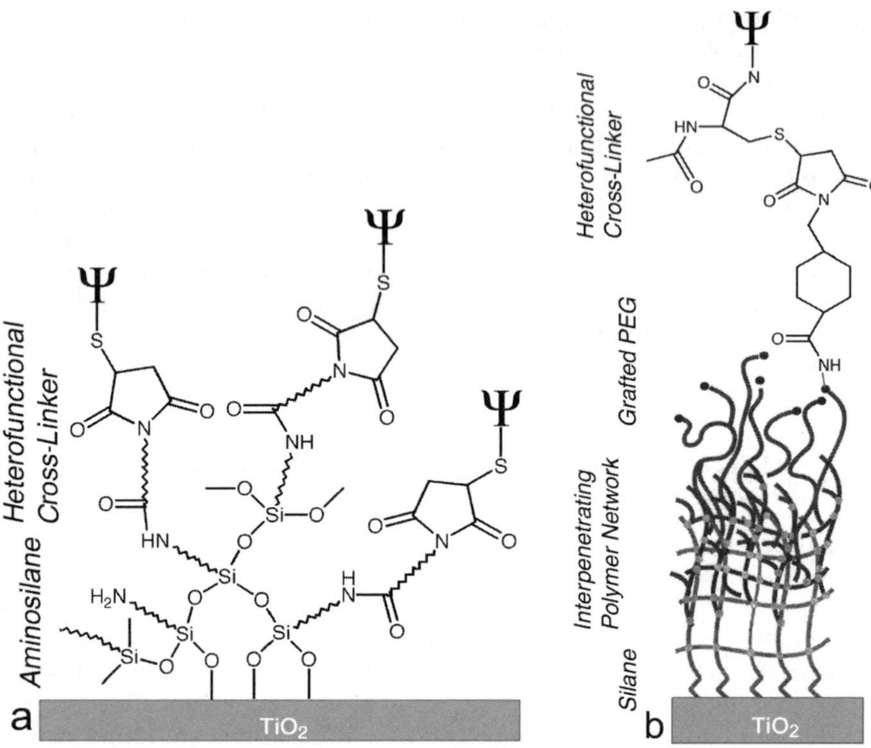

FIGURE 19.2
Structures of biomimetic peptide-modified surfaces following different functionalization concepts described or proposed in the literature: (a) silanization of the titanium oxide/hydroxide surface using (3-aminopropyl)triethoxysilane followed by covalent attachment of maleimide and subsequently of a specific peptide (ψ)[2,15]; (b) silanized surface (allyltrichlorosilane; not shown explicitly) followed by formation of a nonadhesive P(AAM-co-EG/AA) interpenetrating polymer network (IPN), grafting of diamino-PEG to acrylic acid sites in the IPN, and coupling of a peptide (ψ) to the free amine via a linker molecule (AAM = (acrylamide) BIS (N,N-methylene-bis-acrylamide; AA = acrylamide; PEG = poly(ethylene glycol)[11,16]; (c) self-assembled monolayers of long-chain alkane phosphate, partially functionalized at the terminal chain position with a peptide (ψ); the phosphate interacts with the Ti (IV) cations through coordinative complexation[23,28,29]; (d) polycationic poly(amino acid) grafted with PEG side chains for imparting protein resistance to the surface and grafted peptide for specific interaction. The poly(amino acid) has positively charged amino-terminated side chains that bind to the negatively charged titanium oxide surface through multiple-site electrostatic interactions.[45] (*Source:* From Xiao, S.-J. et al., in *Titanium in Medicine*, Brunette, D.M. et al., Eds., Springer, Berlin, 2001, p. 417. With permission.)

raphies have features with sizes >0.1 μm,[20] we can consider molecular assembly systems as tools for tailoring the chemistry of model surfaces and biomedical implant surfaces truly independently of topography. If assembly can be carried out via aqueous solutions at or near room temperature, sensitive biological entities such as proteins and growth factors can be potentially immobilized with little risk of loss of bioactivity in comparison to immobilization schemes that need organic solvents, higher temperatures,

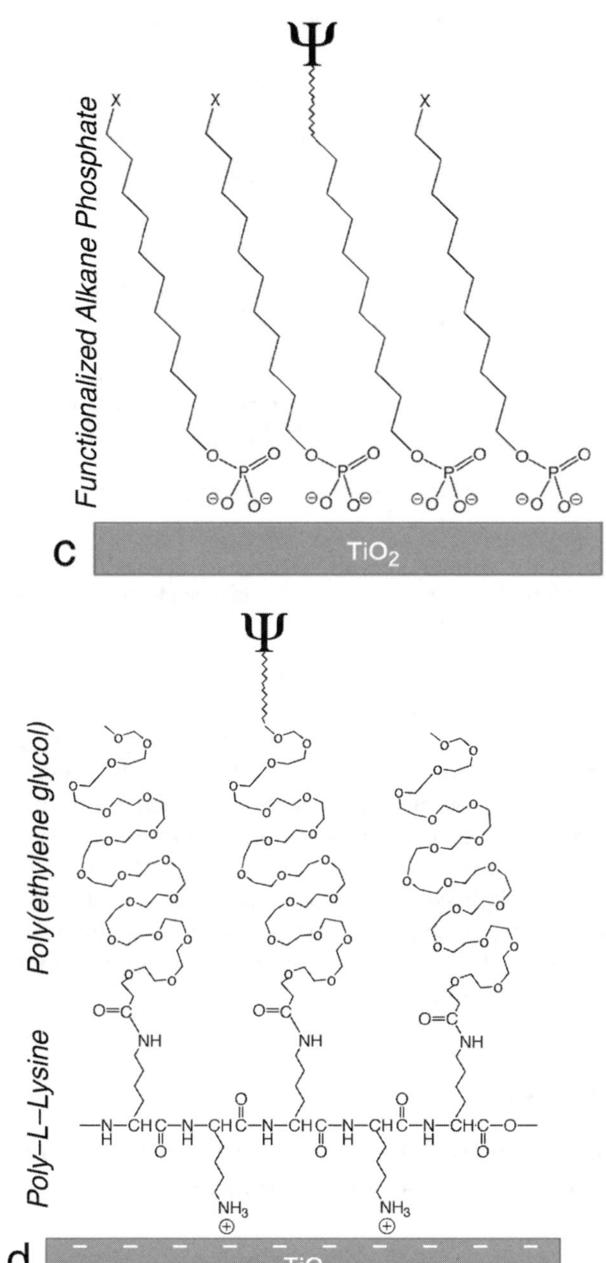

FIGURE 19.2
Continued.

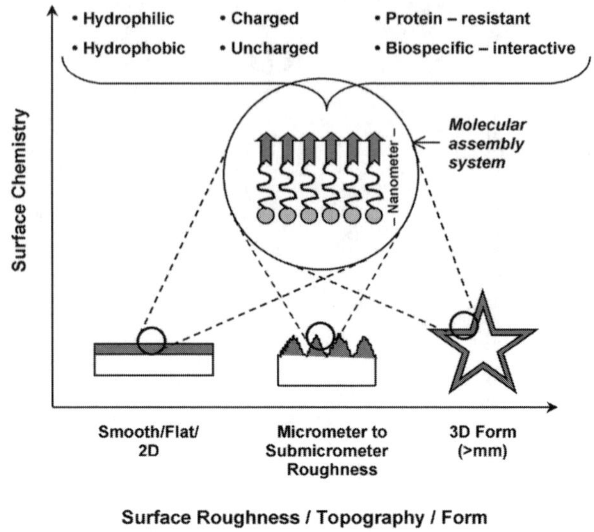

FIGURE 19.3
The ability of molecular assembly systems to tailor the surface chemistry and physicochemical properties (wettability, charge, biointeractiveness) independently of surface roughness, topography, and three-dimensional form.

mechanical actions (such as in print transfer), or ultraviolet light for photochemical coupling reactions.

It is conceivable that molecules with multifunctional properties can be designed and produced. For example, it would be desirable to combine functionalities for immobilization to the surface with functionalities that control interaction with the biological environment to achieve specific targeted interactions with cells and tissues. By combining functionalities in a single step, molecular assembly could emerge as a cost-effective robust technique to produce biologically active novel chemical surfaces on devices with complex shapes such as vascular or cardiovascular stents, osteosynthesis screws, or cages for spinal surgery.

19.2 Surface Modifications of Titanium by Alkane Phosphate Self-Assembled Monolayers to Control Physicochemical Properties

19.2.1 Background and Surface Technologies

Alkane phosphates and phosphonates have received attention for a number of years in view of their strong chemical affinities toward transition metal ions of high (≥3) valence, for example Ti (IV), Zr (IV), Nb (V), Ta (V), and Al (III). Moreover, long alkane chains (C_{12} and longer) tend to form ordered monolay-

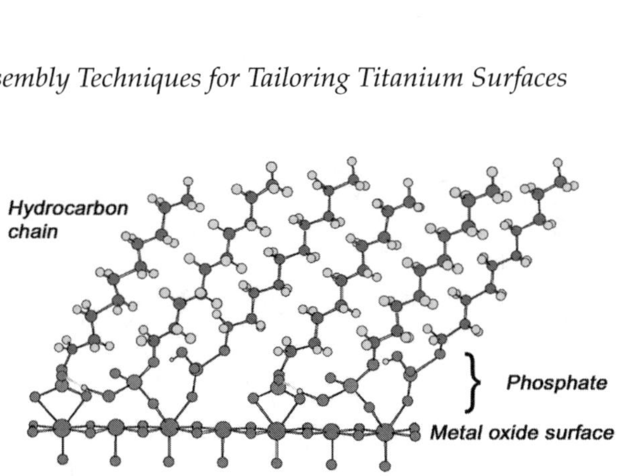

FIGURE 19.4
Model of the structure of octadecylphosphate self-assembled at the tantalum oxide surface, deduced from XPS, NEXAFS, SIMS, and AFM studies.[22,23] Only 10 of the 18 carbon atoms of the hydrocarbon chain are shown for simplicity. Analogous monolayers can be formed at titanium oxide surfaces. (*Source:* From Textor, M. et al., *Langmuir*, 16, 3257, 2000. With permission. Copyright American Chemical Society.)

ers as a consequence of both strong head group–substrate and hydrophobic–hydrophobic chain-to-chain interactions. Several papers deal with the assembly, structure, and properties of alkane phosphates on a variety of metal oxide surfaces.[19,21-26] For example, octadecyl phosphate has been shown to form adlayers spontaneously from heptane/2-propanol solutions on tantalum oxide (Ta_2O_5) surfaces, resulting in highly hydrophobic surfaces with structural and chemical properties resembling those of long-chain alkane thiols on gold.[22]

In particular, the average tilt angle of 30 degrees (relative to the surface normal) and the detection by atomic force microscopy (AFM) of two-dimensional hexagonal patterns of the terminal methyl group with characteristic intermolecular spacing of ca. 0.5 nm (measured parallel to the surface) are very close to the corresponding characteristic values reported for gold–alkane thiol SAMs and results in highly hydrophobic surfaces. Combining information from several surface characterization techniques (x-ray photoelectron spectroscopy, XPS; atomic force microscopy, AFM; time-of-flight secondary ion mass spectrometry, SIMS; and near edge x-ray absorption fine structure spectroscoppy, NEXAFS),[23,27] a model based on direct complexation of the metal cation by the phosphate head group was proposed, as shown in Figures 19.2c and 19.4.

The use of organic solvents to produce surface layers has clear disadvantages if the aim is to use such techniques on an industrial scale. Therefore, a technique based on the deposition of SAMs from purely aqueous alkyl phosphate solutions has been developed and successfully applied to a variety of metal oxide substrates[28] including TiO_2.[29]

19.2.2 Applications to Smooth and Rough Titanium Surfaces

One possible use of alkane phosphates in biomaterials applications is to produce well-defined model surfaces in which properties such as wettability,

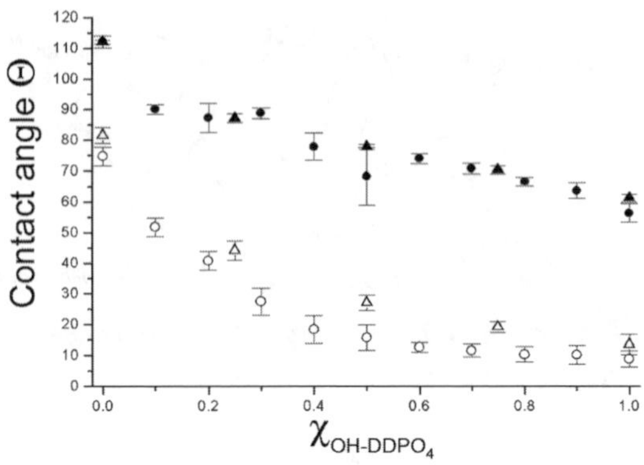

FIGURE 19.5
Advancing and receding contact angles of water on smooth titanium metal-coated glass (• = advancing; o= receding) and silicon wafer (▲ = advancing; △ = receding) surfaces as a function of OH-DDPO$_4$(NH$_4$)$_2$ concentration in SAM-forming solution expressed as a mole fraction, $\chi_{OH-DDPO4}$ = [OH-DDPO$_4$(NH$_4$)$_2$]/{[OH-DDPO$_4$(NH$_4$)$_2$] + [DDPO$_4$(NH$_4$)$_2$]}. (*Source:* From Tosatti, S. et al., *Langmuir*, 18, 3537, 2002. With permission. Copyright American Chemical Society.)

polarity, and surface charge are controlled. Such well controlled surfaces could be used to study the effects of physicochemical properties on cell and extracellular matrix interactions on modified titanium oxide surfaces.

Using mixtures of methyl-terminated (nonpolar, uncharged, hydrophobic) and hydroxy-terminated (polar, uncharged, hydrophilic) dodecyl phosphate, it was shown that the water contact angles could be precisely adjusted between approximately 110 and 55 degrees for the advancing angle and between 90 and 10 degrees for the receding angle[29] as shown in the plot of advancing and receding contact angles versus molar ratios in aqueous self-assembly solution (Figure 19.5). Similarly, carboxy-terminated alkane phosphonic acids with alkane $(CH_2)_n$ chains of length n varying from 2 to 15 were shown to bind to titania powders through the phosphonate group, producing a polar, negatively charged (at physiological pH) surface.[26]

We used the concept of alkane phosphate-based SAMs to produce models on smooth titanium surfaces (silicon wafers coated with thin titanium films) and alumina-particle-blasted and chemically etched (SLA) surfaces commonly used in dental implants by Institut Straumann AG of Waldenburg, Switzerland.[27,29] Figure 19.6 is a scanning electron micrograph of the SLA surface topography. The graph of water contact angle versus composition of the SAM solution in Figure 19.7 illustrates the complex wetting behavior of SAM-covered SLA surfaces. In comparing Figures 19.5 and 19.7, the effects of topography and chemistry on water contact angle can be clearly recognized. For the methyl-terminated SAMs, note an important increase in advancing and receding contact angles, sometimes called the "lotus effect" because lotus leaves use micro- to nano-structured surfaces in combination with hydrophobic surface chemistry to achieve high resistance to particle contamination, i.e., a self-cleaning effect.[30]

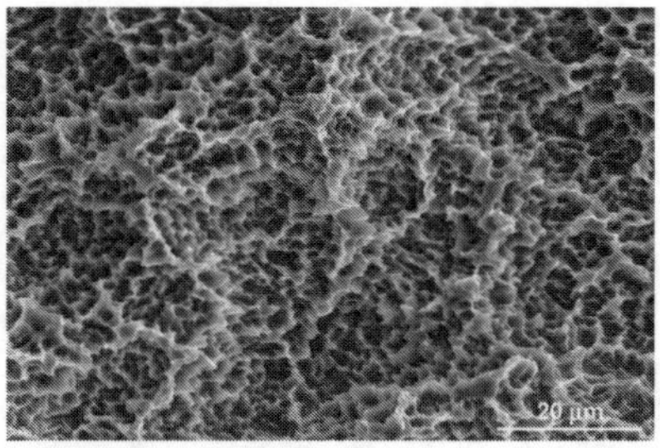

FIGURE 19.6
Scanning electron microscopy image of the topography of a particle-blasted and acid-etched CP titanium (SLA) surface. (*Source:* From Tosatti, S. et al., *Langmuir,* 18, 3537, 2002. With permission. Copyright American Chemical Society.)

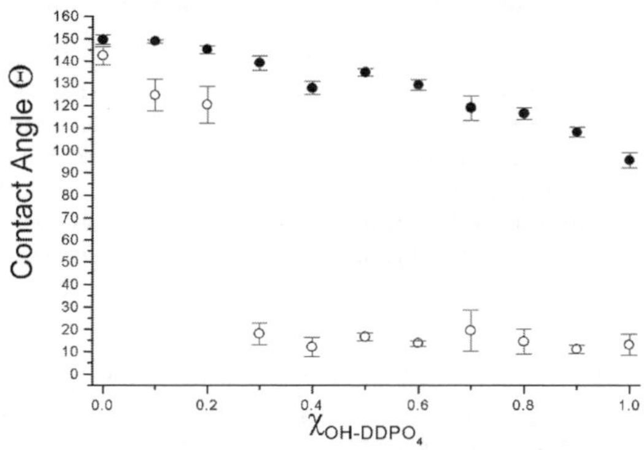

FIGURE 19.7
Advancing (●) and receding (○) contact angles of water on rough particle-blasted and acid-etched (SLA) titanium metal surfaces as a function of OH-DDPO$_4$(NH$_4$)$_2$ concentration in SAM-forming solution expressed as a mole fraction, $\chi_{OH\text{-}DDPO4}$ = [OH-DDPO$_4$(NH$_4$)$_2$]/{[OH-DDPO$_4$(NH$_4$)$_2$] + [DDPO$_4$(NH$_4$)$_2$]}. (*Source:* From Tosatti, S. et al., *Langmuir,* 18, 3537, 2002. With permission. Copyright American Chemical Society.)

XPS studies further confirmed that alkane phosphates indeed assemble on rough (SLA) surfaces with the same or similar density of alkane phosphate molecules per unit effective area.[29] Human gingival fibroblasts were seeded on hydrophobic (methyl-terminated) and hydrophilic (hydroxy-terminated) alkane phosphate SAMs applied to smooth and rough (SLA) titanium substrates with and without serum in cell culture medium. Cell morphology, spreading, and coverage clearly reflected the importance of surface topography or roughness. When cultured for 24 hours in medium containing 15% serum fibroblasts, rough surfaces were covered to a lesser extent than smooth surfaces (Figure 19.8). Moreover, fibroblasts cultured on rough surfaces were less spread, i.e., occupied smaller area (Figure 19.9a) and were significantly thicker compared to fibroblasts cultured on smooth surfaces, as assessed by confocal laser scanning microscopy. Rough surface topography also tended to inhibit actin stress fiber formation.[31,32]

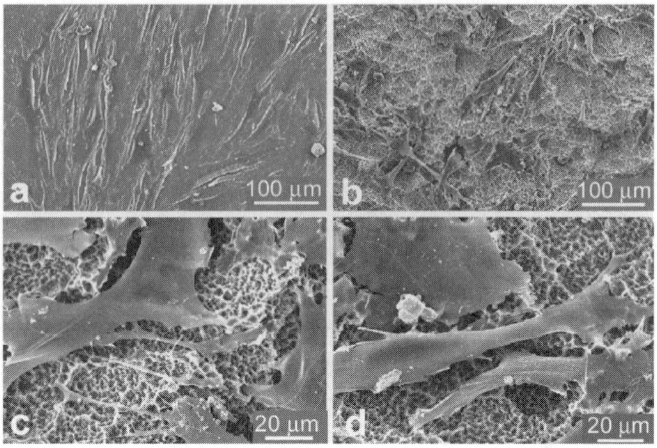

FIGURE 19.8
Scanning electron micrographs of fibroblasts (10,000 cells/ml, cell culture medium with 15% serum, 24-hour culture time, glutaraldehyde-fixed and osmium tetroxide-stained), cultured on smooth and rough (SLA) titanium surfaces, covered by hydrophobic (methyl-terminated) or hydrophilic (hydroxy-terminated) alkane phosphate SAMs. (a) smooth/hydrophobic; (b) rough/hydrophobic; (c) rough/hydrophobic (higher magnification); and (d) rough/hydrophilic (higher magnification). (*Source:* From Vanoni, C., diploma thesis, ETH, Zürich, 2000. With permission.)

Surface wettability was found to be generally less important and only partly influenced cell behavior. When fibroblasts were cultured in media of low serum content (0 to 2%) for 24 hours, cell spreading on hydrophilic smooth surfaces was enhanced compared to cells spread on hydrophobic smooth surfaces. However, the differences became smaller with increasing serum content. At a serum content of 15%, no statistical significant differences in terms of cell attachment, area, shape, or thickness were observed between hydrophilic and hydrophobic surfaces with the same topography (Figures 19.9a and 19.9b). These findings agree with an earlier report[33] noting that fibroblast cell area and spreading were similar for surfaces with different surface energies when cultured in the presence of 15% fetal calf serum.

The fact that chemical composition and hydrophilicity–hydrophobicity of titanium–alkane phosphate SAM surfaces affect fibroblast cell behavior to a lesser degree than surface topography does is likely related to two issues.

First, cells in the *presence of serum* or *single protein* solutions do not interact with the synthetic surface. They generally interact through a proteinaceous layer that develops at the interface due to fast protein adsorption and usually slower exchange processes. Water contact angle is a property that is very sensitive to changes in surface quality, types of functional surface groups, and order of SAMs, but it is much less relevant in the context of protein adsorption. While hydrophobic surfaces always interact strongly with proteins, proteins adsorb to many types of hydrophilic surfaces such as clean metal oxides and hydroxy-terminated SAMs. Although it is likely that initial

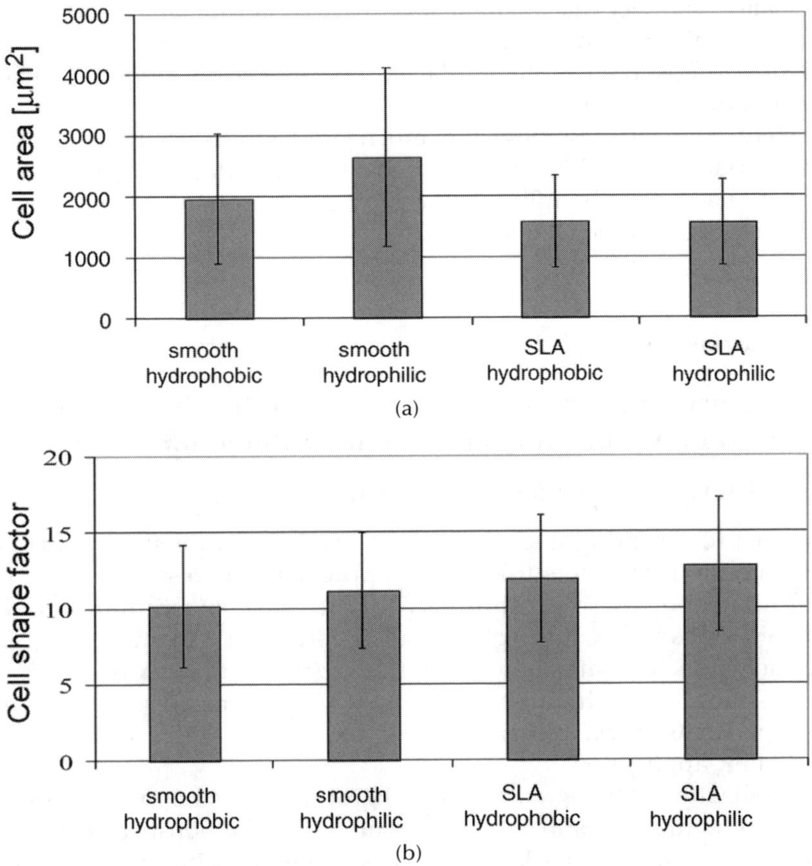

FIGURE 19.9
(a) Projected cell area for fibroblasts cultured on hydrophobic and hydrophilic smooth and rough (SLA) surfaces (same types shown in Figure 19.8). Cells were seeded at concentration of $1.3 \cdot 10^4$ cells/ml and incubated 24 hours (n = 21 for each surface, mean value ± standard deviation). Cell area on hydrophilic, smooth surfaces was significantly statistically different from cell area on rough hydrophobic and hydrophilic (SLA) surfaces but not from cell area on smooth hydrophobic surface (Bonferroni $p = <0.05$). (b) Cell shape factor of fibroblasts cultivated on hydrophobic and hydrophilic smooth and SLA surfaces. Cell shape factor Φ is defined as $\Phi = 4\pi A/P^2$ where A is the projected area and P is the perimeter. A round cell has a shape factor of 1. Increased spreading results in increased Φ. Same cell seeding conditions were used.

differences in composition and conformation exist between protein adlayers on hydrophobic and hydrophilic surfaces, the differences may disappear in the course of exposure of the surface to the cell culture or body fluid medium and under the influence of cellular activity at the interface. The observation that cells react differently to hydrophobic and hydrophilic surfaces *in vitro* in the *absence of serum* is consistent with this view.

Second, alkane phosphate SAMs are not perfectly stable in contact with cell culture media, but show exposure time-dependent changes in contact angle, e.g., decreasing contact angles for hydrophobic, methyl-terminated phosphates. The fact that methyl- and hydroxy-terminated SAMs are not significantly different in terms of short-term fibroblast–surface interaction is likely due to adsorbed protein adlayers and biological properties that are probably not very different.

We were led to the hypothesis that much larger effects of surface chemistry on cell-surface interaction can be expected with surface chemical systems that allow us to directly influence the protein adsorption process. This concept is discussed in the next section.

19.3 Molecular Assembly Systems to Control Non-Specific Protein Adsorption and Specific Interactions with Cells

19.3.1 Background and Surface Technologies

In contrast to accepting uncontrolled adsorption of proteins from plasma or serum onto implanted surfaces, our approach is to design surfaces with chemical properties that eliminate or at least substantially reduce unwanted nonspecific adsorption and incorporate "silent" background components such as attachment peptides, growth factors, or drugs that exert specific effects. Although this approach is recognized as a prerequisite for biospecificity in the biosensor field, it is less common for biomaterial and implant applications.

Immobilization of bioligands on a background that is not protein-resistant is likely to be unsuccessful because the effects of the nonspecific adsorbed proteins may compete, mask, or otherwise interfere with the effects of the specific factor added to the surface by design. Perhaps the simplest approach to controlling protein adsorption at the titania interface is to passivate the surface with a layer of an inert protein such as albumin. In effect, this approach involves the blocking of all or most of the protein-binding sites at the surface with albumin so that subsequent proteins cannot attach. The effectiveness of this method is limited by the fact that albumin binding to titania is often partially reversible, and thus subsequent proteins could replace albumin within the protein layer.

A number of chemistries have been proposed and used to reduce the interactiveness of surfaces, in particular the immobilization of the following molecular entities:

1. Poly(ethylene glycol) or poly(ethylene oxide)
2. Phosphorylcholine (phospholipid polar headgroup of cell membrane)[34,35]
3. Polysaccharides such as dextran derivatives[36,37]

Poly(ethylene glycol) (PEG) is the chemical basis of the most versatile approach to controlling nonspecific adsorption. Of the many models proposed to explain this effect, steric stabilization and excluded-volume effects are the most commonly cited.[38,39] A general approach to the immobilization of PEG onto metal oxide surfaces involves the coupling of PEG to a functional group that has an affinity for or can be covalently bound to the oxide surface.

A common strategy for covalent attachment of PEG to silica or titania surfaces involves a two-stage reaction. In the first stage, an aminosilane or thiosilane can be reacted with a clean oxide surface to form a surface rich in amine or thiol functionalities.[17,40] In the second stage, a PEG polymer that contains a functional group reactive with the modified surface (i.e., with amines or thiols) is covalently coupled to the surface. Irvine et al. showed that for many different PEG polymer lengths and types, the surfaces with the highest PEG-grafting density exhibited the greatest suppression of human serum albumin and cytochrome c adsorption.[41] Sophia et al. showed that the full suppression of protein adsorption requires a PEG-grafting density in which the PEG side chains neighboring at the surface structurally overlap.[42] In general, such modified surfaces involving silanized functionalities are unstable and subject to hydrolytic degradation over time when in contact with aqueous fluids.

In view of the simplicity of molecular assembly processes, scientists have searched for suitable PEG-based chemical systems. One approach involves the assembly of amphiphilic or surfactant-like molecules at the solid titania interface. Generally speaking, amphiphiles are molecules possessing two domains of different properties. As a result, amphiphilic molecules often spontaneously assemble at an interface due to electrostatic or hydrophobic interactions, and their orientations are determined by the relative properties of the domains and the properties of the interface.

A large body of research on Pluronic© products, amphiphilic triblock copolymers containing a hydrophobic domain and two hydrophilic domains, showed that surfaces of hydrophobic materials such as polyethylene demonstrated substantially improved resistance to protein adsorption when treated with Pluronic F-108.[43,44] This approach also requires multistage surface-chemical reactions, since in a first step, the titanium oxide surface must be rendered hydrophobic, e.g., by silanization or application of an alkane phosphate self-assembled monolayer (see Section 19.2.2).

19.3.2 Poly(L-Lysine)-*Graft*-Poly(Ethylene Glycol) (PLL-g-PEG)

Graft copolymers, having a poly-L-lysine backbone (ionic domain) and poly(ethylene glycol) side chains (nonionic domain) (Figure 19.10a), can be spontaneously assembled out of solution to form stable PEG-containing layers on several different metal oxide surfaces including titanium dioxide.[45,46] The polymer layer was shown to orient such that its positively

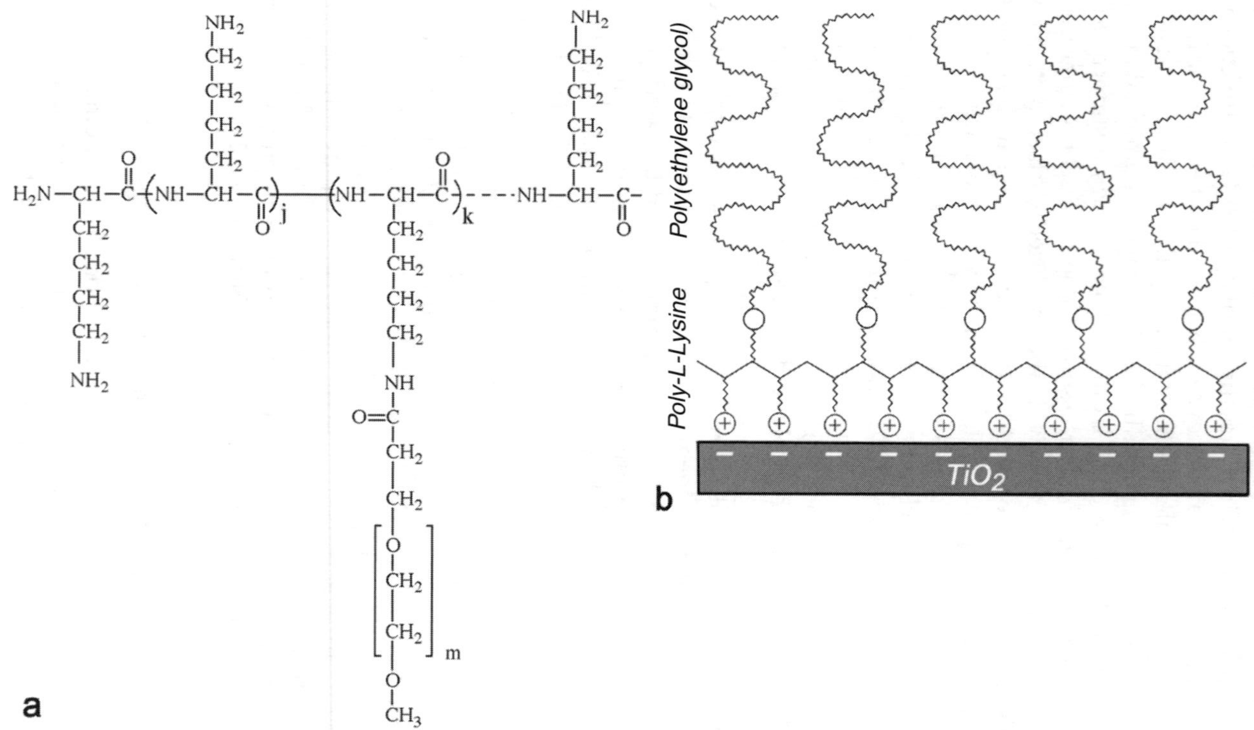

FIGURE 19.10
(a) Molecular structure and (b) schematic model of a PLL-g-PEG layer that spontaneously adsorbed onto a titania surface. The adsorption was driven by electrostatic interaction of the negatively charged titania surface and the positively charged copolymer backbone, producing a PEG-modified titania surface with high resistance to protein adsorption and good chemical stability. (*Source:* From Kenausis, G.L. et al., *J. Phys. Chem. B,* 104, 3298, 2000. With permission. Copyright American Chemical Society.)

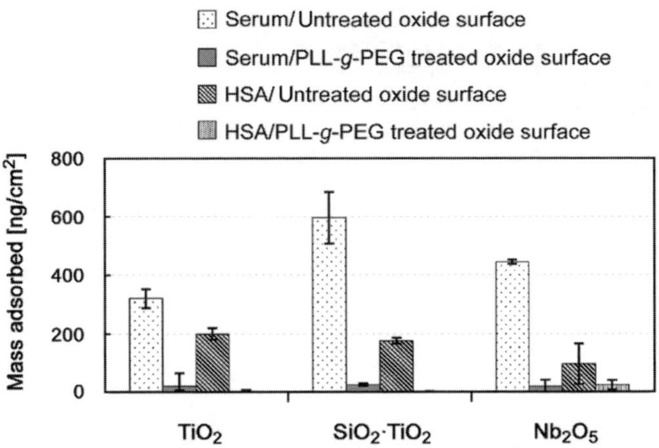

FIGURE 19.11
Effect of PLL-g-PEG pretreatment on adsorption of human serum and human serum albumin onto various metal oxide surfaces. (*Source:* From Kenausis, G.L. et al., *J. Phys. Chem. B*, 104, 3298, 2000. With permission. Copyright American Chemical Society.)

charged backbone was bound to the surface and covered under a layer of PEG side chains in a brush-like structure (Figure 19.10b).

These modified surfaces proved highly resistant to adsorption of albumin, fibrinogen, and whole human serum at a level typically below 5 to 10 ng/ cm^2 (Figure 19.11), with optimized architectures and in buffers of physiological ionic strength below 1 ng/cm^2,[46] which is the lower detection limit of the optical *in situ* sensor technique (optical waveguide lightmode spectroscopy or OWLS)[47] used to evaluate protein adsorption. The degree of protein resistance turned out to be dependent on polymer architecture (i.e., on the molecular weight of the PLL and PEG and on the grafting ratios of PEG chains to lysine monomer units) and could be roughly correlated with the surface areal density of the PEG pendent chains.[45]

In Figure 19.12, the amount of serum adsorption, as determined by OWLS, is plotted as a function of the ratio of the mean distance between the PEG chains and the diameter of gyration. Low protein adsorption is typically found at high surface PEG coverages where substantial compression due to steric repulsion between the PEG moieties is present. This observation is in agreement with the hypothesis that the PEG chains are squeezed out perpendicularly to the surface as judged by the polarization dependence of the infrared reflection–absorption spectroscopy measurements.[46]

19.3.3 Applications of PLL-g-PEG Adlayers with and without Grafted Peptides to Smooth and Rough Titanium Surfaces

PLL-g-PEG was assembled on both smooth titanium surfaces deposited as metal films onto silicon wafers and on alumina-blasted acid-etched (SLA)

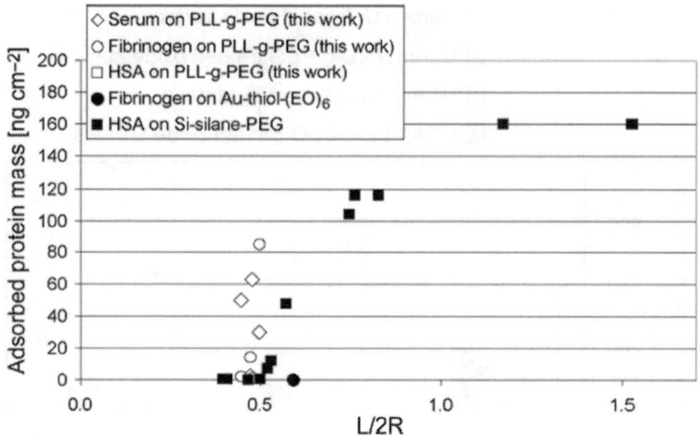

FIGURE 19.12
Dependence of protein adsorption on the extent of surface PEG side chain packing density. The ratio of the mean distance L between surface-immobilized PEG moieties to the diameter of gyration (2R) of the corresponding PEG molecule (L/2R) is calculated as described by Kenausis.[45] Values from our work are compared to published data for which the areal mass density of protein and average PEG spacing (L) are taken from Sofia[42] and Harder.[54] (*Source:* From Kenausis, G.L. et al., *J. Phys. Chem. B*, 104, 3298, 2000. With permission. Copyright American Chemical Society.)

surfaces of bulk titanium specimens (see Section 19.2.2) serving as models for cell-surface studies. In addition to the base polymer, functionalized PLL-g-PEG with peptides grafted to a fraction of the PEG chain was synthesized by Van de Vondele and Hubbell[48] and applied in a spontaneous one-step, molecular assembly process to the titanium surfaces to produce surfaces characterized by independently controlled peptide ligand density and topography.

For the peptide-modified polymer, a peptide of –GCRGYG**RGD**SPG type containing the active peptide sequence RGD (arginine, glycine, aspartic acid) well known to interact specifically with α/β integrin receptors in the membranes of many different types of cells was chosen.[49] RGD sequences are present in a number of cell-adhesive proteins such as fibronectin and vitronectin, proteins involved in the attachment of many type of cells to biomaterial surfaces, including osteoblasts, fibroblasts, and bacteria.

Proof of the concept of employing such peptide approaches requires control surfaces, an integrin-inactive peptide, –GCRGYG***RDG***SPG, was therefore grafted to the PLL-g-PEG with 5% of the PEG as chain-end-functionalized (PLL-g-PEG/PEG-RGD 5%).[48] The R*DG* with inverse-sequence DG has no specific activity toward α/β integrin receptors and therefore serves as proof of the presence or absence of specific interactions in cell surface studies. As a further control, unmodified titanium surfaces characterized by well cleaned titanium oxide and with the same smooth and rough (SLA) surface topographies were used in the cell culture experiments. All surfaces were carefully controlled by surface analytical techniques such as XPS, contact angle, and ellipsometry.[50]

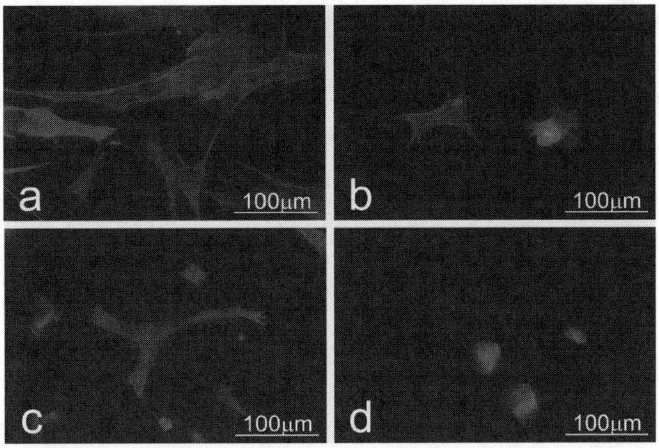

FIGURE 19.13
(See color insert.) Fluorescence microscopy of human foreskin fibroblast cells stained for actin stress fibers on smooth and rough (SLA) titanium surfaces with and without assembled monolayers of poly-L-lysine-g-poly(ethylene glycol) (PLL-g-PEG): (a) smooth/natural oxide film surface; (b) smooth/PLL-g-PEG surface; (c) rough/natural oxide film surface; and (d) rough/PLL-g-PEG surface. Cells were seeded at a concentration of 10^4 cells per mL in culture medium with 10% fetal calf serum and incubated for 24 hours, fixed in 10% formalin solution, and fluorescently stained for actin stress fibers with dissolved phalloidin. (*Source:* From Tosatti, S. et al., in preparation, 2003. With permission.)

Human foreskin fibroblast (HFF) cells at a density of 10,000 cells/ml in standard cell culture medium supplemented with 10% fetal calf serum were seeded onto smooth and rough (SLA) titanium surfaces with the following surface chemistries: (1) uncoated (natural oxide-covered); (2) coated with PLL-g-PEG; (3) coated with PLL-g-PEG/PEG-**RGD** 5%; or (4) coated with PLL-g-PEG/PEG-R*DG* 5%). After 24 hours of incubation, the cells were stained to evaluate spreading and actin stress fiber architecture with a fluorescence microscope.[51]

Figures 19.13 and 19.14 demonstrate that the PLL-g-PEG system indeed allows the design and fabrication of cell-specific surface functionalities on titanium surfaces with both smooth and rough surface topographies. On the smooth, natural oxide film-covered surface, the fibroblasts in the serum-containing culture medium showed the expected extensive spreading (Figure 19.13a); this surface is known to adsorb cell-adhesive proteins from serum (e.g., fibronectin and vitronectin). In contrast, far fewer cells were detected on the surface covered with a monolayer of protein-resistant PLL-g-PEG and they showed limited spreading and poor actin stress fiber organization (Figure 19.13b).

The situation is qualitatively similar on the rough (SLA) surface (Figures 19.13c and d), but in comparison to the corresponding smooth case, less cell spreading and inferior development of stress fibers were noted. The fact that fibroblasts seem to shun rough surfaces, in contrast to macrophages, was observed more than 20 years ago by Rich and Harris and designated *rugo-*

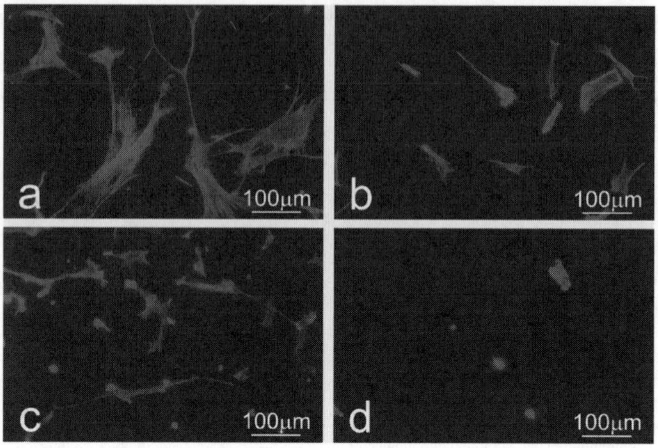

FIGURE 19.14
(See color insert.) Fluorescence microscopy of human foreskin fibroblast cells stained for actin stress fibers on smooth and rough (SLA) titanium surfaces with and without assembled monolayers of poly-L-lysine-g-poly(ethylene glycol) (PLL-g-PEG): (a) smooth PLL-g-PEG/PEG-RGD 5% (active peptide); (b) smooth PLL-g-PEG/PEG-R*DG* 5% (inactive peptide control); (c) rough PLL-g-PEG/PEG-RGD 5% (active peptide); and (d) rough PLL-g-PEG/PEG-R*DG* 5% (inactive peptide control). Cells were seeded at a concentration of 10^4 cells per mL in culture medium with 10% fetal calf serum and incubated for 24 hours, fixed in 10% formalin solution, and fluorescently stained for actin stress fibers with dissolved phalloidin. (*Source:* From Tosatti, S. et al., in preparation, 2003. With permission.)

phobia.[20,52] If, however, the assembled polymeric layer contains grafted RGD–peptide sequences (and remains resistant to nonspecific protein adsorption), the tendency to form well spread and adhering cells with well developed stress fiber architecture is fully restored (Figure 19.14a).

The 5% chain functionalization seems sufficient to provide the necessary density of such adhesive sites normally present in protein adlayers. The observed cell behavior is definitively a consequence of direct interaction of the RGD-type peptide with cells, as the control (PLL-g-PEG/PEG-R*DG* 5% surface with *in*active peptide) shows strongly reduced spreading and a cell morphology more comparable to the nonfunctionalized PLL-g-PEG surface (compare Figures 19.14b and 19.13b). The negative influence of surface roughness on cell attachment and spreading is again obvious (compare Figures 19.14c and 19.14d with Figures 19.14a and 19.14b).

The same types of surfaces were also tested after 72 hours HFF incubation for total mitochondrial activity as a measure of total cell proliferation and viability.[51] The same trends regarding influence of specific peptides and surface roughness were observed (Figure 19.15).

These results serve as good evidence that the PLL-g-PEG technology that can be implemented by simple dipping in aqueous solution at room temperature is applicable to both smooth and rough surfaces and can reduce nonspecific adsorption of proteins. On this background of low nonspecific adsorption, surface peptide moieties able to interact specifically with fibro-

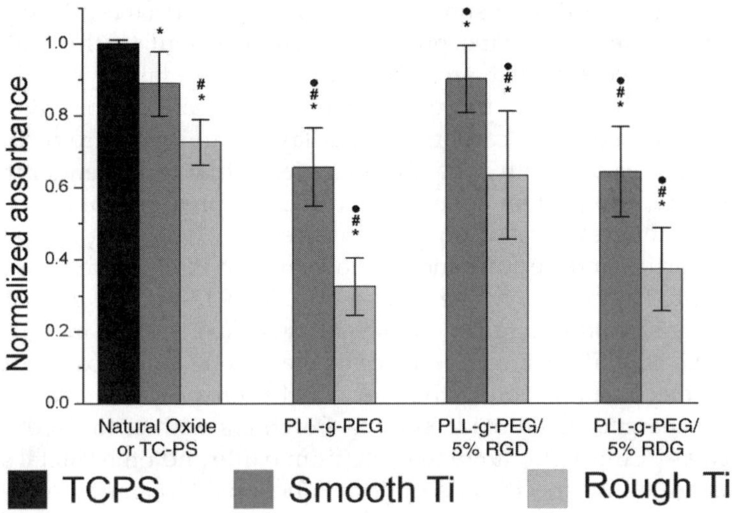

FIGURE 19.15
Cell viability and proliferation of human foreskin fibroblasts determined as total mitochondrial activity using WST-1 kit after 72 hours of culture. Same types of surfaces shown in Figures 19.13 and 19.14 were used. Statistical differences were calculated via ANOVA: *P = <0.05 versus tissue culture plastic; #P = <0.05 versus smooth Ti; ·P = <0.05 versus rough Ti. (*Source:* From Tosatti, S. et al., in preparation, 2003. With permission.)

blast cells can be introduced at the interface in the same assembly step. A further advantage is the fact that the bioligand (peptide in this case) surface areal density can be precisely controlled via assembly from mixed PLL-g-PEG plus PLL-g-PEG/PEG-ψ solutions, as has been successfully demonstrated for ψ = biotin in the context of biosensor chip development based on the biotin/(strept)avidin interface.[53]

19.4 Conclusions and Outlook

Molecular assembly techniques are interesting alternatives to other types of chemical surface reactions for the functionalization of metal oxide surfaces. Alkane phosphates and PLL-g-PEG are two examples successfully applied to titanium surfaces covered with a natural (passive) oxide film. Alkane phosphates can be used to alter physicochemical properties such as wettability (hydrophobicity and hydrophilicity) and surface charge.

The responses of fibroblasts to alterations in these properties were weak when serum was present. More pronounced effects were seen in serum-free cell culture media, but this condition is only of academic interest. The likely explanation is that the physicochemical properties of the interface are modified with time when exposed to biological media and that cell-adhesive proteins finally adsorb in a similar way to all these surfaces. Possible strategies that will render alkane phosphates more useful to the biologically interested surface scientist are: (1) increasing the stability of the phosphate–titanium bond (e.g., through thermal post-treatment or cross-linking within the ordered hydrocarbon chain adlayer), and (2) introducing functionalities such as oligo(ethylene glycol) moieties that could render the oxide surface resistant to protein adsorption at the terminal group, in analogy to the alkane thiol system used on gold surfaces.[54]

The properties and performance of polycationic PEG-grafted copolymers are different. They form, in the course of a 5- to 15-minute assembly step from aqueous solution, rather stable adlayers (>2 weeks in cell culture media). This stability is a consequence of the kinetic inertness produced by the many electrostatic bonds that form between polymer backbone and oppositely charged metal oxide surface. Polymers with optimized architectures such as PLL-g-PEG can render titanium oxide and other metal surfaces very resistant to nonspecific adsorption. Functional bioligands such as peptides can be introduced through covalent grafting to the polymer, allowing the design of both smooth and rough surfaces with almost perfectly controlled bioligand surface densities. RGD-containing peptide moieties attached to PLL-g-PEG were shown to interact specifically with fibroblast cells through peptide–integrin receptor interactions.

RGD peptides, often used for proof-of-concept experiments, are not the only interesting peptides for modification of implant surfaces. Other sequences have been reported in cell-binding domains, for example YIGRS and IKVAV in laminin, RKK in collagen-I,[55-58] and a variety of heparin-binding domains interacting electrostatically with transmembrane proteoglycans such as FHRRIKA and KRSR, which are also present in cell-binding proteins such as fibronectin.[13,59]

The specific interactions of osteoblasts with peptide-functionalized surfaces were carefully reviewed by Healy et al.[11] Heparin-binding motifs of type FHRRIKA and KRSR as ligands to attach osteoblast-like cells have recently attracted increased attention due synergistic action in combination with integrin-binding RGD-type peptides (FHRRIKA)[17] and for the ability to preferentially bind osteoblasts from fibroblast–osteoblast cocultures (KRSR).[60]

In conclusion, using molecular assembly techniques based on PEG-grafted polyionic copolymers, one can imagine introducing at the implant surface one or a combination of several synergistic biofunctionalities such as specific peptides at highly controlled surface densities and combining such designed biochemical surface compositions with preferred surface topographies. Such concepts have potential to be compatible with implants specifically designed for given medical applications.

From an economic perspective, molecular assembly processes are potentially very cost effective. Although the synthesis of multifunctional polymers may be costly, the fact that only about 100 to 200 ng/cm^2 of polymer is needed makes material costs almost negligible (at a rate of 10^4 €/g (Euro/gram) and 10% use of material, the cost is on the order of 1 cent/cm^2). What is generally much more important is the handling cost. In this respect, molecular assembly techniques (simple dipping from aqueous solutions) have clear advantages in terms of costs, scalability, large batch sizes, and compatibility with modern industrial, environmentally acceptable production techniques.

The limitations to the use of the molecular assembly approach should be mentioned here. Monolayers of a few-nanometer thickness have limited lifetimes in friction and wear situations (albeit less so in topographically structured surfaces with large proportions of the surface "protected" from outside mechanical action). Second, the molecular adlayers are likely to be altered and degraded over the longer term due to biological (cellular, chemical, or enzymatic) activity, but this reactivity may not interfere with their usefulness. The relevant consideration is the time span that such adlayers must be present and active in order to exert a positive influence on the direction and kinetics of specific healing and integration pathways. Carefully planned animal experiments based on quantitatively characterized model implants and surfaces are needed to reach a definitive conclusion on the usefulness of the molecular assembly approach in biomedical applications.

Acknowledgments

The authors thank Claudio Vanoni for providing data on surface characterization of and cell interaction with titanium oxide surfaces modified by self-assembled monolayers (diploma thesis, ETH Zurich, 2000). Dr. Michael Horrisberger at Paul Scherrer Institute, Villigen, Switzerland, is thanked for performing titanium and titanium oxide coatings on various substrates.

This work was financially supported by the International Team for Oral Implantology (ITI), Waldenburg, Switzerland (Project 192).

References

1. Ratner, B.D. et al., *Biomaterials Science: An Introduction to Materials in Medicine*, Academic Press, San Diego, 1996.
2. Xiao, S.-J., Kenausis, G., and Textor, M., Biochemical surface treatment of titanium, in *Titanium in Medicine*, Brunette, D.M. et al., Eds., Springer, Berlin, 2001, p. 417.
3. Textor, M. et al., Properties and biological significance of natural oxide films on titanium and its alloys, in *Titanium in Medicine*, Brunette, D.M. et al., Eds., Springer, Berlin, 2001, p. 171.
4. Williams, D.F., Titanium for medical applications, in *Titanium in Medicine*, Brunette, D.M. et al., Eds., Springer, Berlin, 2001, p. 13.
5. Boyan, B.D. et al., The titanium–bone cell interface *in vitro*: the role of the surface in promoting osteointegration, in *Titanium in Medicine*, Brunette, D.M. et al., Eds., Springer, Berlin, 2001, p. 561.

6. Jaeger, N.A.F. and Brunette, D.M., Production of microfabricated surfaces and their effects on cell behavior, in *Titanium in Medicine*, Brunette, D.M. et al., Eds., Springer, Berlin, 2001, p. 343.
7. Esposito, M., Titanium for dental applications (I), in *Titanium in Medicine*, Brunette, D.M. et al., Eds., Springer, Berlin, 2001, p. 827.
8. Buser, D., Titanium for dental applications (II), in *Titanium in Medicine*, Brunette, D.M. et al., Eds., Springer, Berlin, 2001, 875.
9. Massaro, C. et al., Comparative investigation of the surface properties of commercial titanium dental implants. Part i: chemical composition, *J. Mater. Sci. Mater. Med.*, 13, 535, 2002.
10. Tengvall, P., Proteins at titanium interfaces, in *Titanium in Medicine*, Brunette, D.M. et al., Eds., Springer, Berlin, 2001, p. 457.
11. Healy, K.E. et al., Osteoblast interactions with engineered surfaces, in *Bone Engineering*, Davies, J.E., Ed., em squared, Toronto, 2000, p. 268.
12. Dee, K.C. et al., Conditions which promote mineralization at the bone-implant interface: a model *in vitro* study, *Biomaterials*, 17, 209, 1996.
13. Dee, K.C., Andersen, T.T., and Bizios, R., Design and function of novel osteoblast-adhesive peptides for chemical modification of biomaterials, *J. Biomed. Mater. Res.*, 40, 371, 1998.
14. Massia, S.P. and Hubbell, J.A., Covalent surface immobilization of Arg–Gly–Asp-containing and Tyr–Ile–Gly–Ser–Arg-containing peptides to obtain well-defined cell-adhesive substrates, *Anal. Biochem.*, 187, 292, 1990.
15. Xiao, S.J. et al., Covalent attachment of cell-adhesive (Arg–Gly–Asp)-containing peptides to titanium surfaces, *Langmuir*, 14, 5507, 1998.
16. Bearinger, J.P., Castner, D.G., and Healy, K.E., Biomolecular modification of p(AAM-CO-EG/AA) IPNS supports osteoblast adhesion and phenotypic expression, *J. Biomater. Sci. Polymer Ed.*, 9, 629, 1998.
17. Rezania, A. et al., Bioactivation of metal oxide surfaces 1. Surface characterization and cell response, *Langmuir*, 15, 6931, 1999.
18. Scotchford, C.A. et al., Growth of human osteoblast-like cells on alkane thiol on gold self-assembled monolayers: the effect of surface chemistry, *J. Biomed. Mater. Res.*, 41, 431, 1998.
19. Folkers, J.P. et al., Self-assembled monolayers of long-chain hydroxamic acids on the native oxides of metals, *Langmuir*, 11, 813, 1995.
20. Brunette, D.M., Principles of cell behavior on titanium surfaces and their application to implanted devices, in *Titanium in Medicine*, Brunette, D.M. et al., Eds., Springer, Berlin, 2001, 485.
21. Gao, W. et al., Self-assembled monolayers of alkylphosphonic acids on metal oxides, *Langmuir*, 12, 6429, 1996.
22. Brovelli, D. et al., Highly oriented, self-assembled alkane phosphate monolayers on tantalum (V) oxide surfaces, *Langmuir*, 15, 4324, 1999.
23. Textor, M. et al., Structural chemistry of self-assembled monolayers of octadecylphosphoric acid on tantalum oxide surfaces, *Langmuir*, 16, 3257, 2000.
24. Gawalt, E.S. et al., Enhanced bonding of alkanephosphonic acids to oxidized titanium using surface-bound alkoxyzirconium complex interfaces, *Langmuir*, 15, 8929, 1999.
25. Maege, I. et al., Ultrathin organic layers for corrosion protection, *Macromolec. Symp.*, 126, 7, 1998.
26. Pawsey, S., Yach, K., and Reven, L., Self-assembly of carboxyalkylphosphonic acids on metal oxide powders, *Langmuir*, 18, 5205, 2002.

27. Vörös, J. et al., Characterization of titanium surfaces, in *Titanium in Medicine*, Brunette, D.M. et al., Eds., Springer, Berlin, 2001, p. 87.
28. Hofer, R., Textor, M., and Spencer, N.D., Alkyl phosphate monolayers self-assembled from aqueous solution onto metal oxide surfaces, *Langmuir*, 17, 4014, 2001.
29. Tosatti, S. et al., Self-assembled monolayers of dodecyl and hydroxy-dodecyl phosphates on both smooth and rough titanium and titanium oxide surfaces, *Langmuir*, 18, 3537, 2002.
30. Barthlott, W. and Neinhuis, C., Purity of the sacred lotus, or escape from contamination in biological surfaces, *Planta*, 202, 1, 1997.
31. Tosatti, S. et al., unpublished data, 2001.
32. Vanoni, C., Production and Physiochemical Characterization of Self-Assembled Monolayers on Titanium Surfaces and Their Influence on Fibroblast Behavior, diploma thesis, ETH, Zürich, 2000.
33. Schakenraad, J.M. et al., The influence of substratum surface free-energy on growth and spreading of human fibroblasts in the presence and absence of serum proteins, *J. Biomed. Mater. Res.*, 20, 773, 1986.
34. Chapman, D., Biomembranes and new hemocompatible materials, *Langmuir*, 9, 39, 1993.
35. Ishihara, K. et al., Hemocompatibility of human whole-blood on polymers with a phospholipid polar group and its mechanism, *J. Biomed. Mater. Res.*, 26, 1543, 1992.
36. Barie, N. et al., Covalent photolinker-mediated immobilization of an intermediate dextran layer to polymer-coated surfaces for biosensing applications, *Biosensors Bioelectr.*, 13, 855, 1998.
37. Hartley, P.G. et al., Physiochemical properties of polysaccharide coatings as determinants of protein adsorption, in *AVS 48th International Symposium Abstracts*, 2001, p. 198.
38. Claesson, P., Poly(ethylene oxide) surface coatings: relations between intermolecular forces, layer structure and protein repellency, *Colloids Surf. A Physicochem. Eng. Aspects*, 77, 109, 1993.
39. Jeon, S.I. and Andrade, J.D., Protein surface interactions in the presence of polyethylene oxide 2. Effect of protein size, *J. Colloid Interface Sci.*, 142, 159, 1991.
40. Healy, K.E. et al., Kinetics of bone cell organization and mineralization on materials with patterned surface chemistry, *Biomaterials*, 17, 195, 1996.
41. Irvine, D.J. et al., Comparison of tethered star and linear poly(ethylene oxide) for control of biomaterials surface properties, *J. Biomed. Mater. Res.*, 40, 498, 1998.
42. Sofia, S.J., Premnath, V., and Merrill, E.W., Poly(ethylene oxide) grafted to silicon surfaces: grafting density and protein adsorption, *Macromolecules*, 31, 5059, 1998.
43. Amiji, M. and Park, K., Prevention of protein adsorption and platelet-adhesion on surfaces by PEO PPO PEO triblock copolymers, *Biomaterials*, 13, 682, 1992.
44. Amiji, M.M. and Park, K., Analysis on the surface-adsorption of PEO PPO PEO triblock copolymers by radiolabeling and fluorescence techniques, *J. Appl. Polymer Sci.*, 52, 539, 1994.
45. Kenausis, G.L. et al., Poly(L-lysine)-g-poly(ethylene glycol) layers on metal oxide surfaces: attachment mechanism and effects of polymer architecture on resistance to protein adsorption, *J. Phys. Chem. B*, 104, 3298, 2000.
46. Huang, N.P. et al., Poly(l-lysine)-g-poly(ethylene glycol) layers on metal oxide surfaces: surface analytical characterization and resistance to serum and fibrinogen adsorption, *Langmuir*, 17, 489, 2001.

47. Vörös, J. et al., Optical grating coupler biosensors, *Biomaterials*, 23, 3699, 2002.
48. Van de Vondel, S., Vörös, J., Textor, M., and Hubbell, J.A., RGD-grafted poly-L-lysine-*graft*-(polyethylene glycol) copolymers block nonspecific protein adsorption while promoting cell adhesion, *Biotechnol. Bioeng.*, in press, 2003.
49. Pierschbacher, M.D. and Ruoslahti, E., Cell attachment activity of fibronectin can be duplicated by small synthetic fragments of the molecule, *Nature*, 309, 30 1984.
50. Tosatti, S. et al., in preparation, 2003.
51. Tosatti, S. et al., in preparation, 2003.
52. Rich, A. and Harris, A.K., Anomalous preferences of cultured macrophages for hydrophobic and roughened substrata, *J. Cell Sci.*, 50, 1, 1981.
53. Huang, N.P. et al., Biotin-derivatized poly(L-lysine)-g-poly(ethylene glycol): a novel polymeric interface for bioaffinity sensing, *Langmuir*, 18, 220, 2002.
54. Harder, P. et al., Molecular conformation in oligo(ethylene glycol)-terminated self-assembled monolayers on gold and silver surfaces determines their ability to resist protein adsorption, *J. Phys. Chem. B*, 102, 426, 1998.
55. Bowditch, R.D. et al., Integrin-alpha-IIb-beta-3 (platelet gpIIb-IIIa) recognizes multiple sites in fibronectin, *J. Biol. Chem.*, 266, 23323, 1991.
56. Staatz, W.D. et al., Identification of a tetrapeptide recognition sequence for the alpha-2-beta-1-integrin in collagen, *J. Biol. Chem.*, 266, 7363, 1991.
57. Xiao, G.Z. et al., Role of the alpha(2)-integrin in osteoblast-specific gene expression and activation of the Osf2 transcription factor, *J. Biol. Chem.*, 273, 32988, 1998.
58. Ivaska, J. et al., A peptide inhibiting the collagen binding function of integrin alpha I-2 domain, *J. Biol. Chem.*, 274, 3513, 1999.
59. Dee, K.C., Andersen, T.T., and Bizios, R., Enhanced endothelialization of substrates modified with immobilized bioactive peptides, *Tissue Eng.*, 1, 135, 1995.
60. Hasenbein, M.E., Andersen, T.T., and Bizios, R., Micropatterned surfaces modified with selected peptides promote exclusive interactions with ostcoblasts, *Biomaterials*, 23, 3937, 2002.

Section VI

Development and Application of Scientific Data: Regulatory and Commercial Aspects

20

Development and Application of Scientific Data: Do Industry and Academia Have Different Scientific Perspectives?

Björn Delin

Scientific development within the fields of pharmaceutical and medical device applications is one of the most important and resource-consuming activities in modern society. Industry and universities work on their own or in various forms of cooperation to conduct research and develop products.

Historically, academic research was considered superior and had higher status as compared to industry-driven research. This view can actually be traced back to ancient Greece where sciences and arts were the privileges of philosophers who indulged in theoretical reasoning about nature and the laws governing the life of mankind and the world as a whole. Practical application of science, for example, in construction, production, or commercial activities was considered to have extremely low status. Any involvement with money was absolutely unthinkable and applications of science principles conceived by philosophers were left to citizens of low standing, soldiers, and slaves. Much has happened since those days, but traces of these attitudes can be detected on occasion.

Modern industrial and academic research efforts have reached equal status. Academic research has to some extent suffered from isolation and is often performed on an individual basis under the pressures of strong competition among individuals and groups. Limited financial support is also a restricting factor. Today collaboration with industry is encouraged and often a prerequisite for the realization of high quality science. Within the academic world, the goals of and reasons for conducting research are often of short-term perspective and aimed at publication and personal gratification even if the work fits into a long-term perspective at the institution where a researcher is active.

The objective of "purely" academic research is to increase our knowledge base in the life sciences, technology, etc. to benefit mankind in general. The

0-8493-1474-7/03/$0.00+$1.50

results need not be directly applicable as products or disease treatment. The reason for starting a project may be that "it is interesting from a scientific perspective" — a phrase that would be considered as rather suspect in the industrial world, if cited as a motive for starting any form of activity. However, more and more research is done today for the direct benefit of society and is slanted preferably toward industrial exploitation. This is often a condition for obtaining funding for the research; regrettably less so-called "free research" can be conducted.

Industrial research is strongly target-oriented and aims at producing patentable drugs or devices. The primary targets are to generate revenue for shareholders and fund investments in new development projects. The time required for development of a new drug is on average 12 years and the cost is approximately $4.8 billion. Industry often can allocate large amounts of resources and create highly competent multidisciplinary teams to pursue efficient product development. Progress is evaluated frequently and decisions are made from a marketing perspective. This approach can prematurely kill a potentially viable project.

Today's collaboration between industry and academia is more or less a must. Industry is in need of specialists and competence and input in the form of new ideas for development of new product concepts. Academia is in need of resources along with input and guidance to identify projects with potential.

Collaboration generally follows one of two principles. First, an academic institution can act as a contract research organization (CRO) from which industry can buy research. Alternatively, research may focus on a common subject and ideally a win–win situation is created when high quality research produces benefits for the academic scientist by enhancing his or qualifications and reputation. Industry gains scientific results and ideas. Academia contributes work by top scientists, ideas, and results while industry makes available resources and results from its laboratories. The risk of conflict of interest lies in the fact that industry may want to delay publication of results due to patent requirements and marketing and competitive considerations. An individual scientist usually wants to publish results as soon as possible for his or her benefit and gratification.

The potential risk of unsound influence on an academic institution by industry must be considered. The fact that industry sponsors or funds research at an institution must not affect the sound judgment or scientific independence of the scientists involved. Industry should have the right to comment on scientific material before it is published but the final word must be the right of the academic scientist. Scientists who knowingly deviate from the truth or "massage" data for a specific purpose will damage the reputation and credibility of both academia and industry. Anyone working in the scientific field must be aware of the potential for intentional and unintentional bias. Scientists seek results and the risk is always that parameters are chosen on the basis of showing significant results in line with expectations or hopes rather than sound scientific considerations. This situation applies to academia as well as industry. The perspective on science is and should remain the same for both types of organizations. The only fundamental difference is perhaps that while industry applies science to achieve a result in the form of a product, the science is the product in the academic field.

21

Medical Devices: Regulatory Perspectives and Aspects of Regulatory Risk Management

Stina Gestrelius and Arne Hensten-Pettersen

CONTENTS

21.1 Regulation of Medical Devices ... 374
21.1.1 United States ... 374
21.1.2 European Union Member States ... 375
21.1.2.1 New Approach Directives ... 375
21.1.3 Japan ... 376
21.2 Definitions of Medical Devices ... 376
21.3 Classification ... 378
21.3.1 FDA's Three Classes of Medical Devices ... 378
21.3.2 MDD's Four Classes of Medical Devices ... 378
21.3.2.1 CE Marking Related to Risk Classification ... 379
21.3.3 Global Harmonization of Risk Classification ... 380
21.3.4 Other Aspects ... 380
21.3.4.1 Animal-Derived Medical Devices ... 381
21.3.4.2 Growth Factors ... 381
21.4 Regulatory Issues Concerning Medical Devices Used in Dentistry ... 381
21.4.1 History of Quality Assessment of Devices Used in Dentistry ... 382
21.4.1.1 International Aspects ... 382
21.4.1.2 Nordic Dental Materials: Testing and Certification ... 382
21.4.1.3 Practical Implications of NIOM's List of Certified Products ... 383
21.4.1.4 Dental Implants in Nordic Countries ... 383
21.4.1.5 International Product Standards in Dentistry ... 384
21.5 Risk Analysis, Assessment, and Management ... 384
21.5.1 Device Development ... 384
21.5.2 Risk versus Benefit ... 385

0-8493-1474-7/03/$0.00+$1.50

21.5.3 Biological Properties....386
21.5.4 Postmarketing Surveillance....386
21.6 Information Sources....386
21.6.1 Quality Systems....387

21.1 Regulation of Medical Devices

21.1.1 United States

The Food and Drug Administration (FDA) has regulated medical devices in the United States since 1938. The present regulatory framework is based on five statutes:

The Food, Drug, and Cosmetic Act of 1938 (FD&C Act)

The Medical Device Amendments of 1976 (1976 Amendments)

The Safe Medical Devices Act of 1990 (SMDA)

The Medical Device Amendments of 1992 (1992 Amendments)

The Federal Drug Administration Modernization Act of 1997 (FDAMA of 1997)

The original 1938 FD&C Act prohibited the marketing of adulterated or misbranded devices. The 1976 Amendments provided the FD&C Act with new authority expressly designed to ensure the safety and efficacy of devices and gave FDA premarket control over classification, notification, and approval of devices. Additionally, the 1976 Amendments strengthened post-market controls over devices and gave FDA the authority to require, among other things, patient identification, reporting, and record keeping, in addition to following good manufacturing practices (GMPs).

Concerns continued to be expressed, however, about the safety and efficacy of medical devices and the need for still more government controls. As a result, in 1990, the SMDA provided FDA with new enforcement authority over medical devices. SMDA streamlined certain procedures and added authority in others. It also refined the premarket and postmarket controls related to medical devices. The 1992 Amendments included changes to certain provisions of the SMDA.

The FDAMA of 1997 introduced more stringent controls to medical device safety, particularly those pertaining to quality assurance systems, by introducing quality system regulations (QSRs), risk analysis, design verification, and validation. The FDAMA of 1997 also introduced the *authorization of accredited third persons*, independent third party bodies that could evaluate product dossiers up to but not including the final approval of *substantial equivalence* status for some medical devices. The intention is that in the future accredited third persons will be permitted to audit manufacturers for compliance with QSR areas of the FDA regulations.

21.1.2 European Union Member States

21.1.2.1 New Approach Directives

The new European approach aims at ensuring free movement of goods, persons, services, and capital in the internal market (countries of the European Union [EU] and the European Economic Area Agreement [EEA]), without any restricting national regulations that may act as barriers to trade. The measure is regulated mainly by transposition of European community directives to national legislation in each EU/EEA member state.

The new directives encompass many of the traditional national strategies for premarket approval of products and introduced modules for conformity assessment. Compliance with the directives is symbolized by affixing the CE marks to products. The CE symbol on a product signifies that the manufacturer declares that the product meets the essential requirements of the relevant European directive and therefore can be freely moved within the internal market.

21.1.2.1.1 Nonactive Medical Devices

Dental implants and most other devices in contact with patients' bodies are categorized as medical devices. The regulatory situation for nonactive medical devices in EEA/EU member states changed in 1998. All national and regional certification programs on medical devices including dental products ceased to exist on June 14, 1998. The European Economic Community (EEC) council directive concerning medical devices (93/42/EEC), also called the MDD, was transposed to national laws and regulations and was in full effect after June 14, 1998 in all member countries of the EU and the EEA. Applicant countries, the potential new members of the EU, are now actively transposing the EU directives into national legislation, including the directive concerning medical devices (93/42/EEC).

National health authorities such as a ministry of health or national board of health traditionally regulated medical devices. Under the new system, the MDD is primarily in the domain of the Directorate of General Enterprise (formerly DG 3, Industry) with some new assignments of responsibilities. The MDD operates by virtue of *Competent Authority* and *Notified Bodies.*

Competent Authority (CA) — The CA is the national health authority responsible for implementation of the directive. The CA designates notified bodies (see next section) to which it delegates the authority to perform conformity assessment procedures according to requirements of the modules specified in the MDD. The CA has several other responsibilities. It registers all class I products and dental technical laboratories and other manufacturers of custom-made devices, and performs market surveillance of all medical devices. The CA is also responsible for the vigilance system, which is mainly intended to collect reports of deaths and serious injuries associated with medical devices. Any national vigilance activity is also reported to the CAs of other member states.

Notified Bodies — Notified bodies act as third-party certification entities. They are strictly required to maintain their independence of financial and other ties to the manufacturers with which they are in contact. The task of a notified body is to assess whether products in the higher risk classes fulfill the appropriate requirements of the MDD and ensure that a manufacturer has performed adequate risk analyses and can trace its products to end users. Manufacturers are required to have structured systems for postmarketing surveillance and feedback.

21.1.2.1 Practical Consequences

Every product shall be safe to use and fulfill the manufacturer's claims such as its intended use. This provision does not necessarily coincide with the requirements of international or European product standards. However, where devices do not comply with key relevant published standards, a rationale should be stated in the technical documentation for the product. The majority of the medical devices used in dentistry obtain their CE marks based on conformity with the requirements of manufacturers' quality assurance systems.

21.1.3 Japan

The Ministry of Health, Labour, and Welfare handles the Japanese medical device regulations concerning approval of foreign manufacture of medical devices (via an in-country caretaker) and granting product import licenses. Japan recently declared that it intends to harmonize its system by changing to a marketing approval procedure that would allow Japanese importers to handle registrations.

Japanese authorities are strongly safety oriented and may require additional safety studies. It is possible to obtain approvals without clinical studies in Japan, but extensive postmarketing studies may then be required.

21.2 Definitions of Medical Devices

The FD&C defines a medical device as an instrument, apparatus, implement, machine, contrivance, implant, *in vitro* reagent, or other similar or related article, including a component, part or accessory, which is:

1. Recognized in the official *National Formulary* or the *U.S. Pharmacopeia*, or any supplements

2. Intended for use in the diagnosis of disease or other conditions, or in the cure, mitigation, treatment, or prevention of disease in humans or animals
3. Intended to affect the structures or any functions of the bodies of humans or animals which does not achieve any of its primary intended purposes through chemical action within or on the bodies of humans or animals and is not dependent upon being metabolized for the achievement of any of its principal intended purposes.

The MDD defines a medical device as any instrument, apparatus, appliance, material, or other article, whether used alone or in combination, including the software necessary for its proper application, intended by the manufacturer to be used for human beings for:

1. Diagnosis, prevention, monitoring, treatment, or alleviation of disease
2. Diagnosis, monitoring, treatment, alleviation of, or compensation for an injury or handicap
3. Investigation, replacement, or modification of the anatomy or of a physiological process
4. Control of conception

The device must not achieve its principal intended action in or on the human body by pharmacological, immunological, or metabolic means, but may be assisted in its function by such means.

Based on the definitions in the MDD alone, a medical device and a drug can be difficult to distinguish. This issue is expanded upon in the demarcation between the medical device directives and the medicinal products directive in MEDDEV 2.1/3 (Revision 2, July 2001). Products in the following situations can be defined as medical devices:

1. Bone cements containing antibiotics
2. Root canal fillers incorporating medicinal products with secondary actions
3. Bone void fillers intended for the repair of bone defects when the primary action of the device is a physical means or matrix that provides a volume and a scaffold for osteoconduction and an additional medicinal substance is incorporated to assist and complement the action of the matrix by enhancing the growth of bone cells.

The ancillary would be determined by the performance of the matrix on its own and the extent of the enhancement of growth due to the presence of the substance. With reference to the overall purpose of the product, where the medicinal substance has such an effect that its ancillary nature cannot be clearly established, the product should be considered in accordance with the concept of a drug delivery system.

It should be noted that the mere coating of a product with a chemical does not imply that the chemical is a medicinal substance. For example, hydroxyapatite, frequently used as coating for orthopedic and dental implants, is not considered a medicinal substance. Other coatings in use that are not medicinal substances are hydromers and phosphoryl cholines. At present, products incorporating medicinal substances of human origin are excluded from the MDD.

21.3 Classification

The classification of a medical device is strongly linked to the type of risk that conceivably may be associated with its use. Medical devices vary widely in simplicity or complexity and the degree of risk or benefit involved. The regulatory categories or classes are assigned according to the extent of control necessary to assure the safety and efficacy of a device.

21.3.1 FDA's Three Classes of Medical Devices

Class I: General controls — Devices in Class I are those for which general controls alone are sufficient to assure safety and effectiveness. General controls include regulations that govern GMPs, records, reports, and inspections.

Class II: Special controls — Devices in Class II are those for which general controls alone are insufficient to provide reasonable assurance of safety and effectiveness, and for which sufficient information exists to establish special controls to provide this assurance.

Class III — Registration of Class III products may require premarket approval (PMA) or product development protocol (PDP).

Most Class I devices are exempt from notification. Class II devices require 510(k) notification if they are substantially equivalent to existing devices. New products are placed in Class III, but it is possible to submit statements of reasons to reclassify implants, for example, to Class II. Class III includes endosseous implants, including TCP granules, and biology-based products such as Emdogain® Gel.

According to a new draft guidance issued February 2002, resorbable bone void fillers such as calcium carbonate, calcium sulfate, calcium phosphate, and calcium salt additives derived from biological sources (animal or human tissue) are proposed to be placed in Class II.

21.3.2 MDD's Four Classes of Medical Devices

Products subject to the MDD fall into four risk classes, depending on which part of the body they contact and the duration of the contact. Dental restorative materials are considered surgically invasive products for permanent use. This implies that they should be placed in Class IIb. However, the directive includes a special rule stating that permanent products for use in teeth fall into a lower risk Class, IIa, that applies to dental restorative materials.

Dental implants are in Class IIb due to their long-term (>30 days) contact. If the manufacturer claims a biological activity for any coating, the implant is assigned to class III. Biora's Emdogain® Gel is a Class III device due to its animal origin rather than long-term placement.

21.3.2.1 CE Marking Related to Risk Classification

The certification of products (CE marking) is based on a manufacturer's declaration of conformity with the essential requirements (Annex I) of the MDD (Table 21.1). For Class I products, a manufacturer affixes the CE mark and registers the product with the CA. For high-risk products, a notified body performs the conformity assessment according to the MDD to verify the manufacturer's claims. The choice of practical procedure to achieve CE marking for any product is up to the manufacturer.

Class IIa products such as dental restorative materials used as suprastructures for implants have two different routes: (1) certification based on testing

TABLE 21.1

MDD Requirements[a]

Class	Design	Production
Product Approach		
I	Manufacturer's declaration	Manufacturer's declaration
IIa	Manufacturer's declaration	EC verification, production quality assurance, or product quality assurance
IIb	EC type examination	EC verification, production quality assurance, or product quality assurance (Annex VI)
III	EC type examination	EC verification or production quality assurance
Class		**Design and Production**
Quality Approach		
IIa	Full quality assurance without design dossier examination by notified body	
IIb	Full quality assurance without design dossier examination by notified body	
III	Full quality assurance including design dossier examination by notified body	

[a] The MDD contains a number of procedures to be followed for the assessment of conformity of medical devices with the provisions of the MDD. The procedure to be followed is determined by the class of medical device. Class I products presenting low risks are subject to a manufacturer's declaration based on a risk analysis and risk management approach carried out by the manufacturer without intervention of a third party. The procedures for class IIa, IIb, and III devices always require intervention by a notified body, i.e., a public or private organization designated by member states to carry out conformity assessment tasks specified in the MDD.

of batches of the product in accordance with the manufacturer's claims for the product and its intended use (Annex IV); and (2) certification of the manufacturer's quality assurance systems for production of the product (Annex II), the production line (Annex V), or testing and inspection of the final product (Annex VI).

For Class IIb products, for example dental implant systems, the options are (1) design verification (Annex III) plus batch control (Annex IV); (2) certification of the manufacturer's quality assurance systems either for production of the product (Annex II, not including design verification) or the production line (Annexes III and V); and (3) design verification plus a quality assurance system for testing and inspection of the final product (Annexes III and VI).

Class III products include dental implant systems with bioactive coating or containing medicinal substances. The options are (1) design verification (Annex III) plus batch control (Annex IV) or production control (Annex V); and (2) certification of the manufacturer's quality assurance systems for production of the product (Annex II including design verification).

21.3.3 Global Harmonization of Risk Classification

A global harmonization task force consisting of representatives from the U.S. Food and Drug Administration together with European, Japanese, Canadian, Chinese, and Australian authorities proposed a risk-based classification for medical devices (2001):

Class A — Invasive devices for transient use (<60 minutes)

Class B — Invasive devices for short-term use (<30 days)

Class C — Invasive devices for long-term use (>30 days)

Class D — Implantable devices in heart, blood, or CNS; or devices that are life-supporting; or produce biological effects; or have biological origins; or devices that are wholly or mainly absorbed or undergo chemical change (except in teeth); or devices that administer medicines

Human cells and tissues are not proposed to be harmonized by the task force, since they are regulated differently in different markets. It should be noted that Class D includes medical devices with biological effects, which appear to include the immunological and metabolic effects excluded from the present European definition discussed above.

21.3.4 Other Aspects

Products may be regulated differently, based on their applications rather than their types and origins. Future global harmonization might classify some current biological products as medical devices.

21.3.4.1 Animal-Derived Medical Devices

The recent European standard EN-12442 has three parts dealing with different aspects of standardization of production of animal-derived medical devices. Part 1 requires a risk analysis regarding animal species and tissues that can be used for different medical device applications. It also requires an extension of EN-1441 (risk analysis) regarding possible hazards for special categories of patients (e.g., immunocompromised individuals or those with endocrine disorders, malignancies, hypersensitivities, or autoimmunity). Part 2 standardizes the control of sourcing and handling (geographical origin, infection control, veterinary inspections, certification, etc.). Part 3 covers validation of virus elimination or inactivation and requirements for literature reviews and/or experimental proof.

The development and manufacture of Emdogain® Gel in accordance with this standard were approved by the U.S. and Japanese authorities in 2001. Only the French authorities required a special listing of animal-derived devices and additional information. An application must then be submitted to the Agence Francaise de Securité Sanitaire des Produits de Santé.

21.3.4.2 Growth Factors

In October 2001, FDA approved a growth factor under the humanitarian device exemption. It was the OP-1 implant, i.e., recombinant human protein OP-1 on bovine collagen, which may be used for bone formation when an autograft is not a good choice and other treatments have failed. In contrast, recombinant human PDGF-BB (platelet-derived growth factor) was approved as a *pharmaceutical* for treatment of diabetic foot ulcers in 1998. It is now sold under the tradename Regranex®.

21.4 Regulatory Issues Concerning Medical Devices Used in Dentistry

The quality of dental products has been under discussion for more than a century. The discussion has centered on what qualities are important and how they can be assured in design and manufacture. The longevity and efficacy of dental restorative procedures are to a great extent related to the qualities of the products used.

The quality and use of medical devices directly impact health issues and economics. Many dental products are relatively easy to make and most countries formerly imposed few regulatory constraints on design, production, marketing, and sales. For economical and other reasons, products were often manufactured in small quantities and variation in batches was sometimes considerable. Not all manufacturers had the necessary testing equipment to control the batches before release to customers. A Danish market survey and test of products on the market in the late 1950s showed that 50% of the amalgam products guaranteed by the manufacturers to fulfill minimum requirements of the corresponding ADA specification failed to do so.

The increasing focus on consumer protection related to the safety and efficacy of medical devices in general led to a more cautious attitude to accepting new products at face value. Various legislative measures to ensure the safety and efficacy of medical devices including those used in dentistry were introduced in the 20th century

21.4.1 History of Quality Assessment of Devices Used In Dentistry

Certification of products is based on independent third-party assessment of compliance with specified requirements. The certification programs for dental products are voluntary in some countries and regulatory in others.

21.4.1.1 International Aspects

The first certification program for dental products came as a result of standardization activities of the American Dental Association in the 1920s. The Australian Dental Association initiated a corresponding formalized program in the 1930s. Both organizations published lists of approved or certified materials. The development of dental product standards started early in Japan, but certification of products with the JIS (Japanese Industrial Standards) mark followed much later.

Australia, U.S., and Japan based their certifications on compliance with their own developed national product standards. The standards were relatively similar at the outset, but deviated in some areas. The basis for certification was to protect domestic producers.

In Europe, the health authorities of Great Britain and the Nordic countries established formal certification programs for dental products early in the 1970s. The programs were based on British standards in Great Britain and on international standards in the Nordic countries. In Germany, direct filling materials were classified as pharmaceutical products and were subject to legislation regulating pharmaceuticals. Other voluntary national certification programs were also enacted.

21.4.1.2 Nordic Dental Materials: Testing and Certification

The health ministries of Denmark, Finland, Iceland, Norway, and Sweden formed the Scandinavian Institute of Dental Materials (NIOM) in 1972. NIOM's mission was to ensure that dental products on the Nordic market were safe and effective. Its materials testing programs from 1972 to 1998 were based on evaluation of product properties in relation to specifications in international dental standards. For two important product areas that lacked international standards, alloys for porcelain-fused-to-metal and composite materials for use in the molar area (posterior composites), NIOM developed acceptance programs based on national drafts for standards or acceptance programs.

NIOM bought the materials for testing on the open markets in Nordic countries each year and tested them according to standards. The manufacturers already guaranteed that the products fulfilled the requirements of the standard. NIOM's testing showed that 10 to 30% of the products did not comply with the standards.

21.4.1.3 Practical Implications of NIOM's List of Certified Products

The recommendation to use NIOM-certified products in clinical practice was not of a regulatory nature in any country. However, national interests sought quality control for specific product groups. In Sweden, the national health insurance program required that only high noble content gold alloys certified by NIOM be used. Similarly, in Norway, the tariffs for dental treatment agreed to by the health directorate and the Norwegian Dental Association specified that dental treatment procedures should only be performed with materials certified by NIOM. The Danish tariffs for treating children and adolescents in public clinics also had similar requirements. Finland had a similar recommendation for treatment in public clinics.

In Australia, the Therapeutic Goods Administration (TGA) accepted products certified by NIOM as equivalent to those subjected to TGA testing and certification activities. The result was that NIOM-certified products could be freely marketed in Australia without further testing by TGA.

21.4.1.4 Dental Implants in Nordic Countries

The Norwegian Directorate of Health registered and controlled dental implants under authority of the 1981 regulations for registration and control of single-use medical devices as products which, based on their intended use, are assumed to be sterile.

In Sweden, only dental implants with adequate documentation of long-term use as assessed by an advisory expert panel were remunerated under the national health insurance plan.

Finland established a national register of dental implants in 1994. All implant systems were accepted. The register is used for follow-up and evaluation of the safety and usability of dental implants. It records information concerning implant, operation, surgical unit, patient, diagnosis, and possible complications.

After implementation of the European Community directive concerning medical devices (93/42/EEC), also called the MDD, in 1998, the Norwegian and Swedish national systems ceased operations, and all CE-marked dental implants were accepted. The Finnish registry continues to collect information and publish annual reports.

21.4.1.5 International Product Standards in Dentistry

The International Organization for Standardization (ISO) developed more than 110 dental product standards. The work was performed by ISO Technical Committee (TC) 106, Dentistry. These vertical product standards were adopted by CEN, the European Standardization Committee, as EN standards with identical content. As a result of a mandate from the commission responsible for the MDD, the vertical product standards, were combined with horizontal standards for biological evaluation, risk analysis, labeling, etc. and grouped into four semihorizontal European standards concerning dental instruments, materials, equipment, and dental implants (EN 1639 through 1642). Showing compliance with these standards is one of the options for conformity assessment (CE certification) in Europe.

21.5 Risk Analysis, Assessment, and Management

ISO also developed a protocol for methods by which risk analysis, assessment, and management can be performed (ISO 14971, Application of Risk Management to Medical Devices).

21.5.1 Device Development

The classical path of a pharmaceutical from the discovery stage through research and development, preclinical testing, and clinical Phases I, II, and III is followed often for medical devices in classes IIb and III. The quality system regulation of FDAMA (1997) and the ISO 9001 standard require that a design control system be followed. The system emphasizes that development starts with specified user needs and specified detailed input criteria. The design process must be reviewed periodically, and the design output (product) must be verified against the design input and validated against user needs (Figure 21.1).

The use of internationally recognized good practices is an advantage during design development and in the subsequent manufacturing process. Guidelines cover good laboratory practices (GLPs), good clinical practices (GCPs), and good manufacturing practices (GMPs). Some of these are mandatory in the U.S. and Japan.

During the development stage, many devices are tested in animal experiments to assess their properties under conditions of use. Complete study design protocols should encompass full utilization of the animals. Irrespective of the local effects sought, biopsies of all organs should also be taken for later histopathological evaluation. They may be useful in premarket regulatory documentation of biological effects.

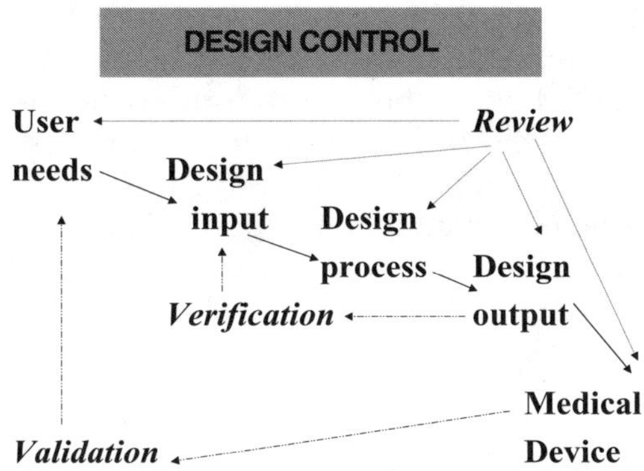

FIGURE 21.1
Design control process according to the U.S. Food and Drug Administration Quality System Regulation and ISO 9001.

21.5.2 Risk versus Benefit

Medical devices should provide patients, users, and third parties with high levels of protection and attain the performance levels attributed to them by their manufacturers. Ideally, biomaterials and medical devices should perfectly fulfill the functions for which they were designed without adverse effects. Practically, however, some minor side effects can be tolerated if outweighed by benefits for the patient. Annex I of the MDD (Essential Requirements) states:

> The devices must be designed and manufactured in such a way that, when used under the conditions and for the purposes intended, they will not compromise the clinical condition or the safety of the patients, or the safety and health of users, or where applicable other persons, provided that any risks which may associated with their use constitute acceptable risks when weighed against the benefits to the patient and are compatible with a high level of protection of health and safety.

This is further elaborated in the requirements covering design and construction. Such devices must be designed and manufactured in such a way as to guarantee the characteristics and performances referred to in Section I (General Requirements). Particular attention must be paid to (1) the choice of materials used, particularly regarding toxicity and, where appropriate, flammability; and (2) compatibility between the materials used and biological tissues, cells, and body fluids, taking into account the intended purpose of the device.

The MDD requires a manufacturer to present documented results of risk analysis. The analysis should address all known or reasonably foreseeable hazards of the product types and technologies involved, together with the likelihood and consequences of occurrence and measures to be taken to reduce all relevant risks to acceptable levels. For example, in the case of devices incorporating a medicinal substance, material of animal origin, or natural rubber latex, the risk analysis should include the additional risks and benefits associated with the incorporation. In the case of devices intended for single use, the risk analysis should address the hazards associated with reuse as an example of foreseeable misuse.

The results must demonstrate that an appropriate risk analysis has been performed and provide a conclusion with appropriate evidence that the remaining risks are acceptable when weighed against the intended benefits to patients.

21.5.3 Biological Properties

Assessment of biological properties of the individual components and the complete device may comprise literature surveys, characterization, and evaluation of substances leachable from the devices, biological testing under simulated laboratory conditions, and clinical testing in humans. The CEN and ISO standardization bodies developed standard ISO 10993-1 for selecting relevant test methods for biological evaluation of medical devices. The ISO 10993 series detailed in Table 21.2 describes the biological test methods and their rationales for use. These tests do not cover all biocompatibility aspects and should be used with due caution. The methods described in the standards generally do not include pass/fail criteria.

The final risk assessment needs to be performed in a structured manner by a knowledgeable person (expert). The final responsibility for the safety and performance of the product remains with the manufacturer.

21.5.4 Postmarketing Surveillance

Severe limitations are inherent in extrapolation of biological laboratory studies in relatively few animals to human use situations involving large numbers of persons. According to the MDD, a manufacturer is required to have a structured system for postmarketing surveillance and feedback of complaints. Used properly, the system is a valuable tool for periodic review of the design of a device to ensure high levels of safety and efficacy.

21.6 Information Sources

Changes and developments are continuous in the regulatory field. Updated information is available from the following sources:

U.S. Food and Drug Administration, Center for Devices and Radiological Health: http://www.fda.gov/cdrh

European Union Council Directive 93/42/EEC (MDD) concerning medical devices: http://europa.eu.int/comm/dg03/directs/dg3d/d2/meddev/md/dirmd/dirmd/htm

Information about new approach to technical harmonization and standardization: http://europa.eu.int/comm/enterprise/newapproach/standardization/index.html

http://europa.eu.int/comm/enterprise/newapproach/standardization/harmstds/index.html

References to harmonized standards (New Approach Directives): http://europa.eu.int/comm/enterprise/newapproach/standardization/harmstds/index.html

Overview of all healthcare sector standards: http://www.cenorm.be/sectors/healthcare.htm

Guidance documents:

http://europa/eu.int/comm/dg03/directs/dg3d/d2/meddev/md/dirmd/dirmd/html

Japan: *Guide to Medical Device Registration*, 5th ed., Yakuji Nippon, Ltd., 1994.

21.6.1 Quality Systems

Good Laboratory Practices (GLPs), European Union and Organisation for Economic Cooperation and Development (OECD)

Principles of Good Laboratory Practice, Nonclinical Laboratory Studies, Good Laboratory Practice Regulations, U.S. Food and Drug Administration

Good Clinical Practices (GCPs), European Union, U.S., and Japan, ICH Harmonised Tripartite Guideline for Good Clinical Practice

Good Manufacturing Practices (GMPs), European Union EEC Commission Directive 91/356/EEC, Principles and Guidelines of Good Manufacturing Practices for Medicinal Products for Human Use, Eudralex Volume 4

U.S. Food and Drug Administration, Current Good Manufacturing Practices (cGMPs) for Medical Devices, Volume 21, Code of Federal Regulations, Section 821

TABLE 21.2

Standards for Evaluation of Biological Properties and Clinical Investigations of Medical Devices[a]

Technical committees involved in preparing standards of biological and clinical evaluation procedures

ISO/TC 194, Biological evaluation of medical devices
CEN/TC 206, Biocompatibility of medical and dental materials and devices
CEN/TC 258, Clinical investigation of medical devices
CEN/TC 55, Dentistry
ISO/TC 106, Dentistry

Standards for biological evaluation

EN ISO 10993-1, 1997, Biological evaluation of medical devices, Part 1: Evaluation and testing
ISO/DIS 10993-17.2, 1999, Biological evaluation of medical devices, Part 17: Methods for the establishment of allowable limits for leachable substances using health-based risk assessment
EN ISO 10993-2, 1998, Biological evaluation of medical devices, Part 2: Animal welfare requirements
EN 30993-3, 1993, Biological evaluation of medical devices, Part 3: Tests for genotoxicity, carcinogenicity, and reproductive toxicity (revision of ISO 10993-3, 1992)
ISO/CD 10993-3.2, 1998, Biological evaluation of medical devices, Part 3: Tests for genotoxicity, carcinogenicity, and reproductive toxicity (revision of ISO 10993-3, 1992)
EN 30993-4, 1993, Biological evaluation of medical devices, Part 4: Selection of tests for interactions with blood (revision of ISO 10993-4, 1992)
EN ISO 10993-5, 1999, Biological evaluation of medical devices, Part 5: Tests for *in vitro* cytotoxicity
EN 30993-6, 1994, Biological evaluation of medical devices, Part 6: Tests for local effects after implantation (revision of ISO 10993-6, 1994)
EN ISO 10993-7, 1995, Biological evaluation of medical devices, Part 7: Ethylene oxide sterilization residuals
ISO/DIS 10993-8, 1999, Biological evaluation of medical devices, Part 8: Guidance on the selection and qualification of reference materials for biological tests
ISO 10993-9, 1999, Biological evaluation of medical devices, Part 9: Framework for identification and quantification of potential degradation products
EN ISO 10993-10, 1996, Biological evaluation of medical devices, Part 10: Tests for irritation and sensitization
prEN ISO 10993-10, 2000, Biological evaluation of medical devices, Part 10: Tests for irritation and delayed-type hypersensitivity (revision of ISO 10993-10, 1995)
EN ISO 10993-11, 1995, Biological evaluation of medical devices, Part 11: Tests for systemic toxicity
EN ISO 10993-12, 1996, Biological evaluation of medical devices, Part 12: Sample preparation and reference materials
EN ISO 10993-13, 1998, Biological evaluation of medical devices, Part 13: Identification and quantification of degradation products from polymeric medical devices
ISO/DIS 10993-14, 1999, Biological evaluation of medical devices, Part 14: Identification and quantification of degradation products from ceramics
EN ISO 10993-15, 2000, Biological evaluation of medical devices, Part 15: Identification and quantification of degradation products from metals and alloys
EN ISO 10993-16, 1997, Biological evaluation of medical devices, Part 16: Toxicokinetic study design for degradation products and leachables
prEN ISO 10993-17, 1999, Biological evaluation of medical devices, Part 17: Methods for the establishment of allowable limits for leachable substances using health-based risk assessment

TABLE 21.2 (CONTINUED)

Standards for Evaluation of Biological Properties and Clinical Investigations of Medical Devices[a]

ISO/CD 10993-18.2, 1998, Biological evaluation of medical devices, Part 18: Chemical characterisation of materials
ISO/NWIP (ISO/TC 194 WG 15 TF1), 1999, Biological evaluation of medical devices, Part 20: Principles and methods for immunotoxicology testing of medical devices
ISO 7405, Preclinical evaluation of biocompatibility of medical devices used in dentistry: test methods for dental materials
Standards for clinical investigations of medical devices
EN 540, 1993, Clinical investigation of medical devices for human subjects
ISO 14155, 1996, Clinical investigation of medical devices
ISO and CEN are working on a harmonized standard to replace the two above

[a] The CEN and ISO standardization bodies developed a series of standards for biological evaluation of medical devices that may be of help in selecting relevant test methods. These tests do not cover all biocompatibility aspects and should be used with due caution. The test methods described in the standards generally do not include pass/fail criteria. The final risk assessment must be performed in a structured manner by a knowledgeable person (expert). The selection of test methods and the rationales for their use shall be documented in the manufacturer's technical file (dossier) for each medical device.

Section VII

Inventive Forward Looks: Where Do We Go from Here?

22

Self-Assembling and Biomimetic Biomaterials

Samuel I. Stupp, Elia Beniash, Jeffrey D. Hartgerink, and Eli D. Sone

CONTENTS

22.1 Introduction 393
22.2 Tissue Engineering 397
22.3 Design and Synthesis of an Extracellular Matrix 398
22.4 Mineralization of Nanofibers 400
22.5 Chemically Customized Extracellular Matrices 402
22.6 Conclusions 404
Acknowledgments 404
References 405

22.1 Introduction

A fundamental mechanism to achieve function in biology is the interaction among nanoscale objects that have both defined shapes and surface chemistries. The most important nanostructures are, of course, proteins that can engage in molecular recognition events of high fidelity with small molecules, with segments of macromolecules, or with other proteins forming complexes that range from dimers to polymers. An interesting example of shape and surface chemical map versus function is offered by the complex known as α-hemolysin shown in Figure 22.1. This complex is formed by the self-assembly of seven polypeptide chains into a mushroom-shaped structure produced by a human pathogen, *Staphylococcus aureus*.[1]

The chemical map on the surface of this "nanomushroom" consisting of a hydrophobic stem and a hydrophilic cap allows the complex to insert itself into the external bilayer lipid membranes of human cells, keeping the

0-8493-1474-7/03/$0.00+$1.50

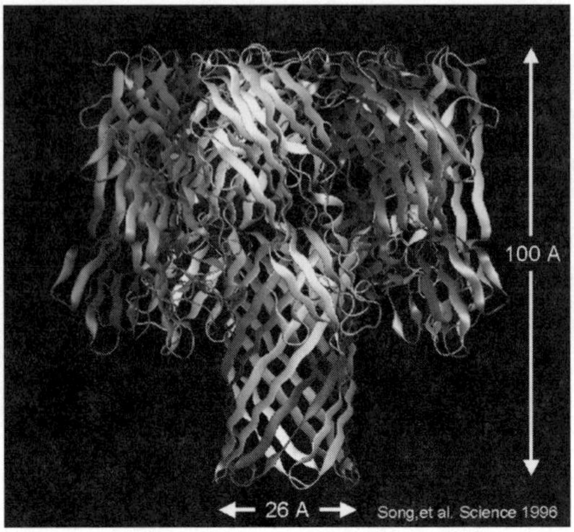

FIGURE 22.1
(See color insert.) Complex of seven polypeptide chains known as α-hemolysin, synthesized by the human *Staphylococcus aureus* pathogen. This mushroom-shaped nanostructure has a pore parallel to the long axis and inserts itself into the bilayer membranes of cells. (*Source:* From Song, L. et al., *Science*, 274, 1859, 1996. With permission.)

stem within the hydrophobic compartment and the cap in the more hydrophilic external environment. Along the long axis of this mushroom-shaped object is a cylindrical cavity roughly 16 Å in diameter that the pathogen uses to deliver ions or molecules into cells targeted for destruction. Thus, shape and surface chemistry of this nanostructure are key elements in its efficient function.

The macromolecules of common polymers lack the defined three-dimensional shapes and chemical sites of proteins. We hypothesized earlier that new functional materials could emerge from the introduction of such features in synthetic organic structures.[2] This biomimetic approach to materials could lead to novel biomaterials or novel designs for the interfaces of permanent implants and biological tissues. Our laboratory targeted supramolecular self-assembly among synthetic molecules as a strategy to generate designed nanostructures.[2-8] Figure 22.2 illustrates some of the nanostructures of interest.

Two different families of molecules that yield nanostructures by self-assembly in organic solvents were discovered in our laboratory over the past few years. One family consists of short triblock polymers containing one segment that is identical in all molecules of the system and is the driver of self-assembly. Self-assembly proceeds as a result of crystallization of these segments. However, these crystallizable segments are covalently bonded to two others that are incapable of crystallizing. These segments also have a greater specific volume per structural unit relative to the crystallizable segments, and therefore steric forces arise as nanocrystals begin to form.[2]

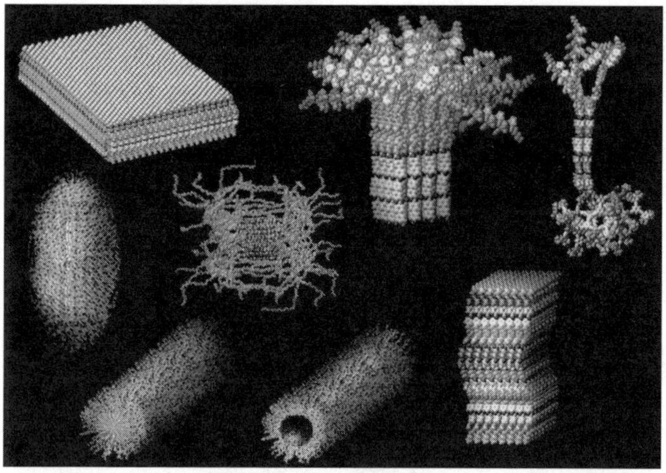

FIGURE 22.2
Molecular graphics renditions of supramolecular nanostructures formed by self-assembly of organic molecules. (*Source:* From Stupp, S.I. et al., *Mater. Res. Sci. Bull.*, 25, 42, 2000. With permission.)

This stops crystallization after only dozens or hundreds of molecules have formed a supramolecular structure and thus results in the formation of nanostructures in the size range of proteins. Figure 22.3 (left) shows a molecular model of these triblock molecules and the mushroom-shaped aggregate they form, as well as a transmission electron micrograph of the aggregates. Figure 22.3 (right) also shows another family of molecules we have termed dendron rodcoils (DRCs). DRCs are also triblock molecules but the structurally defined segments that could crystallize are unable to do so for geometrical reasons. Such segments are rigid and dendritic and therefore cannot form dense clusters of molecules arranged parallel to each other. These dendritic segments have termini with hydrogen bond-forming functions (phenolic groups in the Figure 22.3 example). Thus, these molecules aggregate head-to-head through hydrogen bonding and create one-dimensional, ribbon-shaped structures only 10 nm wide and about 2 nm thick.[9] However, their length can be 100 to 1000 times greater than their width reaching micron scale.

Creating nanostructures by self-assembly of organic molecules results in the formation of interesting materials. The mushroom-shaped nanostructures yielded thin films in which the nanostructures were arranged in layers and stacked in head-to-tail polar fashion. This led to films that had two parallel surfaces, one exposing the tops and the other the bottoms of the nanostructures. These films, therefore, have hydrophobic and hydrophilic surfaces and very different properties on opposite surfaces.[2] In fact, this particular characteristic would be useful in designing biomaterial interfaces. For example, one could produce a thin film by self-assembly that would bond to a permanent implant material on one side and expose to the bio-

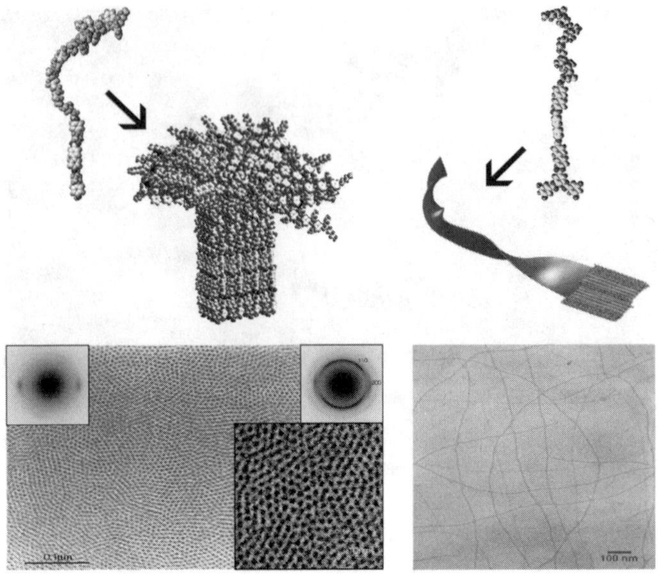

FIGURE 22.3
Triblock molecule containing one rigid segment and two flexible segments that self assemble into mushroom-shaped nanostructures (left). Triblock molecule containing one rigid segment, a dendritic segment at one terminus, and a flexible segment at the opposite terminus (right). The molecule on the right side self-assembles into a ribbon structure of nanoscale dimensions and lengths of several microns (see text). Transmission electron micrographs at the bottom of the figure correspond to each type of nanostructure and electron diffraction patterns for the mushroom-shaped nanostructures. (*Sources:* From Stupp, S.I. et al., *Science*, 276, 384, 1997, and Zubarev, E.R. et al., *J. Am. Chem. Soc.*, 23, 4105, 2001. With permission.)

logical environment a chemically different surface with useful biological properties such as specific cell recruitment ability, blood compatibility, or cell differentiation signals. The polar assembly of nanostructures also results in films that exhibit piezoelectricity[10] or second harmonic generation.[11-12]

The formation of nanoribbons is useful in other ways, for example, in forming gels from dilute solutions[9] and modifying physical properties of polymers.[13-14]

Another important mechanism to achieve biological function in the context of materials is the formation of mineral phases with diverse forms using organic structures as templates.[15-18] In our previous research, we demonstrated the use of one-dimensional nanoribbons described above as templates for the formation of inorganic nanostructures. In a recent publication, we reported on the formation of a helix of cadmium sulfide with nanoscale thickness and pitch using an organic helical template as the nucleation surface for the mineral (see Figure 22.4).

The possibility of nucleating mineral crystals with shapes and sizes that can be designed would be an extremely important capability for materials to be used in hard tissue repair, particularly repair of bone. Later in this

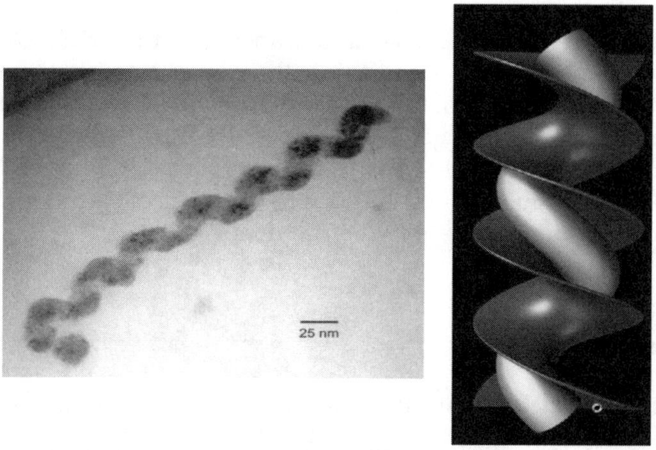

FIGURE 22.4
Transmission electron micrograph of a cadmium sulfide nanohelix (left) templated on a helical organic nanoribbon substrate. Templating of the nanohelix is shown (right). (*Source:* From Sone, E.D. et al., *Angew. Chem.*, 41, 1705, 2002. With permission.)

chapter, we demonstrate this possibility using a nanofiber substrate to nucleate hydroxyapatite crystals.

22.2 Tissue Engineering

The necessary strategies for complete regeneration of adult human tissues, in spite of genetics and clinical variables, should be the ultimate endpoint for the field of regenerative medicine. This field has been labeled over the past 20 years as tissue engineering.[19-24] The achievement of this goal may not be possible for many decades, but a number of related targets could be reached earlier. One target is the development of biomaterials that form ideal interfaces with tissues, for example, materials that prevent avascular encapsulation or, in the case of bone implants, materials that lead to immediate mechanical fixation because of rapid tissue regeneration around them.

The ultimate goal of regenerative medicine will require extracellular matrix engineering — a task that will require learning more about self-assembly, supramolecular chemistry, nanoscience, and biomimetic chemistry. The effectiveness of synthetic extracellular matrices (ECMs) for tissue regeneration will also increase with advances in genomics, proteomics, and stem cell biology.

The engineering of a synthetic ECM is necessary because tissue engineering requires tailored biodegradable matrices. Peptides that mimic epitopes in ligands must be part of the design, as well as the ability of these matrices to carry growth factors for local release. At the same time, the matrices need to integrate the right mechanical and transport properties, and must be amenable to facile clinical delivery with minimal trauma, for example through simple injection. Finally, an ideal synthetic ECM will probably have to carry drugs and possibly genes to mediate local response. With regard to synthetic matrices, the field of tissue engineering is dominated by the use of simple biodegradable polyesters such as poly(L-lactic acid), poly(glycolic acid), and copolymers of these two structures.[25-30]

22.3 Design and Synthesis of an Extracellular Matrix

We designed an extracellular matrix that mimics the nanoscale architecture of collagen fibrils, possibly the most common components of biological ECMs. As illustrated in Figure 22.5, the model system utilized relatively small molecules that could self-assemble into fibers having dimensions similar to those of the smallest collagen fibrils, around 10 nm. The first molecule synthesized for this purpose was the peptide amphiphile shown in Figure 22.6 which, upon assembly, yields fibers with diameters of approximately 7 to 8 nm. The nanofibers tend to have very large aspect ratios, reaching lengths on the order of several microns, and thus as they form in dilute solutions of the peptide amphiphile in water, they lead to the formation of gels.[31]

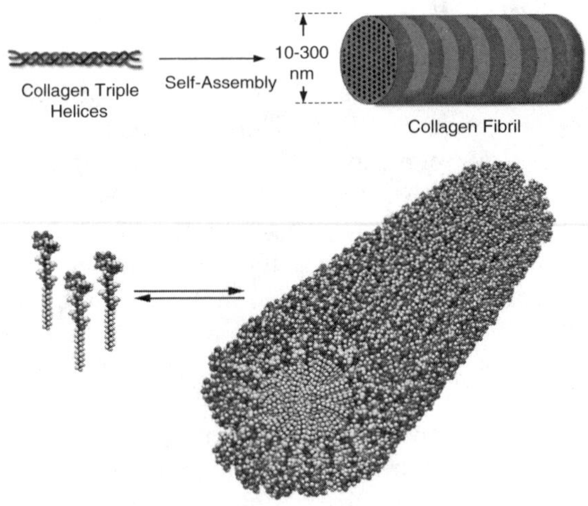

FIGURE 22.5
(See color insert.) Schematic showing how small molecules (bottom left) self-assemble into solid fibers with nanoscale diameters (bottom right). Self-assembly produces nanostructures that mimic the morphology of collagen fibrils — common constituents of extracellular matrices formed through the aggregation of polypeptide triple helices (top).

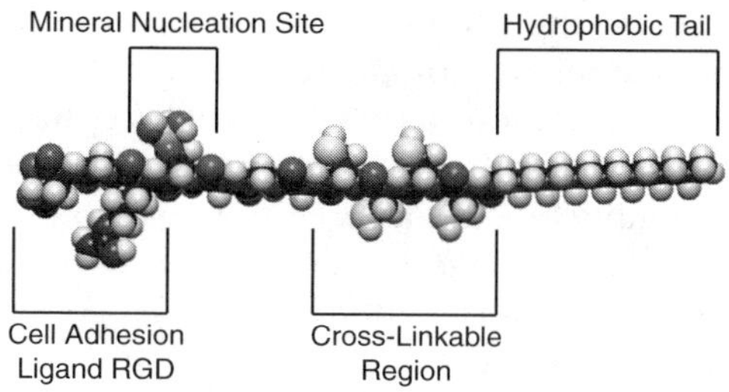

FIGURE 22.6
(See color insert.) Molecular graphics of a molecule designed to generate a synthetic extracellular matrix by self-assembly. The molecule has four important regions: a bioactive tripeptide at one terminus for cell adhesion, a phosphorylated serine residue to generate in the supramolecular structure an array of mineral nucleation sites, a tetrapeptide of cysteine residues to capture covalently the supramolecular nanofiber through disulfide bonds, and a hydrophobic alkyl segment to impart a large amphiphilic moment to the molecule backbone.

This property is of course useful for clinical delivery. The molecules that form the gels consist of two blocks: a peptide segment and a hydrophobic alkyl chain that causes them to self-assemble in water into nanofibers, provided their charges are neutralized. Charge neutralization can be carried out by changes in pH or by introduction into the water of metal ions that will screen charges. The molecules are synthesized by solid phase peptide chemistry in an automated synthesizer using standard fluorenylmethoxycarbonyl chemistry. After the peptide segments of these molecules are prepared, the N-termini are capped with fatty acid segments. Further details of the synthesis of these peptide amphiphiles can be found elsewhere.[31,32] Figure 22.7 is a transmission electron micrograph of nanofibers obtained after self-assembly.

The molecule shown in Figure 22.6 has a number of structural features that should allow it to form a bioactive synthetic ECM. First, the overall

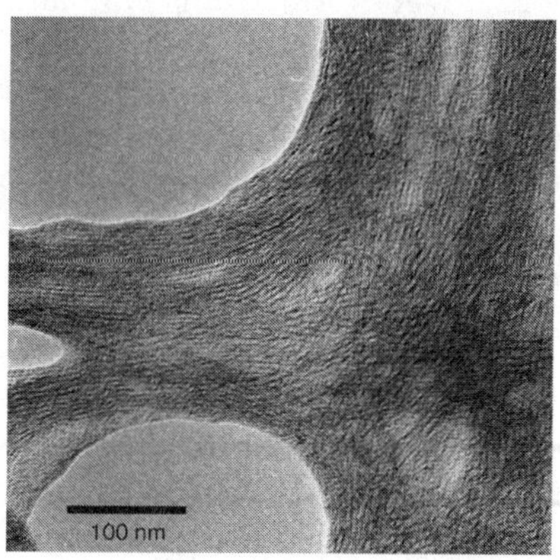

FIGURE 22.7
Transmission electron micrograph showing arrays of nanofibers formed by self-assembly.

shape of the molecule is slightly tapered — a feature that should result in curved rather than flat arrays of packed molecules once self-assembly occurs.[33] The peptide segment at the N-terminus begins with four cysteine residues used to polymerize the supramolecular assemblies into covalent structures. This is possible by oxidation of the assemblies with either iodine or oxygen, and interestingly the polymerization is reversible with the introduction of reducing agents such as dithiothreitol. A sequence of three glycine residues follows the cysteines as a spacer that should facilitate the polymerization of the structure through disulfide bond formation.

The last four amino acid residues, depending on molecular dynamics in the supramolecular structure, should be exposed on surfaces of the nanofibers and were selected to induce nucleation of hydroxyapatite mineral (phosphoserine) and recruit cells to the fibers once formed (arginine, glycine, and aspartic acid). Phosphoserine residues are present in proteins such as phosphophoryn[34-36] found in bone matrix and are believed to participate in mineralization. The tripeptide RGD, on the other hand, is known to be present in extracellular proteins such as fibronectin and involved in cell adhesion through binding to integrin receptors in mammalian cells.[37] Once nanofibers form, their surfaces may recruit cells and in the presence of suitable calcium and phosphate concentrations may nucleate hydroxyapatite crystals. The nucleation of such crystals is possibly important in the recruitment of osteogenic cells for bone repair.[38]

22.4 Mineralization of Nanofibers

The nanofibers described above can form by simple drying of peptide amphiphile solutions on solid surfaces. Nanofibers composed of the molecules shown in Figure 22.5 were formed this way and also by exposing the peptide amphiphile solution to HCl vapor to lower pH and neutralize charge. In this key experiment designed to mineralize nanofibers, the peptide amphiphile solution (1 mg/ml) was placed on one surface of a copper grid covered on its opposite side with a perforated carbon film. The opposite surfaces of this grid were treated with 5 μl of 10 mM $CaCl_2$ on one side and 5 μl of 5mM $NaHPO_4$ on the other side. This experiment is shown schematically in Figure 22.8.

The two solutions could mix only by passing through the holes of the carbon film. After 30 minutes, crystals of hydroxyapatite grew on the surfaces of nanofibers. They had the expected atomic ratios of Ca and P found in hydroxyapatite, and interestingly the c-axes of these crystals had a preferred orientation parallel to the long axes of the nanofibers.[32]

This same relationship existed between the c-axes of hydroxyapatite crystals and the long axes of collagen fibrils.[37,40-42] Thus, our system recreated

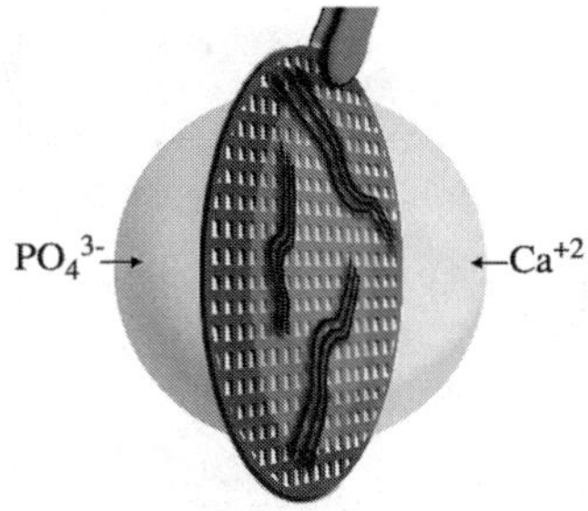

FIGURE 22.8
Nanofiber mineralization experiment. Nanofibers form on one surface of a copper grid coated on the opposite side with a perforated carbon film. The nanofibers are exposed to the precursor ions of the mineral by first placing a droplet of a calcium ion-containing solution on one side of the grid, and then treating the opposite side with a droplet of phosphate ion-containing solution.

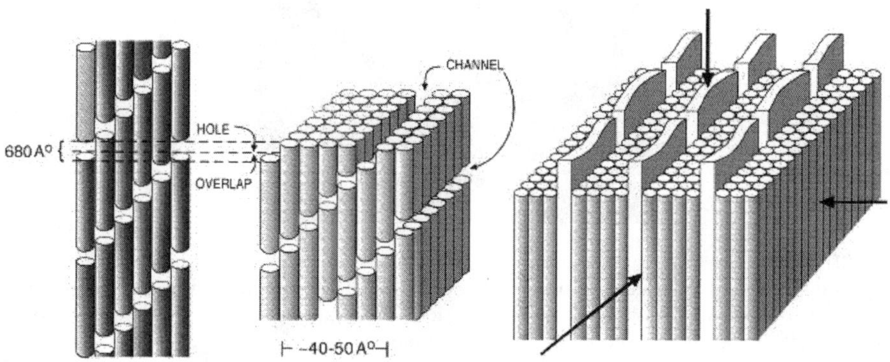

FIGURE 22.9
Nanoscale architecture of bone matrix showing cylindrical collagen fibrils with their long axes parallel to the c-axes of flat hydroxyapatite crystals (*Source:* From Weiner, S. and Wagner, H.D., *Annu. Rev. Mater. Sci.*, 28, 271, 1998. With permission.)

this aspect of the nanoscale structures of bone and dentin. Based on tilting experiments with an electron microscope, the crystals formed in our nanofiber networks were found to have flat shapes similar to those that occur in biology. Figure 22.9 shows a previously published schematic of the geometrical relationship of collagen fibrils and mineral crystals in the bone family of materials.[40] Figure 22.10 is a transmission electron micrograph of mineralized nanofibers along with our model describing one possible way the crystals could be oriented with respect to the supramolecular structures. Even though the c-axis of the nanoscale crystals has a preferential orientation parallel to the organic nanofibers, the a- and b-axes of the crystals can have many different orientations.

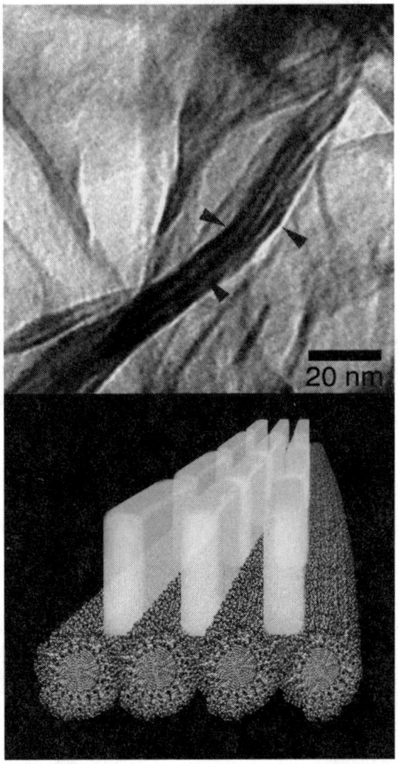

FIGURE 22.10
(See color insert.) Top: transmission electron micrograph of peptide amphiphile nanofibers covered by hydroxyapatite crystals (darkest regions indicated by arrows). Bottom: hydroxyapatite crystals growing on nanofibers. (*Source:* From Service, R.F., *Science*, 294, 1635, 2001. With permission.)

22.5 Chemically Customized Extracellular Matrices

Our laboratory synthesized a large variety of peptide amphiphiles varying in amino acid sequences in their hydrophilic segments.[33] Figure 22.11 shows molecules found to self-assemble into the nanofiber supramolecular architecture in spite of their differences in peptide sequences. This observation suggests that synthetic ECMs can be customized to different types of tissues. For example, one of the molecules shown in the figure contains the sequence IKVAV known to be an epitope in the extracellular laminin protein that promotes neurite growth.[43,44]

This particular amphiphile forms nanofibers as well, but relative to those discussed earlier, they are shorter and appear more rigid as well. Nonethe-

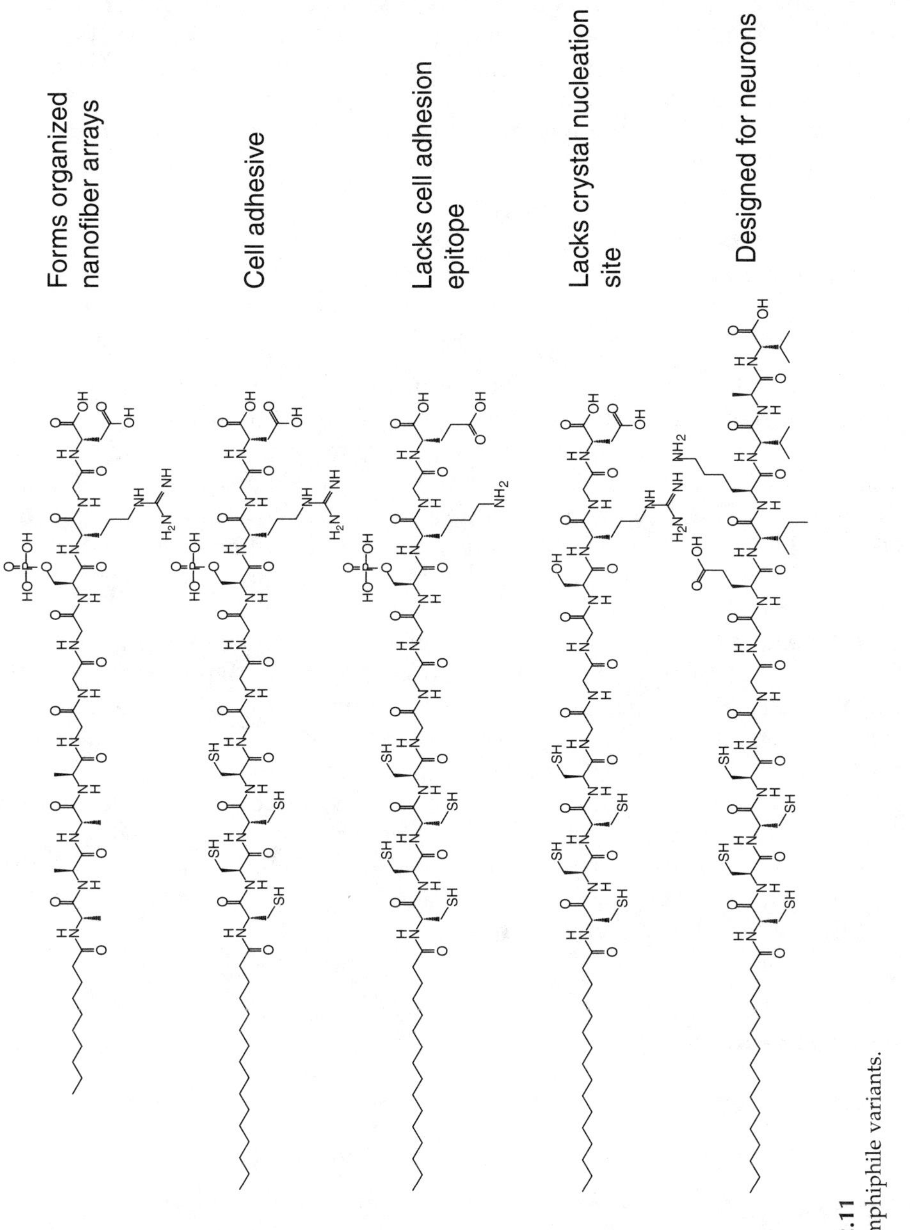

FIGURE 22.11
Peptide–Amphiphile variants.

less, these nanofibers also lead to gel formation, presumably because of their ability to create a three-dimensional structure.

The observed chemical versatility of these systems indicates that the strong amphiphilic nature of the molecules drives self-assembly, and so relatively hydrophobic peptide sequences such as IKVAV are still able to form nanofiber structures in aqueous environments. Many other epitopes and combinations of molecules within the supramolecular structures could lead to customized ECMs to mediate the regeneration of both soft and hard tissues. Combinations of two different molecules have been recently shown to form nanofibers containing two different epitopes.[45]

22.6 Conclusions

The regeneration of hard and soft tissues should be the ultimate goal in biomaterials design. This regeneration might occur around permanent implants or the new tissue could completely replace a biodegradable synthetic ECM scaffold. The implementation of this goal is likely to require delivery of ECMs that carry cells, possibly stem cells, and the role of the ECM will be to deliver suitable signals for differentiation and proliferation of cells. These cells would in turn synthesize the necessary extracellular matrix to produce the new tissue.

The greatest challenge will be to integrate other functions into such synthetic ECMs. For example, in the fixation of bone implants, the synthetic ECM would ideally behave as a mechanically sound adhesive allowing immediate fixation of the implant before cell-mediated processes take over for tissue regeneration. The transition from one set of functions to another poses the greatest challenge. The ability of the synthetic ECM to sustain cell viability and proliferation and blood vessel network formation with proper kinetics are, of course, parts of the challenge as well. Preliminary work in our laboratory indicates the synthetic ECMs described here have potential to meet some of these requirements.

Acknowledgments

The work in S.I. Stupp's laboratory described in this chapter was supported by the U.S. Department of Energy, the National Science Foundation, the Air Force Office of Scientific Research, the Office of Naval Research, and the Army Research Office. Mark Seniw of our laboratory helped with the preparation of figures.

References

1. Song, L. et al., Structure of staphylococcal alpha-hemolysin, a heptameric transmembrane pore, *Science*, 274, 1859, 1996.
2. Stupp, S.I. et al., Supramolecular materials: Self-organized nanostructures, *Science*, 276, 384, 1997.
3. Stupp, S.I. et al., Self-assembly of organic nano-objects into functional materials, *Mater. Res. Sci. Bull.*, 5, 42, 2000.
4. Zubarev, E.R. et al., Conversion of supramolecular clusters to macromolecular objects, *Science*, 4, 523, 1999.
5. Tew, G.N., Pralle, M.U., and Stupp S.I., Supramolecular materials from triblock rodcoil molecules containing phenylene vinylene, *J. Am. Chem. Soc.*, 121, 9852, 1999.
6. Tew, G.N., Pralle, M.U., and Stupp, S.I., Supramolecular materials with electroactive chemical functions, *Angew. Chem.*, 112, 527, 2000.
7. Radzilowski, L.H. and Stupp, S.I., Nanophase separation in monodisperse rodcoil diblock polymers, *Macromolecules*, 27, 7747, 1994.
8. Radzilowski, L.H., Carragher, B.O., and Stupp, S.I., Three-dimensional self-assembly of rodcoil copolymer nanostructures, *Macromolecules*, 30, 2110, 1997.
9. Zubarev, E.R. et al., Self-assembly of dendron rodcoil molecules into nanoribbons, *J. Am. Chem. Soc.*, 23, 4105, 2001.
10. Pralle, M.U. et al., Piezoelectricity in polar supramolecular materials, *Angew. Chem.*, 112, 1546, 2000.
11. Li, L.M. and Stupp, S.I., Effects of substrate micropatterning on nonlinear optical properties of polar self-assembling films, *Appl. Phys. Lett.*, 78, 4127, 2001.
12. Li, L.M., Zubarev, E.R., and Stupp, S.I., Chemical structure versus nonlinear optical properties in self-assembling materials, *Macromolecules*, 35, 2560, 2002.
13. Zubarev, E.R. et al., Scaffolding of polymers by supramolecular nanoribbons, *Adv. Mater.*, 14, 198, 2002.
14. Stendahl, J.C. et al., Toughening of polymers by self-assembling molecules, *Adv. mater.*, in press.
15. Braun, P.V., Osenar, P., and Stupp, S.I., Semiconducting superlattices templated by molecular assemblies, *Nature*, 41, 1705, 1996.
16. Stupp, S.I. and Braun, P.V., Molecular manipulation of microstructures: biomaterials, ceramics, and semiconductors, *Science*, 277, 1242, 1997.
17. Braun, P. et al., Nanostructure templating in inorganic solids with organic lyotropic liquid crystals, *J. Am. Chem. Soc.*, 121, 7302, 1999.
18. Sone, E.D., Zubarev, E.R., and Stupp, S.I., Semiconductor nanohelices templated by supramolecular ribbons, Angew. Chem., 41, 1705, 2002.
19. Langer, R. and Vacanti, J.P., Tissue engineering, *Science*, 260, 920, 1993.
20. Griffith, M. et al., Functional human corneal equivalents constructed from cell lines, *Science*, 286, 2169, 1999.
21. Baum, B.J. and Mooney, D.J., The impact of tissue engineering on dentistry, *J. Am. Dent. Assn.*, 131, 309, 2000.
22. Burg, K.J.L., Porter, S., and Kellam, J.F., Biomaterial developments for bone tissue engineering, *Biomaterials*, 21, 2347, 2000.
23. Hwang, J.J., Harrington, D.A., and Stupp, S.I., in *Methods of Tissue Engineering*, Atala, A. and Lanza, R., Eds., 2001, p. 65.

24. Hwang, J.J. et al., Self-assembling biomaterials: liquid crystal phases of cholesteryl oligo(L-lactic acid) and their interactions with cells, *Proc. Natl. Acad. Sci. U.S.A.*, 99, 9662, 2002.
25. Peter, S.L. et al., Polymer concepts in tissue engineering, *J. Biomed. Mater. Res.*, 43, 422, 1998.
26. Ma, P.X. and Langer, R., Morphology and mechanical function of long-term *in vitro* engineered cartilage, *J. Biomed. Mater. Res.*, 44, 217, 1999.
27. Isogai, N. et al., Formation of phalanges and small joints by tissue engineering, *J. Bone Joint Surg. Am.*, 81A, 306, 1999.
28. Evans, G.R.D. et al., *In vivo* evaluation of poly (L-lactic acid) porous conduits for peripheral nerve regeneration, *Biomaterials*, 20, 1109, 1999.
29. Marra, K.G. et al., *In vitro* analysis of biodegradable polymer blend/hydroxyapatite composites for bone tissue engineering, *J. Biomed. Mater. Res.*, 47, 324, 1999.
30. Hutmacher, D.W., Scaffolds in tissue engineering bone and cartilage, *Biomaterials*, 21, 2529, 2000.
31. Hartgerink, J.D., Beniash, E., and Stupp, S.I., Peptide-amphiphile nanofibers: A versatile scaffold for the preparation of self-assembling materials, *Proc. Natl. Acad. Sci. U.S.A.*, 99, 5133, 2002.
32. Hartgerink, J.D., Beniash, E., and Stupp, S.I., Self-assembly and mineralization of peptide-amphiphile nanofibers, *Science*, 294, 1684, 2001.
33. Israelachvili, J.N., *Intermolecular and Surface Forces*; 2nd ed., Academic Press, London, 1992.
34. Burke, E.M. et al., Influence of polyaspartic acid and phosphophoryn on octacalcium phosphate growth kinetics, *Col. Sur. B Biointerfac.*, 17, 49, 2000.
35. Butler, W.T., Dentin matrix proteins, *Eur. J. Oral. Sci.*, 106, 204, 1988.
36. Veis, A., Mineral matrix interactions in bone and dentin, *J. Bone Min. Res.*, 8, S493, 1993.
37. Pierschbacher, M.D. and Ruoslahti, E., Cell attachment activity of fibronectin can be duplicated by small synthetic fragments of the molecule, *Nature*, 309, 5963, 1984.
38. Spoerke, E.D. and Stupp, S.I., Colonization of organoapatite–titanium mesh by pre-osteoblastic cells, *J. Biomed. Res.*, in press.
39. Weiner, S. and Traub, W., Bone structure: from angstroms to microns, *FASEB J.*, 6, 879, 1992.
40. Weiner, S. and Wagner, H.D., The material bone structure: mechanical function relations, *Annu. Rev. Mater. Sci.*, 28, 271, 1998.
41. Traub, W., Arad, T., and Weiner, S., Three-dimensional ordered distribution of crystals in turkey tendon collagen fibers, *Proc. Natl. Acad. Sci. U.S.A.*, 86, 9822, 1989.
42. Landis, W.J. et al., Structural relations between collagen and mineral in bone as determined by high voltage electron microscopic tomography, *Microsc. Res. Tech.*, 33, 192, 1996.
43. Chalazonitis, A. et al., The alpha-1 subunit of laminin-1 promotes the development of neurons by interacting with LBP-110 expressed by neural crest-derived cells immunoselected from the fetal mouse gut, *J. Neurobiol.*, 33, 118, 1997.
44. Tashiro, K. et al., A synthetic peptide containing the IKVAV sequence from the a-chain of laminin mediates cell attachment, migration, and neurite outgrowth, *J. Biol. Chem.*, 264, 16174, 1989.
45. Hartgerink, J.D., Niece, K.L., and Stupp, S.I., Self-assembly of peptide–amphiphile nanofibers by electrostatic attraction, *J. Am. Chem. Soc.*, in press.

23

The Inert–Bioactivity Conundrum

David F. Williams

CONTENTS

23.1 Introduction 407
23.2 Inertness and Bioactivity: How Materials Control Host Response 409
23.3 Clinical Experience with Implanted Medical Devices 411
 23.3.1 Joint Replacements 412
 23.3.2 Prosthetic Heart Valves 412
 23.3.3 Cardiovascular Devices 413
 23.3.4 Inertness and Bioactivity in Long-Term Implantable Devices 414
23.4 Bioactive Surfaces 415
 23.4.1 Bioactivity and Bone Bonding 416
 23.4.2 Bioactivity and Control of Long-Term Tissue Response 417
 23.4.3 Bioactivity for Avoidance of Specific Tissue Responses 418
 23.4.4 Bioactivity in Tissue Engineering 419
23.5 General Discussion and Conclusions 421
References 421

23.1 Introduction

This chapter is primarily concerned with the analysis of the requirements of long-term implantable devices, their biocompatibility, and especially with the implicit material selection dilemma of whether inert or so-called biomaterials represent the best choices. It was written in outline before the start of the workshop on which this book is based, restructured after most of the presentations were given, and finalized after the workshop ended. The ratio-

0-8493-1474-7/03/$0.00+$1.50

nale for this chapter is based on the need to improve the interfacial reactions between implants and tissues.

The workshop was primarily concerned with dental implants, which represent one of the more important areas of clinical practice in which interfacial reactions between implants and the host control behavior. This chapter is directed to phenomena associated with dental implants but addresses these issues from a broader perspective, drawing upon experience in other clinical areas.

It should be emphasized that the discussion relates to implantable devices that are intended to replace tissues or organs that have become diseased or damaged or are congenitally absent. It is not directly concerned with other implantable or invasive devices, although the conclusions may well be relevant to other situations. Indeed, it will be seen that bioactivity is of greatest relevance in medical devices other than long-term implants. The specific objectives of these replacement implantable devices obviously vary from one clinical situation to another, but the generic objectives are always the same: to replace or augment the affected tissues, to provide a clinically effective mechanical, cosmetic, or other function from the replacement, to provide sufficient and appropriate anchorage or fixation of the device in the host, and to maintain this anchorage and functionality as long as required. The latter point subsumes the requirement that the material is neither toxic nor unintentionally degraded in the body.

The requirement for functionality in a long-term implantable device is usually concerned with mechanical functionality, whether structural or fluid mechanical functionality. This requirement has been one of the more important mediators of material selection and will be discussed later. For the moment, attention will be paid to the interface between implant and host. The establishment and subsequent maintenance of this interface have attracted attention for many years with respect to implants in many different clinical situations.

It is important to recognize that in many devices, this interface establishes the attachment or fixation to the host, so that the desired interfacial reactions must encompass both the criteria for attachment and those for long-term biocompatibility. In other situations, where attachment is achieved by some other mechanism, for example, a suture in soft tissue or a screw in hard tissue, the interface itself can concentrate on the nonattachment aspects of biocompatibility. Thus, an endosseous dental implant must command the characteristics that facilitate fixation to the mandibular or maxillary bone while ensuring the long-term maintenance of a stable bone–implant interface and adequate mucosal interface. On the other hand, a prosthetic heart valve achieves its fixation via the sewing ring so the hemodynamically functioning parts of the valve are not encumbered by the requirement for fixation and their surfaces can address the issues of blood compatibility alone.

Whatever the functions of the devices, several approaches have been made to the selection of the materials for the construction and design of their surfaces. These have broadly followed the two apparently opposite approaches of *inertness* and *bioactivity.* This chapter is concerned with the rationales for and experiences with both approaches.

23.2 Inertness and Bioactivity: How Materials Control Host Response

Inertness is a rather undefinable quality that alludes to the inability of one substance to react with any other substance. From a purely chemical view, it is not too difficult to characterize substances based on their inertness since chemical reactions can be described from thermodynamic and kinetic considerations and it is possible to determine quite precisely the conditions under which any one substance can react with other substances.

In the context of biomaterials, this is not so easily achieved because the physiological environment is not a simple chemical entity. It is a complex biochemical milieu that changes constantly in constitution and activity (albeit within well defined limits) and contains complex cascades of reactions (e.g., complement activation and coagulation) with powerful nonlinear amplification mechanisms. Moreover, biomaterials can influence various processes within the physiological environment without undergoing any apparent chemical change, most obviously by adsorption or a surface-initiated activation process.

The origins of this currently controversial conundrum relating to the conflicting values of inertness and bioactivity can be traced back to confusion about the mediators and mechanisms of interfacial reactions and the meaning of *inertness.* Over the years, many attempts have been made to identify the most important material and especially its surface — characteristics that control biocompatibility. Two major difficulties have impeded this analysis: the mutual interdependence of many materials and material surface variables that make it impossible to vary one parameter without simultaneously varying many others, and the multiplicity of events and mechanisms that contribute to biocompatibility. Table 23.1 lists material characteristics that may be relevant to biological performance and the features of tissue responses that may contribute to overall biocompatibility. The mutual interdependence of factors is readily seen. It is difficult to vary surface chemistry without affecting (although not necessarily in a linear manner) hydrophobicity, surface energy, surface molecular mobility, and so on. Many physiological responses are dependent on each other, as protein adsorption precedes cell attachment, platelet activation interacts with the clotting cascade, and so on.

If we now consider the mechanisms by which the host tissue responds to the implantation of a device, it is possible to identify processes for which most of the material variables (i.e., processes on the left side of Table 23.1) are responsible, or at least may influence most of the responses of tissues (listed on the right side of Table 23.1). For example, experimental evidence

TABLE 23.1

Material Variables that Can Influence Host Response and Key Features of Host Response

Variables of Materials and Material Surfaces	Key References	Features of Host Response	Key References
Bulk material composition	1–3	Protein adsorption and desorption (general)	65–67
Bulk material microstructure or morphology	4	Protein conformational change and activation (general)	68–70
Bulk material elastic constants/ compliance	5	Protein binding to material constituent	8, 71,
Surface chemical composition	6–9	Complement activation	72–74
Subsurface chemistry or chemical gradient	10, 11	Platelet adhesion, activation, and aggregation	19, 75
Surface topography or roughness	12–16	Leukocyte behavior	76–78
Implant material, particle size, and shape	17, 18	Fibrous tissue capsule	79–81
Isolated surface electrical charge/ dielectric constant	19, 20	Red cell behavior/hemolysis	82, 83
Imposed electrical charge or charge transfer process	21–23	Neutrophil activation	84, 85
Water content	24, 25	Fibroblast behavior and fibrosis	86, 87
Hydrophobic–hydrophilic balance	26–28	Antibody production	88, 89
Surface energy	29–31	Humoral phase of inflammatory response	90, 91
Surface molecular mobility	32, 33	Macrophage activation	92–94
Surface crystallography and crystallinity	34, 35	Foreign body giant cell production	95–97
Rate of metal ion release (for metals and alloys)	36, 37,	Lymphocyte behavior	98, 99
Cytotoxicity/biological reactivity of released metal ions	38–41	Activation of intrinsic clotting cascade	100–102
Oxide film breakdown parameters (for passivated metals and alloys)	42, 43	Osteoblast/osteoclast behavior (materials in contact with bone)	6, 13, 104
Cytotoxicity/biological reactivity of corrosion products	44–47	Endothelial proliferation	105–107
Dissolution rate (for ceramics and glasses)	48, 49	Microvascular changes	7, 103
Rate of leaching and composition of leached additives, residual monomers, or catalysts (for plastics)	50, 51	Acute hypersensitivity/ anaphylaxis	108, 109
Cytotoxicity/biological reactivity of leached additives, monomers, or catalysts	52, 53	Delayed hypersensitivity	110, 111
Cytotoxicity/biological reactivity of degradation products	54, 55	Infection	112–114
Rate of release of debris by nondegradation processes (e.g., wear)	56, 57	Tumor formation	115, 116

TABLE 23.1 (CONTINUED)

Material Variables that Can Influence Host Response and Key Features of Host Response

Variables of Materials and Material Surfaces	Key References	Features of Host Response	Key References
Cytotoxicity/biological reactivity of debris particles	58–61	Necrosis	117, 118
Sterility of product and sterilization procedure	62, 63	Genotoxicity	119–121
Presence of endotoxins	59, 64		
Presence of surface contaminants	11		

indicates that surface topography influences fibroblast behavior[15]; that the equilibrium water content of hydrogels influences neutrophil behavior[122]; that an imposed electrical charge can influence inflammatory response[20]; that the cytotoxicity of polymer degradation products influences macrophage behavior[123]; and that surface energy has some influence on cell attachment.[124]

In terms of establishing how materials and their surfaces may be designed to optimize tissue response in relation to a particular application, however, three major difficulties must be faced. The first is that in most cases linking a material as the cause and the host response as the effect, the relationship is indirect rather than direct and cannot be established in an objective or quantifiable manner. Thus, there is no predictable and quantitative way to causally relate topography to cell behavior, surface energy to cell attachment, or electrical properties to the inflammatory response, and so on.

Second, biocompatibility consists of two-way processes that evolve over time, with host affecting material and material affecting host, in processes that are usually dependent on each other. Thus, a material that degrades in the body will affect host response, and the nature of that response will influence the stability of the material. For example, intracellular enzymes released from a macrophage that is activated as a result of the presence of a foreign material may exert damaging effects on the material. This makes interpretation of the events that occur at an interface very difficult with respect to the evolving response. Third, any attempt to correlate material properties with host response must be capable of extrapolation from the experiment to the clinical experience. This point is crucial and deserves close examination.

23.3 Clinical Experience with Implanted Medical Devices

If we consider this from the perspective of how the material characteristics listed on the left side of Table 23.1 control the characteristics of the responses listed on the right side of the table, some interesting observations may be made with respect to data and observations related to the successes or failures of devices in clinical practice.

23.3.1 Joint Replacements

Considering first the experiences with total joint replacement, it is well known that after some early setbacks concerned with the toxicity of methylmethacrylate and the poor wear resistance of polytetrafluoroethylene, Charnley identified the best materials to be stainless steel and polyethylene for the femoral and acetabular components respectively, cemented in place with polymethylmethacrylate bone cement.[125] His judgment was based on the desire to have the best mechanical properties coupled with the least irritating and most degradation-resistant characteristics.

Since then, changes to the polyethylene were introduced in order to improve degradation resistance, and cobalt–chromium alloys have largely replaced stainless steel, often with a harder ceramic such as alumina or zirconia as the bearing surface on the femoral head.

Attempts have been made over the years to mprove performance, but often had the opposite effect, with poorer performance derived from fiber reinforcement of polyethylene and variable quality performance with developments such as hydroxyapatite-coated prostheses for cementless fixation, diamond-like carbon coatings for wear resistance, ion-implanted and anodized surfaces, and some of the modular systems. The main problem with joint replacements that limits their clinical performance involves loosening of the prostheses arising from the release of wear debris —a situation that appeared to get worse, not better, as the quality of the polyethylene or the oxidative effects of gamma sterilization caused a deterioration of wear characteristics. This is a significant point since the situation was addressed by introducing modifications to the polyethylene, for example, by cross-linking, to make it more resistant to oxidation and wear, i.e., to make it more inert. The most significant attempt to introduce bioactivity into orthopedic practice has involved the use of hydroxyapatite coatings for use in cementless fixation. The experience here has been varied. Dissolution of the HA layer was a barrier to clinical effectiveness in some cases.

The joint replacement experience, therefore, indicates that the best results are achieved by optimizing the inertness of the materials and maximizing mechanical performance. The recent reintroduction of metal-on-metal systems follows this pattern. Attempts to move away from this principle of inertness, including the introduction of surface modifications directed at bioactivity, have generally not met with success.

23.3.2 Prosthetic Heart Valves

Turning now to prosthetic heart valves, two major categories have dominated the field for 30 years: mechanical and bioprosthetic valves. The mechanical valves are typically constructed with either a tilting disc or bileaflet configuration, but each type essentially has a metal frame of titanium or cobalt–chromium alloy, a moving part that is almost universally made from or coated with carbon, and a sewing ring fabricated from an expanded PTFE fluorocarbon polymer or a Dacron polyester medical textile.[126]

There are two points of interest here. First, the choice of materials was based on inertness combined with functionality, and generally this has been an excellent policy. Even with these materials, however, it is impossible to eliminate the chance of foreign surface-induced thrombogenicity. All prosthetic valve patients require continuous anticoagulation therapy for the rest of their lives. It has been impossible to improve materials or material surfaces to eliminate this effect.

The second point is that attempts to induce other functionalities into heart valves of this type have not been successful, as exemplified by the ill-fated attempts to reduce the risks of infective endocarditis in valves by surface modification of the sewing ring by a thin layer of silver.[127]

The second major type of prosthetic heart valve is the bioprosthetic valve, typically derived from porcine aorta. The rationale here is to combine more natural hemodynamics and materials in order to obviate the tendency toward blood clotting. While this goal has been achieved, there has been a price to pay. The collagenous material is not completely inert and suffers from both degradation and calcification, thus limiting the lifetime of the prosthesis.[128] Again, experience shows that inertness and mechanical functionality usually combine to yield very good long-term results and deviation from this principle must be undertaken with caution.

23.3.3 Cardiovascular Devices

Similar experiences were found with cardiovascular devices. Replacement of major arteries following atherosclerosis can be achieved by the use of Dacron and e-PTFE.[129] Their functionality is derived from their porosity that allows tissue in-growth such that the surface in contact with flowing blood works as a tissue lining while providing good mechanical performance. The e-PTFE gives slightly better performance, and can be used in smaller arteries than Dacron, possibly because Dacron is not quite as inert.[130] The performance and utilization of synthetic artificial arteries are limited. They cannot be used for arteries much less than 6 mm in diameter because of the effects of the slow accumulation of tissue on the intimal surface. This is important because it precludes the use of synthetic materials in the replacement of coronary arteries, for which transposed vascular grafts remain the only alternatives.

These significant limitations for vascular replacement led to the adoption of different technologies to treat atherosclerotic lesions. Once again we can see the issues that arise with respect to deviations from inertness and the effects of irritating tissues. Angioplasty is the basis of this technology, in which a balloon catheter is inserted into the affected blood vessel and the plaque deposits are interrupted, dislodged, or compressed by a mechanical force exerted via the balloon.[131] This can be very effective in alleviating the condition, but often the effect is only short-lived as the damage caused to the endothelium by the angioplasty stimulates inflammation that leads to intimal hyperplasia (a further thickening of the vessel wall), clinically giving rise to restenosis.[132] In order to prevent this, or at least to reduce or delay its effects, most angioplasty techniques are accompanied by the deployment of an implantable intravascular stent, usually an expandable metallic tubular frame that compresses the vessel wall and maintains patency.[133] These devices have been successful, but success is limited because the combination of mechanical compression and the presence of the material causes chronic irritation to the endothelium such that the endothelium is able to grow over the stent, again causing restenosis.[134]

Many stents are now augmented by components intended to limit restenosis. Typically, a radioactive structure emits gamma or beta radiation that reduces proliferation or a drug-releasing structure delivers an antirestenosis compound.[135,136] This whole process can be seen as one in which tissue irritation by a device produces an undesirable response. Every successive technological approach is aimed at minimizing the adverse effect of the previous step. The final measure cited above, the drug-eluting stent, represents the dichotomy at the heart of this discussion. Since there is no inert solution to the intravascular stent which will irritate the endothelium by its very presence, the release of a bioactive compound is an attempt to reduce the damage so caused.

23.3.4 Inertness and Bioactivity in Long-Term Implantable Devices

There are many other examples of implantable medical devices in which the inherent inertness of the selected material provides the optimal biocompatibility, and only under exceptional circumstances does a need to deviate from this principle arise. The intraocular lens is a good case in point, since many consider that the best lenses are made from highly inert polymethylmethacrylate. Meticulous surgical technique is necessary to minimize inflammation that could compromise performance. In some cases, for example, in patients such as diabetics with predispositions to inflammation, lenses with so-called bioactive surfaces, for example, heparin, may be used.[137]

Experience with implantable medical devices therefore indicates almost invariably that inertness is the best option for producing adequate long-term performance. Moreover, most attempts to introduce bioactivity to surfaces for such long-term devices have not been successful, although short-term interventions and possibly tissue engineering applications have much better chances of success.

23.4 Bioactive Surfaces

Taking into account the requirements for an implantable device outlined in the first part of this chapter, it is a logical deduction that if the functionality is mechanical or physical, and if the fixation of the device is achieved separately (as with the sewing ring of a heart valve, the anastomoses of vascular prostheses, the haptic of an intraocular lens, or the screw of a bone plate), the most effective performance will be achieved when the device minimally interferes with the tissue repair process of the host. This is why inert materials generally perform so well under these circumstances.

The question arises as to why any other approach, involving less inert or even deliberately active materials or surfaces, should be considered. Before answering this question, it is necessary to consider what type of activity may be involved, or more specifically, what is meant by *bioactivity* in this context. Much discussion has focused on this term in the biomaterials literature over the years. Many contributions were intended to limit the use of the *bioactivity* term to a specific situation, most commonly, in the contexts of bioactive ceramics and bone bonding. Since the *bio* prefix has a very general meaning, it does not seem sensible to limit use of *bioactive* in this way. The *Williams Dictionary of Biomaterials*[138] defines *bioactivity* as "the phenomenon by which a biomaterial elicits or modulates biological activity." Therefore, a bioactive material may be defined as a biomaterial designed to elicit or modulate biological activity. Since biological activity in this context is usually controlled by the surface of a device, and since the features determining biological activity are unlikely to be the same as those that determine mechanical performance, bioactive coatings or surface modifications (rather than bulk bioactive materials) are usually involved in attempts to modulate biological activity.

A bioactive surface is therefore any surface of a material designed and produced to induce or control the response of the host tissue to the material. This is in contrast to an inert surface designed to do nothing. The features of a surface that impart bioactivity may be physicochemical characteristics of the solid surface, any attached molecules, or any molecules intended to be released from the surface into the local tissues of the host. It is emphasized that the term *inert* is used here in the sense that it qualifies a material as "not readily being changed by chemical means"[138] rather than implying an absolute lack of interaction with anything.

At least four generic features or processes of bioactivity of medical devices can be identified:

1. Modulating local tissue response to produce faster or more effective bonding between implant and host, where no other form of attachment is possible

2. Modifying host response to a long-term implantable device where inertness alone is insufficient
3. Avoiding adverse reactions to a material that could cause a patient harm, especially reactions involving amplification mechanisms such as complement activation or contact phase activation
4. Facilitating a specific cellular response to promote tissue regeneration rather than repair, especially in the context of tissue engineering

Each of these areas will now be discussed separately.

23.4.1 Bioactivity and Bone Bonding

This topic is covered in detail elsewhere in this volume and is discussed here only from the conceptual view. In contrast to most other tissues, bone has a remarkable capacity to repair through regeneration of new functional tissue. In many situations, either after trauma or surgical intervention, complete bone regeneration may occur. This leads to full and effective fracture healing in the former case and full bony adaptation to a prosthesis in the latter case.

Only two problems arise in an otherwise healthy individual. First, this process takes time, which may be clinically inconvenient. Second, it is possible, if local conditions are adverse, for fibrous tissue to form instead of or in addition to bone. In the context of implantable devices in orthopedic and dental/maxillofacial surgery, provided the surgical technique is of good quality and the patient has no concurrent diseases that affect bone healing, it should be possible to achieve excellent adaptation of new bone to a prosthesis through the use of inert materials that will have a minimal tendency to irritate the tissue. In the vast majority of circumstances, it is not possible to improve on the quality of bone adaptation to a device that is achieved through appropriate design and technique and the use of an appropriate inert biomaterial, such as titanium, polyethylene, polymethylmethacrylate, or alumina ceramic.

Once new bone has adapted itself to a material surface, it is important for the continued functionality of the device that the adaptation is mechanically robust. This is the reason for the texturing of titanium surfaces, discussed elsewhere in this volume, to provide a degree of micromechanical interlocking. It is generally accepted that no chemical attachment of bone to a titanium surface will occur.[139] Suggestions were made to induce chemical bonding by surface treatments involving, for example, phosphonic acid[140] or hydrogen peroxide.[141] Available data show only marginal benefits *in vitro* and no benefits *in vivo*. It is contended here that in agreement with much clinical literature,[142] only optimization of the surface roughness of titanium is of any clinical benefit, and no effective bioactive titanium surface exists.

Much attention has been paid to the possibility of coating devices with some type of calcium phosphate with the intention of producing a faster or stronger bond to bone; hydroxyapatite is the most frequently used coating. Some hydroxyapatite-coated devices have worked well clinically,[143,144] and the rate of bone apposition may be greater than with a titanium surface, although the quality of the bone on reaching maturity is no different between the two systems.[145] Evidence indicates that hydroxyapatite can dissolve over time,[146,147] although this issue has been debated thoroughly.[148]

It may be concluded from this analysis that limited advantages related to the speed of bone apposition accrue from utilizing hydroxyapatite-based bioactive coatings on long-term implantable devices that require fixation to bone, but equally good long term results are achieved generally with textured titanium (especially for endosseous dental implants) and with cemented fixation in the case of most total joint replacement prostheses.

23.4.2 Bioactivity and Control of Long-Term Tissue Response

In the area of soft tissue replacement prostheses or soft tissue-contacting devices, the usual tissue response is that acute inflammation leads to mild chronic inflammation, which resolves over time, leaving a thin fibrous capsule around the material.[149] If the material degrades over time, the inflammation can be restimulated, which may give rise to a granuloma or only to excessive fibrosis.

Fibrosis can also be stimulated by other features of an implant. For example, excessive movement can stimulate fibroblasts to produce more collagen. A quite common feature with large breast implants is an extensive fibrous capsule, most likely caused by relative movement between the implant and the breast tissue.[150] Significant fibrosis can also occur at the tip of a pacemaker electrode within the myocardium due to both the relative movement as the heart beats and to the electrical charge delivered by the pacemaker.

In these situations, the increase in fibrous tissue is clinically significant. The increase is painful in the case of the breast implant and leads to an increase in stimulating threshold in the pacemaker. In other applications, the inflammation itself is troublesome, for example, with intraocular lenses where it interferes with light transmission.

It is not surprising that under these circumstances attempts have been made to control inflammation and fibrosis by the introduction of what might be termed *bioactivity*. Thus, pacemaker electrodes have been designed to elute antiinflammatory agents to control fibrosis and minimize the effects on the stimulation threshold. The release of steroids from these electrodes has been found to produce beneficial effects in some but not all patients.[151] Heparin has been attached to polymethylmethacrylate intraocular lenses to reduce inflammatory cell attachment and resulting opacification of the lens, but with conflicting results.[137,152]

In general, the introduction of surface bioactivity has not been very successful when the aim was to control long-term tissue reaction to a device. While beneficial effects occasionally appeared, such effects in the main were not reproducible nor of statistical significance, bearing in mind the natural range of patient responses to any device. This is not a surprising conclusion. When any material is placed in the body, it is immediately covered by a layer of proteins adsorbed from the blood or extracellular fluid, and a subsequent exchange of different proteins within this layer will occur over time. If the surface of the biomaterial is designed to have a specific functionality, perhaps described as *bioactivity*, the molecules that impart that functionality are soon covered by these proteins, and it may be impossible for them to fulfill their desired effect despite this layer. Such functionality is not impossible, but it is difficult to guarantee and especially difficult to maintain. Equally important, surface bioactivity introduced by the addition of a surface layer that is quite different from the substrate may not be maintained very long. The tissues of the body are extremely effective in degrading organic molecules attached to surfaces, and it is probable that most surface functionality will be lost over time. Bioactivity intended to control the long-term response to medical devices is therefore unlikely to succeed.

23.4.3 Bioactivity for Avoidance of Specific Tissue Responses

Some responses of the human body to medical devices are dramatic, highly undesirable, and easy to identify. They are not generally associated with the development of a tissue response over time, as discussed in the previous section, but instead involve the activation of a potent cascade process. Two specific processes involving the coagulation and complement systems are of special relevance. Both systems are integral parts of the body's defense mechanism responding to injury. While their actions are normally very beneficial, they can be very damaging, and indeed fatal, if initiated by a biomaterial acting as a foreign body and allowed to continue unimpeded.

The real significance is that the material surface may be able to interact with one or more plasma proteins of the clotting cascade or complement pathway, with subsequent enzymatic-controlled amplification processes that are unrelated to the material. This could result in the rapid formation of a blood clot in the former case and possibly an anaphylactic reaction in the latter. Both may occur with biomaterial surfaces. The association of the clotting process with biomaterials surfaces is well known.[153,154] Anaphylaxis is rare but possible.[155]

Under these circumstances, it is entirely logical to consider how a material surface could be designed to minimize these effects. Inertness of materials, in the context of the definition used earlier, is not the key to minimizing the risk of activating such a cascade process because the initiation mechanism is not a chemical reaction involving the surface. Taking the clotting cascade as the better example, the manner in which the various plasma proteins are adsorbed onto the surface is the important issue since a conformational change in a critical adsorbed protein can initiate enzymatic cleavage of the molecule, which is the key starting point of the cascade. It may not matter that the material is chemically inert if adsorption is able to take place by virtue of morphological or physicochemical characteristics. However, because the processes are complex and influenced by so many variables, it is not a trivial process to design a surface that eliminates this possibility.

Among the strategies employed to minimize the tendency to clot are some that employ *bioactivity*. These include attachment to the surface of a biomaterial that minimizes protein adsorption generically, including hydrogel-like materials such as polyethylene glycol[156] and phospholipids that mimic cell membranes, which have no intrinsic affinity for plasma proteins.[157] Other methods employ molecules that interfere with some part of the clotting cascade, minimize adhesions and/or activation of platelets that play integral roles in the build-up of a blood clot, or attempt to destroy or lyse a clot as it is being established.[158-165] Probably the most common substance used to minimize clot-forming tendencies on biomaterials is heparin,[166] a polysaccharide that has multiple effects on the blood clotting process and is effective as a coating on devices such as blood-contacting catheters.[167,168] This is probably one application of bioactivity that is demonstrably successful under some circumstances. It is clear, however, that these effects are essentially confined to short-term devices, for example angioplasty equipment and central venous catheters, and it is extremely unlikely that their effects will be long-lasting. If an activity is dependent on continuous elution of a bioactive molecule, the effect may last only while a sufficient amount of that molecule is in the reservoir. If, on the other hand, the effect is surface-controlled, it will last only as long as the relevant molecules remain attached to the surface and remain capable of exerting their antithrombogenic effects through the protein layer that almost inevitably builds up.

Anaphylaxis is rare and no serious attempts have been made to modify surfaces to make them resistant to this rare event. It is important to note, however, that some attempts to modify the surfaces of catheters for other reasons, for example to improve lubricity, could adversely affect the interaction with these cascade-inducing molecules, as noted with some polyvinylpyrrolidone-coated central venous catheters.[155]

23.4.4 Bioactivity in Tissue Engineering

Finally, it is necessary to discuss the role of bioactivity in tissue engineering. It is obvious from the foregoing that many implantable medical devices provide reasonable performance in the replacement of structure and function with respect to a variety of tissues. Provided that the sound principles of biomaterials science are followed, decades of performance can be expected from joint replacements, intraocular lenses, and artificial arteries.

It may be argued, however, that this approach to the treatment of disease and trauma is pragmatic rather than scientifically logical. The replacement of a joint that normally consists of bone, cartilage, and synovial fluid — all of which are viable natural components — with a combination of a metal and a thermoplastic polymer — synthetic, nonviable, monolithic structures — cannot represent ideal medical therapy.

In view of this, a profound change of emphasis occurred in recent years with respect to the concepts of tissue or organ replacement. Tissue engineering is effectively a compromise between treatment through the use of implantable medical devices and direct tissue transplantation, both of which have serious clinical and logistics limitations. Tissue engineering does not involve the replacement of diseased or injured tissues by synthetic medical devices, nor does it involve the transplantation of intact living tissue from donors. Instead, tissue engineering, defined as "the persuasion of the body to heal itself through the delivery to the appropriate site of cells, biomolecules and supporting structures,"[138] involves providing patients with the means to regenerate their own tissues.

One of the major problems with mammalian physiology with respect to the treatment of disease and trauma is the loss of the ability of mature individuals to produce new tissue. Obviously a fetus and an embryo have the capacity to produce new tissue. After birth, an individual will continue to grow tissues and organs developed within the embryo. However, the individual generally loses the power to generate new tissue, or more specifically to regenerate compromised tissue. The main exceptions are skin and bone, both of which can regenerate when injured, but healing in most tissues involves nonspecific repair (typically with fibrous connective tissue, or scar) rather than regeneration.

Tissue engineering involves temporary reversion to the state where regeneration is possible in order to produce a healing process through the generation of the correct tissue rather than a scar. A typical tissue engineering process will involve the sourcing of appropriate cells, their incorporation into a biomaterial scaffold or matrix, the manipulation of this material–cell construct in a suitable bioreactor in which correct molecular and mechanical signals are applied, and the delivery of the tissue produced to the appropriate site in the individual.[169-175]

In most tissue engineering processes developed to date, the biomaterial has been in the form of a biodegradable polymer, which is degraded or dissolved concurrently with tissue regeneration, although this is by no means a specific requirement. It will become obvious that such processes are unlikely to be successful if the biomaterials selected for the scaffold or matrix are inert; indeed it is fully expected that in most circumstances, the materials used in tissue engineering will possess highly specific bioactivity naturally or acquire it.

Thus, the requirements of tissue engineering biomaterials are likely to be quite different from those for medical device biomaterials. Nevertheless, and this is not surprising because the underlying science of tissue engineering is only emerging, it is far from clear what type of bioactivity is required. It is generally thought that the material substrate must be able to support cell adhesion and growth, but the precise requirements in this respect are unclear. It is also probable that the biomolecules necessary to stimulate the cells to do exactly what is required will have to be delivered very carefully and precisely, implying local delivery processes.

In light of the definition of *bioactivity* given earlier and the specific objectives of tissue engineering, there is no doubt that bioactive materials and surfaces will be of crucial significance in this newly emerging therapeutic modality. It remains to be seen how this bioactivity will be delivered. Although the concepts and scientific principles are quite different from those underpinning classical medical devices, it is important that the fundamental lessons of biocompatibility learned over decades are not forgotten as a new approach takes over.

23.5 General Discussion and Conclusions

This chapter attempted to rationalize the various attempts to produce so-called bioactive surfaces on medical devices in terms of their objectives and the available evidence concerning their clinical success. Without in any way undermining the scientific basis for the development of bioactive surfaces, that is, the search for molecular or microstructural features able to control how tissue responds to the device in question, it must be concluded that the overwhelming majority of clinical evidence suggests that in most circumstances, bioactivity is doomed to failure and the best that can be achieved is the design of even more inert surfaces.

The reason almost certainly is that any structure that is sufficiently active to have a theoretical chance of modulating cellular behavior at the device–tissue interface will either become covered by host proteins so that the activity cannot be realized, otherwise will become inactivated by host physiology, or will be removed from the surface by dissolution, delamination, or other means. Only when the bioactivity is so profound or when the desired influence of the bioactivity is so short-lived, can the concept of bioactivity supersede that of inertness whenever a synthetic biomaterial is presented to host tissues. It is better to avoid influencing host response than to compromise biocompatibility by attempting to introduce an active surface that cannot possibly be achieved. Possibly the conundrum ends here.

References

1. Williams, D.F., Ed., *Biocompatibility of Clinical Implant Materials*, CRC Press, Boca Raton, Vols. I and II, 1982.
2. Ronneberger, B. et al., The *in vivo* biocompatibility study of ABA triblock copolymers consisting of poly(L-lactic co glycolic acid) A blocks attached to central poly(oxyethylene) B blocks, *J. Biomed. Mater. Res.*, 30, 31, 1996.

3. Campoccia, D. et al., Semisynthetic resorbable materials from Hyaluronan esterification, *Biomaterials*, 19, 2101, 1998.
4. Long, M. and Rack, H.J., Titanium alloys in total joint replacement: a materials science perspective, *Biomaterials*, 19, 1621, 1998.
5. Seifalian, A.M. et al., Noncompliance: the silent acceptance of a villain, in *Tissue Engineering of Vascular Prosthetic Grafts*, Zilla, P. and Greisler, H.P., Eds., G.G. Landes Co., Austin, TX, 1999, p. 45.
6. Mustafa, K. et al., Electrochemical impedance spectroscopy and x-ray photoelectron spectroscopy analysis of titanium surfaces cultured with osteoblast-like cells derived from human mandibular bone, *J. Biomed. Mater. Res.*, 59, 655, 2002.
7. Sanders, J.E., Baker, A.B., and Golledge, S.L., Control of *in vivo* microvessel ingrowth by modulation of biomaterial local architecture and chemistry, *J. Biomed. Mater. Res.*, 60, 36, 2002.
8. Scotchford, C.A. et al., Protein adsorption and human osteoblast-like cell attachment and growth on alkylthiol on gold self assembled monolayers, *J. Biomed. Mater. Res.*, 59, 84, 2002.
9. Textor, M. et al., Properties and biological significance of natural oxide films on titanium and its alloys, in *Titanium in Medicine*, Brunette, D.M. et al., Eds., Springer, Berlin, 2001, p. 171.
10. Sul, Y.T. et al., Qualitative and quantitative observations of bone tissue reactions to anodised implants, *Biomaterials*, 23, 1809, 2002.
11. Kasemo, B. and Lausmaa, J., Surface science aspects of inorganic biomaterials, *CRC Crit. Rev. Biocompat.*, 2, 335, 1986.
12. Klinge, U. et al., Impact of polymer pore size on the interface scar formation in a rat model, *J. Surg. Res.*, 103, 208, 2002.
13. Bannister, S.R., Shear force modulates osteoblast response to surface roughness, *J. Biomed. Mater. Res.*, 60, 167, 2002.
14. Curtis, A.S.G. and Wilkinson, A., Topographical control of cells, *Biomaterials*, 18, 1573, 1997.
15. Oakley, C. and Brunette, D.M., The sequence of alignment of microtubules, focal contacts and actin filaments in fibroblasts spreading on smooth and grooved titanium substrates, *J. Cell Sci.*, 106, 343, 1993.
16. McDevitt, T.C. et al., *In vitro* generation of differentiated cardiac myofibres on micropatterned laminin surfaces, *J. Biomed. Mater. Res.*, 60, 472, 2002.
17. Hirabayashi, K. et al., Influence of fibril length upon ePTFE graft healing and host modification of the implant, *J. Biomed. Mater. Res.*, 26, 1433, 1992.
18. Shanbhag, A.S. et al., Macrophage/particle interactions: effect of size, composition and surface area, *J. Biomed. Mater. Res.*, 28, 81, 1994.
19, Lee, J.H. and Oh, S.H., MMA/MPEOMA/VSA copolymer as a novel blood compatible material: effect of PEO and negatively charged side chains on protein adsorption and platelet adhesion, *J. Biomed. Mater. Res.*, 60, 44, 2002.
20. Hunt, J.A. et al., Effect of biomaterial surface charge on the inflammatory response; evaluation of cellular infiltration and TNF alpha production, *J. Biomed. Mater. Res.*, 17, 963, 1996.
21. Supronowicz, P.R. et al., Novel current-conducting substrates for exposing osteoblasts to alternating current stimulation, *J. Biomed. Mater. Res.*, 59, 499, 2002.
22. Kotwal, A. and Schmidt, C.E., Electrical stimulation alters protein adsorption and nerve cell interactions with electrically conducting biomaterials, *Biomaterials*, 22, 1055, 2001.

23. Kobayashi, T., Nakamura, S., and Yamashita, K., Enhanced osteobonding by negative surface charges of electrically polarised hydroxyapatite, *J. Biomed. Mater. Res.*, 57, 477, 2001.
24. Bryant, S.J. and Anseth, K.S., Hydrogel properties influence ECM production by chondrocytes photoencapsulated by poly(ethylene glycol) hydrogels, *J. Biomed. Mater. Res.*, 59, 63, 2002.
25. Corkhill, P.H., Fitton, J.H., and Tighe, B., Towards a synthetic articular cartilage, *J. Biomat. Sci. Polymer Ed.*, 4, 615, 1993.
26. Rabinow, B.E. et al., Biomaterials with permanent hydrophilic surfaces and low protein adsorption properties, *J. Biomat. Sci. Polymer Ed.*, 6, 91, 1994.
27. Collier, T.O. et al., Adhesion behaviour of monocytes, macrophages and foreign body giant cells on poly(N-isopropylacrylamide) temperature-responsive surfaces, *J. Biomed. Mater. Res.*, 59, 136, 2002.
28. Williams, R.L., Hunt, J.A., and Tengvall, P., Fibroblast adhesion onto methyl–silica gradients with and without pre-adsorbed protein, *J. Biomed. Mater. Res.*, 29, 1545, 1995.
29. Kanno, M. et al., Biocompatibility of fluorinated polyimide, *J. Biomed. Mater. Res.*, 60, 53, 2002.
30. Kilpadi, D.V. and Lemons, J.E., Surface energy characterisation of unalloyed titanium implants, *J. Biomed. Mater. Res.*, 28, 1419, 1994.
31. Han, D.K. et al., Surface characteristics and blood compatibility of polyurethanes grafted with perfluoroalkyl chains, *J. Biomat. Sci. Polymer Ed.*, 3, 229, 1992.
32. Irvine, D.J. et al., Comparison of tethered star and linear polyethylene oxide for control of biomaterials surface properties, *J. Biomed. Mater. Res.*, 40, 498, 1998.
33. Ji, J. et al., Stearyl poly(ethylene oxide) grafted surfaces for preferential adsorption of albumin. Part 2: the effect of molecular mobility on protein adsorption, *Polymer*, 41, 3713, 2000.
34. ter Brugge, P.J., Wolke, J.G.C., and Jansen, J.A., Effect of calcium phosphate coating crystallinity and implant surface roughness on differentiation of rat bone marrow cells, *J. Biomed. Mater. Res.*, 60, 70, 2002.
35. Kawamoto, N. et al., Blood compatibility of polypropylene surfaces in relation to the crystalline–amorphous microstructure, *J. Biomat. Sci. Polymer Ed.*, 8, 859, 1997.
36. Ku, C.H. et al., Effects of different Ti-6Al-4V surface treatments on osteoblast behaviour, *Biomaterials*, 23, 1447, 2002.
37. Uo, M. et al., Tissue reaction around metal implants observed by x-ray scanning analytical microscopy, *Biomaterials*, 22, 677, 2001.
38. Messer, R.L.W. and Lucas, L.C., Localisation of metallic ions within gingival fibroblast subcellular fractions, *J. Biomed. Mater. Res.*, 59, 466, 2002.
39. Shih, C.C. et al., Growth inhibition of cultured smooth muscle cells by corrosion products of 316L stainless steel wire, *J. Biomed. Mater. Res.*, 57, 200, 2001.
40. Wagner, M. et al., Mechanisms of cell activation by heavy metal ions, *J. Biomed. Mater. Res.*, 42, 443, 1998.
41. Schmalz, G., Langer, H., and Schweikl, H., Cytotoxicity of dental alloy extracts and corresponding metal salt solutions, *J. Dent. Res.*, 77, 1772, 1998.
42. Schenk, R., The corrosion properties of titanium and titanium alloys, in *Titanium in Medicine*, Brunette, D.M. et al., Eds., Springer, Berlin, 2001, p. 145.

43. Williams, D.F., Electrochemical aspects of corrosion in the physiological environment, in *Fundamental Aspects of Biocompatibility*, Vol. 1, Williams, D.F., Ed., CRC Press, Boca Raton, 1981, p 11.
44. Hallab, N.J. et al., Concentration and composition-dependent effects on metal ions on human MG-63 osteoblasts, *J. Biomed. Mater. Res.*, 60, 420, 2002.
45. Shih, C.C. et al., The cytotoxicity of corrosion products of Nitinol stent wire on cultures smooth muscle cells, *J. Biomed. Mater. Res.*, 52, 395, 2000.
46. Messer, R.L.W. and Lucas, L.C., Cytotoxicity of nickel–chromium alloys: bulk alloys compared to multiple ion salt solutions, *Dent. Mater.*, 16, 207, 2000.
47. Tracana, R.B., Sousa, J.P., and Carvalho, G.S., Mouse inflammatory response to stainless steel corrosion products, *J. Mater. Sci. Mater. Med.*, 5, 596, 1994.
48. Langstaff, S. et al., Resorbable bioceramics based on stabilised calcium phosphates. Part II: evaluation of biological response, *Biomaterials*, 22, 135, 2001.
49. Butler, K.R., Benghuzzi, H.A., and Puckett, A., Morphometric evaluation of tissue implant reaction associated with ALCAP and TCP bioceramics *in vivo*, *J. Invest. Surg.*, 14, 139, 2001.
50. Geursten, W., Spahl, W., and Leyhausen, G., Residual monomer additive release and variability in cytotoxicity of light curing glass ionomer cements and copolymers, *J. Dent. Res.*, 77, 2012, 1998.
51. Koda, T. et al., Leachibility of denture base acrylic resins in artificial saliva, *Dent. Mater.*, 6, 13, 1990.
52. Granchi, D. et al., Effects of bone cement extracts on the cell-mediated immune response, *Biomaterials*, 23, 1033, 2002.
53. Loff, S. et al., Polyvinylchloride infusion lines expose infants to large amounts of toxic plasticisers, *J. Paed. Surg.*, 35, 1775, 2000.
54. Mathur, A.B. et al., *In vivo* biocompatibility and biostability of modified polyurethanes, *J. Biomed. Mater. Res.*, 36, 246, 1997
55. Anderson, J.M. and Shive, M.S., Biodegradation and biocompatibility of PLA and PLGA microspheres, *Adv. Drug Delivery Rev.*, 28, 5, 1997.
56. Kobayashi, A. et al., Number of polyethylene particles and osteolysis in total joint replacements, *J. Bone Joint Surg.*, 79, 844, 1997.
57. Green, T.R. et al., Effect of size and dose on bone resorption activity of macrophages by *in vitro* clinically relevant ultrahigh molecular weight polyethylene particles, *J. Biomed. Mater. Res.*, 53, 490, 2000.
58. Lohmann, C.H. et al., Phagocytosis of wear debris by osteoblasts affects differentiation and local factor production in a manner dependent on particle size, *Biomaterials*, 21, 551, 2000.
59. Akisue, T. et al., The effect of particle wear debris on NFkB activation and proinflammatory cytokine release in differentiated THP-1 cells, *J. Biomed. Mater. Res.*, 59, 507, 2002.
60. Shanbhag, A.S. et al., Composition and morphology of wear debris in failed uncemented total hip replacements, *J. Bone Joint Surg.*, 76B, 60, 1994.
61. Vermes, C. et al., The effects of particulate wear debris, cytokines and growth factors on the functions of MG-63 osteoblasts, *J. Bone Joint. Surg.*, 83, 201, 2001.
62. Muller, T. and Kaufer, H., Influence of sterilization procedures on thermoplastics, with special regard to modified surfaces, *Biomed. Technik*, 44, 2, 1999.
63. Parola, P. et al., Vascular graft infections: diagnostic and therapeutic problems, *J. Malad. Vascul.*, 24, 194, 1999.
64. Nelson, S.K. et al., Lipopolysaccharide affinity for titanium implant biomaterials, *J. Prosthet. Dent.*, 77, 76, 1997.

65. Tengvall, P. and Askendal, A., Ellipsometric *in vitro* studies on blood plasma and serum adsorption to zirconium, *J. Biomed. Mater. Res.*, 57, 285, 2001.
66. Norde, W., Adsorption of proteins from solution at the solid–liquid interface, *Adv. Colloid Interface Sci.*, 25, 267, 1986.
67. Williams, R.L. and Williams, D.F., The characteristics of albumin adsorption on metal surfaces, *Biomaterials*, 9, 206, 1988.
68. Andrade, J.D., Hlady, V.L., and van Wagenen, R.A., Effects of plasma protein adsorption on protein conformation and activity, *Pure Appl. Chem.*, 56, 1345, 1984.
69. Weber, N., Wendel, H.P., and Ziemer, G., Hemocompatibility of heparin-coated surfaces and the role of selective plasma protein adsorption, *Biomaterials*, 23, 429, 2002.
70. Paynter, R.W. et al., XPS studies on the organisation of adsorbed protein films on fluoropolymers, *J. Colloid Interface Sci.*, 191, 233, 1984.
71. MacDonald, D.E. et al., Adsorption and dissolution behaviour of human plasma fibronectin on thermally and chemically modified titanium dioxide particles, *Biomaterials*, 23, 1269, 2002.
72. Wettero, J. et al., On the binding of complement to solid artificial surfaces *in vitro*, *Biomaterials*, 23, 981, 2002.
73. Chenoweth, D.E., Complement activation in extracorporeal circuits, *Ann. N.Y. Acad. Sci.*, 516, 306, 1987.
74. Black, J.P. and Sefton, M.V., Complement activation by PVA as measured by ELISA for SC5b-9, *Biomaterials*, 21, 2287, 2000.
75. Spijker, H.T. et al., Platelet adhesion and activation on a shielded plasma gradient prepared on polyethylene, *Biomaterials*, 23, 757, 2002.
76. Rosenson-Schloss, R.S. et al., Alteration of leukocyte motility on plasma-conditioned prosthetic biomaterial, ePTFE, via a flow-responsive cell adhesion molecule, CD43, *J. Biomed. Mater. Res.*, 60, 8, 2002.
77. Sapatnekar, S., Kao, W.J., and Anderson, J.M., Leukocyte–biomaterial interactions in the presence of *Staphylococcus epidermidis*: flow cytometric evaluation of leukocyte activation, *J. Biomed. Mater. Res.*, 35, 409, 1997.
78. Sefton, M.V. et al., Does surface chemistry affect thrombogenicity of surface modified polymers? *J. Biomed. Mater. Res.*, 55, 447, 2001.
79. Kidd, K.R. et al., A comparative evaluation of the tissue responses associated with polymeric implants in the rat and mouse, *J. Biomed. Mater. Res.*, 59, 682, 2002.
80. Clubb, F.J. et al., Surface texturing and coating biomaterial implants: effects on tissue integration and fibrosis, *ASAIO J.*, 45, 281, 1999.
81. Stokes, K. et al., The encapsulation of polyurethane-insulated transvenous cardiac pacemaker leads, *Cardiovasc. Pathol.*, 4, 163, 1995.
82. Hill, H.R. et al., The effects of polyvinyl chloride and polyolefin blood bags on red blood cells stored in a new additive solution, *Vox Sanguin.*, 81, 161, 2001.
83. Toth, K., Wenby, R.B., and Meiselman, H.J., Inhibition of polymer-induced red cell aggregation by poloxamer 188, *Biorheology*, 37, 301, 2000.
84. Gorbet, M.B., Yeo, E.L., and Sefton, M.V., Flow cytometric study of *in vitro* neutrophil activation by biomaterials, *J. Biomed. Mater. Res.*, 44, 298, 1999.
85. Hunt, J.A., Remes, A., and Williams, D.F., The effect of metal ions on neutrophil degranulation, *J. Mater. Sci. Mater. Med.*, 3, 160, 1992.
86. Goldstein, A.S. and DiMilla, P.A., Effect of adsorbed fibronectin concentration on cell adhesion and deformation under shear on hydrophobic surfaces, *J. Biomed. Mater. Res.*, 59, 665, 2002.

87. Hu, W.J., Eaton, J.W., and Tang, L.P., Molecular basis of biomaterial-mediated foreign body reactions, *Blood*, 98, 1231, 2001.
88. Zippel, R. et al., Antigenicity of polyester vascular prostheses in an animal model, *Eur. J. Vasc. Endovasc. Surg.*, 21, 202, 2001.
89. de Jong, W.H. et al., Study to determine the presence of antipolymer antibodies in a group of Dutch women with a silicone breast implant, *Clin. Exper. Rheumatol.*, 20, 151, 2002.
90. Hunt, J.A., Rhodes, N.P., and Williams, D.F., Analysis of the inflammatory exudates surrounding implanted polymers using flow cytometry, *J. Mater. Sci. Mater. Med.*, 6, 839, 1995.
91. Elves, M.W., Immunological aspects of biomaterials, in *Fundamental Aspects of Biocompatibility*, Vol. ll, Williams, D.F., Ed., CRC Press, Boca Raton, 1981, p. 159.
92. Bosetti, M., Hench, L., and Cannas, M., Interaction of bioactive glasses with peritoneal macrophages and monocytes *in vitro*, *J. Biomed. Mater. Res.*, 60, 79, 2002.
93. Rhodes, N.P., Hunt, J.A., and Williams, D.F., Macrophage sub-population differentiation by stimulation with biomaterials, *J. Biomed. Mater. Res.*, 37, 481, 1997.
94. McNally, A.K. and Anderson, J.M., Interleukin-4 induces foreign body giant cells from human monocytes/macrophages, *Am J. Pathol.*, 147, 1487, 1995.
95. Anderson, J.M., Multinucleated giant cells, *Curr. Opin. Hematol.*, 7, 40, 2000.
96. von Knoch, M. et al., Polyethylene loading of foreign body giant cells in aseptic loosening of hip arthroplasty, *Zeit. Orthop. Grenzgeb.*, 138, 522, 2000.
97. Neale, S.D. and Athanasou, N.A., Cytokine receptor profile of arthroplasty macrophages, foreign body giant cells and mature osteoclasts, *Acta Orthop. Scand.*, 70, 452, 1999.
98. van Luyn, M.J.A. et al., Modulation of the tissue reaction to biomaterials. II: the function of T cells in the inflammatory response to crosslinked collagen implanted in T cell-deficient rats, *J. Biomed. Mater. Res.*, 39, 398, 1998.
99. Thomssen, H. et al., Cobalt-specific T lymphocytes in synovial tissue after an allergic reaction to a cobalt alloy joint prosthesis, *J. Rheumatol.* 28, 2001, 1121.
100. Grunkemeier, J.M., Tsai, W.B., and Horbett, T.A., Haemocompatibility of treated polystyrene surfaces; contact activation, platelet adhesion and procoagulant activity, *J. Biomed. Mater. Res.*, 41, 657, 1998.
101. Vanderkamp, K.W.H.J. and Vanoeveren, W., Factor XII fragment and kallikrein generation in plasma during incubation with biomaterials, *J. Biomed. Mater. Res.*, 28, 349, 1994.
102. Rhodes, N.P. and Williams, D.F., Plasma recalcification as a measure of contact phase activation and heparin efficiency after contact with biomaterials, *Biomaterials*, 15, 35, 1994.
103. Kidd, K.R., Nagle, R.B., and Williams, S.K., Angiogenesis and neovascularisation associated with extracellular matrix-modified porous implants, *J. Biomed. Mater. Res.*, 59, 366, 2002.
104. Dean, D.D. et al., Ultrahigh molecular weight polyethylene particles have direct effects on proliferation, differentiation and local factor production of MG63 osteoblast-like cells, *J. Orthop. Res.*, 17, 9, 1999.
105. Risbud, M.V., Bhonde, M.R., and Bhonde, R.R., Effect of a chitosan–polyvinyl pyrrolidone hydrogel on proliferation and cytokine expression of endothelial cells, *J. Biomed. Mater. Res.* 57, 300, 2001.

106. Cenni, E. et al., Production of growth factors by *in vitro* cultured human endothelial cells after contact with carbon coated polyethylene terephthalate, *J. Biomat. Sci. Polymer Ed.*, 10, 989, 1999.
107. Feldman, L.J. et al., Differential expression of matrix metalloproteinases after stent implantation and balloon angioplasty in the hypercholesterolemic rabbit, *Circulation*, 103, 3117, 2001.
108. Stephens, R. et al., Two episodes of life threatening anaphylaxis in the same patient to a chlorhexidine–sulphadiazine-coated central venous catheter, *Brit. J. Anaesth.*, 87, 306, 2001.
109. Tang, L.P., Jennings, T.A., and Eaton, J.W., Mast cells mediate acute inflammatory responses to biomaterials, *Proc. Natl. Acad. Sci. U.S.A.*, 95, 8841, 1998.
110. Hallab, N., Jacobs, J. J., and Black, J., Hypersensitivity to biomaterials: a review of leukocyte migration inhibition assays, *Biomaterials*, 21, 1301, 2000.
111. Murakami, Y. et al., Interaction of poly(2-acrylamido 2-methylpropane sulfonate)p-grafted polystyrene beads with cationic complement proteins, *J. Biomater. Sci. Polymer Ed.*, 12, 451, 2001.
112. An, Y.H. and Friedmann, R.F., Concise review of mechanisms of bacterial adhesion to biomaterial surfaces, *J. Biomed. Mater. Res.*, 43, 338, 1998.
113. Oosterbos, C.J.M. et al., Osseointegration of hydroxyapatite coated and noncoated Ti-6Al-4V implants in the presence of local infection, *J. Biomed. Mater. Res.*, 60, 339, 2002.
114. Janatova, J., Activation and control of complement, inflammation, and infection associated with the use of biomedical polymers, *ASAIO J.*, 46, S53, 2000.
115. Kirkpatrick, C.J. et al., Biomaterial-induced sarcoma, *Amer. J. Pathol.*, 156, 1455, 2000.
116. Vahey, J.W., Simonian, P.T., and Conran, E.U., Carcinogenicity and metallic implants, *Am. J. Orthop.*, 24, 319, 1995.
117. Gough, J.E. and Downes, S., Osteoblast cell death on methacrylate polymers involves apoptosis, *J. Biomed. Mater. Res.* 57, 497, 2001.
118. Granchi, D. et al., Cell death induced by metal ions: necrosis or apoptosis, *J. Mater. Sci. Mater. Med.*, 9, 31, 1998.
119. Yamamoto, A., Kohyama, Y., and Hanawa, T., Mutagenicity evaluation of 41 metal salts by the umu test, *J. Biomed. Mater. Res.*, 59, 176, 2002.
120. Bosetti, M. et al., Silver-coated materials for external fixation devices: *in vitro* biocompatibility and genotoxicity, *Biomaterials*, 23, 887, 2002.
121. Chauvel-Lebret, D.J. et al., Evaluation of the capacity of the SCGE assay to assess the genotoxicity of biomaterials, *Biomaterials*, 22, 1795, 2001.
122. Cadee, J.A. et al., *In vivo* biocompatibility of dextran based hydrogels, *J. Biomed. Mater. Res.*, 50, 397, 2000.
123. Lescure, F. et al., Long term histopathologic study of new polypeptidic polymer for implantable drug delivery systems, *Biomaterials*, 13, 1009, 1992.
124. Jenney, C.R. et al., Human monocyte/macrophage adhesion, macrophage motility and IL-4 induced foreign body giant cell formation on silane-modified surfaces *in vitro*, *J. Biomed. Mater. Res.*, 41, 171, 1998.
125. Charnley, J., Arthroplasty of the hip in a new operation, *Lancet*, i, 1129, 1961.
126. Westaby, S., Development of surgery for valvular heart disease, in *Landmarks in Cardiac Surgery*, Westaby, S., Ed., Isis Medical, Oxford, 1997, chap. 4.
127. Schaff, H.V. et al., Paravalvular leak and other events in Silzone-coated mechanical heart valves: a report from AVERT, *Ann. Thorac. Surg.*, 73, 785, 2002.

128. Vesely, I., Barber, J.E., and Ratliff, N.N., Tissue damage and calcification may be independent mechanisms of bioprosthetic heart valve failure, *J. Heart Valve Dis.*, 10, 471, 2001.
129. Bos, G.W. et al., Small diameter vascular graft prostheses: current status, *Arch. Physiol. Biochem.*, 106, 100, 1998.
130. Davids, L., Dower, T., and Zilla, P., The lack of healing in conventional vascular grafts, in *Tissue Engineering of Vascular Prosthetic Grafts*, Zilla, P. and Greisler, H.P., Eds., G.G. Landes Co., Austin, TX, 1999, p. 3.
131. Topol, E.J. et al., A comparison of directional atherectomy with coronary angioplasty in patients with coronary artery disease, *New Engl. J. Med.*, 329, 221, 1993.
132. Durand, E. et al., Time course of apoptosis and cell proliferation and their relationship to arterial remodelling and restenosis after angioplasty in an atherosclerotic rabbit model, *J. Amer. Coll. Cardiol.*, 39, 1680, 2002.
133. Martinez-Elbal, L. et al., Direct coronary stenting versus stenting with balloon pre-dilatation: immediate and follow-up results of a multicentre, prospective, randomised study: the DISCO trial, *Eur. Heart J.*, 23, 633, 2002.
134. Weissman, N.J. et al., Extent and distribution of in stent intimal hyperplasia and edge effect in a non radiation stent population, *Am. J. Cardiol.*, 88, 248, 2001.
135. New, G. et al., The effect of 17 beta-estradiol coated stents on the endothelial cell repair, intimal hyperplasia and restenosis, *Eur. Heart J.*, 22, 483, 2001.
136. Fox, R.A., Intravascular brachytherapy of the coronary arteries, *Phys. Med. Biol.*, 47, R1, 2002.
137. Versura, P. et al., Adhesion mechanisms of human lens epithelial cells on four intraocular lens materials, *J. Cataract Refract. Surg.*, 25, 527, 1999.
138. Williams, D.F., *The Williams Dictionary of Biomaterials*, Liverpool University Press, Liverpool, 1999.
139. Brunette, D.M., Principles of cell behaviour on titanium surfaces and their application to implanted devices, in *Titanium in Medicine*, Brunette, D.M. et al., Eds., Springer, Berlin, 2001, p. 485.
140. Viornery, C. et al., Surface modification of titanium with phosphonic acid to improve bone bonding, *Langmuir*, 18, 2582, 2002.
141. Wu, J.M. et al., *In vitro* evaluation of bone bonding of chemically modified titanium, *Key Eng. Mater.*, 218, 141, 2002.
142. Korovessis, P.G., Deligianni, D.D., and Lenke, L.G., Role of surface roughness of titanium versus hydroxyapatite on human bone marrow cell response, *J. Spinal Disorders Tech.*, 15, 175, 2002.
143. Tonino, A.J. and Rahmy, A.I.A., The hydroxyapatite ABG hip system: 5- to 7-year results from an international multicentre study, *J. Arthroplasty*, 15, 274, 2000.
144. Bauer, T.W. and Schils, J., The pathology of total joint arthroplasty. I: mechanisms of fixation, *Skel. Radiol.*, 28, 423, 1999.
145. Larsson, C. et al., The titanium–bone interface, in *Titanium in Medicine*, Brunette, D.M. et al., Eds., Springer, Berlin, 2001, p. 587.
146. Gross, K.A., Ray, N., and Rokkum, M., The contribution of coating microstructure to degradation and particle release in hydroxyapatite coated prostheses, *J. Biomed. Mater. Res.*, 63, 106, 2002.
147. Gledhill, H.C., Turner, I.G., and Doyle, C., *In vitro* dissolution behaviour of two morphologically different thermally sprayed hydroxyapatite coatings, *Biomaterials*, 22, 695, 2001.

148. Proussaefs, P., Lozada, J., and Ojano, M., Histologic evaluation of threaded HA-coated root form implants after 3.5 to 11 years of function, *Int. J. Periodont. Rest. Dent.*, 21, 21, 2001.
149. Williams, D.F., Tissue–biomaterial interactions, *J. Mater. Sci.*, 22, 3421, 1987.
150. Caffee, H.H., Textured silicone and capsular contracture, *Ann. Plast. Surg.*, 24, 197, 1990.
151. Schuchert, A., Kuck, K.H., and Meinertz, T., Do steroid-eluting pacemaker electrodes allow programming at lower pacing amplitudes? *Deut. Med. Woch.*, 120, 593, 1995.
152. Lardenoye, C.W.T.A. et al., A retrospective analysis of heparin surface-modified intraocular lenses versus regular polymethylmethacrylate intraocular lenses in patients with uveitis, *Doc. Ophthalmol.*, 92, 41, 1996.
153. Ziats, N.P. et al., Adsorption of Hageman factor and other human plasma proteins to biomedical polymers, *J. Lab. Clin. Med.*, 687, 116, 1990.
154. Vroman, L., The life of an artificial device in contact with blood: initial events and their effect on its final state, *Bull. N.Y. Acad. Med.*, 64, 352, 1988.
155. Myers, G.E. et al., Latex versus iodinated contrast media anaphylaxis in the cardiac cath lab, *Cath. Cardiovasc. Diag.*, 35, 228, 1995.
156. Ahmed, F. et al., The ability of poloxamers to inhibit platelet aggregation depends on their physicochemical properties, *Thromb. Haemostasis*, 86, 1532, 2001.
157. Lewis, A.L. et al., Crosslinkable coatings from phosphorylcholine based polymers, *Biomaterials*, 22, 99, 2001.
158. Favia, P. and d'Agostino, R., Plasma treatments and plasma deposition of polymers for medical applications, *Surf. Coating Tech.*, 98, 1102, 1998.
159. Hill-West, J.L. et al., Inhibition of thrombosis and intimal thickening by *in situ* photopolymerisation of thin hydrogel barriers, *Proc. Nat. Acad. Sci. U.S.A.*, 91, 5967, 1994.
160. Boyd, K.L. et al., Endothelial cell seeding of ULTI carbon coated small diameter vascular graft, *ASAIO Trans.*, 33, 631, 1987.
161. Abraham, G.A., de Queiroz, A.A.A., and San Roman, J., Immobilisation of a non steroidal anti-inflammatory drug onto commercial segmented polyurethane surface to improve haemocompatibility properties, *Biomaterials*, 23, 1625, 2002.
162. Zhang, H.P. et al., Nitric oxide-releasing silicone rubbers with improved blood compatibility: preparation, characterization and *in vivo* evaluation, *Biomaterials*, 23, 1485, 2002.
163. Klement, P. et al., Blood-compatible biomaterials by surface coating with a novel antithrombin–heparin covalent complex, *Biomaterials*, 23, 527, 2002.
164. Lee, H.J. et al., Platelet and bacterial repellence on sulfonated poly(ethylene glycol)-acrylate copolymer surfaces, *Coll. Surfaces B Biointerfac.*, 18, 355, 2000.
165. Han, H.J and Chung, D.J., Synthesis of novel blood compatible copolymers containing pendent oligosaccharide group, *Polymer Kor.*, 22, 722, 1998.
166. Nemets, E.A. and Sevastianov, V., The interaction of heparinized biomaterials with human serum, albumin, fibrinogen, antithrombin III and platelets, *Artific. Org.*, 15, 381, 1991.
167. Bassmadijan, D. and Sefton, M.V., Relationship between release rate and surface concentration for heparinized materials, *J. Biomed. Mater. Res.*, 17, 509, 1983.
168. Yuan, S. et al., Immobilization of high affinity heparin oligosaccharide to radio frequency modified polyethylene, *J. Biomed. Mater. Res.*, 27, 811, 1993.

169. Hubbell, J.A., Biomaterials in tissue engineering, *Biotechnology,* 13, 565, 1995.
170. Langer, R. and Vacanti, J.P., Tissue engineering, *Science*, 260, 920, 1993.
171. Yannas, I.V. et al., Wound tissue can utilize a polymeric template to synthesise a functional extension of skin, *Science*, 215, 174, 1982.
172. Langer, R., Biomaterials: status, challenges and perspectives, *Amer. Inst. Chem. Eng. J.*, 46, 1286, 2000.
173. Sodian, R. et al., Tissue engineering of a trileaflet heart valve: early *in vitro* experiences with a combined polymer, *Tissue Eng.*, 5, 489, 1999.
174. Laurencin, C.T. et al., Tissue engineered bone regeneration using degradable polymers, *Bone*, 19, 93S, 1996.
175. West, J.L. and Hubbell, J.A., Polymeric biomaterials with degradation sites for proteases involved in cell migration, *Macromolecules*, 32, 241, 1999.

24

Enhancing the Processes of Discovery and Innovation for Optimal Host Response at Implant Surfaces

Malcolm L. Snead

CONTENTS

24.1 Introduction 431
24.2 Methods and Materials 433
24.3 Data and Discussion 434
Acknowledgments 437
References 437

24.1 Introduction

This chapter addresses a series of questions and potential solutions gained from advances in genomics and proteomics that can be used to optimize implant surfaces for better host integration. The availability of the nucleotide sequence for the complete human genome and comparable advances with the genomes of pertinent animal models suggest that reevaluating implant development in light of these advances may allow additional enhancements of the implant–host interface.

Interactions of host and implant surface are the lynch pins of a successful implant. Technologic advances suggest new ways to manipulate animal models to examine implant surfaces for specific patterns of gene expression in host cells responding to implants. We can sample selected time intervals after placement of an implant. Gene expression profiles can be obtained for a material or surface modification across appropriate time intervals during healing response. "Snapshots" of host responses can be created for a variety

0-8493-1474-7/03/$0.00+$1.50

of implants. The snapshots can then be correlated to implant integration and allow selection of gene expression profiles associated with optimal outcomes. The gene expression assay can identify the host cellular pathway leading to optimal outcome. Such information may be helpful also in optimizing implant outcomes for systemically compromised hosts.

A team of specialists from the biomedical sciences used their understanding of materials science and device design to create implants that perform as fully functional devices for prosthetic reconstruction in a variety of patients.[1-4] Such a desirable outcome was achieved by an empirical approach to clinical research coupled with the redesign of an implant to achieve an optimal outcome (see Chapters 2, 3, 6, 8, 9, 10, 14, 16, 17, 18, this volume). What remains is the elucidation of cell responses and gene expression profiles that yield an endpoint identified as a suitable intrabony implant device for humans.

In addition, the use of bioactive materials such as amelogenin or ameloblastin, also known as amelin (see Chapter 15, this volume), and chemically engineered self-assembling micelles or fibers (see Chapter 22, this volume) suggests that a variety of proteins or surface topologies can provide instructional information leading to an optimized host response, including the creation of bone. Moreover, it may be possible to intercept and reuse information imparted in the cascade of signals during normal development of bone to drive stem cells (see Chapter 11, this volume) toward osteogenic lineages that would improve host response to an implant. Finally, it is also possible to utilize gene therapy techniques to cause expression of pro-osteogenic growth factors locally by host cells.[5]

These possibilities suggest that knowing the gene expression profiles for the host cells responding to the implant surface may allow us to optimize the final outcome by promoting intermediary steps that are more favorable to cell viability or to gene expression profiles that result in optimal integration of the implant into host tissues. Knowing the gene expression profiles for host cells responding to various implant surfaces or materials may allow us to to identify gene expression profiles that lend themselves to more favorable outcomes. By working as a consortium of laboratories with specific expertise in biomedical research, we will be able to design better experimental strategies and gather more information about optimal responses and outcomes in a time- and cost-efficient manner. We may also be able to design implants that respond more favorably in compromised hosts such as the immune-deficient, the aged, and those who suffer from systemic diseases such as diabetes. Thus, the processes of innovation and discovery may allow us to design better implant materials, surface properties, or bioactive contents optimized for specific outcomes in selected hosts.

The first constraint is defining what is meant by success.[3,4,6] For the moment, we can avoid a definition for a successful implant because it is not required to describe the process of discovery. Ideally, a consortium of investigators would define their optimal final outcomes and then gather data correlating gene expression profiles from various treatments that resulted in favorable outcomes. For our purpose and this exercise, we describe the process of discovery in terms of a titanium implant with a mirrored surface (Ti-MS) or a textured oxide surface (Ti-TS).[7] Other designs are possible and limited by the need to obtain sufficient sample size to provide reasonable power for the final analysis, the size of the research team, and the financial underpinnings of the team.

24.2 Methods and Materials

A variety of approaches could be used for the discovery phase of this project. These include analysis based on nucleic acid biochemistry such as differential display, serial analysis of gene expression, representational display, and cDNA library construction.[8-13] Alternatively, equally powerful but perhaps more demanding approaches would be based on protein biochemistry, for example, two-dimensional gel electrophoretograms, protein chip arrays, and high performance liquid chromatography (HPLC) coupled to mass spectroscopy.[14-18]

While any of these techniques can serve as a useful alternative or compelling corroborative technique, the methodology that may be best suited to the task of discovery is DNA chip analysis.[19-21] Indeed, once markers are identified as proactive in the steps leading to a successful outcome,[22] more directed methods such as immunologic detection methods[23] could be used for assessment. In this chapter, we will consider the application of DNA chip technology only. We further restrict our attention to the use of complementary DNAs to messenger RNA expressed by cells adherent to or in close physical association with the implant surface.

In preliminary experiments, we used Affymetrix DNA chips (U74) for the analysis of gene expression profiles of ameloblast-like cells that were stably transfected with a strong transcription activator for the amelogenin gene in mice. The U74 chip set contains probes that can interrogate for the expression of 36,000 full-length mouse genes and EST clusters (http://www.affymetrix.com/products/arrays/specific/mgu74.affx). Alternatively, a corresponding chip set that would interrogate the complete human genome (U133) could be employed if these experiments received institutional review board approval for execution in human subjects.

In brief, cells were harvested and total nucleic acid was recovered and isolated using standard cell biology techniques, with the RNA isolated and recovered by differential centrifugation through CsCl.[24,25] First-strand cDNA was prepared enzymatically from purified RNA and hybridized to the selected chip set according to manufacturer's suggestions (*Gene Chip Expression Analysis*, Affymetrix 701021, Revision 2). Analysis was performed using Affymetrix software to detect two-fold changes in gene expression magnitude based on parental control cell lines.

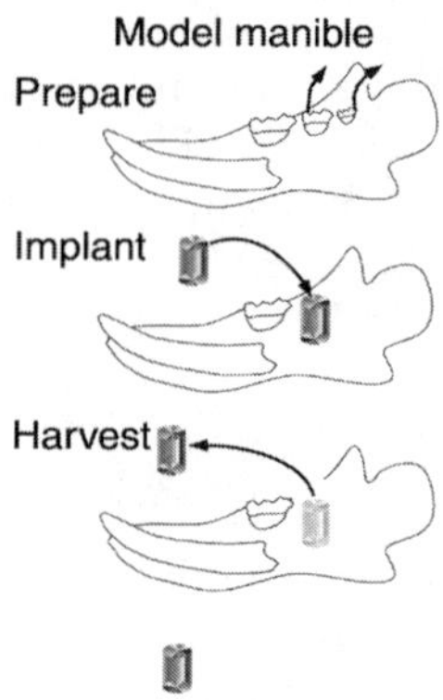

FIGURE 24.1
Recovered implant with adherent tissues for DNA chip analysis.

24.3 Data and Discussion

What seems particularly exciting about the approach outlined herein is the possibility of performing these analyses at various centers and creating a combined pool of information far greater than any single research team could compile in a reasonable length of time. Perhaps through shared design, shared protocols for execution, calibration among surgeons, and shared approaches to gene analysis, a consortium of groups could produce a first-generation product in a modest period (3 to 5 years) and for a reasonable budget ($1 million to $1.5 million) using four to six interacting groups in America, Europe, and Asia.

Figure 24.1 illustrates one model for implant surface analysis. A cylinder of specific design would be implanted in alveolar bone following extraction of the second and third molar teeth in a rodent model. Other animal models are possible, as is varying the time for implant placement after removing the teeth. These details would be established by the principal investigators from the consortium.

As many markers favorable for bone differentiation are already known,[34] it may be possible to shorten the time line by using array profiles gained from surfaces that better approximate pro-osteogenic markers. Gene expression profiles would be recovered from cells adherent to the implant as shown in Figure 24.2 using standard cell and molecular biology techniques. By calibrating surgical procedures, sampling intervals, material properties, and other potential variables, data from members of the consortium could be pooled to create a robust set of pro-integration and anti-integration gene expression profiles.

A potential windfall from the efforts of this consortium would be the creation of a rather complete lexicon for gene expression profiles for selected

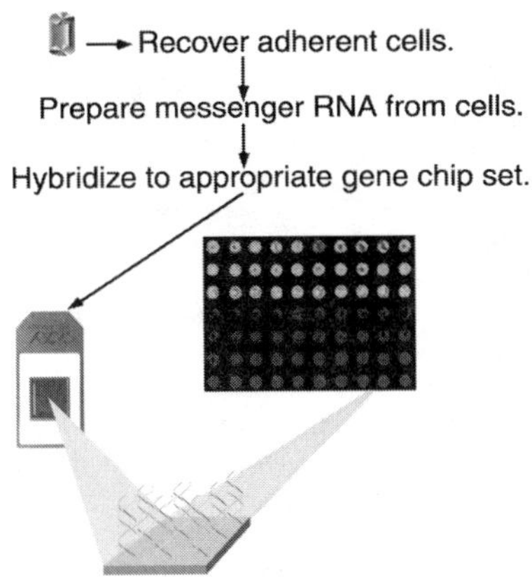

FIGURE 24.2
Gene expression analysis.

implants across wide temporal intervals following implant placement. Information from these studies could be mined to permit the leverage of innovation and discovery for the enhancement of patient care. This may be achieved without sacrificing productivity among individual laboratories that contributes to the success of the whole if the consortium chooses to publish its findings as a whole. Success among many laboratories working on shared themes and resources has contributed to significant biomedical advances,[35,36] while producing a wide body of scientific publications for contributing members. The workshop that led to the creation of this volume took the first steps in developing such a framework for a collective process of discovery for implants.

One significant area of concern resides around the potential to register cellular responses from an animal model that may not sufficiently mimic the human condition to permit extrapolation of design features.[37] This pitfall cannot be overcome in the absence of data. However, the process of discovery for gene expression responses cannot be achieved ethically in human subjects because it is based on retrieving implants at selected times — a strategy that would be difficult to execute in human subjects. The final outcome assessment for an implant is predicted to involve functional test parameters such as pull-out strength and histomorphometric analysis of implant surfaces. Again, such analyses could not be carried out readily in humans for ethical reasons. However, several opportunities exist for corroboration of data from animal models to a human host.[37,38] For example, it should be possible to analyze early response intervals to compare human and animal responses. Based on previous success, it is anticipated that members of the consortium can identify a suitable animal model for these studies.[38,39] Pilot studies could be undertaken to provide data suggesting the usefulness of a specific animal model. Nonetheless, the success of the endeavor could be compromised by a poor fit between a human and animal model although this seems unlikely.

TABLE 24.1

Changes in Gene Expression Recorded for LS8 Cells[a]

Fold Change	Gene Detail/Description
~11.2	U72032: *Mus musculus* eosinophil secondary granule ribonuclease-1
~9.7	D49544: Mouse mRNA for KIFC1
4.2	D87908: *Mus musculus* mRNA for nuclear protein np95
~3.6	M63695: CD1d1 antigen
3.3	L17076: HnRNP-associated with lethal yellow
2.8	M83218: *Mus musculus* intracellular calcium-binding protein (MRP8) mRNA
2.8	AF017258: *Mus musculus* ribonuclease 3 precursor (mR-3) gene
~2.7	D01034: TATA box binding protein
~2.7	AV361373: *Mus musculus* cDNA, 3 end
~2.7	AB006141: *Mus musculus* mRNA for IGFBP-like protein
2.5	X89998: *Mus musculus* mRNA for 17 beta-hydroxysteroid dehydrogenase type IV
2.1	X15052: Neural cell adhesion molecule
~2.1	K02782: Mouse complement component C3 mRNA, α and β subunits
2	M33988: Mouse histone H2A.1 gene

[a] Expression of the transcription activator for amelogenin was induced in ameloblast-like cells and a threshold of greater than two-fold increase in selected mouse gene recorded by DNA chip analysis.

It would also be plausible to explore surface modifications that promoted gene expression profiles associated with successful outcomes. In one experimental strategy, selected surface modifications that promote cell adhesion, cell proliferation, and cell differentiation markers could be examined. For example, the chemical micelles and fibers described by Dr. Stupp (Chapter 22, this volume) could be examined for their ability to promote gene expression profiles in host cells known to be linked with optimal outcomes and contained in the lexicon of host responses discovered by the consortium.

Table 24.1 shows an example of the analysis depicting changes in gene expression in ameloblast-like cells that express high levels of the transcription activator C/EBP-α. In subsequent experiments, we will determine whether changes in the gene expression profile are linked with signaling pathways that are altered (in this case, pathways that are activated, e.g., AB006141, M83218, X15052) and whether changes in mRNAs encoding transcription proteins (e.g., D01034, D49544) are sufficient or necessary for activation of the amelogenin gene.

Similarly, data for genes whose mRNA levels are reduced can also be identified and their significance to biological pathways assessed.[26,27] The latter step of assessing significance to biological pathways is the most difficult. Work on the networks that regulate protein-to-protein interactions and hence alter gene expression profiles is still in its infancy,[28-30] although breakthroughs in model organisms such as sea urchins suggest that significant progress is being achieved.[31] Clearly, the relatively recent discovery of a novel protein, osteoprotegerin, and its seminal role in osteoclast behavior[32,33] is one example of how primitive our discovery process remains despite immense gains in computational and gene analysis power.

Acknowledgments

The support of the organizers and participants in the workshop on which this book is based was extremely important to shaping the ideas expressed in this chapter. We thank the anonymous reviewers for critiques that were instrumental in improving this manuscript. This work was supported by the National Institutes of Health, National Institute for Dental and Craniofacial Research Grant DE-13045, DE-06988.

References

1. Stanford, C.M., Biomechanical and functional behavior of implants, *Adv. Dent. Res.*, 13, 88, 1999.
2. Bryant, S.R. and Zarb, G.A., Outcomes of implant prosthodontic treatment in older adults, *J. Can. Dent. Assn.*, 68, 97, 2002.
3. Esposito, M. et al., Biological factors contributing to failures of osseointegrated oral implants. I: success criteria and epidemiology, *Eur. J. Oral Sci.*, 106, 527, 1998.
4. Esposito, M. et al., Biological factors contributing to failures of osseointegrated oral implants. II: etiopathogenesis, *Eur. J. Oral Sci.*, 106, 721, 1998.
5. Franceschi, R.T. et al., Gene therapy for bone formation: *in vitro* and *in vivo* osteogenic activity of an adenovirus expressing BMP7, *J. Cell Biochem.*, 78, 476, 2000.
6. Branemark, R. et al., Biomechanical characterization of osseointegration during healing: an experimental *in vivo* study in the rat, *Biomaterials*, 18, 969, 1997.
7. Larsson, C. et al., Bone response to surface-modified titanium implants: studies on the early tissue response to machined and electropolished implants with different oxide thicknesses, *Biomaterials*, 17, 605, 1996.
8. Zhang, J.S. et al., Differential display of mRNA, *Mol. Biotechnol.*, 10, 155, 1998.
9. Fend, F. and Raffeld, M., Laser capture microdissection in pathology, *J. Clin. Pathol.*, 53, 666, 2000.
10. Yamamoto, M. et al., Use of serial analysis of gene expression (SAGE) technology, *J. Immunol. Methods*, 250, 45, 2001.
11. Riggins, G.J. and Strausberg, R.L., Genome and genetic resources from the Cancer Genome Anatomy Project, *Hum. Mol. Genet.*, 10, 663, 2001.
12. Korneev, S., Blackshaw, S., and Davies, J.A., cDNA libraries from a few neural cells, *Prog. Neurobiol.*, 42, 339, 1994.
13. Cooper, L.F. et al., Incipient analysis of mesenchymal stem-cell-derived osteogenesis, *J. Dent. Res.*, 80, 314, 2001.

14. Peng, J. and Gygi, S.P., Proteomics: the move to mixtures, *J. Mass Spectrom.*, 36, 1083, 2001.
15. Nordhoff, E. et al., Large-gel two-dimensional electrophoresis–matrix assisted laser desorption ionization–time of flight mass spectrometry: an analytical challenge for studying complex protein mixtures, *Electrophoresis*, 22, 2844, 2001.
16. Hubbard, M.J. and McHugh, N.J., Human ERp29: isolation, primary structural characterisation and two-dimensional gel mapping, *Electrophoresis*, 21, 3785, 2000.
17. Honore, B., Genome- and proteome-based technologies: status and applications in the postgenomic era, *Expert Rev. Mol. Diagn.*, 1, 265, 2001.
18. Fung, E.T. et al., Protein biochips for differential profiling, *Curr. Opin. Biotechnol.*, 12, 65, 2001.
19. Werner, T., Target gene identification from expression array data by promoter analysis, *Biomol. Eng.*, 17, 87, 2001.
20. Lee, P.S. and Lee, K.H., Genomic analysis, *Curr. Opin. Biotechnol.*, 11, 171, 2000.
21. Hacia, J.G., Brody, L.C., and Collins, F.S. Applications of DNA chips for genomic analysis, *Mol. Psychiatry*, 3, 483, 1998.
22. Cooper, L.F., Biologic determinants of bone formation for osseointegration: clues for future clinical improvements, *J. Prosthet. Dent.*, 80, 439, 1998.
23. Rosengren, A., et al., Immunohistochemical studies on the distribution of albumin, fibrinogen, fibronectin, IgG and collagen around PTFE and titanium implants, *Biomaterials*, 17, 1779 1996.
24. Sambrook, J., Fritsch, E.F., and Maniatis, T., Molecular cloning: a laboratory manual, 2nd ed., Cold Spring Harbor Laboratory, Cold Spring Harbor, NY, 1989.
25. Snead, M.L. et al., *De novo* gene expression detected by amelogenin gene transcript analysis, *Dev. Biol.*, 104, 255, 1984.
26. Rebhan, M. et al., GeneCards: a novel functional genomics compendium with automated data mining and query reformulation support, *Bioinformatics*, 14, 656, 1998.
27. Lee, H.S., DNA chip data mining, *Exp. Mol. Med.*, 33, 151, 2001.
28. de Jong, H., Modeling and simulation of genetic regulatory systems: a literature review, *J. Comput. Biol.*, 9, 67, 2002.
29. Tong, A.H. et al., A combined experimental and computational strategy to define protein interaction networks for peptide recognition modules, *Science*, 295, 321, 2002.
30. Schacherer, F. et al., The TRANSPATH signal transduction database: a knowledge base on signal transduction networks, *Bioinformatics*, 17, 1053, 2001.
31. Davidson, E.H. et al., A genomic regulatory network for development, *Science*, 295, 1669, 2002.
32. Feige, U., Osteoprotegerin, *Ann. Rheum. Dis.*, 60, 81, 2001.
33. Simonet, W.S. et al., Osteoprotegerin: a novel secreted protein involved in the regulation of bone density, *Cell*, 89, 309, 1997.
34. Keller, J.C. et al., Characterizations of titanium implant surfaces III, *J. Biomed. Mater. Res.*, 28, 939, 1994.
35. Xu, J., Combined analysis of hereditary prostate cancer linkage to 1q24-25: results from 772 hereditary prostate cancer families from the International Consortium for Prostate Cancer Genetics, *Am. J. Hum. Genet.*, 66, 945, 2000.

36. Burke, W. et al., Recommendations for follow-up care of individuals with an inherited predisposition to cancer II: BRCA1 and BRCA2, Cancer Genetics Studies Consortium, *JAMA*, 277, 997, 1997.
37. Abron, A. et al., Evaluation of a predictive model for implant surface topography effects on early osseointegration in the rat tibia model, *J. Prosthet. Dent.*, 85, 40, 2001.
38. Masuda, T. et al., Cell and matrix reactions at titanium implants in surgically prepared rat tibiae, *Int. J. Oral Maxillofac. Implants*, 12, 472, 1997.
39. Cooper, L. et al., A multicenter 12-month evaluation of single-tooth implants restored 3 weeks after one-stage surgery, *Int. J. Oral Maxillofac. Implants*, 16, 182, 2001.

Index

A

Acid etching, 4, 20, 50, 66–67
Acrylamide, 346
Actin, 316, 351, 359
Adaptive immune system, 294
Adenovirus, 129
Adipocytes, 306
Adlayers, 345
Adaptive responses, 294
Advisory expert panel, 383
Albumin, 90, 286, 354–357
Alkaline phosphatase, 127, 144–149, 171, 249, 306
Alkane phosphate SAMs, 351
Alkane phosphates, 348–349, 351
Alkane phosphonic acids, 350
Alkane thiols, 292
Alkyl chain, 399
Aluminium oxide, 147, 191
Aluminum, 291, 296–297, 412, 416
Alveolar bone, 271–272
Amalgam, 295, 382
Ameloblastin, 275
Amelogenesis, 274
Amelogenin, 240, 271–272, 274, 432–433
Aminosilane, 355
Amphiphilic molecules, 355
Amplitude parameters, 63
Anaphylaxis, 418
Angiogenesis, 127, 227, 270
Angioplasty, 413
Animal models, 431, 435
Animal–Derived Medical Devices, 381
Anisotropy, 65
  anisotropic surfaces, 64
Anticoagulant, 289
Antiproperdin, 297–299
Antithrombogenic, 419
Apatite, 233, 239–240, 310–312, 324, 331
  coatings, 143
Arginine-glycine-aspartic acid (RGD), 270, 308
Acetyl Salisylic Acid (ASA), 290
Ascorbic acid, 314
Autocrine regulation, 178

B

Bacteria, 358
β-glycerophosphate, 314
Bioactivity, 92, 409, 412, 415, 421
Biocompatibility, 184, 262, 385, 407, 409
Biodegradation, 328
Biofilm, 46, 265
Bioglass, 287
Bio-inertness, 198
Biologic width, 46
Biological properties, 386
Biomimicry, 393, 269, 397
Bioprosthetic valve, 413
Biosynthesis, 315
Biotin, 361
Blood, 167–170, 289–295, 413
  α-hemolysin, 394
  α-lactalbumin, 286
  albumin, 355, 286
  anticoagulant, 289
  antithrombogenic, 419
  cells, 221, 299
  clot, 222, 300, 418–419
  complement factors, *see* Complement system
  plasma coagulation factors, 290
  plasma proteins, 289
  thrombin, 222, 289
  thrombomodulin, 270, 289
  thrombospondin-2, 287
  von Willebrand factor, 290
Bone, 227, 234, 368, 271, 306, 401
  adsorption, 343–344
  alveolar, 248
  bone acidic glycoprotein (BAG-75), 237
  bonding, 226–227, 416
  canaliculi, 317
  cancellous bone, 30, 326

cement, 295, 412
cortical, 326
densities, 253
formation, 49, 175, 219-220, 227, 255, 305
healing, 227
integrity, 270
loss, 234, 344
marrow, 306
matrix, 153, 212, 222
mineralization, 270, 326
remodelling, 219, 227
trabeculae, 255
trabecular bone, 276
thrombomodulin, 270, 289
thrombospondin-2, 287
woven, 145

C

Calcifying carcinomas, 235
Calcium phosphate (CaP), 51, 233, 263, 309, 314, 343, 416
amorphous coatings, 314
apatite, 312
brushite, 90, 233
calcein, 328
calcification, 225, 314
calcium, 235, 329
calcium deposition, 251, 254, 257
calcium hydroxyapatite, 232
calcium–phosphate binding, 329
calvarial bone critical defects, 257
ceramics, 314
coatings, 50, 264
degradation, 317
dissolution, 317
mineralization, 225
precipitation, 312, 314, 329
pyrophosphate, 233
Capsule, 287
Carbonate apatite, 317
Carbonate, 232–233, 235, 263
Cardiovascular device, 413
Cartilage, 237, 271
hypertrophic, 235
cbfa-1, 275
cDNA, 433
Cells, 313
adhesion, 106, 265, 307
adipocytes, 306
ameloblasts, 274, 432
ameloblast stem cells, 207
attachment, 315
cell-specific surface, 359
chondroblasts, 326
contact guidance, 105
differentiation, 105, 315
epidermal stem cell, 207
fibroblasts, 306, 326, 358, 352, 358–362
hematopoietic, 206, 307, 313
human gingival fibroblasts, 112, 351
leukocyte, 222, 294
macrophage, 117, 170, 174
mesenchymal cells, 274
mesenchymal stem cells (MSCs), 207, 306
migration, 106–107, 114, 135, 222, 227
monocytes, 117, 170, 175
neutrophils, 222, 227
non-collagenous molecules, 235
odontoblast stem cells, 215
octadecyl phosphate, 469
orientation, 115
osteogenic, 222, 227, 313
osteoblast, 114, 127–128, 131, 144, 235, 248, 254, 257, 306, 326, 358, 362
osteoclasts, 117, 306
osteoprogenitors, 307, 309
population density, 107
preadipocytes, 307
preodontoblasts, 274
preosteoblast, 131, 307
proliferation, 315, 360
rat bone marrow (RBM), 314
rugofile, 327
rugophobe, 359
selection, 105, 117
signalling, 265
stem cells, 206–207, 287, 432
viability, 360
Cementum, 232, 234, 263, 271–272
cement line matrix, 220, 222
cement lines, 226–227
cementogenesis, 274
root cementum, 271
Certification, 375, 380
Charge density, 235
Chemical binding, 343
Chemical foci, 234
Chromium, 296
Chronic inflammation, 300
Cloning, therapeutic, 209
Clustering, 232
Coating, 4, 309, 312
resorbable, 76
crystalline CaP coatings, 316
Cobalt–chromium, 412
Cochrane Collaboration, 6

Collagen, 127, 135, 226, 234–238, 269–271, 417
bovine, 381
collagen-I, 144, 234, 307
fibrils, 257, 400
hole zones, 234
sponge, 257
tropocollagen, 234–235
Competent authority, 375
Complement system, 294, 295, 418
activator, 296
antiproperdin, 297–299
contact activation, 290
factor 1q (C1q), 286
factor 3b (C3b), 286
factor 3bi (iC3b), 286
factor 3dg/three-dimensional (C3dg C3d), 286, 299
factor-1q (C-1q), 290
factor Xa, 289
factor-XII(FXII), 290
Cross-link, 234, 344
Crystal, 316, 327, 235
faces, 234
inhibition, 234
initiation, 232–234
growth, 225
growth modulation, 234
morphology, 232, 234
nucleation, 153, 225, 235, 275, 313, 325, 398
size, 232, 234
ultrastructure, 233
Cytochrome, 355
Cytokine, 221, 267, 273, 313
Cytoskeleton, 267
Cytotoxicity, 388, 410–411

D

Dacron, 413
Dehydration, 232
Delamination, 324, 421
Dendron rodcoil, 395
Dentin, 232, 234, 238, 271, 401
Design control system, 384
Design studies, 20
Devices, 370
Dexamethasone, 314
Dextran, 289, 534
Dielectric constant, 324
Differential display, 433
Differentiation factors, 210
Dimers, 393
Discovery, 435
Dithiothreitol, 400
DNA
chip markers, 433
microarray analysis, 133
Dodecyl phosphate, 350

E

Electrical charge, 411
Electrochemical oxidation, 324
Electrodischarge, 4
Enamel, 232, 234, 240, 274
crystals, 232
extracellular matrix, 270, 276
matrix-derived proteins, 131, 241
Enamelin, 240
Enthalpy, 289
Entropy, 289
Enzymes
α-amylase, 286
alkaline phosphatase, 144, 171, 149, 251, 306
Ecto-ADPase, 289
focal adhesion kinase (p125FAK), 268
metalloproteinases (MMPs), 270
Epigenetic signal, 265, 267, 269
Epithelial root sheath, 274
Excluded-volume effect, 355
Extracellular matrix, 106, 108 226, 323, 248, 254, 265, 269, 307, 398, 420
ameloblastin, 274–275, 432
amelogenin, 240, 271–272, 274, 432–433
bone sialoprotein (BSP), 153, 225, 235–237, 251, 270, 273, 307
components, 234
dentine phosphoprotein (DPP), 234, 238,400
dentine sialoprotein (DSP), 270, 238–239
deposition, 326
enamelin, 240
engineering, 397
fibronectin, 127, 135, 174, 267–270, 286, 318, 358, 362, 400
laminin, 127, 269–270, 402
lumican, 270
MMP (metalloproteinases), 270
non-collagenous molecules, 225, 235
phosphophoryn, 238, 400
proteins, 145, 268
synthetic, 397
TIMP (tissue inhibitors of metalloproteinases), 270
vitronectin, 154, 270, 358

F

Fibrillogenesis, 235
Fibrin, 222, 234–235,
  clot, 168
  retention, 222
  scaffold, 222
Fibrosis, 175, 417
Fibrous encapsulation, 262, 285, 287, 300, 417
Finite element analyses, 47, 54
Flammability, 385
Fluoride, 232
Focal adhesion kinase (p125FAK), 268
Focal adhesions, 307
Force
  compressive, 51
  shear, 31,51
  tensile, 35–38, 51
Foreign body reaction, 262
Fracture, 334
  healing, 222, 416
  lines, 334
Free surface energy, 288
Frustrated phagocytosis, 300

G

Gene expression, 432–433
Gene therapy, 129
Genomics, 431
Gibbs free energy (G), 288
Glutamic acid, 236
Glycoproteins, 307
Glycosylaminoglycans (GAGs), 234, 266, 270
Gold, 295
Good Clinical Practices (GCP), 384
Good Laboratory Practices (GLP), 384
Good Manufacturing Practices (GMPs), 374, 384
Granuloma, 417
Graft
  autografts, 248
  synthetic, 248
Grinding, 4
Grit blasting, 50, 152
Growth factors, 210, 221, 267, 268, 269, 381
  BMP (Bone Morphogenic Protein), 129, 170, 212, 258, 264, 268, 270
  BMP-2, 251, 268
  BMP-4, 251
  BMP-6, 171
  BMP-7, 129
  expression of, 269
  FGF-1 (fibroblast growth factor-1), 132
  HGF (hepatocyte growth factor), 254
  OCN (osteocalcin), 249–251
  ON (osteonectine), 270
  OP-1 (osteogenic protein-1), 381
  OPN (osteopontin), 118, 225, 237, 251, 270, 307–308
  OPG (osteoprotegerin), 436
  PDGF-AB (platelet derived growth factor AB), 273
  PDGF-BB, 381
  TGF-β (transforming growth factor beta), 129, 172, 264, 268, 273, 326

H

Hafnium, 195
Hemostasis, 299
Heparan sulphate, 270
Heparin, 289–290, 414, 419
Heparin-like molecules, 289
High molecular weight kininogen (HMWK), 286, 290
Hirudin, 290
Hybrid parameters, 62–63
Hydrogen peroxide, 416
Hydroxides, 288, 320
Hydroxyapatite, 51, 233, 235, 271, 328, 343, 400, 412, 417
  coatings, 4, 75–76, 90
  crystals, 241
  plasma-sprayed, 86, 90
  poorly crystalline, 90
Hypersensitivity, 294
  type I, 294
  type II, 294
  type III, 294
  type IV, 294

I

Ilmenite, 124
Immune System
  immune-deficiency, 432
  immunoglobulin (IgG, IgM), 286, 290, 294, 299
  reactions, 294
  recognition, 294
  rejection, 294
  suppression, 295

Implant, 4, 261–262, 326, 408
  bone-to-implant interface, 132, 227
  bone-to-metal retention, 325
  breast, 417
  dental, 383
  devices, 408
  failures, 5, 15
  neck, 31
  oral, 4, 308
  osteoinductive, 269
  root-formed, 19
  stability, 49
  subcutaneous, 316
  subperiosteal, 316
  surfaces, 11, 44, 222, 269, 285, 408, 431
Inertness, 198, 409
Inflammation, 299, 414, 417
Integrelin, 290
Integrin, 127, 174, 178, 267–268, 307, 358, 400
  expression, 316
  receptors, 270, 273
Interface, 264, 299, 395, 408
  dissolution, 315
  matrix, 226
  precipitation, 315
  reactions, 408–409
Interferons, 294
IL-6 (Interleukin 6), 273
Intrafibrillar mineral, 235
Intraocular lens, 414
Intravascular stent, 414
Ion beam, 312, 328
Ion implantation, 327
Isotropy, 62–68

J

Joint replacements, 262, 412

L

Lamina limitans, 315, 317
Lectin, 299
Ligands, 265–267, 398–399
  bioligands, 344
  matrix, 127, 174, 307
  presentation, 267
  integrin ligands (RGD), 127, 174, 307
  RGD, 358, 360, 400
Loading, 29, 262
  early, 29
  immediate, 29, 74
Lotus effect, 350
Lysozyme, 286

M

Magnesium, 232–233
Marginal bone losses, 66
Marketing, 370, 374
Material variables, 410
Mercaptoethanol, 299
Microarrays, 134
Microcracking, 45
Microparticles, 221
Molecular assembly, 345, 358
Molecular recognition, 393

N

Nanofibers, 389–399
Nanohelix, 397
Nanoribbons, 396
Nanospheres, 241
Nanostructures, 393
Niobium, 191–192
Nitric oxide, 289
Nucleic acid, 170, 433
  mRNA, DNA, cDNA, 267, 436

O

Octacalcium phosphate, 233
Oligo(ethylene glycol) (OEG), 297–298
Organogenesis, 214
Osseointegration, 48, 126, 167, 263, 268, 305
Osteoblast, 235, 254, 306
  adhesion, 128
  cbfa-1, 275
  cultures, 248, 257
  differentiation, 131, 127–128
  migration, 114
  orientation, 109
  phenotype, 126–128
  proliferation, 127, 131
  shape, 144
Osteocalcin (OCN), 170, 251, 307, 314–315
Osteocapacity, 313–314
Osteoclast, 117, 306, 436

Osteoconduction, 50, 219–221, 227, 257–263, 328
Osteodentine, 275
Osteogenesis, 227
Osteogenic, 262, 313
Osteoid, 232
Osteoinduction, 169, 174, 178, 257
Osteopontin, 118, 225, 237, 270, 307–308

P

Pacemaker, 417
Parathyroid hormone (PTH), 133
Periodontal ligament, 213, 271–272
Perovskite, 124
Phospholipids, 419
Phosphonates, 348
Phosphonic acid, 416
Phosphorylcholine, 534
Plasma spraying, 4, 47, 263, 328
Platelets, 221, 289, 299
  activation, 222, 227
  glycoprotein GP-IIb, 290
  glycoprotein GP-IIIa, 290
  microparticle formation, 222
  platelet-activating factor (PAF), 289
Polymers, 393
  fluorenylmethoxycarbonyl, 399
  methylmethacrylate, 412
  poly(ethylene glycol) (PEG), 344, 346, 355, 357, 534
  poly(ethylene oxide), 344, 534
  poly(glycolic acid), 398
  poly(L-lactic acid), 298
  poly(L-lysine)-g-poly(ethylene glycol) (PLL-PEG), 292, 355–357
  poly(L-Lysine)-Graft-Poly(Ethylene Glycol), 355
  polycationic PEG-grafted copolymer adlayers, 345
  polydimethylsiloxane, 287, 295
  polyethylene glycol, 289, 419
  polyethylene, 412, 416
  polymethylmethacrylate (PMMA), 295, 412, 414, 416–417
  polypropylene, 287
  polytetrafluoroethylene (PTFE), 285, 412–413
Polysaccharides, 534
Prekallikrein (PKK), 290
Prostacyclin, 289
Prostaglandins, 144
Prostheses, 261–262
Prosthetic heart valves, 412
Proteins, 233, 266, 432
  adlayers, 253
  adsorption, 288, 300
  biochemistry, 433
  chip arrays, 433
  films, 290
Proteoglycans, 270, 362
Proteomics, 431
P-selectin, 222, 286

R

Radiopacity, 253
Randomized controlled clinical trial, 4
Regulatory
  510(k), 378
  animal-derived medical devices, 381
  approval, 374
  assessment analysis, 384
  authorization, 374
  batch control, 380
  British standards, 382
  CE mark, 375, 379
  certification, 375, 380
  competent authority, 375
  conformity, 379
  consolidated standards of reporting trials, 20
  consumer protection, 382
  design control system, 384
  design input, 384
  design output, 384
  design studies, 20
  design verification, 374, 380
  directorate of general enterprise, 375
  European Economic Area Agreement [EEA], 375
  European Standardization Committee, 384
  European Union [EU], 375
  Federal Drug Administration Modernization Act, 374
  Food and Drug Administration (FDA), 374
  Food Drug and Cosmetic Act, 374
  Good Clinical Practices(GCP), 384
  Good Laboratory Practices (GLP), 384
  Good Manufacturing Practices (GMPs), 374, 384
  information sources, 386
  ISO (International Organization for Standardization), 384

international standards, 382
Japanese Industrial Standards, 382
medical device, 369, 375–377
medical device amendments, 374
notified bodies, 375–376
PDP, 378
pharmaceuticals, 369, 381
risk analysis, 374, 384–385
risk classes, 378, 380
Safe Medical Devices Act, 374
substantial equivalence, 374
therapeutic goods administration (TGA), 383
user needs, 289
validation, 374
Relative movement, 48
Removal torque, 325, 331
Representational display, 433
Restenosis, 414
Revascularization, 285
Rutile, 325

S

Scaffold, 235, 248, 420
Self-assembled monolayers (SAMs), 292, 298, 346, 350, 393, 397–398,
Self-cleaning, 350
Serine, 236
Serum, *see* Blood
Silanization, 344, 346
Silicone, 295
Sintering
beads, 143
porous-surfaced, 47
technologies, 142
Spacing parameters, 63
Sputter-coated, 314
Stainless steel, 412
Stem cells, *see also* Cells, 206–207, 287, 432
Steric stabilization, 355
Stress distribution, 326
Stroma, 306
Supersaturation, 232–233, 235
Surface, 11, 44, 222, 226, 269, 285, 408, 431
anisotropic, 64, 69
biochemical modification, 343
blasting, 4, 32, 60–65, 75
charge, 308
composition, 308, 323
contact angle, 350–351
electropolished, 188
energy, 308, 411
geometry, 44
machined, 4, 113, 332
microstructure, 326
microtextured, 221–222
modifications, 4, 14, 50
molecular recognition, 265
oxide, 324
polished, 4
pore size, 326
porous, 47, 325
properties, 4, 288
reactive ion-etched (RIE), 192
recognition molecules, 267
roughness, 11, 13, 33, 75, 60–69, 113, 193, 309, 316, 326–327, 330
smooth, 152, 316
SLA surface, 143
structure, 309, 324
threaded, 50
titanium dioxide (TiO_2) grit-blasted, 169
topography, 60–61, 64,105, 115, 227, 262, 342, 411, 432
ultrastructure, 326
wettability, 352
Surfactant, 355

T

Tantalum, 189
oxide, 349
Telopeptide, 234
Templates, 396
Thin films, 345
Threads, 142
profiles, 34
Thrombin, 222, 289
Thrombomodulin, 270, 289
Thrombospondin-2, 287
Ticlopidine, 290
Tissue, 232
damage, 265
engineering, 261, 397, 414, 419
factor, 290
fibrous, 253
repair, 262
Titanium, 136, 184, 2668, 290, 296, 309, 314, 316, 323, 342, 416
alloy, 187, 342
amorphous, 325
amorphous titanium oxide, 325
anastase, 325
anodic oxidation, 188, 287, 324–325
anodic oxides, 125

c.p. titanium, 177
dioxide, 124
dioxide as blasting particle, 32
discs, 316
fluoride-modified oxide, 328
implants, 274
plasma spray (TPS), 143
rutile, 325
Ti-6Al-4V, 136,188
turned, 4, 64, 69, 325
Toxicity, 385
Transcription factors, 436
Triblock molecules, 395

U

Urokinase, 289

V

Vanadium, 187
Vinculin, 267
Virus elimination, 381
Vitallium, 196
Vitamin D, 144, 326
Vitronectin, 154, 270, 358
von Willebrand factor, 290

W

Waviness, 61–62
Wear debris, 412
Wound
contraction, 222
healing, 222, 262, 265, 299

Z

Zirconium, 195